Physiotherapy in

Obstetrics and Gynecology

(A Comprehensive Textbook on Women's Health)

Physiotherapy in
Obstetrics and Gynecology
(A Comprehensive Textbook on Women's Health)

Second Edition

Megha Sandeep Sheth MPT PhD (Guide)
Lecturer
SBB College of Physiotherapy
Ahmedabad, Gujarat, India

Anu Arora MPT (Gold Medalist) PhD
Professor
DY Patil Deemed to be University
School of Physiotherapy
Navi Mumbai, Maharashtra, India

Priyasingh Rangey MPT PhD (Scholar)
Assistant Professor
LJ Institute of Physiotherapy, LJ University
Ahmedabad, Gujarat, India

Neeta Jayprakash Vyas PT PhD
Professor Emerita
Ahmedabad Institute of Physiotherapy
Ahmedabad, Gujarat, India

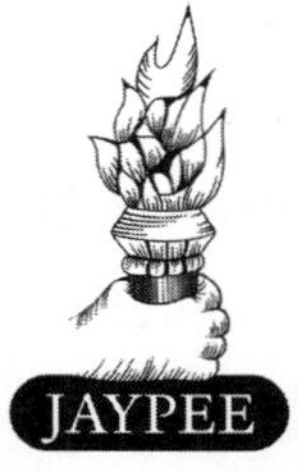

JAYPEE BROTHERS MEDICAL PUBLISHERS
The Health Sciences Publisher
New Delhi | London

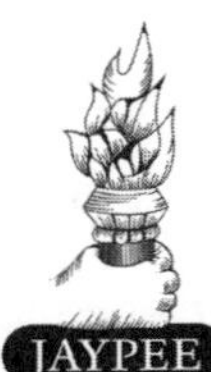

Jaypee Brothers Medical Publishers (P) Ltd

Headquarters
EMCA House
23/23-B, Ansari Road, Daryaganj
New Delhi - 110 002, India
Landline: +91-11-23272143, +91-11-23272703
+91-11-23282021, +91-11-23245672
E-mail: jaypee@jaypeebrothers.com

Corporate Office
4838/24, Ansari Road, Daryaganj
New Delhi - 110 002, India
Phone: +91-11-43574357
Fax: +91-11-43574314
E-mail: jaypee@jaypeebrothers.com

Overseas Office
J.P. Medical Ltd
83 Victoria Street, London
SW1H 0HW (UK)
Phone: +44 20 3170 8910
E-mail: info@jpmedpub.com

EU GPSR Authorised Representative
Logos Europe, 9 rue Nicolas Poussin
17000, La Rochelle, France
Phone: +33 (0) 6 67 93 73 78
E-mail: contact@logoseurope.eu

Website: www.jaypeebrothers.com
Website: www.jaypeedigital.com

Inquiries for bulk sales may be solicited at: jaypee@jaypeebrothers.com

Physiotherapy in Obstetrics and Gynecology: A Comprehensive Textbook on Women's Health

First Edition: 2023

Second Edition: **2026**

ISBN: 978-93-6616-261-4

Printed at: Samrat Offset Pvt. Ltd.

Dedicated to

The Woman

Who is a daughter...

A wife...

A mother...

A grandmother...

Who is an individual...

Who is intelligent, courageous, passionate, generous, powerful, ...yet kind....

Who gives you life and nurturing, love and care...

Who deserves nothing but the very best of life!!!

To her healthy living...

Contributors

Ajay Junnarkar DCP MD (Pathology)
Consultant Pathologist
Dr Junnarkar's Laboratory
Kailash Cancer Hospital and Research Centre
Vadodara, Gujarat, India

Ami Vishal Mehta MD DGO Fetal Medicine Fellow
Associate Professor
Department of Obstetrics and Gynecology
SVP Hospital
Smt NHL Municipal Medical College
Ahmedabad, Gujarat, India

Amruta Nerurkar MPTh MA C/NDT Certified Arts based Therapy Practitioner
Professor and Head
Department of Neurophysiotherapy
DY Patil Deemed to be University
School of Physiotherapy
Navi Mumbai, Maharashtra, India

Anshumi Desai MBBS MS
Breast Surgical Oncology Fellow
University of Miami/Jackson Memorial Hospital
Miami, Florida, USA

Anu Arora MPT (Gold Medalist) PhD
Professor
DY Patil Deemed to be University
School of Physiotherapy
Navi Mumbai, Maharashtra, India

Anuprita Thakur PT PhD
Professor
DY Patil Deemed to be University
School of Physiotherapy
Navi Mumbai, Maharashtra, India

Apurv Shimpi MPTh PhD (Scholar)
Director and Professor
Symbiosis College of Physiotherapy
Symbiosis International (Deemed University)
Pune, Maharashtra, India

Archana Shah MD DCH
Professor
Department of Pediatrics
LG Hospital, Narendra Modi Medical College
Ahmedabad, Gujarat, India

Ava Desai MD DGO
Gynecologic Oncologist
Senior Consultant
Zydus Cancer Centre
Ahmedabad, Gujarat, India

Daxa Mishra PT PhD
Professor and IQAC Director
BN Patel College of Physiotherapy
Ex-Professor
KM Patel Institute of Physiotherapy
Anand, Gujarat, India

Deepali N Hande MPT PhD (Scholar)
Professor and Head
Department of Community Physiotherapy
Dr APJ Abdul Kalam College of Physiotherapy
Pravara Institute of Medical Sciences
Ahmednagar, Maharashtra, India

Gopi Contractor MPT PhD (Scholar)
Lecturer
Ahmedabad Institute of Medical Sciences
Ahmedabad, Gujarat, India

Hiran Pandya MPT
Ex-Assistant Professor
SKUM College of Physiotherapy
Ahmedabad, Gujarat, India

Kiransha R Velingkar
MPT (Obstetrics & Gynecology)
Women's Health Physiotherapist
IAP, HCPC, CSP, POGP Registered
NHS Foundation Trust
United Kingdom

Komal Shah MPT
Lecturer
Ahmedabad Institute of Medical Sciences
Ahmedabad, Gujarat, India

Kruti Oza Modi PT PRPC ASTYM Cert 3DMAPS PCES
Women's Health Physiotherapist
Chicago, USA

Manisha A Rathi PT PhD
Vice Principal and Professor
Dr DY Patil College of Physiotherapy
Dr DY Patil Vidyapeeth
Pune, Maharashtra, India

Mariya P Jiandani MSc (PT) FAIMER Fellow
Professor
Seth Gordhandas Sunderdas Medical College
King Edward Memorial (KEM) Hospital
Mumbai, Maharashtra, India

Mayur Revadkar MPT PhD (Scholar)
Associate Professor
Department of Community Physiotherapy
KJ Somaiya College of Physiotherapy
Mumbai, Maharashtra, India

Megha Sandeep Sheth MPT PhD (Guide)
Lecturer
SBB College of Physiotherapy
Ahmedabad, Gujarat, India

Mohammed Sabir Shaikh Masters in Yogashastra
Founder—Chairman
Chief Yoga Teacher
YSM Institute of Yoga and Research Foundation
Assistant Professor
Department of Yogashastra
KJ Somaiya Bharatiya Sanskriti Peetham
Mumbai, Maharashtra, India

Neeta Jayprakash Vyas PT PhD
Professor Emerita
Ahmedabad Institute of Physiotherapy
Ahmedabad, Gujarat, India

Nipa Atul Shah MPT
Lecturer
SBB College of Physiotherapy
Ahmedabad, Gujarat, India

Nupoor Kulkarni MPT PhD
Professor
Marathwada Mitra Mandal's College of Physiotherapy
Pune, Maharashtra, India

Nupur Shah MPT
Assistant Professor
LJ Institute of Physiotherapy
LJ University
Ahmedabad, Gujarat, India

Parul R Agrawal PT PhD
Principal
HIMS College of Physiotherapy
Heritage Institute of Medical Sciences
Varanasi, Uttar Pradesh, India

Payal P Gahlot MPT
Lecturer
SBB College of Physiotherapy
Ahmedabad, Gujarat, India

Pothiraj Pitchai
Diploma in Gerontology PhD (Scholar)
Professor and Head
Department of Community Physiotherapy
KJ Somaiya College of Physiotherapy
Mumbai, Maharashtra, India

Preetha Ramachandra
PT PhD (Women's Health Physiotherapy)
Associate Professor
Department of Physiotherapy
Manipal College of Health Professions
Manipal Academy of Higher Education
Manipal, Karnataka, India

Priyasingh Rangey MPT PhD (Scholar)
Assistant Professor
LJ Institute of Physiotherapy
LJ University
Ahmedabad, Gujarat, India

Pushpa Yadava MD DGO
Professor
Department of Obstetrics and Gynecology
SVP Hospital
Smt NHL Municipal Medical College
Ahmedabad, Gujarat, India

R Harihara Prakash PT PhD
Principal and Head
KM Patel Institute of Physiotherapy
Anand, Gujarat, India

Reena Kumari BSc BPT MPT (Neurology) COCMT
Professor and Head
Department of Physiotherapy
SBS University
Dehradun, Uttarakhand, India

Sakshi P Arora MPT (Community Health Physiotherapy)
Founder and Director
TheoRapy LLP
Nagpur, Maharashtra, India

Shefali Desai MS
Consultant Breast Surgeon and Director
Breast Care Clinic, Samved Hospital
Ahmedabad, Gujarat, India

Shivani Sheth MPT DPT
Physical Therapist, Results, Physiotherapy
North Raleigh, NC, USA
Ex- Assistant Professor
Khyati Institute of Physiotherapy
Ahmedabad, Gujarat, India

Shyam Ganvir PT PhD
Principal and Professor
DVVPF's College of Physiotherapy
Ahmednagar, Maharashtra, India

Smita Amit Mehta PT DPT PRPC
Brooke Army Medical Center
Women's Health Department
Fort Sam Houston, Texas, USA

Suroshree Mitra MPT PhD (Scholar)
Professor and Head
Department of Community Physiotherapy
Sancheti Institute College of Physiotherapy
Pune, Maharashtra, India

Suvarna Ganvir PT PhD
Professor
Dr Vithalrao Vikhe Patil Foundation's College of Physiotherapy
Ahmednagar, Maharashtra, India

Waqar M Naqvi PT PhD
Founder Director and CEO
AD Vivum Education and Research
Nagpur, Maharashtra, India

Preface to the Second Edition

The warm reception of the first edition of *Physiotherapy in Obstetrics and Gynecology* has been both, gratifying as well as humbling, for us as editors.

While we were initially putting together this work, our primary intention was to provide a focused, clinically relevant resource that would support students, academicians and clinicians in understanding and applying key concepts in Physiotherapy within this specialty. The encouraging feedback from readers across universities and clinical settings has reaffirmed our belief in the need and utility of this book, as both, a learning companion, and a practical reference.

For this second edition, we have chosen not to substantially alter the fundamental structure, scope, and approach of the book. The major new feature in this edition, is the inclusion of multiple choice questions (MCQs), at the end of each chapter. We sincerely hope that this addition will make the book more learner-friendly and a valuable tool for the teachers designing assessments, tutorials, and revision sessions.

We remain grateful to all our readers for their continued interest, constructive suggestions, and encouragement, which have paved the path for this improved edition. We also warmly acknowledge the contribution of all chapter authors and reviewers, whose expertise and commitment have shaped the quality of this work.

We sincerely hope that this second edition meets the expectations of our readers and continues to be a reliable guide in their academic journey and clinical practice.

HAPPY READING!!!

Editors of Physiotherapy in Obstetrics and Gynecology

Megha Sandeep Sheth
Anu Arora
Priyasingh Rangey
Neeta Jayprakash Vyas

Preface to the First Edition

Physiotherapy in Obstetrics and Gynecology is not just a book but a heartfelt endeavor dedicated to all women across age groups, and beyond geographical boundaries. It is not an individual but a collaborative effort by several esteemed professionals belonging to a diversity of specialties like Gynecology and Obstetrics, Surgery, Biochemistry, Physiotherapy and Yoga to name a few. The vision behind developing this book was simple—to fill the knowledge gap that exists in the literature to understand the health of a woman from the perspective of experts from various specialties and address the concerns with appropriate and evidence-based physiotherapeutic approaches.

The very essence of human existence is deeply entrenched in the variances on the basis of gender, stated in terms of both biological structures and functions. Women contribute almost 50% to the total world population, truly representing the significant half that deserves our due attention to its healthcare and well-being.

The life of a woman has several aspects to it. A woman's health, not only concerns her alone, but also the health and welfare of the entire family since she is the primary care-taker. The journey of a woman from womb to tomb is not simple, but filled with many complexities. Right from conception, through adolescence and motherhood, to menopause and old age, a woman has to go through diverse life-changing events due to hormonal changes that occur with age and social influences. A woman is not only an individual but a daughter, a wife, a mother, a care-giver and a strong pillar of the society.

In spite of playing such a humongous and vital role in the family and the society, there is dearth of knowledge regarding a woman's health. It is common perception that women's health includes only the phase of motherhood and child care, but it is not so. Women's health includes much more than that. It includes the conditions that may occur during the intrauterine period, diseases occurring during pediatric age, problems faced by women during adolescence, early and late adulthood and old age, care required during antepartum and postpartum phases and menopause, early child care and several other pathologies that may more commonly occur in women. Therefore, it encompasses a woman's life from the point of conception in womb till her body travels to the tomb.

The book, though titled *Physiotherapy in Obstetrics and Gynecology*, includes not only physiotherapy but several other specialties too. This is what differentiates it from the other books available in the market. The editors felt a need to create a book that not only included the physiotherapist's perspective in detail, but also tried to look at a woman's health from the perspective of a gynecologist, an obstetrician and a breast surgeon, among other professionals. The editors of the book have tried to identify the role of a woman not just as a homemaker, but also as a professional working in office spaces, in sports and other areas.

The editors are strong believers of equality and hence, even with a book where the main highlight is woman's health, they have tried to introduce the upcoming and lesser known topic of men's pelvic health. Even though men's health has always taken priority over women's health, the male pelvic floor has been ignored up till now, which actually plays a really important role in the function of the core musculature, spinal stability, continence, and ultimate health of a male.

The sole purpose of developing this book was to provide a platform to readers, where they can gain knowledge about each and every health problem that may be faced by a woman during her life and its physiotherapy management. Development of this book has been a golden opportunity and we thank the publishers from the bottom of our hearts for this. We wish the reader also experiences the same enrichment that we had while writing and compiling this book.

HAPPY READING!!!
Editors of Physiotherapy in Obstetrics and Gynecology

Megha Sandeep Sheth
Anu Arora
Priyasingh Rangey
Neeta Jayprakash Vyas

Acknowledgments

Physiotherapy in Obstetrics and Gynecology is a collaborative effort by several noteworthy esteemed contributors. This endeavor would not have been a possibility without the blessings of Almighty God. A heartfelt gratitude towards all the contributors who have devoted their time, knowledge and hard work to this book. Each chapter has turned out to be a source of clinically and academically enriching insight. It was sheer hard work and perseverance by the authors that has made the book such a bountiful reservoir of knowledge. We would like to extend our gratitude towards all the patients who have provided their time and their experience for this endeavor. Without them, our profession is a void. We want to thank all the subjects and models for providing images for the book. It was the constant support, motivation and determination provided by Dr Neeta Jayprakash Vyas (PT) that this book could achieve the potential it has.

I am very grateful to the whole team of M/s Jaypee Brothers Medical Publishers (P) Ltd, New Delhi, India, who helped and guided me, Shri Jitendar P Vij (Group Chairman), Mr Ankit Vij (Managing Director), Mr MS Mani (Group President), Dr Madhu Choudhary (Director-Educational Publishing), Ms Pooja Bhandari [Director-Production (Books and Journals)], Mr Ajay Kumar Sharma [Deputy General Manager (Books and Journals)], Ms Sunita Katla (Executive Assistant to Group Chairman and Publishing Manager), Ms Samina Khan (Executive Assistant to Director-Educational Publishing), Dr Upma Tomar (Managing Editor), Mr Vijay Kumar Bhatia (Manager-Production), Mr Bishan Singh (Production Manager-Press), Ms Seema Dogra (Cover Visualizer), Ms Neha Verma (Graphic Designer-Cover), Ms Geeta Barik (Quality Controller), Mr Kuldeep Dobriyal (Typesetter), Mr Gopal Singh Kirola (Graphic Designer) and their team members, for all their support to work in this project and make it a success. Without their cooperation, I could not have completed this project.

I am thankful to my parents, Mr Navnit Desai and Mrs Aruna Desai, my in-laws—Mr Bachubhai Sheth and Mrs Veenaben Sheth for their constant support and encouragement in all endeavors. I would like to thank my husband—Dr Sandeep Sheth who has been a continuous source of inspiration. I want to acknowledge my children, my son—Siddharth, my daughter—Shivani, my daughter-in-law—Shivani and my son-in-law—Tej, who have been my pillars of strength through the crucial phases of writing. I thank my postgraduate students—who have always supported me and inspired me to never give up. My heartfelt appreciation towards the work done by my undergraduate and postgraduate students. A special note of thanks to Ridham, Sonal, Sangita, Paresh and Sachi for always being there. I am thankful to the entire team of SBB College of Physiotherapy, AMC Medical Education Trust. I appreciate the endeavors made by my co-editors—Dr Neeta Jayprakash Vyas, Dr Anu Arora and Dr Priyasingh Rangey.

Megha Sandeep Sheth

I acknowledge with gratitude and devotion to The Almighty for giving me the power and motivation to be a part of this endeavor.

I would like to express my deepest and most sincere gratitude to my mentor and guide, Prof. Sujata Yardi for always being there to inspire me. I gratefully acknowledge the support and encouragement of the Director of my institute, and my dear friend Dr Unnati Pandit. While working on a book is an arduous journey, it was made pleasant by some unstinting support from my colleagues Dr Esha Shetty and Dr Kirti Jadhav who assisted me with the photographs for various chapters.

This book would not have reached its current form, without the kind acceptance and contribution of authors, of my learned colleagues, from across not just India but the world over. I am greatly obliged to all of you, for your time and sincere efforts.

A special thanks to my co-editor, Dr Megha Sandeep Sheth for not just initiating this project, but also being the driving force who made the timely execution of this work possible. It has been an enriching learning experience and a great pleasure working with our team of editors: Dr Neeta Jayprakash Vyas, Dr Megha Sandeep Sheth, and Dr Priyasingh Rangey.

It is my mother who has taught me to follow my passions: to dream about things worth pursuing and then to go for them. My passion to write professionally, would not have been possible without the unconditional love and wholehearted support of my parents. Most importantly, I wish to thank my husband and my lovely daughter for their understanding and emotional support. An extra special thanks to my daughter—Soumya, who lent an attentive ear to all my late-night thought processes and helped curate the grammar of my work.

Last but not the least, my sincere gratitude to all my teachers and my patients who have been the source of all knowledge and clinical expertise that has formed the foundation of this book.

Anu Arora

I would like to extend my gratitude towards my parents—Mr Bhagirath Singh Rangey and Mrs Mina Rangey, my brother—Mr Devrath Rangey, my mother-in-law—Mrs Tara Thakur and my husband—Mr Pradeep Singh Thakur. They have always been a constant support for me, throughout difficult times. I thank Dr Priyanka Sharma for being a pillar of strength for me. I wish to extend my regards to Dr Megha Sandeep Sheth, Dr Nehal Shah and Dr Srishti Sharma for the constant pushing in life. I am obliged to my colleagues, especially Dr Nupur Shah for their help and support. I am thankful to all my students who contributed for photos. I appreciate the hard work and toil by my co-editors Dr Megha Sandeep Sheth, Dr Neeta Jayprakash Vyas, and Dr Anu Arora, that made this book a reality.

Priyasingh Rangey

I would like to thank my parents who have been the reason of my existence and my achievements in life. I am indebted to my husband—Dr Jayprakash Vyas, for being a constant support throughout my life. Heartfelt thanks to Khushbu and Jiya who have been the source of my smiles. I thank all the authors who have contributed towards this book.

Neeta Jayprakash Vyas

Contents

Section 4: Mother and Childcare

Section 5: Cancer in Women

Plate 1

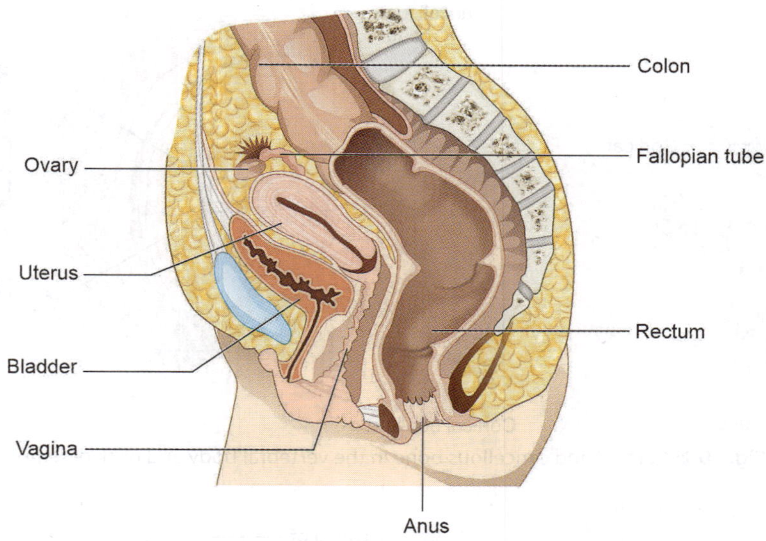

Fig. 3.4: Female pelvic cavity.

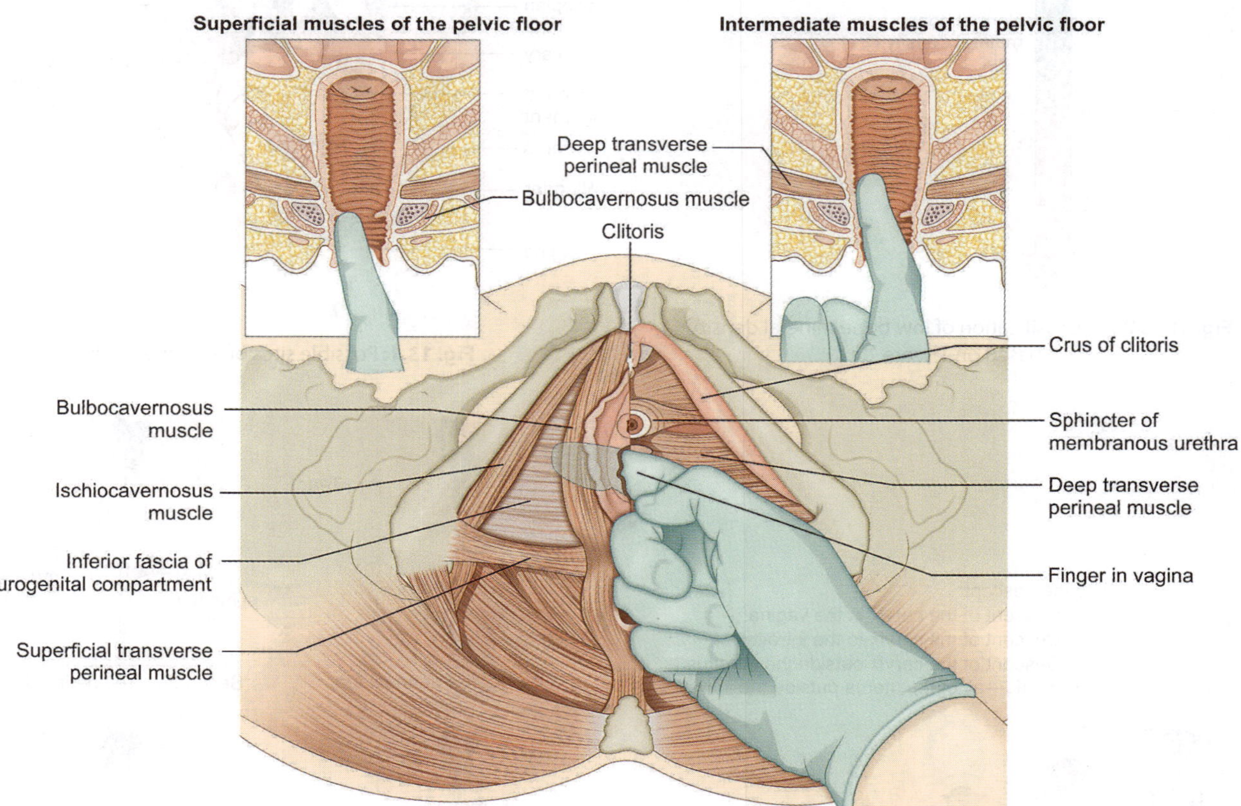

Fig. 4.2: Digital examination of pelvic floor muscles.

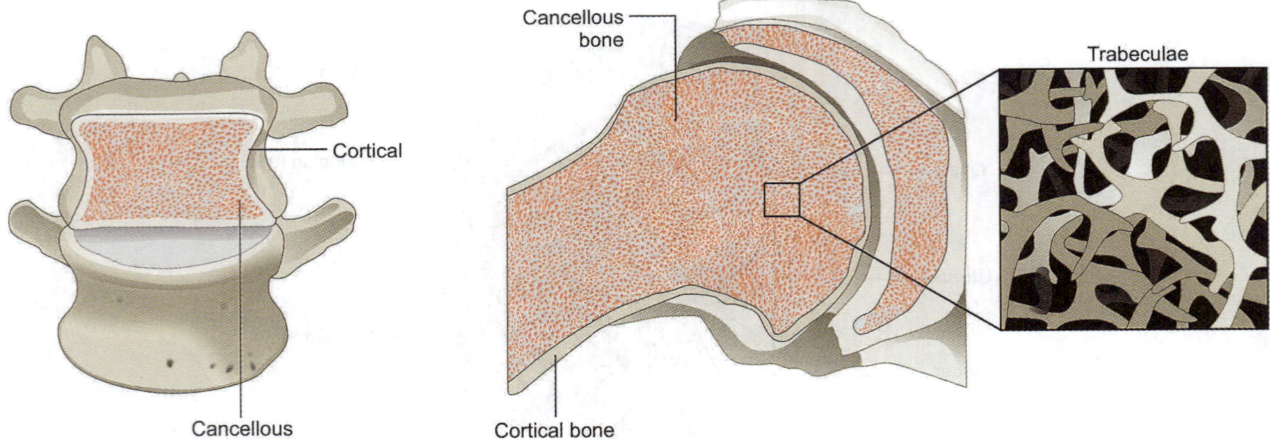

Fig. 10.2: Cortical and cancellous bone in the vertebral body and neck of femur.

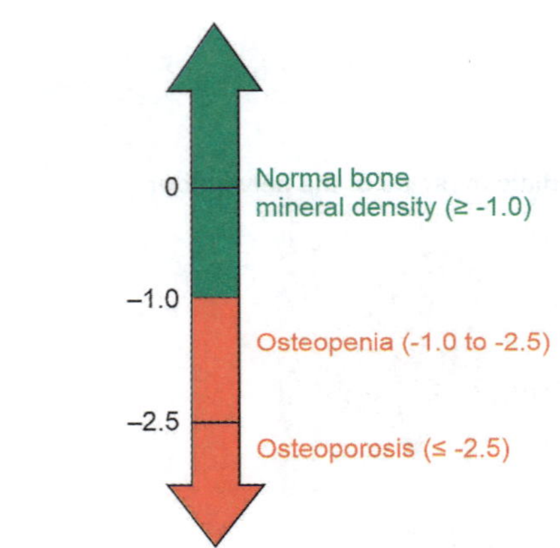

Fig. 10.9: WHO classification of low bone mineral density based on T-score.

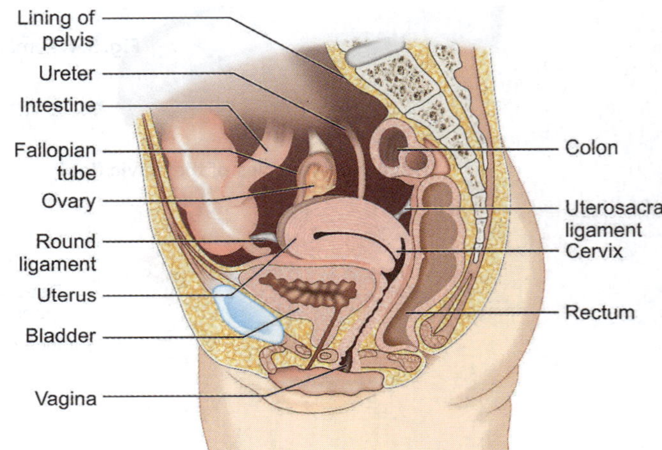

Fig. 13.1: Possible sites of endometriosis.

Uterine descent:
1°↔ Descent of the cervix in the vagina
2°↔ Descent of the cervix to the introitus
3°↔ Descent of the cervix outside the introitus
Procidentia—all of the uterus outside the introitus

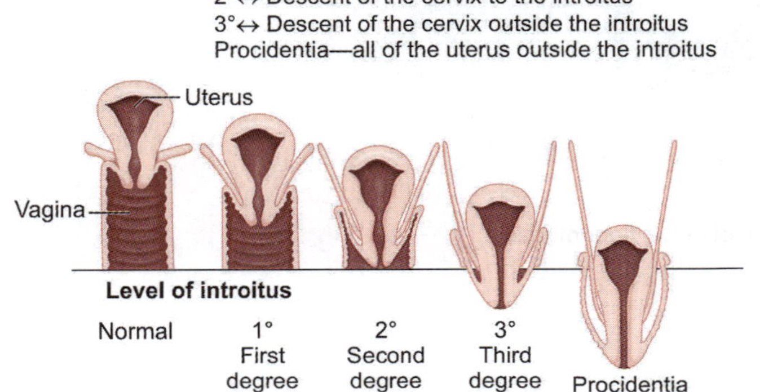

Fig. 13.5: Degrees of uterine prolapse.

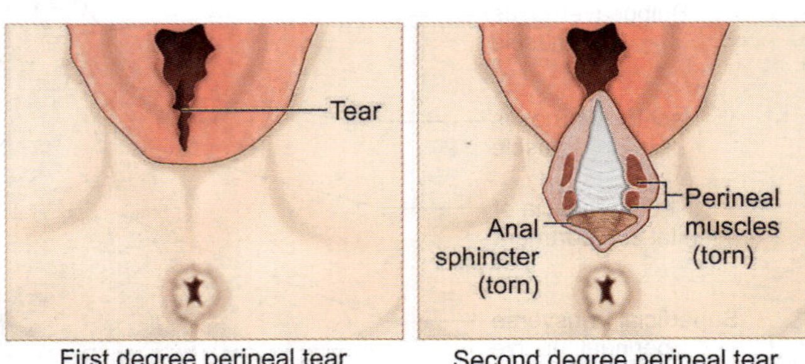

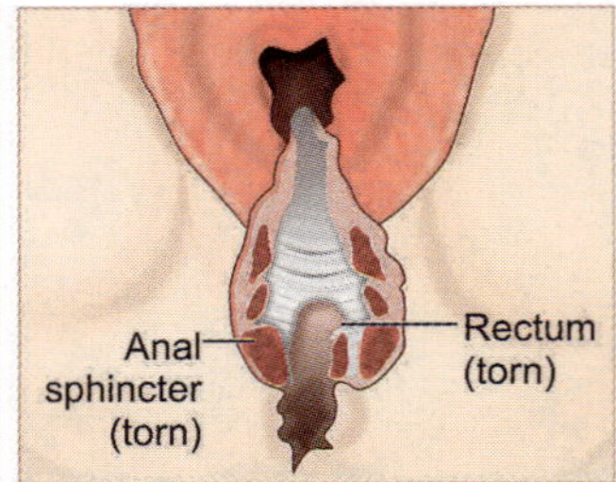

Fig. 13.8: Classification of perineal tears.

Plate 3

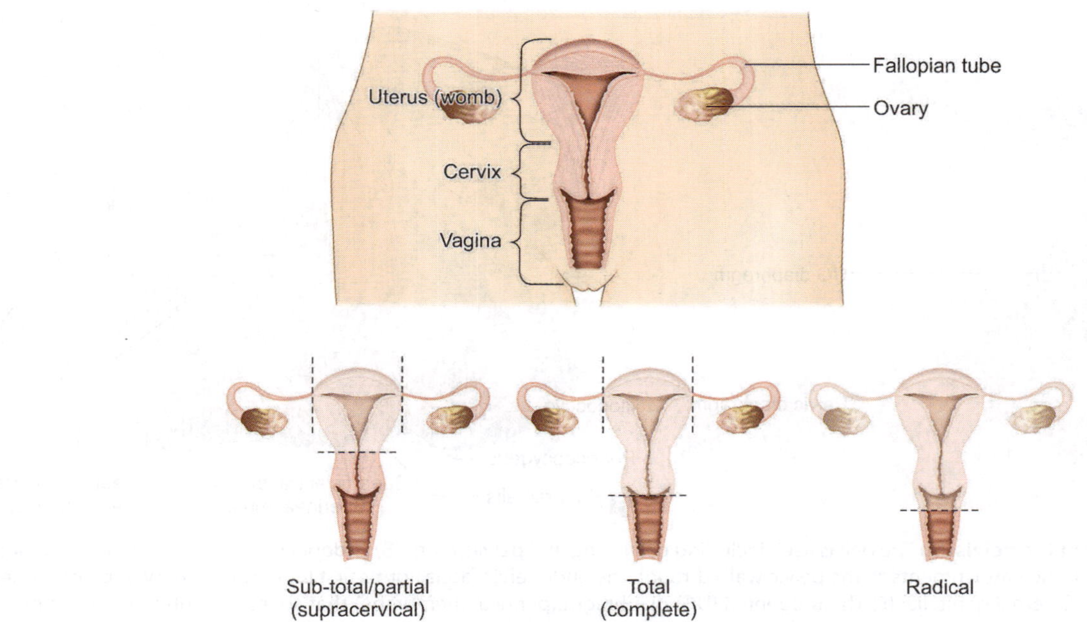

Fig. 13.10: Types of hysterectomy.

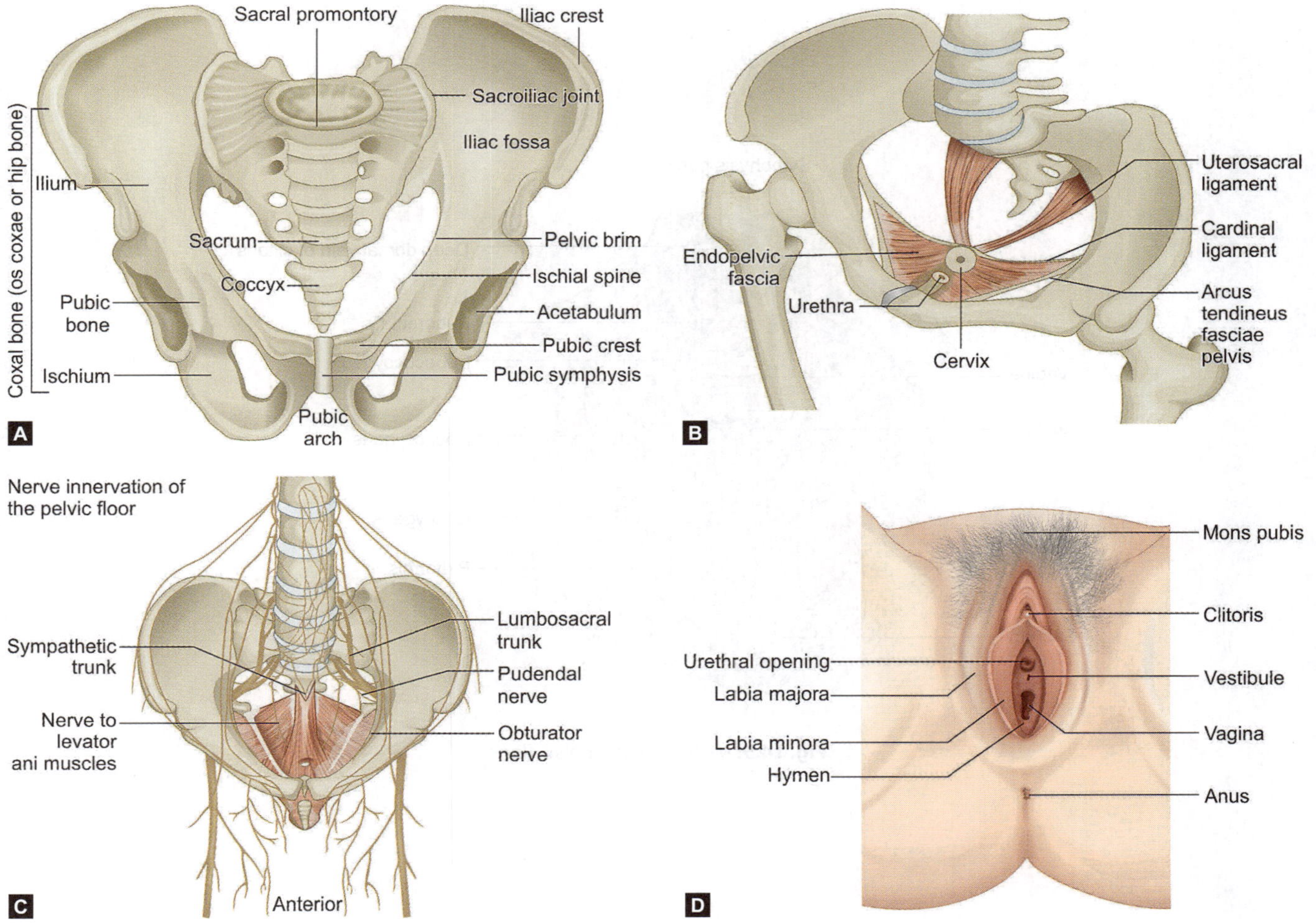

Figs. 14.1A to D

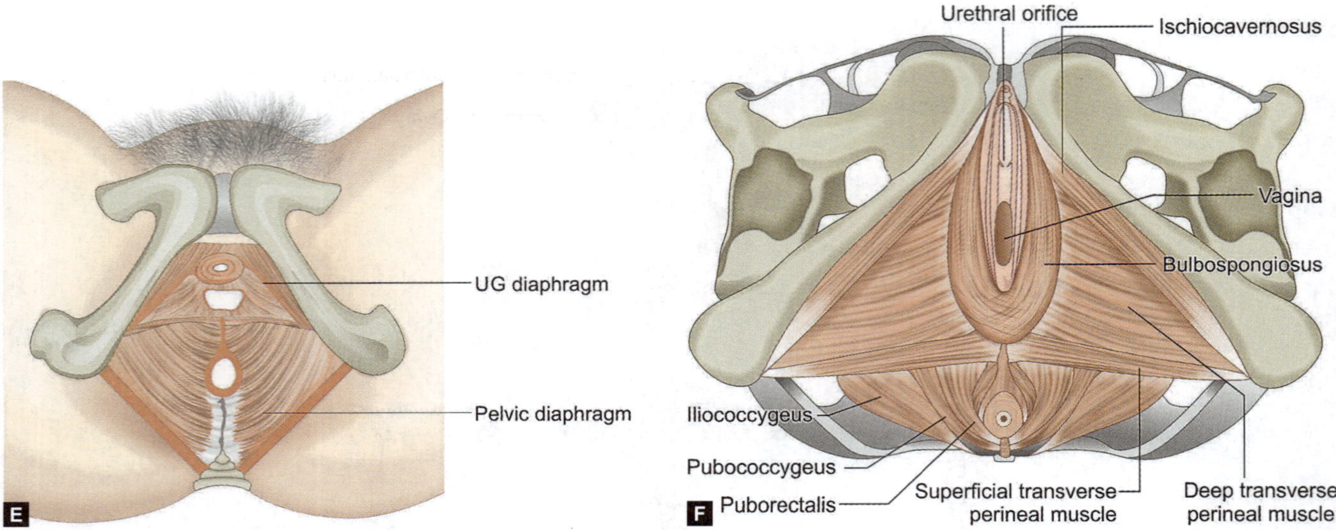

Figs. 14.1A to F. Organs in the pelvis: (A) The pelvis itself including pelvic ring and pelvic joints; (B) Endopelvic fascia and connective tissues (pelvic viscera), along with their attachments to the pelvic walls through the endopelvic fascia, forms first layer; (C) The nerves, blood vessels and lymphatic tissue; (D) External genitalia; (E) The urogenital (UG) diaphragm (perineal membrane) that spans the anterior portion of the pelvic outlet and connects the perineal body to the ischiopubic rami; (F) The bulbocavernosus, ischiocavernosus, and superficial transverse perineal muscles lie in superficial area of anterior outlet (urogenital hiatus) and posterior outlet (anal hiatus).

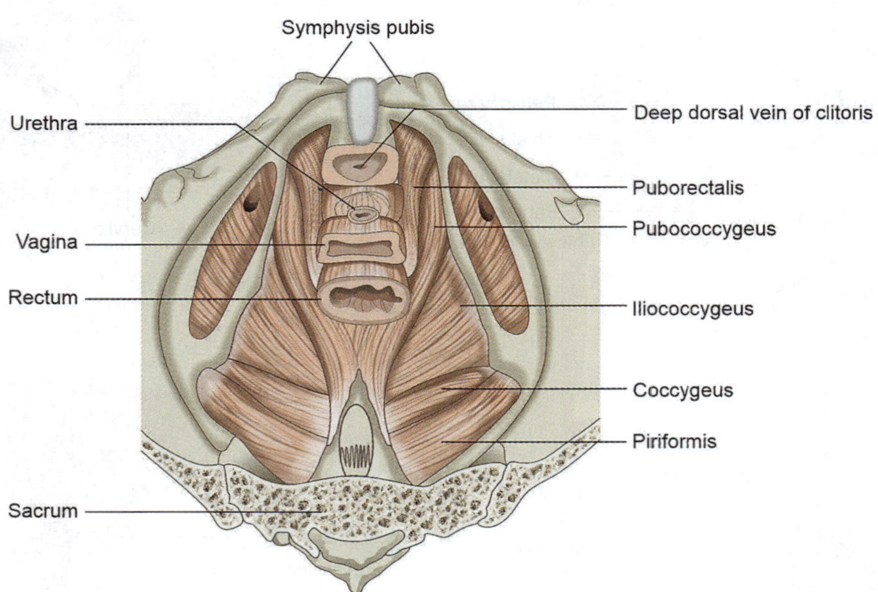

Fig. 14.5: Muscles of the pelvic floor.

Plate 5

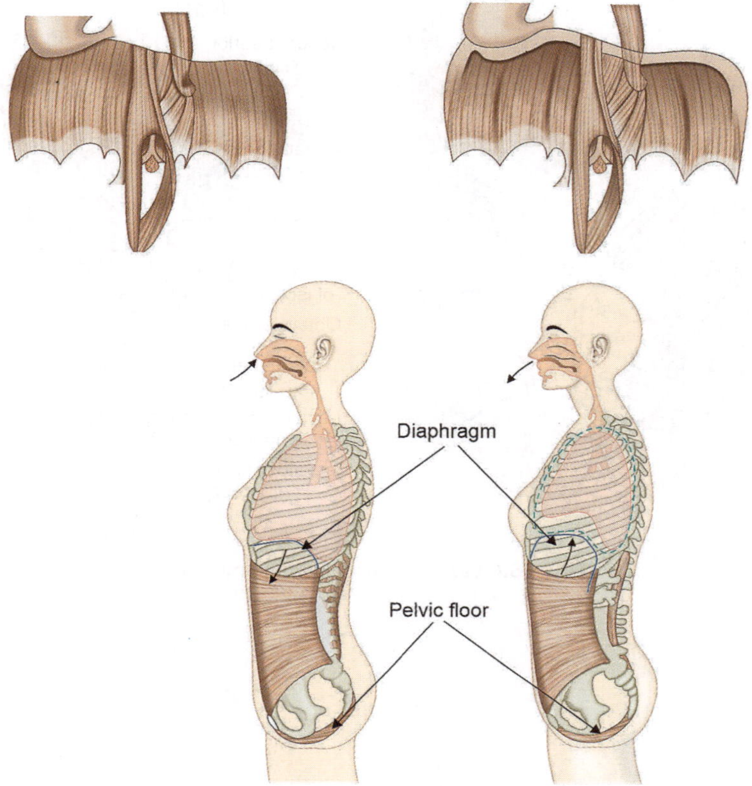

Fig. 15.1: Pelvic floor and respiratory diaphragm.

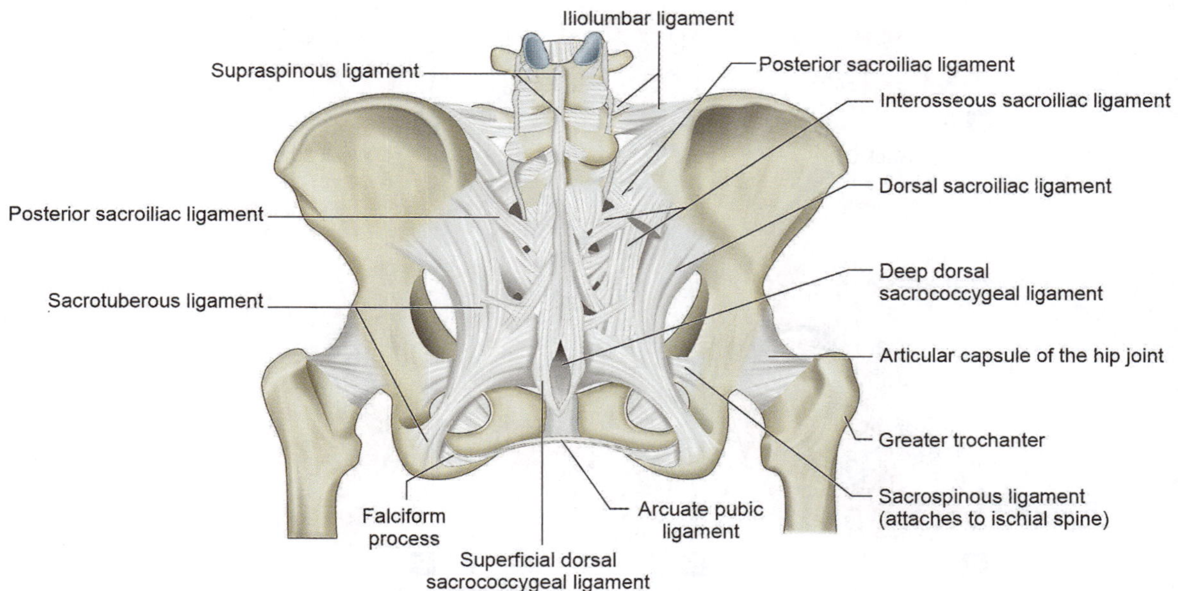

Fig. 15.2: Ligamentous support of bony pelvis.

Plate 6

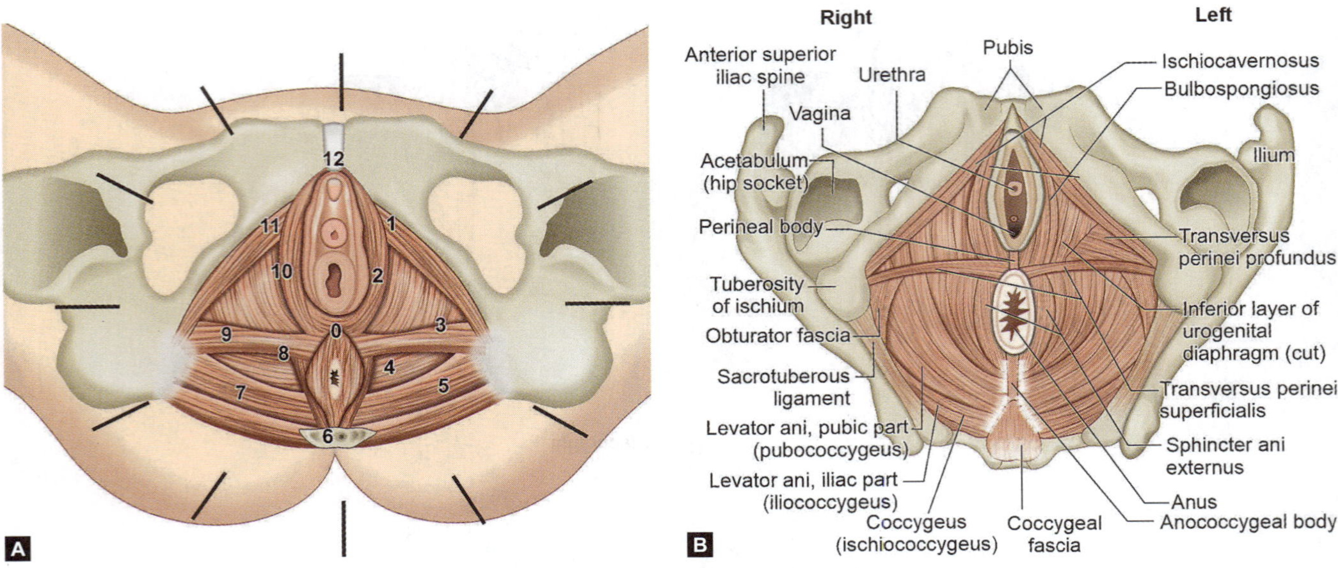

Figs. 15.6A and B: Pelvic clock and muscles.

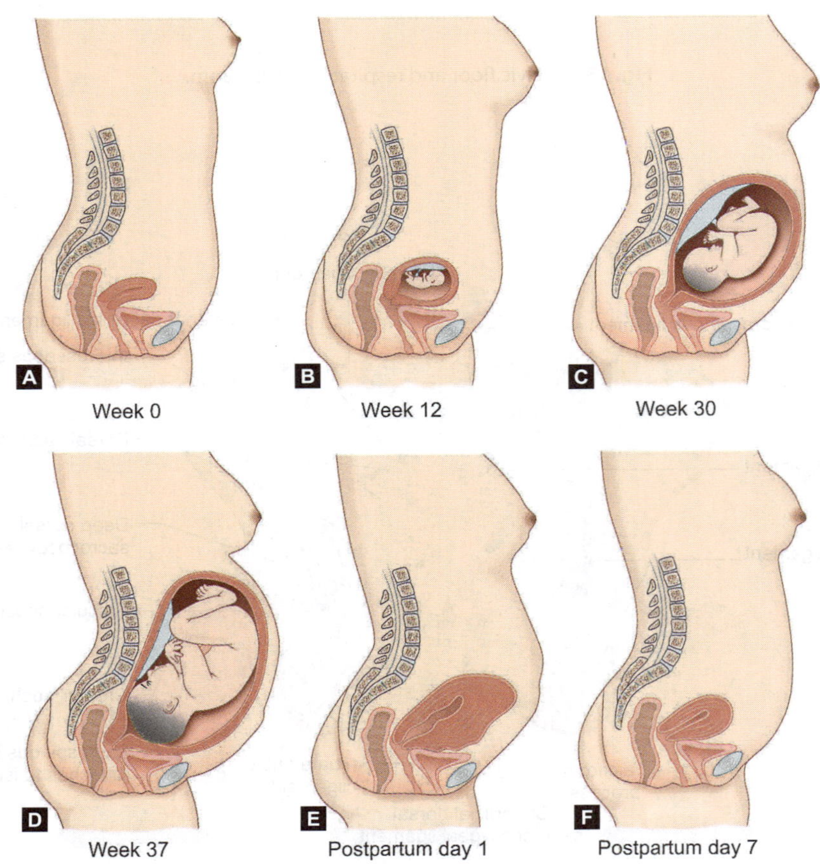

Figs. 19.1A to F: Physical changes with pregnancy.

Plate 7

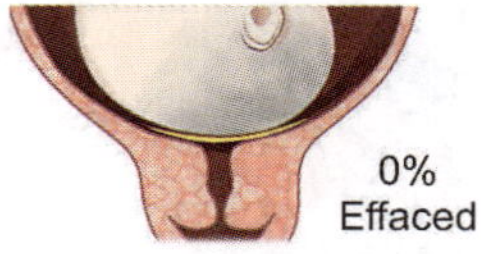

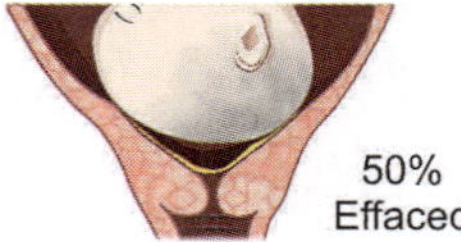

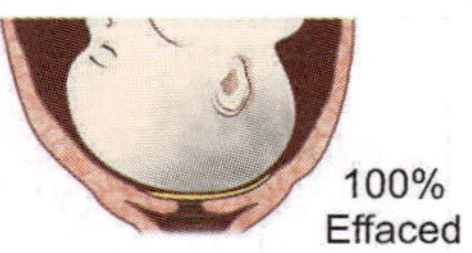

Dilatation—the gradual opening of the cervix measured in centimeters from 0 to 10 cm

Fig. 21.3: Cervical effacement and dilatation.

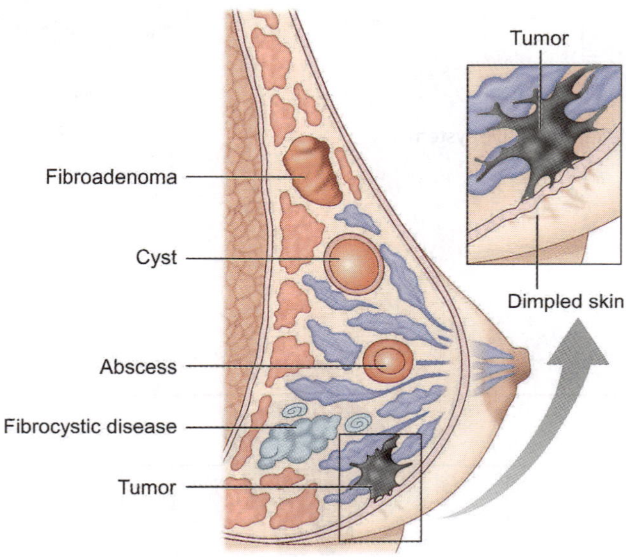

Fig. 26.4: Breast diseases.

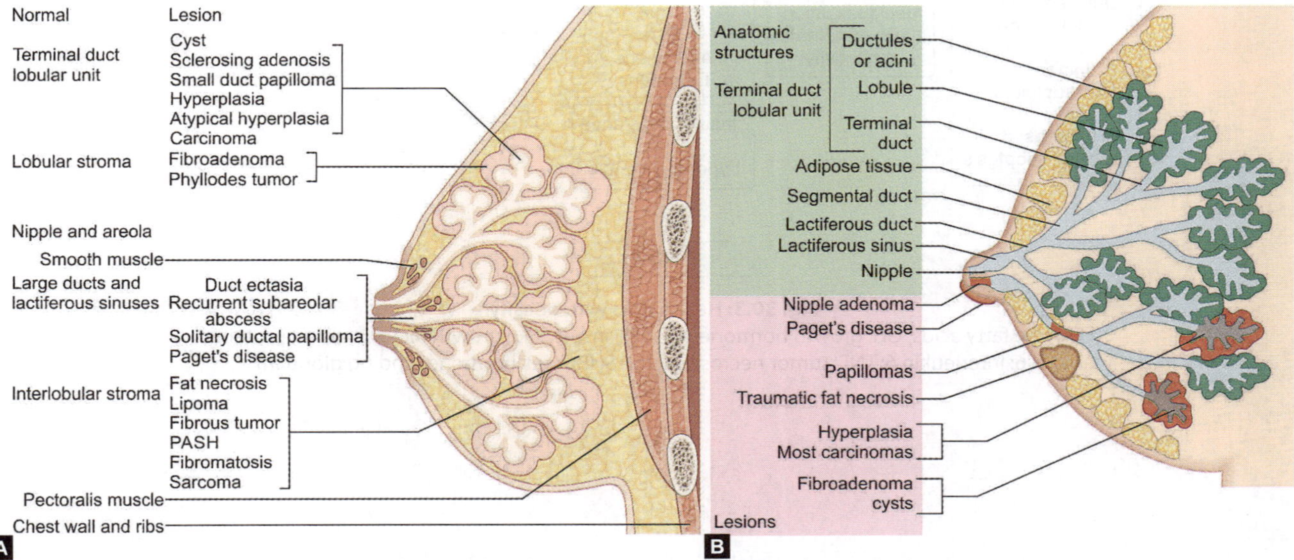

Figs. 26.5A and B: Lesions that are commonly seen according to the breast structure.

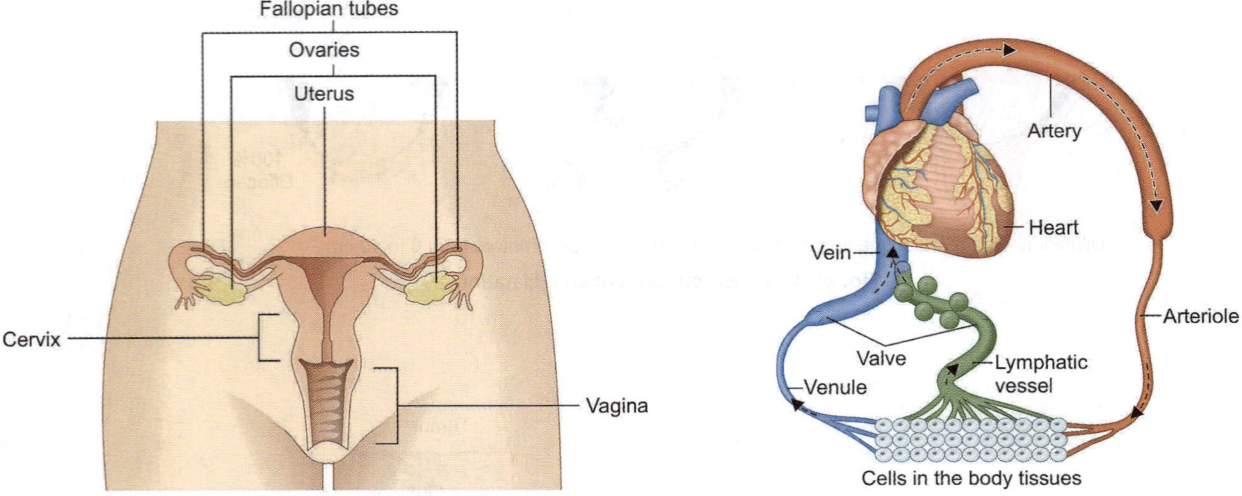

Fig. 27.1: Organs of the female reproductive system.

Fig. 29.1: Lymphatic system.

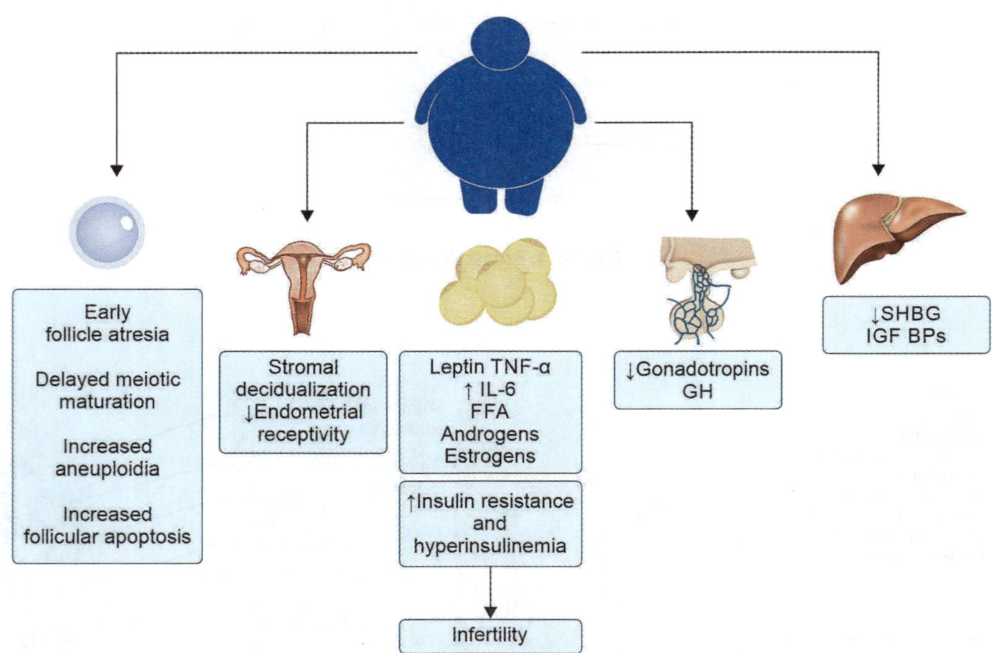

Fig. 30.3: Health risks with obesity.
(FFA: free fatty acids; GH: growth hormone; IGF BPs: insulin-like growth factor binding proteins; IL-6: interleukin 6; TNF: tumor necrosis factor; SHBG: sex hormone binding globulin)

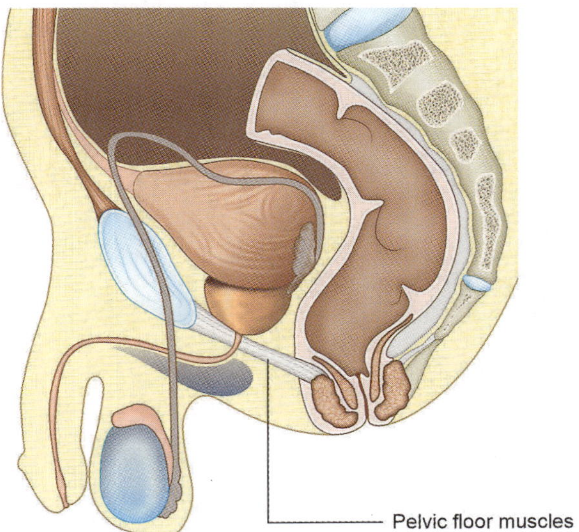

Fig. 36.1: Male urinary system.

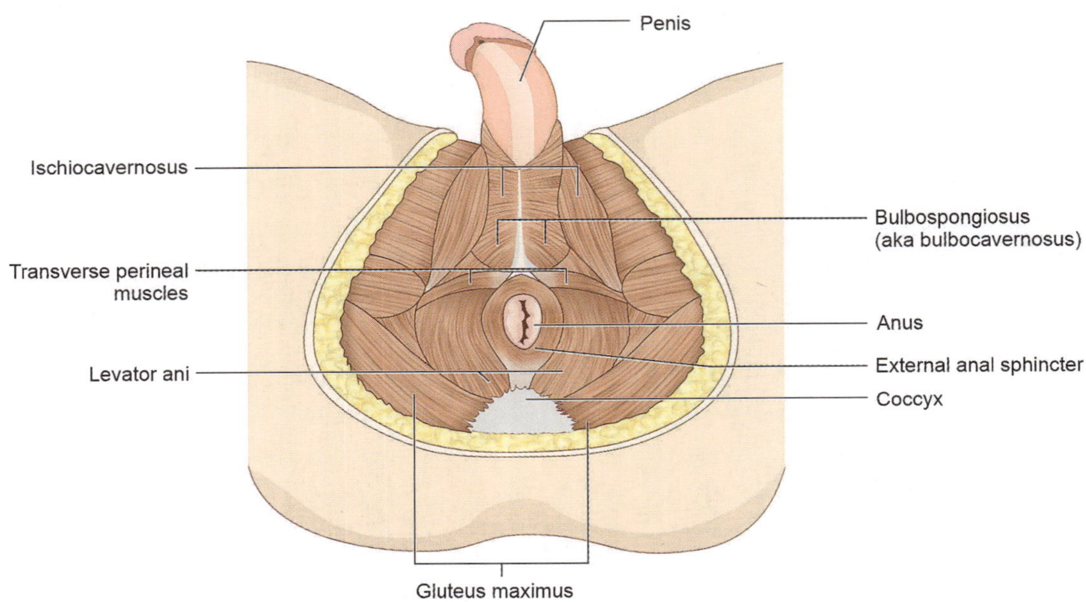

Fig. 36.2: Pelvic floor muscles in males.

Section 1

Basics and Foundational Concepts of Women's Health

Section Outline

Chapter 1

Introduction to Physiotherapy in Women's Health

✍ *Megha Sandeep Sheth, Anu Arora, Priyasingh Rangey, Neeta Jayprakash Vyas*

LEARNING OBJECTIVES

At the end of the chapter, the reader will be able to:
- Understand the importance of women's health.
- Gain knowledge about the stages in life cycle of a woman and the continuum of life.
- Have an understanding of women's problems and the importance of women's health.
- Learn the history of development of women's health as a branch in physiotherapy.
- Discuss various organizations working for women's health.
- Explore the role of physiotherapy in women's health.

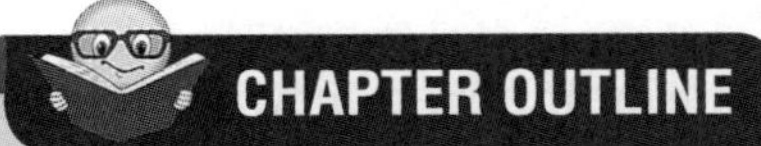

INTRODUCTION

The lifespans of men and women have increased. Women are different from men—physically, mentally, emotionally. Though the fight for superiority may be inconclusive, the fact remains that men and women differ in their behavior and physiology.

The journey of life of a woman from the womb to the tomb has many stages. Physiological, hormonal, anatomical, psychological and emotional changes are seen throughout the life cycle.

STAGES IN THE LIFECYCLE OF A WOMAN

The stages in the life of a woman are generally divided into:
- **Prenatal and infancy:** This stage begins before the birth. The well-being of the mother has a crucial role to play in the development of this stage.
- **Childhood:** Exposure to positive factors forms the basis of healthy adulthood. Games, sports and weight-bearing develop the bone bank reserves and strong bones to fight osteoporosis. Healthy childhood can also prevent obesity and diabetes.
- **Adolescence/puberty:** This is the stage of transition to adulthood. Menarche is the start of the menstrual cycle, where hormonal factors play a crucial role.
- **Reproductive age:** Child-bearing and pregnancy are life events during the reproductive phase which change the life of a woman completely. Pregnancy and motherhood are considered as events which are unique to women.
- **Climacteric period:** Menopause leads to physical and cognitive changes.
- **Elderly years:** There is a decline in the physical strength, memory and cognition. Along with this, social changes like the loss of spouse are also present.

Continuum of Life through a Woman's Lifespan (Fig. 1.1)

The females spend a great proportion of their time preparing for and understanding pregnancy and birth, but often neglect understanding and consideration for

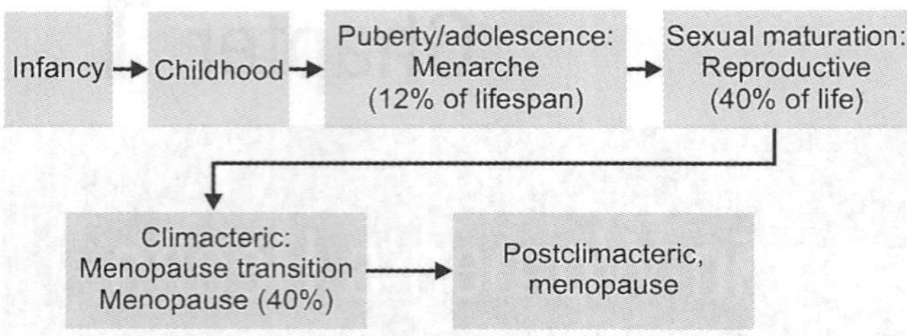

Fig. 1.1: Continuum of life through a woman's lifespan.

the other aspects of their health, including menarche and menstrual abnormalities and menopause transition. They are not diseases that require medical treatment, but transitional phases that may need functional assessment and symptomatic management.

The **goal of physiotherapy in women's health is to understand the special needs of the female population and facilitate the women to attain a good quality of life from the womb to the tomb**. While the skeletal structure, the body composition, the physiological differences, and the hormonal milieu of a female sets her apart from her age-matched male counterpart, it becomes imperative that females be treated as an exclusive entity with unique problems and therefore be provided tailor-made gender-specific solutions for their healthcare needs.

Social and cultural factors also influence the health status. It is necessary to understand the psychosocial aspects and apply them into physiotherapy practice. Education and changes in the concept of marriage delay events in the life stages. The understanding of the role of the woman in each stage is important to assess, diagnose and manage the health issues. A comprehensive view including the medical aspect along with all the above factors helps discover the potential problems and the possible solutions to these issues leading to a better quality of life.

WOMEN'S PROBLEMS

Women's health focuses on several areas related to the health of women. Some among them include:

- Pregnancy and childbirth
- Sexual health
- Menopause
- Osteoporosis and arthritis
- Heart diseases
- Cancer related to the breast, female reproductive organs and other systems of the body
- Benign conditions affecting the female reproductive system
- Contraception
- Sexually transmitted diseases (STDs)
- Pelvic diseases
- Urinary tract infections
- Irregular menses
- Abnormal vaginal bleeding

Common problems seen in women are shown in **Box 1.1** and common conditions seen are enlisted in **Box 1.2**.

Gender discrimination is seen in the following ways:

- Female children are often not sent to school and educated; instead they are forced to do household chores.
- The use of sanitary napkins during menstruation is limited in several rural and underdeveloped regions of the world. This leads to infections of the pelvic organs, which in the long run may even lead to death.
- Several menstrual problems go about unacknowledged, since most of the females are not aware that it is abnormal or they do not vocalize these problems or are not heard. Pain during menses is considered normal and hence, abnormal pain goes unnoticed. Girls are not educated about the normal duration or flow of menstrual blood and hence, increased flow or duration goes unreported. These increase morbidities related to abnormal vaginal bleeding and irregular menses.

Education about contraception, sexually transmitted infections (STIs) and healthy sexual practices is never provided as talking about these topics is usually frowned upon. Unsafe sexual practices lead to STI and unwanted pregnancies. This again increases the morbidity among women. Unwanted pregnancies at young age cause excessive mental and emotional trauma, resulting in several mental health disorders.

Health care received during the antenatal and postnatal period also causes significant impact on maternal and fetal morbidity and mortality. Pregnancy at an early age, malnourished mother, inappropriate guidance during pregnancy, improper care during pregnancy, physical labor during pregnancy, etc., lead to fetal and maternal deaths. Home births under supervision of untrained individuals, unavailability of proper care and equipment at the hospital for the mother and the delivered fetus, lack of timely action on part of the parents and the doctors, etc., lead to intrapartum

Box 1.1: Common problems seen in women.

- Painful or heavy menstruation
- Vaginal itching, discharge, dryness
- Urinary and fecal incontinence
- Pelvic/vaginal pain
- Prenatal and postpartum musculoskeletal pain
- Chronic pain
- Psychosocial concerns
- Conditions specific to the female athlete
- Work-related problems in females
- The elderly female and her concerns

Box 1.2: Common conditions seen in women.

- Dysmenorrhea
- Endometriosis
- Organ prolapse
- Pregnancy and maternal health issues
- Gynecological and breast cancer, lymphedema
- Health concerns like heart disease, diabetes, stroke, urinary tract infections, anemias, osteoporosis, gestational diabetes, preeclampsia

and postpartum complications. These are all avoidable events.

In addition, women are prone to develop certain conditions more than men. Incidence of breast cancer, osteoporosis, arthritis, etc., is higher in females than males. Due to lack of education about various female cancers and lack of screening, many such conditions go undiagnosed resulting in high morbidity and mortality.

Females are not aware about the various possibilities available to them for managing menopausal symptoms. Even if they speak to other members of the family or the society about these problems, they are disregarded saying it occurs to all women and is normal. Osteoporosis is a common complication following menopause and women should be educated about strategies to prevent and manage it. The incidence of heart diseases and cancer increases post-menopause, which the woman should be made aware of.

Women do not get equal representation at occupational practices and hence, it becomes difficult for them to make other people aware of their problems. This can be seen in offices, sports, entertainment, manual labor sector, etc. Menstrual problems, gender discrimination, pay gaps, familial issues, etc., impact a woman negatively and can cause serious health concerns.

IMPORTANCE OF WOMEN'S HEALTH

It is a well-perceived notion among majority of the people that women's health simply means women's reproductive health. However, women's health includes vast list of other conditions and situations that may affect a woman differently than a man. There have been urges to replace the term 'Women's health' with 'The health of women' to encompass and enlighten other aspects of the health of a woman.

Health experiences differ between men and women due to a range of biological, sociocultural and behavioral factors. There are certain issues that are unique for females like pregnancy and menopause. There are conditions which may manifest differently in men and women. The condition may be the same, but the care necessary may differ, e.g., anxiety and depression. There are also conditions that may be more prevalent in females than males, e.g., osteoporosis. **Box 1.3** enlists some of the conditions that may manifest differently among males and females.

Box 1.3: Conditions that manifest differently among males and females.

- **Alcohol abuse:** The effects of alcoholism and alcohol abuse i.e., increased risk of breast cancer, heart disease, etc., are more severe in women compared to men
- **Heart disease:** Death due to heart disease is commoner in females than males
- **Mental health problems:** Women show signs of anxiety and depression more compared to males
- **Osteoporosis and osteoarthritis:** The prevalence of both these conditions is more among females
- **Stroke:** Certain risk factors for stroke like consumption of contraceptives or hormonal medications, pregnancy, etc., are more common in females than males
- **Sexually transmitted infections (STIs):** Symptoms of STI are milder among females and may be confused with other conditions like fungal infections leading to delay in diagnosis and management and may lead to infertility in the long run, thereby causing graver consequences than in men

Women's health also holds more importance since the women are at a disadvantage due to the social discrimination against them.

- The society that a woman lives in dictates the value that the woman holds.
- Cultural influences also determine the health of a woman.
- Domestic abuse, rape, sexual harassment and abuse and other forms of violence against women ensue if the society does not hold women in high regard and does not care for their safety.
- Access to healthcare and health insurance and rights provided by the constitution also determine the health of a woman. Most of the countries now have legislations in place to allow maternal benefits of various kinds. This has reduced the maternal burden and the maternal mortality rate (MMR). Good health practices and better medical practices have allowed the mothers to conceive and deliver without complications and have led to better maternal and neonatal outcomes.
- There are certain countries which have banned free access to birth control or have criminalized abortion. This leads to younger pregnancies and unhealthy practices to get abortion which affects the health of the woman.

Approximately 75% of the maternal deaths that occurred in 2017 were due to the following complications:

- Infections
- Unsafe abortion
- Complications from the delivery
- Severe bleeding
- High blood pressure during pregnancy leading to eclampsia or preeclampsia

Preventing these deaths is rather simple and involves:

- Better quality health care during pregnancy and during and after childbirth
- Prompt medical attention and care
- Easy availability of medications
- Good hygiene
- Better access to contraception and safe abortion practices

It is the duty of the society to consider females as a special population and take care of them since they are the ones that give birth to the new generation and a healthy community.

PHYSIOTHERAPY IN WOMEN'S HEALTH: EVOLUTION OF PERSPECTIVE

Contemporary physiotherapy practices have taken a quantum leap from their concepts and applications at the time of their inception. In view of the gender-based differences between the males and the females of the human species, there was always a much-needed concerted effort in the field of Women's Health.

The archaic belief that women do not have the physical or mental capacity to withstand certain workloads and the stress that such workloads impose; the fear of maternity leave; or the notion that women are not good negotiators and are less likely to seek positions of power due to insecurities or personal situations, no longer carry any weight in the global perspective, where women have come to hold the highest echelons of power with great elan and efficiency. With the growing significance of the roles played by the females of the species, the colloquial boundaries between the importance of the genders have further blurred. Alongside has arisen this need, to emphasize the consequence of being a woman and strengthen the efforts to pave the path of her health, her fitness, and her disability-free enabled life **(Fig. 1.2)**.

Historically, physiotherapy in women's health has been identified with physiotherapy in Obstetrics and Gynecology. This refers to physiotherapeutic care of women encompassing the antenatal and postnatal periods. As per the American Physical Therapy Association (APTA), the section on Women's Health **(Fig. 1.3)** served as a resource for physical therapists, were interested in the healthcare of women before, during, and after pregnancy.

The popularity of the domain of Women's Health specialty grew in 1995, when a group of orthopedic physical therapists recognized that their clinics were crowded with women whose health concerns were beyond the obstetric issues and were not being adequately addressed. These females had no idea that their problems like pelvic pain or incontinence could be managed successfully through a tailor-made, structured exercise regime. They were ignorant of the role of PFM in the problems of sexual intercourse, urination, fertility, pregnancy preparedness, postpartum recovery, and cancer recovery.

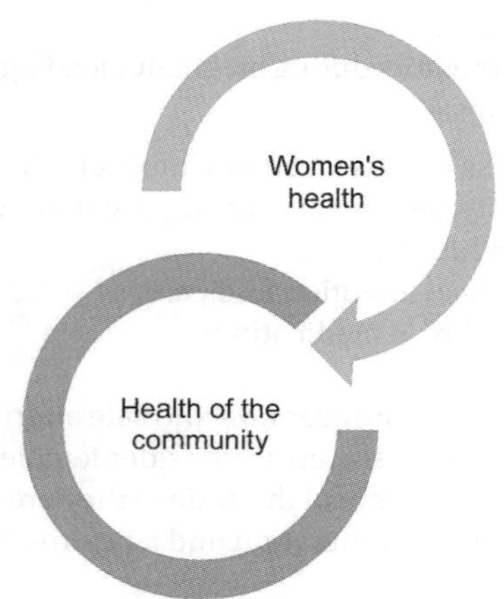

Fig. 1.2: Evolution of the healthy community.

From the times of Janet Campbell, Vaughan, and Helen Heardman, there has been a recognition of the importance of flexible hips and spines being conducive to easy labor. Events of labor and the postnatal period had their precursors in the pre-pregnancy, antenatal, and postnatal care that a female receives. These were the foundation stones for modern-day physiotherapy in Obstetrics and Gynecology.

Organizations Working Towards the Cause of Women's Health

The development of the role of physiotherapy in women's health has seen a change over the years. Various associations have come into existence to improve health care in women's health, to advance the practice and education in pelvic and women's health. Support networks include the following:

- ***Association of Chartered Physiotherapists in Women's Health*** (ACPWH) is a network group of the Chartered Society of Physiotherapy (CSP). It is one of the oldest associations, formed in 1948 as the Obstetric Physiotherapists Association.
- ***International Organization of Physical Therapists in Women's Health*** (IOPTWH) is an official subgroup of World Confederation of Physical Therapy (WCPT) which is now World Physiotherapy since 1999.
- ***American Physical Therapy Association (APTA) Pelvic Health*** (name approved in 2019) is an academy of the American Physical Therapy Association which promotes the role of physical therapy in the field of pelvic and abdominal health and wellness in women, men and children. It was founded by Elizabeth Noble in 1977, under the Section on Obstetrics and Gynecology, which later became Section on Women's Health (SoWH) (1995).
- ***Women's Health Division (WHD)*** is a division of the Canadian Physiotherapy Association (CPA) for advancement of physiotherapy practice in women's health.

Diverse Roles of the Physiotherapist

Over the years, the role of physiotherapy in women's health **(Fig. 1.4)** has diversified from antenatal and postnatal care.

- With female sportspersons putting some stellar performances on the world stage, the role of physiotherapists in training, as well as injury prevention has been brought into the limelight. To meet up with the needs of women returning to physical activity and exercise postpartum, is a task that can be efficiently brought to fruition by therapists working in the domain of women's health, guided by **accurate, research-based, and appropriate information on return to exercise post-childbirth.**

Consideration of Women's Health as being limited to pregnancy and childbirth → Formulation of section on Women's Health of the American Physical Therapy Association in 1977 → Growth of the concept of Women's health beyond Gynecology and Obstetrics

Fig. 1.3: Evolution of the concept of women's health.

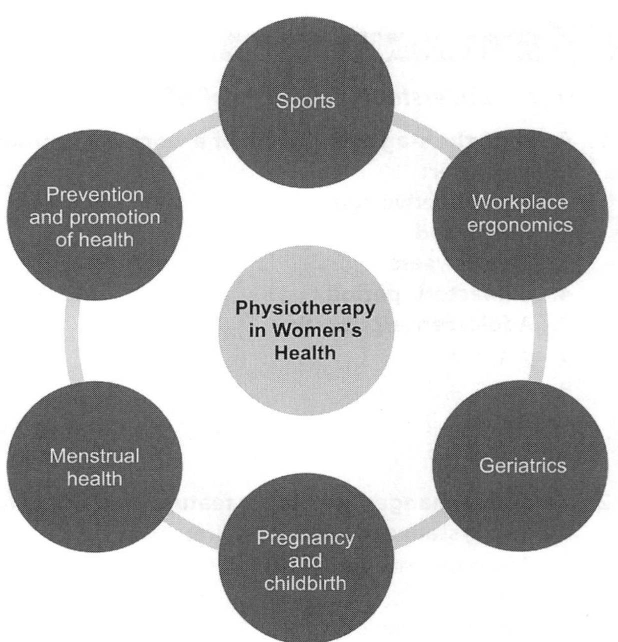

Fig. 1.4: Role of physiotherapy in women's health.

- Exercise is considered one of the strongest pillars of physiotherapy practice, and physiotherapists are the creative scientists who are involved in the battle against **sedentary behavior**. Exercise not only serves to counter the ill effects induced by hypokinesia but along with electrotherapeutic measures and ergonomic advice, can help ameliorate the risk of hypokinetic diseases like osteoporosis and help manage the existing decline in bone mineral density.
- **Geriatric physical therapy**, applied through hydrotherapy, mechanotherapy, and kinesiotherapy (biomechanical movements) has proven to be an important evidence-based method for older adults to improve mobility and balance, build strength—mental as well as physical, boost their confidence in their physical abilities, and nonetheless, remain active throughout the years.
- The gender-based difference does exist in symptom severity, in **work-related health conditions**, pre-existing risk factors at work (repetitive work, poor ergonomic equipment due to anthropometric mismatch), and at home (having less opportunity to relax and exercise outside of work). All these factors ensure that women in the workforce are vulnerable and efforts are needed to identify the unique job descriptions, demand analysis, anthropometric measures, ergonomic evaluation, and appropriate remedies for the same so that the female workforce can continue to work efficiently in an injury-free manner.
- The physical therapy profession has slowly but steadily progressed towards **preventive and promotive roles** instead of solely being focused on the management and remediation of disability. This has been achieved through measures aimed at preventing or reducing risk factors that may lead to disability while considering the external environmental and internal personal factors that impact each person's individualistic response to their health condition. In addition, there is a growing need to explore barriers such as fear and collaboratively look at potential solutions that can increase the engagement of women with exercise.

The ever-expanding active role being played by women in all spheres of life has shifted the focus of healthcare to the fitness and well-being of the female population and has brought to notice, a need to pay closer attention to their bodies during recreation, work, and throughout life.

Scope of Physiotherapy Practice

Physiotherapy in women's health is rarely a hot topic of discussion. This can be attributed to the fact that many issues that women face are delicate topics and many people do not like to discuss their incontinence or sexual dysfunction problems. In addition, information on these topics is not easily found and most women are not aware of the role of a Women's Health Physiotherapist in preventive, promotive, restorative, and rehabilitative aspects of their health.

However, the evidence in the literature is strongly supportive of the scope of practice in all health concerns of women: incontinence, pelvic/vaginal pain, prenatal and postpartum management, osteoporosis, rehabilitation following breast surgery, lymphedema, education, prevention, wellness, and exercise.

Women's health is a complex and multifaceted area of study. This book is our attempt at a passionate take on the uniqueness of being a woman and its implications on the healthcare being offered for the various concerns at different milestones of a women's chronological age.

Females across the life span, right from the young athlete, the childbearing woman, the working woman, the menopausal and elderly woman stand to receive life-long benefit from physical therapy.

Summary

Physiotherapy in women's health is an evolving field dealing with the various issues faced by women related to their health and well-being and the role of physiotherapy in managing them. The field has evolved from being just a subset of Obstetrics and Gynecology to dealing with almost all major problems related to a woman's health. Males have now started giving equal priority to females which has led to strengthening of their social position and standing. The role of a women's health physiotherapist involves creating awareness about the various problems of a woman and managing these problems effectively and efficiently through physiotherapeutic skills.

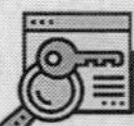

Review Questions

1. What are the stages in the lifespan of a woman?
2. Enlist the various problems faced by a female at various stages of the continuum of life.
3. What is the goal of physiotherapy in women's health?
4. What is the importance of women's health?
5. Write a short note on evolution of physiotherapy in women's health.
6. What is the scope of physiotherapy in women's health?

Bibliography

1. Baranitharan R, et al. Physiotherapy Care for Women's Health, 1st edition. New Delhi: Jaypee Brothers Medical Publishers Ltd.; 2010.
2. Konar H. DC Dutta's Textbook of Gynecology, 8th edition. New Delhi: Jaypee Brothers Medical Publishers Ltd; 2020.
3. Konar H. DC Dutta's Textbook of Obstetrics, 9th edition. New Delhi: Jaypee Brothers Medical Publishers Ltd; 2018.
4. Polden M, Mantle J. Physiotherapy in Obstetrics and Gynaecology, 1st edition. Oxford: Butterworth-Heinemann Publishers. 2018.
5. Sapsford R. Women's Health: A Textbook for Physiotherapists, 1st edition. Bailliere Tindall Publishers; 1997.
6. Sheth M, et al. Physiotherapy in General Medical and Surgical Conditions, 1st edition. New Delhi: Jaypee Brothers Medical Publishers Ltd; 2022.
7. Takeda Y. Understanding the life stages of women to enhance your practice. JMAJ. 2010;53(5): 273-8.

Multiple Choice Questions (MCQs)

To test your understanding and recall of key concepts.

1. Arrange the stages in the life of a woman in chronological order:
   1. Reproductive age
   2. Childhood
   3. Elderly years
   4. Climacteric period
   5. Adolescence/puberty

   A. 2, 5, 1, 4, 3
   B. 1, 2, 5, 4, 3
   C. 2, 5, 4, 1, 3
   D. 1, 2, 3, 4, 5

2. Cognitive changes are a usual feature of which of the following stages of a woman's life:

   A. Reproductive age
   B. Childhood
   C. Climacteric period
   D. Adolescence/puberty

ANSWERS

1. A	2. C

Chapter 2

Ethical Considerations in Women's Health

Megha Sandeep Sheth, Shivani Sheth

LEARNING OBJECTIVES

At the end of the chapter, the reader will be able to:
- Gain awareness about general ethical principles in physiotherapy.
- Gain knowledge about ethical considerations specific to women's health.
- Become aware of the ethical considerations for research on women.
- Understand the approaches to resolve ethical situations and dilemmas.

CHAPTER OUTLINE

INTRODUCTION

Ethics are the moral principles that guide a person's behavior or action. Ethical guidelines help the person to make a choice between right and wrong decisions.

Many ethical issues surround a woman and her health worldwide. Violence against women is condemned by all, whether it is at a societal level (female genital mutilation) or at a domestic level. Major issues include:

- Freedom from violence
- Independence in choices especially in reproduction
- Contraception, diagnosis and fetal abortion
- Sex selection

With an increasing role of physiotherapy in women's and men's pelvic health, the onus of ethical practice lies with the physiotherapist (PT).

Physiotherapists have a basic knowledge of the anatomy and physiology of sexual and reproductive health of women. They have a duty and role to play based on this knowledge. Women are a vulnerable population, more so, because of their function and role in reproduction and the social, economic and cultural circumstances. Gender-based discrimination is also seen socially and family health usually takes a precedence over the woman's individual health which increases the risk of her problems being ignored.

The importance of ethics for therapists dealing with women's health is to increase the sensitivity towards the issues of women and the cultural set-up they are living in.

PRINCIPLES OF ETHICS IN PHYSIOTHERAPY

The guiding ethical principles for physiotherapy practice are as follows:

Autonomy

Autonomy emphasizes the important role that women have in making decisions about their health. PTs should always seek woman's choices and respect their views and ideas.

- The woman should be provided all information about the management, the alternatives, risks and benefits. Consent or dissent should be an ongoing, repeated process through the assessment and management process.
- Because of the personal and intimate nature of the field, confidentiality of the patient needs to be specially protected.

CLINICAL EXAMPLE 1

Ms A who is 65-year-old, comes to the physiotherapy department with knee pain that she has for 10 years. She should be provided with complete information about physiotherapy and surgical options, scope and limitations of physiotherapy, so that she can decide the management strategy *(Autonomy)*.

Beneficence

All treatment should be based on best available evidence and should not be influenced by socioeconomic or other factors.

Non-maleficence

No assessment or treatment techniques should lead to harm including increased pain or emotional trauma.

CLINICAL EXAMPLE 2

Ms P, 37-year-old, came with a complaint of urinary incontinence. She should be assessed for pelvic floor muscle strength, so that appropriate exercises can be suggested *(Beneficence)*. However, if she is apprehensive or embarrassed in having the exam performed, it may be attempted later once she is comfortable *(Non-maleficence)*. The whole process can be explained, videos can be shown so she can make a decision to allow the pelvic floor (PF) exam *(Autonomy)*.

Justice

All women should be treated equally, irrespective of age, marital, religious, socioeconomic or racial status.

ETHICAL CONSIDERATIONS IN WOMEN'S HEALTH

The profession of physiotherapy focuses on interventions based on a complete evaluation and in women this includes the evaluation of pelvic floor muscle (PFM) function and dysfunction. Here, one deals with intimate issues and there maybe embarrassment and humiliation in discussing symptoms like urine or bowel leaks or incontinence and pelvic floor examination and so difficulties may be involved. These specifically create privacy and ethical issues in the field of urogynecology.

Clinical Pointer

A chaperone can be kept at all times to accompany a female patient and take care of her needs.

Strict boundaries need to be maintained in the relationship between patients and therapists because of the imbalance that exists in knowledge and power. This is also one of the factors which increases the vulnerability and so the need to promote independent and informed decisions made by patients.

Clinical Pointer

Any violation of boundaries destroys the trust which is necessary in health care and healing. A sexual or romantic relationship cannot be accepted between a therapist who is actively involved in the treatment and the patient. It can be accepted only if no residual dependency exists from the patient perspective. This is the principle of *fidelity*.

Maternal and fetal risks—recognizing abnormal or warning signs in the woman or fetus and early referral are the moral responsibility of a treating PT for which complete knowledge is necessary.

Code of Ethics

Various associations have their codes of conduct to guide ethical practice. For physiotherapy, the following may be referred to:

World Physiotherapy

The principles advocated by World Physiotherapy include:

- Respect the rights, privacy and personal dignity of all. Provide all information to encourage informed consent.
- Follow the code of ethics by the professional body in the country of practice.
- One should be responsible to exercise sound professional judgment.
- All patients should be equally treated with quality services.
- The remuneration charges should be appropriate.
- Accurate information should be provided to all clients.
- One should contribute to the development of the profession.

The Indian Association of Physiotherapists

The Indian Association of Physiotherapists provides the rules and guidelines among others as shown in **Box 2.1**.

Core Values by the American Physical Therapy Association

Core values by the American Physical Therapy Association (APTA) are shown in **Table 2.1**.

Box 2.1: Rules and guidelines by the Indian Association of Physiotherapists.

- Provide honest quality care to benefit the patient
- Respect the dignity and basic rights of the patients
- Maintain secrecy and confidentiality
- Take prior informed consent
- Comply with laws governing patient's rights and code of ethics
- Shall not indulge in activity that goes against the dignity and honour of the profession

Table 2.1: Core values by the American Physical Therapy Association.

Value	*Description*
Accountability	It is accepting the responsibility for the roles, actions, obligations of the physiotherapist that affects the outcomes of the patient and health needs of the society.
Altruism	It is keeping the interest or needs of the patient ahead of the therapist's needs or goals.
Collaboration	The therapist should work together with the patient, family and other professionals to achieve shared goals.
Compassion and caring	Compassion is the desire to identify with another person and caring is the concern and consideration for the needs and values of the other person.
Duty	The therapist should be committed to providing effective physical therapy services to their clients and positively contribute to the health of the society.
Excellence	The therapist should use current, updated knowledge and skills for assessment and management.
Integrity	It is the steadfast adherence to maintain high ethical practice standards including truthfulness, following through commitments, and verbalizing to others the rationale for actions.

Informed Consent

To prevent medicolegal issues in obstetrics and gynecology, informed consent for evaluation and treatment should be taken.

- It is a communication and interaction process which should be obtained:
  - Freely
  - Without threat
  - Without improper inducement
  - After complete information in understandable language has been provided
- Possible pain or discomfort, risks and side effects need to be described, and consent needs to be taken within treatment sessions to know if patient has any discomfort.
- Consent can be withdrawn at any time.
- Intimate partner consent is not ethically justified and may be taken only where indicated.

Elements of informed consent are described in **Box 2.2**.

Exceptions to informed consent include:

- **Emergency doctrine:** In case of life-threatening situation e.g., cardiopulmonary resuscitation (CPR) to a road traffic accident patient.
- **Therapeutic privilege:** This can be on bequest of family, and if it is the physician's decision. For example, if an old frail woman is diagnosed with cancer where revealing the diagnosis may worsen her cognitive and psychological status, physician can take the decision to waive off the informed consent. Competent patients retain the right to refuse treatment and must be given as much information as necessary to help them make informed decisions about consent or refusal.
- **Pediatrics:** In case of children below 18 years of age, that is if a 16-year old girl comes for treatment for primary dysmenorrhea to a male therapist, consent of parent/ guardian is of utmost importance. Presence of a staff or caregiver in the treatment room is also essential.
- **Waiver of information by patient with capacity:** For example, a patient who is rational, with proper cognition and is well-educated chooses to waive off, "I am busy, let's just begin with the treatment" or "I trust your decision about the treatment choices, do what's best for me".

Box 2.2: What elements should the informed consent include?

- A description of the proposed care, treatment, service, medication, intervention, or procedure
- An explanation of all potential benefits, risks, or side effects
- The likelihood of achieving care goals (curative or palliative)
- A description of any reasonable alternatives to the proposed intervention, as well as the potential benefits, risks, or side effects associated with these alternatives
- When necessary, any limitations on the confidentiality of patient information

Clinical Example 3

Ms T is an 80-year-old patient, diagnosed with low back pain and osteoporosis. After a week of intensive therapy, there is no relief in pain. Magnetic resonance imaging (MRI) and other radiological examinations are then done, which reveal cancer that has metastases in bone.

- The physician has invoked therapeutic privilege and decided not to reveal the diagnosis to her
- Her family also has requested for the same

After a month of her therapy, she asks the physiotherapist "What is my diagnosis, I have never had such a pain."

This now requires critical thinking and ethical decision-making by the therapist which is described later in this chapter.

Confidentiality and Privacy

These are two critically important and sensitive concepts in women's healthcare, which includes:

- **Decisional:** The right to make choices which supports autonomy
- **Physical:** The right to allow or deny examination and treatment, and also includes protection from unnecessary or embarrassing bodily contact or exposure
- **Informational:** Includes issues of confidentiality and access to records.

Clinical Pointer

Women can be exposed to personal harm or discrimination very easily from breeches in medical confidentiality. Therefore, the obligation to ensure strict confidentiality in women's health is even greater than usual.

Female Genital Mutilation

World physiotherapy opposes all forms of female genital mutilation (FGM) or female genital cutting (FGC). FGM is a fundamental violation of the rights of a girl or woman including:

- The right to physical integrity
- The right to health
- The right to life

FGM violates the principle of 'maleficence'. A therapist should be aware that the practice of FGM has serious physical and mental consequences.

Spread of HIV in Women

This is more common because of sexual violence and unprotected sex. It results in spread to the unborn fetus.

Clinical Pointer

A physiotherapist should be careful during treatment of patients with HIV and other easily communicable diseases like sexually transmitted diseases. Use universal precaution methods at all times.

Sexual Assault and Battery

- Battery is an intentional and offensive touching that violates the patient's bodily integrity. Battery in any form means unlawful and unpermitted physical contact with another person.
- Assault means the wrongful act of causing someone to reasonably fear imminent harm.

For example, if a physiotherapist inappropriately touches a patient without consent, it is battery. But if the therapist threatens to forcefully bend the knee joint, and thus creating fear of pain, it is assault.

Transgender Issues

Transgender describes a person whose experienced gender identity differs from that assigned at birth. In healthcare one needs to recognize and respect the fact that all patients may not fit into the binary gender description. The same principles of ethics can help eliminate disparities in healthcare.

Ethical Considerations during COVID-19 Pandemic

Social distancing has led to an increase in the suffering of women with pelvic floor dysfunction and a negative impact on quality of life. This is due to stress, physical inactivity, increase in obesity and difficulty in access to safe physiotherapy care. Some recommendations following COVID-19 are:

- To provide care through telephysiotherapy. Remote monitoring and feasibility need to be considered. Cultural, technological and personal limitations of therapist and patient need to be considered. Privacy, especially in storage of data, should be ensured. Complete information, confidentiality and consent are important.
- For assessment, mobile-based applications assessing voiding can be used. Remote PFM assessment can be avoided. Video or images of exposure of women's bodies should be avoided. Alternate tests like the stop test can be used.
- Health education regarding general health issues and their influence on PFD is recommended. Counseling and making women aware about these topics using various resources should be done.
- In person consultation is recommended based on government rules.

Clinical Pointer

If video or photos are needed, it should be on the facility's device and not on personal device of the therapist.

ETHICAL CONSIDERATIONS FOR RESEARCH ON WOMEN

The research on the use of thalidomide and its adverse effects on the children born, is one of the path breakers for need of consent in research. National Institute of Health (NIH) requires inclusion of women in all funded research unless inappropriate. Many researches are being conducted on women alone. This is necessary as some conditions are seen in women alone, are more commonly seen in women or women respond differently to the condition or treatment strategy. It may not be correct to conclude inferences from studies on men as the generalization may be erroneous due to the biological differences between men and women.

Pregnant women are considered to be a 'vulnerable population'. In fact, they should be considered as 'scientifically complex' as they have the capacity for autonomous decisions but are physiologically and ethically complex.

Issues in Research

- **Informed consent:** The woman should be explained in detail the need of the research, complete method, benefits and risks and then allowed to make a decision to take part in the research.
- Minimal risk should be weighed against the potential benefits before inclusion or exclusion of women in a research protocol.
- Intimate partner consent may not ethically be justified as a woman can decide for herself regarding participation in research. However, in certain situations it may be needed.
- Maternal and fetal risks need to be balanced as they are interconnected.

- One of the hurdles to participation is adequate childcare so that a woman can find time to participate in research.

Testing for genetically based diseases is growing. These are mostly done prenatally. In adults, testing for breast and ovarian cancer associated (BRCA) genes is increasing. Here consent is not considered, and also issues of benefit or harm arise. The harmful effects include emotional trauma, loss of child, stigmatization, financial losses, loss of opportunities and loneliness.

Clinical Pointer

Clinical ethics demands attention to learning practical approaches that can be used to promote trust and enhance the professional relationship between health provider and patient.

Summary

Major ethical issues in healthcare regarding women are patients' rights, equity of resources, confidentiality of the patients, patient safety, conflict of interests, informed consent, dealing with the opposite sex and fetus health. Following the principles of ethics autonomy, beneficence, non-maleficence and justice should be the constant goals. High ethical standards should be set to avoid distress and disrespect to the patient.

CLINICAL EXAMPLE

F, a physiotherapist works with J in a clinic owned by M. F finds out that J is having a consensual relationship with a female patient of the clinic. The next day F tells M about the incident. M calls J, tells him his behavior was unprofessional, and takes a promise that it won't happen again. M tells F there's no need for stronger action given this one-time lapse of judgment. F is unhappy with M's decision.

Applicable Principles of the Code of Ethics for the Employee (J)

- Respect the dignity and rights of all individuals.
- Do not exploit persons over whom they have a supervisory, evaluative, or other authority (e.g., patients/clients, students, supervisees, research participants, or employees).
- Physical therapists shall not engage in any sexual relationship with any of their patients/clients, supervisees, or students or harass anyone verbally, physically, emotionally, or sexually.

Applicable Principles of Code of Ethics for the Employer (M)

- Exercise sound professional judgment.
- Discourage misconduct by health care professionals and report illegal or unethical acts to the relevant authority, when appropriate.
- Protect the public and the profession from unethical, incompetent, and illegal acts.

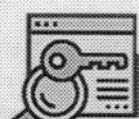

Review Questions

1. Why is ethics important in women's health?
2. What are the ethical problems in women?
3. What are the principles of ethics?

Bibliography

1. Cain JM. A global overview of ethical issues in women's health. International Journal of Gynecology & Obstetrics. 2000;70(1): 165-72.
2. Glantz LH, Annas GJ, Grodin MA, Mariner WK. Research in developing countries: taking benefit seriously. The Hastings Center Report. 1998,28(6):38.
3. Holm S. Principles of biomedical ethics, 5th edition. Journal of Medical Ethics. 2002;28:332.
4. Holub P. Clinical ethics: Somewhere between absolutism and relativism. The Internet Journal of Allied Health Sciences and Practice. 2010;8(4), Article 2.
5. https://bioethics.jhu.edu/about/what-is-bioethics/
6. https://collegeofphysiotherapy.com/the-iap-ethical-rulesregulations/
7. https://ethicsunwrapped.utexas.edu/glossary/moral-absolutism
8. https://plato.stanford.edu/entries/moral-relativism/
9. https://www.apta.org/siteassets/pdfs/policies/core-valuesendorsement.pdf
10. https://www.apta.org/your-practice/ethics-and-professionalism/clinical-decision-making/rips-model
11. https://www.glowm.com/pdf/english%20ethical%20issues%20in%20obstetrics%20and%20gynecology.pdf
12. https://www.sciencedirect.com/science/ar ticle/pii/B9780123739322003859
13. Kabira WM, Gachukia EW, Matiangi FO. The effect of women's role on health: the paradox. International Journal of Gynecology & Obstetrics. 1997;58(1):23-34.
14. Kim TH, Choi SD, Woo SH. An ethical issue in medical education of obstetrics and gynecology. J Menopausal Med. 2015;21(3):130-2. doi: 10.6118/jmm.2015.21.3.130. Epub 2015 Dec 25. PMID: 26793677; PMCID: PMC4719086.
15. Kirsch NR. Ethics in Practice: Practical matters, applying the new ethics documents to clinical scenarios. PT in Motion. 2009;1(3):48-50.
16. Kirsch NR. New and improved. PT in Motion. 2009;1(2):50-55.
17. Larson EL. United Nations Fourth World Conference on Women: Action for Equality, Development, and Peace (Beijing, China: September 1995). Emory Int'l L. Rev. 1996;10:695.
18. Shah P, Thornton I, Turrin D, et al. Informed Consent. [Updated 2021 Jun 14]. In: StatPearls [Internet]. Treasure Island (FL): StatPearls Publishing; 2022 Jan-. Available from: https://www.ncbi.nlm.nih.gov/books/NBK430827/
19. Svoboda JS. Promoting genital autonomy by exploring commonalities between male, female, intersex, and cosmetic female genital cutting. Global Discourse. 2013;3(2) 237-55.
20. Turner L. Medical ethics in a multicultural society. Journal of the Royal Society of Medicine. 2001; 94(11):592-94. https://doi.org/10.1177/014107680109401114

21. World Health Organization, United Nations Population Fund, Key Centre for Women's Health in Society. Mental health aspects of women's reproductive health: a global review of the literature. 2009.

Multiple Choice Questions (MCQs)

To test your understanding and recall of key concepts.

1. **Which of the following ethical principles refers to the right of a patient seeking treatment to the information about the management, the alternatives, risks and benefits:**
   A. Autonomy
   B. Beneficence
   C. Non-maleficence
   D. Justice
2. **Which of the following is *not* a principles of ethics in physiotherapy?**
   A. Autonomy
   B. Beneficence
   C. Non-maleficence
   D. Social welfare
3. **What is the primary goal of informed consent in physiotherapy?**
   A. To ensure the therapist's safety from medicolegal issues
   B. To provide financial clarity for the patient undergoing the treatment
   C. To respect the patient's autonomy and right to make informed decisions
   D. To comply with legal requirements of the governing body of the region
4. **During a session, a patient reveals she is a victim of domestic violence. How should the physiotherapist respond?**
   A. Respect confidentiality but encourage the patient to seek appropriate support services
   B. Confront the perpetrator of violence as you are privy to the information
   C. Share the information with the patient's employer or family members
   D. Ignore the information as it is outside the scope of practice
5. **A physiotherapist is conducting a research study on pelvic floor dysfunction in pregnant women. The study involves a per vaginal assessment that may cause mild discomfort. A 26-year-old pregnant participant who consented to the procedure but seems visibly distressed during the assessment. How should the physiotherapist handle this situation?**
   A. Continue the procedure since the patient has already provided a written informed consent
   B. Pause the procedure, address the participant's concerns, and reconfirm consent before proceeding
   C. Discontinue the participant's involvement in the study immediately
   D. Complete the procedure and address the participant's concerns after the assessment has been completed

ANSWERS

1. A	2. D	3. C	4. A	5. B

Chapter **3**

Anatomy and Biomechanics of the Female Body

Deepali N Hande, Nupoor Kulkarni

The female body is a chthonian machine, indifferent to the spirit who inhabits it.

—Camille Paglia

LEARNING OBJECTIVES

At the end of the chapter, the reader will be able to:
- Understand the normal anatomy of the female body.
- Know the anatomical changes after menarche.
- Know the anatomical changes during pregnancy.
- Know the anatomical changes after menopause.
- Understand the biomechanical changes during puberty, pregnancy, and postmenopause.

CHAPTER OUTLINE

INTRODUCTION

From birth, the female body undergoes various changes. During puberty, the female body undergoes tremendous anatomical and physiological changes like breast development, pubic and axillary hair growth, growth in height, and menstruation. Menarche (onset of first menstruation in life) can happen anywhere from 10–16 years, the peak time being 13 years.

ANATOMY OF THE FEMALE PELVIS

The pelvic cavity is enclosed by a bony, ligamentous and muscular wall and contains the urinary bladder, ureters, pelvic genital organs, rectum, blood vessels, lymphatics and nerves.

The pelvis is made up of pair of innominate bones which are called hip bones (ilium, ischium and pubis), sacrum and coccyx. These two hip bones are joined anteriorly at pubic symphysis and posteriorly at sacrum by sacroiliac joint **(Fig. 3.1)**. The female pelvis is wider than male pelvis to accommodate growing fetus during pregnancy. A wider pelvis in females could possibly be the reason for a greater carrying angle of the elbow (cubitus valgus) in females as compared to their male counterparts **(Fig. 3.2)**.

The Caldwell-Moloy's classification traditionally classifies the female pelvis into four parent types, based on the shape of the inlet **(Fig. 3.3 and Table 3.1)**:

1. Gynecoid
2. Anthropoid
3. Android
4. Platypelloid

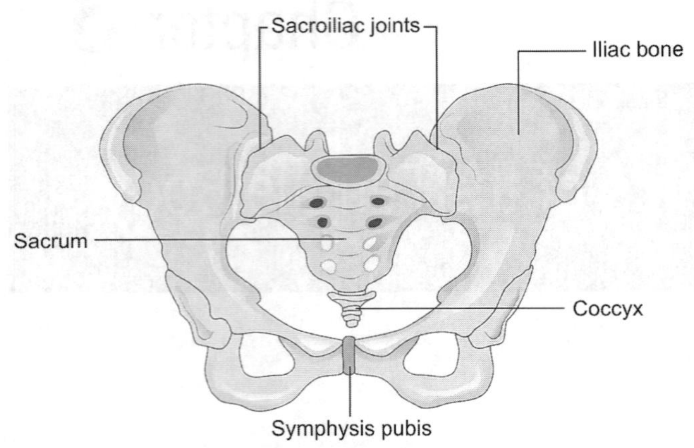

Fig. 3.1: Anatomy of the female pelvis.

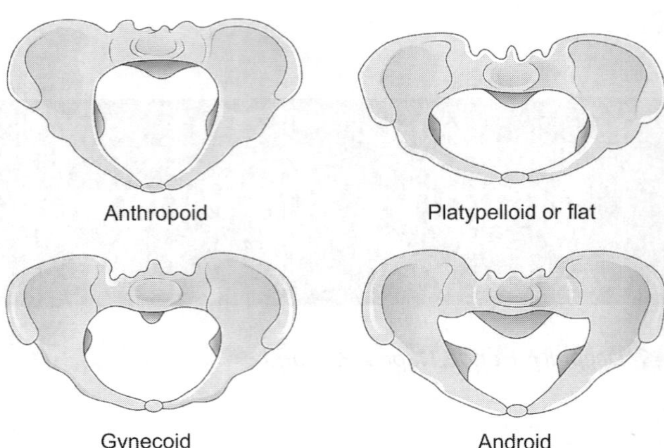

Fig. 3.3: Different types of female pelvis.

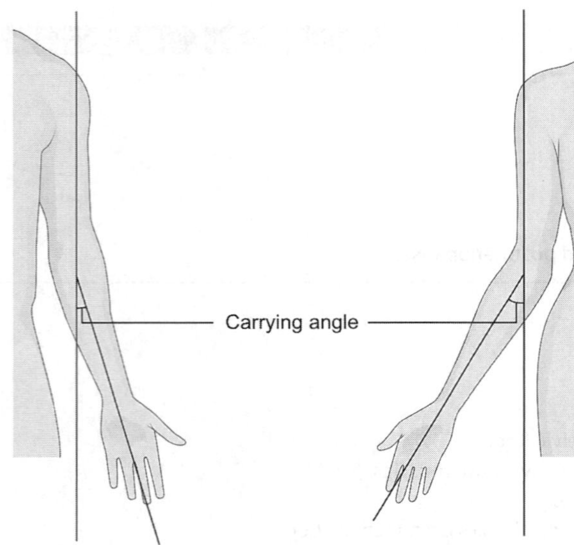

Fig. 3.2: Carrying angles in males and females.

> **Clinical Pointer**
>
> The *Gynecoid pelvis* is considered as an ideal pelvis for childbirth as recognized by its well-rounded oval inlet and similarly uncluttered outlet.

OVERVIEW OF THE FEMALE REPRODUCTIVE SYSTEM

Pelvic cavity contains following pelvic viscera **(Figs. 3.4 and 3.5)**:

- Bladder
- Urethra
- Uterus
- Vaginal canal
- Rectum
- Anal canal

Table 3.1: Characteristics of four parent types of the female pelvis.

Characteristics	*Gynecoid*	*Anthropoid*	*Android*	*Platypelloid*
Shape	Round	Oval anteroposteriorly	Triangular	Oval transversely
Anterior and posterior segment	In both segments almost same	Both segments increased with slight narrowing anteriorly	Anterior segment narrow and posterior segment short	Both segments reduced
Sacrum	Sacral angle more than 90°, anterior/posterior and up/down margins are well defined	Sacral angle more than 90°	Sacral angle less than 90°	Sacral angle more than 90°
Sacrosciatic notch	Broad (85°)	Little narrow	Narrow	Very broad, more than 90°
Side walls	Straight or slightly varying	Straight or varying	Conjoining	Varying
Pubic arch	Curved	Curved and long	Straight and long	Curved and short
Subpubic angle	Broad	Slightly small	Small	Very broad
Bituberous diameter	Standard	Standard or less	Less	Broad

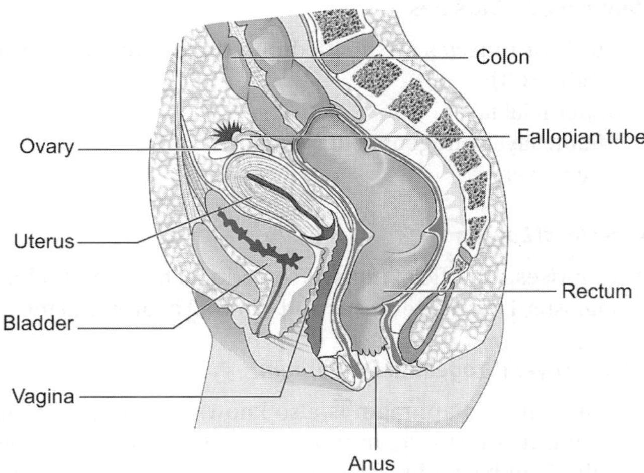

Fig. 3.4: Female pelvic cavity *(For color version, see Plate 1).*

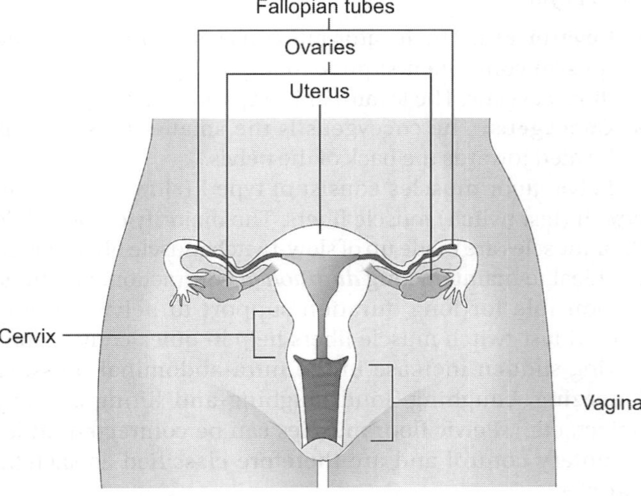

Fig. 3.5: Female reproductive system.

Bladder and Urethra

- Bladder is situated behind the pubic symphysis and it stores urine which is filtered by kidneys.
- The average capacity of bladder is 400–600 mL but can retain as much as 3–4 liters of urine.
- Bladder is made up of detrusor muscle.

Uterus

- The uterus **(Fig. 3.5)** is a pear-shaped organ located in the female pelvis between the urinary bladder anteriorly and the rectum posteriorly.
- Its average weight is 50–80 g.
- The uterus is divided into three main parts:
  1. Body
  2. Isthmus
  3. Cervix
- Uterus consists of the following three tissue layers from inside outwards **(Table 3.2)**:

Table 3.2: Layers of the uterine wall.

Layer	*Characteristics*
Endometrium	The inner layer, called the endometrium, is the most active layer and responds to cyclic ovarian hormone changes; the endometrium is highly specialized and is essential to menstrual and reproductive function.
Myometrium	The middle layer, or myometrium, makes up most of the uterine volume and is the muscular layer, composed primarily of smooth muscle cells.
Perimetrium	The outer layer of the uterus, the serosa or perimetrium, is a thin layer of tissue made of epithelial cells that envelops the uterus.

  1. Endometrium
  2. Myometrium
  3. Perimetrium

The uterus is an important female reproductive organ. In a female's whole lifespan several important physical functions, including menses, implantation, gestation, labor, and delivery are carried out by uterus. It is responsive to the hormonal milieu within the body, which allows adaptation to the different stages of a woman's reproductive life. The uterus adjusts to reflect changes in ovarian steroid production during the menstrual cycle and displays rapid growth and specialized contractile activity during pregnancy and childbirth. It can also remain in a relatively quiescent state during the prepubertal and postmenopausal years.

Blood Supply

- Main blood supply to the uterus is by the uterine artery which is a paired artery that arises from the internal iliac artery.
- This artery is found only in females, supplying the uterus and other parts of the female reproductive system like cervix, vagina, ovaries and uterine tube.

Nerve Supply

- The nerve supply to the pelvis is autonomic.
- Sympathetic nerve supply:
  - The inferior hypogastric plexus (T10–L1) supplies the uterus and cervix.
  - Labor pains are therefore referred to areas of skin supplied by these nerves, e.g., lumbosacral region, lower abdomen and loins.
- Parasympathetic nerve supply: The pudendal nerve (S2-S4) supplies the vagina and pelvic outlet.

Fallopian Tube

- These are the paired tube-like structures on either side of the uterus; each has two openings.

  One communicating with the lateral angle of the uterine cavity and other is on the lateral end of the tube called pelvic opening.
- It has the following functions:
  - Transport of gametes
  - To facilitate fertilization
  - Survival of zygote through its secretion

Ovary

- These are paired sex glands.
- The ovaries are the female pelvic reproductive organs containing ova and responsible for the production of sex hormones.
- There are two ovaries located on either side of the uterus within the broad ligament underneath the uterine (fallopian) tubes.

Vagina

- The vagina is a fibromusculomembranous sheath communicating the uterine cavity with the exterior at vulva.
- It gives channel to uterine secretion and menstrual blood.
- It has great distensibility which is essential during childbirth.

PELVIC FLOOR

The woman's pelvic floor is traditionally defined as a ligament-muscular apparatus that provides dynamic support to the urethra, bladder, vagina and rectum. The pelvic floor can be divided into suspensory and supporting parts.

- The pelvic floor forms a sling across the outlet of the pelvis to support the abdominal and pelvic visceral organs.
- The supporting part is formed by muscles (coccygeus and levator ani) that create a thin funnel. The funnel tapers into a hole that establishes a corridor for the above-mentioned organs. Levator ani is directly in connection with the vaginal muscle.
- The suspensory part, called the endopelvic fascia, is a fibrous component.

The aforementioned muscles and ligaments work in harmony for proper function of the pelvic floor. When the function is unbalanced, it may lead to dysfunctions of the pelvic floor.

Pelvic Floor Muscles

Pelvic floor muscles are divided into three layers **(Fig. 3.6 and Table 3.3)**:

1. Superficial layer
2. Middle layer (urogenital diaphragm)
3. Deep layer

Superficial Layer

It comprises superficial transverse perineal muscles, bulbospongiosus, ischiocavernosus and external anal sphincter.

Middle Layer (Urogenital Diaphragm)

The urogenital diaphragm is also known as the triangular ligament. It is a strong, muscular membrane between the symphysis pubis and ischial tuberosities and extends up to the triangular anterior portion of the pelvic outlet.

Deep Layer

- **Levator ani:** The levator ani consists of three separate muscle components: pubococcygeus, puborectalis and iliococcygeus. The levator ani wraps around the pelvis.
- **Coccygeus:** The coccygeus is the smaller muscle. It is located towards the back of the pelvis.

Pelvic floor muscles consist of type I (slow twitch) and type II (fast twitch) muscle fibers. The majority of the pelvic floor muscles are made up of slow-twitch muscle fibers which are ideal to maintain long *duration* of contraction, and thus, responsible for long duration support to pelvic viscera. Type II fast-twitch muscle fibers help in quick contractions during sudden increase in the intra-abdominal pressure (sneezing, coughing, loud laughing and lifting a heavy object, etc.). Pelvic floor muscles can be contracted under voluntary control and are therefore classified as skeletal muscles.

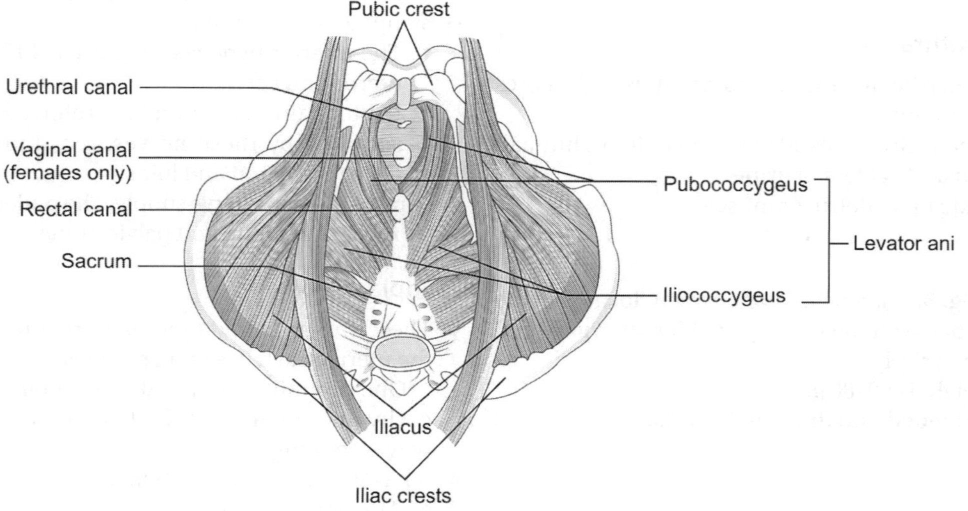

Fig. 3.6: Muscles of the female pelvic floor.

Table 3.3: Anatomy of pelvic floor muscles.

Muscle	Origin	Insertion	Action
Bulbospongiosus	Perineal body then divides to wrap around vagina	Fascia of corpus cavernosa	Empties urethra, acts as a sphincter to reduce lumen of vagina and assists erection of clitoris
Ischiocavernosus	Ischial ramus and tuberosity	Crus of clitoris	Maintains erection of clitoris by compression of outflow veins
Superficial transverse perineal	Ischial tuberosity	Perineal body	Stabilizes perineal body
External anal sphincter	Perineal body and encircles anal canal	Coccyx	Part of voluntary sphincter of anal canal
Levator ani (pubococcygeus)	Dorsal surface of pubis and fascia of obturator internus	Anococcygeal body between tip of coccyx and the anal canal	Voluntary sphincter of the anal canal
Levator ani (puborectalis)	Dorsal surface of pubis and fascia of obturator internus	Unites with its partner to make a U-shaped sling around the rectum	Controls defecation by pulling anorectal junction forward
Levator ani (iliococcygeus)	Posterior aspect of arcus tendinous levator ani and the ischial spine	Anococcygeal body and the coccyx	Helps to support pelvic viscera and lateral coccyx
Coccygeus	Ischial spine	Lower two sacral and upper two coccygeal spinal segments, blends with sacrospinous ligament on its external surface	Supports pelvic viscera, flexion of coccyx, stabilizes sacroiliac joint

 **Clinical Pointer**

Type II muscle fibers reduce with advancing age, which may be a probable reason for accidental leakage of urine droplets on sudden increase in intra-abdominal pressure and increased prevalence of incontinence in postmenopausal women.

Blood Supply

The pelvis receives its blood supply from branches of the anterior division of the internal iliac artery namely inferior vesical, pudendal, inferior gluteal.

Nerve Supply

It has nerve supply from perineal branch of the pudendal nerve (S2–S4).

Functions of Pelvic Floor Muscles

- **Support to pelvic viscera:** The pelvic floor muscles support the bladder, uterus, rectum, and important abdominal organs against gravity and any added downward pressure due to gravity.
- **Lumbo-pelvic stability:**
  - The pelvic floor is one of four muscles making up the inner 'core', which stabilizes the pelvis and lower back.
  - The pelvic floor is a part of the **abdominal capsule/ lumbopelvic cylinder/core muscles (Fig. 3.7)** with the diaphragm, transversus abdominis, multifidus. All these muscles function in coordination, their synergistic working pattern is important in maintenance of posture through intra-abdominal pressure regulation and thoracolumbar fascial tension.

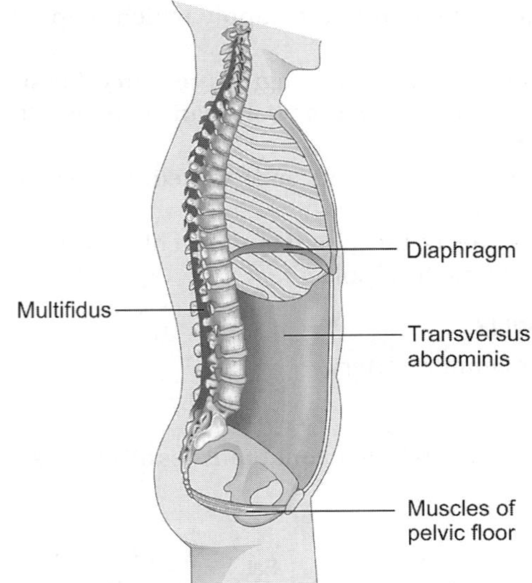

Fig. 3.7: Muscles of the abdominal capsule.

  - Recent studies have shown pelvic floor muscle asymmetry is related to lumbopelvic complex malalignment.
- **Sphincteric function:**
  - These are the muscles which control both the opening of the urethra and rectum. Thus, pelvic floor muscles play important role in urinary and anal continence.
  - During certain activities like sneezing, vomiting, coughing, lifting a heavy object, or forced expiration, these muscles unconsciously contract at rest and can be consciously contracted during times of raised intra-abdominal pressure to maintain continence.
- **Sexual function:** The pelvic floor plays a role in orgasm.

Clinical Pointer

Pelvic floor muscle dysfunction will lead to genital prolapse and incontinence, etc., (anal and urinary) which can be prevented and rehabilitated by physiotherapy treatment.

BREAST

Female breast consists of fat and glandular tissues and it lays on the pectoralis major muscle **(Fig. 3.8)**. Anatomically breasts are called as *mammary gland.*

- It is an important accessory organ of female reproductive system.
- Unlike male breasts, female breasts have milk ducts and glandular tissue, due to which females can do lactation (breastfeeding).
- Shape of the breast is determined by connective tissues and ligaments, which also provide support.
- The size is determined by amount of fat stored in the breast.

Nipples

- Nipples are conical projections present at the level of 4th intercostal space, 10 mm from the midline.
- Nipples have rich nerve supply which helps in sexual arousal.
- Minimal 7 mm nipple length is required for successful breastfeeding, so that the baby can latch onto the breast properly.
- Nipples can be flat, short, and inverted, which may hamper breastfeeding.
- The areola is the circular dark-colored area of skin surrounding the nipple.

Blood Supply

Internal mammary artery

Nerve Supply

Anterior and lateral cutaneous branches of intercostal nerves T3-T5.

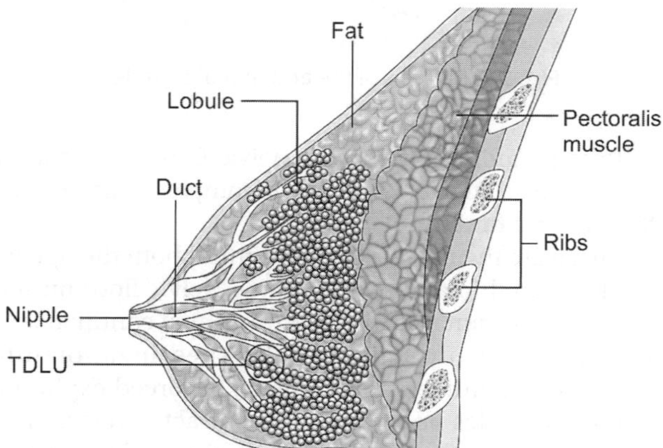

Fig. 3.8: Structure of the breast. (TDLU: terminal ductal lobular unit)

Changes in the Breasts during Lifespan

In a lifespan the breast undergoes hormone mediated growth changes two times, i.e., during puberty and during pregnancy. Females sometimes may feel fullness and tenderness in breast during different stages of menstrual cycle.

Changes in Breasts during Puberty

- Development of breast buds
- It becomes more rounded and bigger
- The areola becomes bigger and darker and the nipples may stick out.

Changes in Breasts during Pregnancy

- Outer margins of areola are rich in modified sebaceous glands, which are enlarged during pregnancy and lactation to form raised tubercles of Montgomery.
- Oily secretions from these sebaceous glands lubricate nipples and areola, helps to prevent cracking of nipples during lactation.
- Breast size increases.
- Veins on breasts become darker.

BIOMECHANICS OF THE FEMALE BODY

Biomechanics is the mechanics of the human body.

Biomechanical Changes during Puberty

After menarche, the female body undergoes changes due to hormonal and other variations.

- Significant changes are observed in lower limb biomechanics due to adolescent growth spurt.
- Wider pelvis affects the lower limb biomechanics, especially, knee joint biomechanics.
- The body undergoes the greatest amount of growth in height and weight. The adolescent growth spurt is associated with rapid growth and hormonal changes, thought to contribute to the increased anterior cruciate ligament injury risk in girls.
- Gender-based differences in anatomical structure play a large role in biomechanical alignment and function **(Table 3.4)**.

Table 3.4: Anatomical differences based on gender.

	Men	*Women*
Height	Taller than women	Shorter than men
Long bones	Longer than women	Shorter than men
Carrying angle	Less	Greater
Center of gravity	Higher than women	Lower than men
Vertebral body	Bigger than women	25% smaller than men
Lordosis angle	Less than women	Greater compared to men
Pelvis	Narrow	Wider
Q angle	Less	Increased
Femoral anteversion	Less	Increased
Tibial torsion	Less	Increased

- Evolutionary adaptation of having wider hips has led to the females having a greater Q angle. In terms of function this implies a tendency for the knees to shift medially during hip flexion, resulting in greater adduction and internal rotation at the hip as well as abduction at the knee and ankle eversion during the stance phase of running.

This vulnerable position of the joints of lower extremity kinematic chain, imposes increased valgus stress on the knee and abnormal forces on the ligaments and other supporting structures, putting the female subjects at a greater risk of injury.

Biomechanical Alterations during Pregnancy

Pregnancy is associated with changes in musculoskeletal system, cardiovascular system, respiratory system and reproductive system with minor changes in gastrointestinal system, urinary system and nervous system, etc. Pregnancy is a natural process that produces a number of physiological changes in a woman's body. Biomechanical and hormonal profile changes during pregnancy can alter musculoskeletal alignments due to variations in spinal curvature, balance, and gait patterns. The hormones chiefly secreted during pregnancy are progesterone, estrogen and relaxin. Among these hormones relaxin is responsible for gradual replacement of collagen in target tissues (e.g., pelvic joints, joint capsules and cervix) with a remodeled modified form that has greater extensibility and pliability which ultimately leads to generalized joint laxity. Over 38 to 42 weeks, women experience several changes in the body's morphology, physiology, and hormonal system.

The changes of pregnancy are due to effect of the interaction of four factors:

1. Changes in collagen and involuntary muscles due to secretion of certain pregnancy-induced hormones.
2. The increased total blood volume.
3. The growth of the fetus leading to enlargement and displacement of the uterus.
4. Increase in body weight and adaptive changes in the center of gravity and posture.

Pregnant women tend to rely on feedforward mechanism instead of feedback mechanism with predominant:

- Increase in postural sway
- Increased base of support
- Increased reliance on visual cues
- Ankle joint strategy

Biomechanical Alterations in Pregnancy Leading to Change in Posture and Gait

A number of *hormonal and biomechanical changes* occur during pregnancy.

- Increased levels of relaxin hormone are thought to be responsible for ***increased ligament laxity*** and thus changes in the musculature of the body, mainly in the lower trunk.
- Growing uterus changes the body's center of gravity (COG), which shifts forward and upwards. To maintain the upright posture, there occur changes in the spinal curvature in terms of both increase in lordosis and kyphosis **(Box 3.1)**.

Box 3.1: Series of adaptation in spine during pregnancy.

- Increased weight and growing uterus, shifts COG forwards and upwards
- To maintain upright position lumbar lordosis increases.
- Compensatory thoracic kyphosis will occur (increased breast mass also leads to thoracic kyphosis)
- Forward tipping of scapula will lead to rounded shoulder
- Head shifts forward
- Posterior neck activity increases to maintain the head position
- Extension at neck to maintain eye horizontal (as per optic righting reflex), results in extension at upper cervical spine
- Scapular adductors and upward rotators undergo stretch weakness because of thoracic kyphosis

- Due to ***shift in the COG***, there is tendency of an increased anterior displacement of line of gravity (LOG). This anterior displacement is counterbalanced by increased activation of gastrocnemius and soleus, extension of hip or posterior displacement of upper trunk. This eventually leads to increase in the lumbosacral angle and an increased lumbar lordosis.
- The effects of these differences during pregnancy are associated with ***alterations in sitting and standing posture.*** This also influences the static and dynamic balance as well as causes changes in the kinematics of the limbs during gait. These kinematic changes include the altered hip, knee, and ankle movements in all planes, as well as alterations in the kinematics of the trunk relating to the relationship between the trunk and the pelvis.
- In terms of balance, ***changes to the center of pressure (COP)*** are used as an indicator of stability. Evidence in literature shows that spatiotemporal parameters of gait during pregnancy demonstrate significantly increased path length, an increase in step width and reduced gait velocity.
- ***Changes to kinematics of the joints during gait*** are also reported. These include reduced flexion and extension in the hip, amongst other effects.
- Weight gain during pregnancy challenges the musculoskeletal system to adapt accordingly. The changes are visible especially in increased weight and skeletal alignment. Other less visible changes are the increased joint laxity and change in the COG. Altogether, these changes affect the balance and body stability and can cause discomfort and pain.
- Change in the COG is compensated by ***hyperextension of knees*** to maintain balance and upright posture. This puts pressure on the anterior cruciate ligaments throughout the pregnancy and may lead to lengthening which results in impingement against the femoral notch. This laxity decreases significantly in the postpartum period.
- Many of the biomechanical changes occur in the pelvis or in adjacent joints. Very few changes occur during late pregnancy, and most of these changes are related to angular motion of pelvis and hip, especially anterior tilting of pelvis. Weight of the uterus, fetus and placenta on the anterior part of the body and weak force production by the rectus abdominis result in the position of the pelvis seen during late pregnancy. However, this anterior tilt of

pelvis and increased lumbar lordosis help in maintenance of the trunk in upright position. However, the function of this anterior tilt and the increase of the lumbar lordosis are related to the maintenance of the trunk in an upright position. Studies have stated that postural changes during pregnancy include increased lordotic angles.

- ***Lordosis*** is seen in the lumbar and cervical regions of the spine and kyphosis in the thoracic and sacral regions of the spine. Studies have shown that pregnancy significantly increases the lordotic angle of the spine as well as the kyphotic angle in the developing pregnancy between 2nd and 3rd trimesters. These changes during pregnancy are attributed to the growing abdomen as it is located closest to the lumbar spine, and thus influencing the lordosis the most.
- Based on previous studies, there are individual variations in the spinal curvature, which could be due to factors like body weight and tendency to exercise.
- ***Anterior pelvic tilt:*** The accumulated literature discusses that pelvic tilt may be associated with alterations in the spine. Increased anterior tilt is attributed to weakened abdominal muscles during pregnancy as a result of increased levels of relaxin and progesterone or overstretching of the muscles due to increased abdominal muscle length, the pelvis is connected to the lumbar spine via hip flexors, and hence, an anteriorly-tilted pelvis shortens the hip flexors and increases lordosis of the spine **(Fig. 3.9)**. This increased anterior pelvic tilt can be a cause of instability in posture of the pregnant female, especially during the third trimester.
- Several studies have assessed the association of spinal curvature with ***pain*** in pregnancy and stated that levels of low back pain increase with the developing pregnancy which correlates with increased lordosis.
- Gait speed is decreased during pregnancy compared to prepregnancy. Other changes in spatial and temporal parameters of gait are shown in **Table 3.5**.

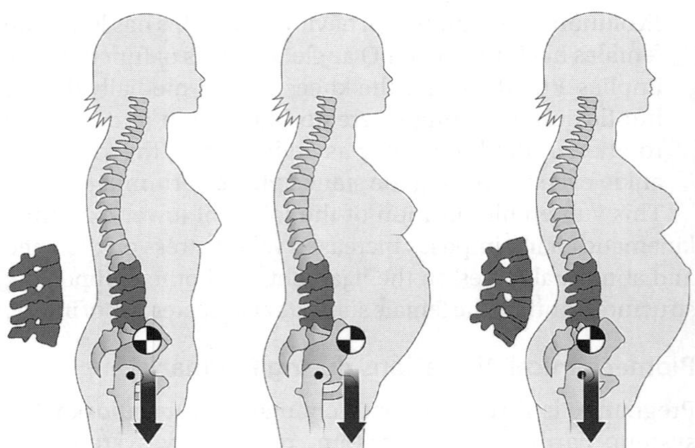

Fig. 3.9: Increased lordosis in pregnancy.

Table 3.5: Changes in gait during pregnancy.

Parameters	*Changes*
Step length	Decreases
Step width	Increases with advancing pregnancy
Stride length	Decreases with advancing pregnancy
Stride width	Normal
Single support time	Decreases
Double support time	Increases with advancing pregnancy
Base of support	Increases
Ground reaction forces	Decreases in late pregnancy

Clinical Pointer

As the changes in posture and gait during pregnancy are individualized and also determined by prepregnancy fitness, it is important to assess pregnant women in early phase of antenatal period for application of preventive measures.

Anthropometric Changes

- Body mass increases with the developing pregnancy, with increased size of trunk and abdominal girth, most significantly observed in the third trimester.
- Increases can also be observed in the width of the thorax, girth of the gluteals, girth of the calves, and biceps and triceps skin folds during pregnancy. Furthermore decreased muscle mass of calves and increased fat deposition can be seen.
- Foot arches are significantly reduced, along with a significant increase in the width of the foot. This results in an increased area of contact between the middle of the foot predominantly second metatarsal and the floor. Studies have reported that pregnant women have higher recorded Foot Posture Indices (FPI) in the third trimester.
- During pregnancy ankle and feet are more prone to water retention. This is a likely explanation for the increase in foot width and contact with the floor. Also, higher relaxin levels may play a role in relaxing the plantar fascia, the ligament on the sole of the foot that supports the arch. A weakened plantar fascia combined with increased weight from pregnancy pushing downwards is a likely explanation for a reduced arch height, and thus an increase in foot contact with the floor. In terms of quality of life, associations have been made between higher reported foot pain levels in women with flat feet in the general population.
- Reduced trunk motion, static and dynamic stability, gait velocity, hip extension/flexion, foot arch height and increased step width, risk of falls and double support time are significantly seen in the third trimester.
- Conflicting results are explained in many cases by reasoning that each woman shows individual pregnant morphologies that have varying effects on the biomechanics of the body. Furthermore, each woman adopts unique methods to minimize risk. Therefore, it might be important to assess the individual changes in a pregnant woman, including ankle stiffness, particularly in her late pregnancy, to understand her own individual risks. Also, studies could investigate whether other individual differences play a role in the effects of pregnancy like number of previous pregnancies,

position of fetus within the uterus, or perhaps even foot size, since it is known that contact of feet with the floor is changed during pregnancy. Further studies could also explore frontal spinal curvature, as well as any associations between quality of life and a reduced trunk range of motion and altered joint kinematics.

Biomechanical Changes with Menopause

The World Health Organization (WHO) defines natural menopause as the permanent cessation of menstruation resulting from loss of ovarian follicular activity. Menopause leads to remarkable change in overall health of a female.

- Changes in body composition seem to be influenced by the menopausal transition; mainly in terms of increase in fat mass and decreased lean body mass and changes in fat distribution from a more peripheral pattern to a central pattern.
- Significant associations have been observed between increased fat mass, waist circumferences, and decreased skeletal muscle mass and increasing follicle-stimulating hormone (FSH) levels, independent of age, indicating a self-regulating and considerable effect of menopause.
- Muscle and bone mass decline with aging, further increasing the risk for sarcopenia and osteoporosis. The contribution of menopause-related hormonal changes, especially estrogen deficiency leads to increased osteoclast activity with a net deficit in osteoblastic activity which leads to bone formation. There may be a loss of 2% of cortical bone and 9% of cancellous bone per year and an overall bone loss of 0.7% per year. Cancellous part of vertebral bone is affected first, which in turn reduces the vertebral height, leading to dowager's hump **(Box 3.2 and Fig. 3.10)**. In addition, there is thinning of the cortex. Hip and distal end of wrist also show similar changes.
- Previous studies have shown a progressive decline in hip bone mineral density (BMD) from premenopausal to postmenopausal status and a significant association between BMD decline and either an increase in FSH or a decline in estradiol levels.
- The age-related deterioration in muscle strength is attributed to the decline in muscle mass. However, that decline in muscle strength may be up to three times greater than the decline in muscle mass suggesting that neural and muscle quality-related factors have a significant effect on muscle strength in old age.

  Bone metabolism constantly takes place through osteoblastic activity of bone formation and osteoclastic activity leading to bone resorption. Deficiency of estrogen hormone leads to deterioration of bone microarchitecture with a decreased bone formation compared to resorption and thus bone loss. Trabecular bone, in the femoral neck, appears sensitive to menopause-related hormonal changes.
- Research reported that menopause transition is associated with balance impairment. There is a close association between postural instability and risk of falling, and stabilometric parameters are predictors of fall in postmenopausal women. In menopause, there is an increase in intra-abdominal fat and total body weight and age-related loss of muscle mass and strength which may be the probable cause affecting functional mobility.

Box 3.2: Dowager's hump.

Dowager's hump is also known as hyperkyphosis or Gibbus deformity which may develop from either muscle weakness and degenerative disc disease, leading to vertebral fractures and worsening hyperkyphosis, or from initial vertebral fractures that precipitate its development. It may lead to difficulty while performing daily activities, a reduced balance, slower gait, respiratory problems and higher postural sway which also adds to risk for falls.

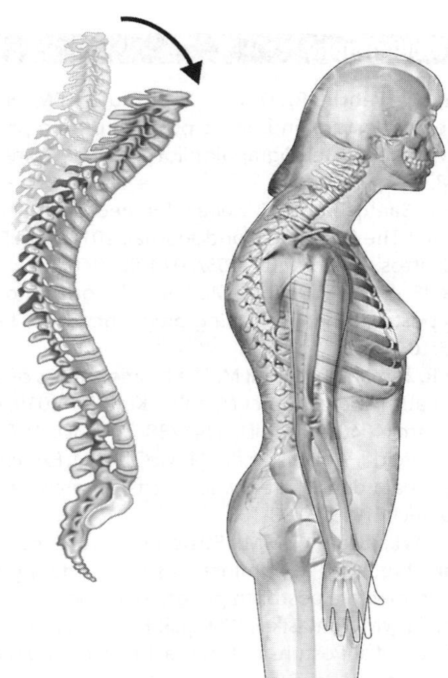

Fig. 3.10: Dowager's hump.

Summary

The *Gynecoid pelvis* is considered as an ideal pelvis for childbirth. Female pelvis is wider than male pelvis. A woman's body undergoes tremendous change in the puberty and during childbearing year. Muscle and bone mass decline with aging, further increasing the risk for sarcopenia and osteoporosis.

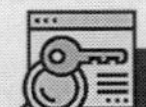

Review Questions

1. Explain anatomy of pelvic floor muscles.
2. Write functions of pelvic floor muscles.
3. Explain biomechanical changes during pregnancy.
4. Describe the biomechanical problems during menopause.
5. Explain postural changes associated with menopause.

Bibliography

1. Betsch M, Wehrle R, Dor L, Jungbluth RW, Hakimi PM, et al. Spinal posture and pelvic position during pregnancy: A prospective rasterstereographic pilot study. Eur Spine J. 2015;24: 1282-88.
2. Branco M, Santos-Rocha R, Vieira F. Biomechanics of gait during pregnancy. The Scientific World Journal. 2014;2014:5. Article ID 527940. https://doi.org/10.1155/2014/527940
3. Bullock JE, Jull GA, Bullock MI. The relationship of low back pain to postural changes during pregnancy. Aust J Physiother. 1987;33:10-17.
4. Conder R, Zamani R, Akrami M. The biomechanics of pregnancy: A systematic review. J Funct Morphol Kinesiol. 2019;4(4):72. doi: 10.3390/jfmk4040072. PMID: 33467386; PMCID: PMC7739277.
5. Dumas G, Reid J, Wolfe L, Griffin M, McGrath M. Exercise, posture, and back pain during pregnancy: Part 1. Exercise and posture. Clin Biomech. 1995;10:98-103.
6. Gilleard WL, Brown JMM. Structure and function of the abdominal muscles in primigravid subjects during pregnancy and the immediate postbirth period. Phys Ther. 1996;76:750-62.
7. Glinkowski WM, Tomasik P, Walesiak K, Głuszak M, Krawczak K, Michoński J, et al. Posture and low back pain during pregnancy—3D study. Ginekol Pol. 2016;87:575-80.
8. Hay O, Dar G, Abbas J, Stein D, May H, Masharawi Y, et al. The lumbar lordosis in males and females, Revisited. PLoS ONE. 2015;10(8):e0133685. doi:10.1371/journal.pone.0133685
9. Desai H. HET's Manual of Pelvic Floor Rehabilitation, 1st edition, New Delhi. Jaypee Brothers Medical Publisher Ltd. 2020.
10. Jelen K, Lopot F, Hadraba D, Herman H, Lopotova M. The Women's Pelvic Floor Biomechanics. In: Goswami T, (Editor). Injury and Skeletal Biomechanics [Internet]. London: IntechOpen; 2012. [cited 2022 Jun 29]. Available from: https://www.intechopen.com/chapters/38121 doi: 10.5772/47773.
11. Katzman WB, Wanek L, Shepherd JA, Sellmeyer DE. Age-related hyperkyphosis: Its causes, consequences, and management. The Journal of Orthopaedic and Sports Physical Therapy. 2010;40(6):352. https://doi.org/10.2519/jospt.2010.3099
12. Konar H. DC Datta's Textbook of Gynecology, 8th edition, New Delhi. Jaypee Brothers Medical Publisher Ltd; 2020.
13. Krkeljas Z. Changes in gait and posture as factors of dynamic stability during walking in pregnancy. Hum Mov Sci. 2018;58: 315-20.
14. McCrory JL, Chambers AJ, Daftary A, Redfern MS. The pregnant "waddle": An evaluation of torso kinematics in pregnancy. J Biomech. 2014;47:2964-68.
15. Moore K, Dumas G, Reid J. Postural changes associated with pregnancy and their relationship with low-back pain. Clin Biomech. 1990;5:169-74.
16. Moore KL, Dalley AF, Agur AMR. Clinically Oriented Anatomy, 7th edition. Philadelphia, PA: Lippincott Williams & Wilkins; 2014.
17. Moore KL, Dalley AF. Essential Clinical Anatomy, 5th edition. Baltimore: Lippincott Williams and Wilkins; 2006.
18. Rivard AB, Laura Galarza-Paez L, Peterson DC. StatPearls [Internet]. StatPearls Publishing; Treasure Island (FL): Service of the National Library of Medicine, National Institutes of Health. 2021. (PMID: 30137859)
19. Santo E, AibarAlmazan J, Martinez-Amat A, de Loureiro NEM A, BrandaoLoureiro V, Lavilla-Lerma ML, et al. Menopausal symptoms, postural balance, and functional mobility in middle-aged postmenopausal women. Diagnostics. 2021;11:2178. https://doi.org/10.3390/diagnostics11122178.
20. Schroder G, Kundt G, Otte M, Wendig D, Schober H-C. Impact of pregnancy on back pain and body posture in women. J Phys Ther Sci. 2016;28:1199-1207.
21. Sipila S, Tormakangas T, Sillanpaa E, Aukee P, Kujala U, Kovanen V, et al. Muscle and bone mass in middle-aged women: role of menopausal status and physical activity, Journal of Cachexia, Sarcopenia and Muscle. 2020;11:698-709.https://doi.org/10.1002/jcsm.12547.
22. Sternfeld B, Dugan S. Physical activity and health during the menopausal transition. Obstet Gynecol Clin North Am. 2011;38(3):537-66. doi: 10.1016/j.ogc.2011.05.008. PMID: 21961719; PMCID: PMC3270074.

Multiple Choice Questions (MCQs)

To test your understanding and recall of key concepts.

1. What is the average capacity of the female bladder?
- A. 200–300 mL
- B. 400–600 mL
- C. 800–1,000 mL
- D. 1–2 liters

2. Which type of pelvis is considered most ideal for childbirth?
- A. Android
- B. Anthropoid
- C. Gynecoid
- D. Platypelloid

3. What is the main function of the endometrium layer of the uterus?
- A. To support pelvic organs
- B. To maintain the structure of the uterus
- C. To respond to cyclic ovarian hormone changes
- D. To provide lubrication

4. Which hormone is primarily responsible for joint laxity during pregnancy?
- A. Estrogen
- B. Progesterone
- C. Relaxin
- D. Oxytocin

5. If a woman presents with stress urinary incontinence during menopause, which type of muscle fiber reduction might be a contributing factor?
- A. Type I (slow-twitch)
- B. Type II (fast-twitch)
- C. Smooth muscle
- D. Cardiac muscle

6. A pregnant woman complains of lower back pain due to changes in posture. Which compensatory mechanism is most likely observed in her gait?
- A. Decreased lumbar lordosis
- B. Increased anterior pelvic tilt
- C. Reduced base of support
- D. Elevated center of gravity

7. **What distinguishes the gynecoid pelvis from the platypelloid pelvis in terms of structure?**
   A. Gynecoid pelvis is round compared to an oval platypelloid pelvis
   B. Shorter pubic arch in the gynecoid pelvis
   C. Greater anterior and posterior segments in the platypelloid pelvis
   D. Smaller subpubic angle in the gynecoid pelvis

8. **During pregnancy, which biomechanical alteration could explain the increased risk of knee injury?**
   A. Decreased Q angle
   B. Increased valgus stress on the knee
   C. Reduced adduction at the hip
   D. Increased tibial torsion

9. **Which of the following gender-based differences in anatomical structure is *true*?**
   A. Tibial torsion is more in females
   B. Femoral anteversion is less in females
   C. Pelvis is narrower in females
   D. Center of gravity is higher in females

ANSWERS

1. B	2. C	3. C	4. C	5. B
6. B	7. A	8. B	9. A	

Section 2

Evaluation in Women's Health

Section Outline

Chapter 4

Assessment in Women's Health

Payal P Gahlot

LEARNING OBJECTIVES

At the end of the chapter, the reader will be able to:

- Describe salient points of physiotherapy assessment to be included in various gynecological and obstetric conditions.
- Assess women with menstrual problems.
- Perform assessment of women in the antenatal and postnatal periods.
- Assess diastasis recti during the postnatal period.
- Understand the importance and method of assessment of pelvic floor muscles.
- Understand the details about transvaginal and transrectal pelvic floor muscle examination.
- Understand the details about different assessment methods for urinary incontinence.
- Perform physiotherapy assessment of women suffering from breast cancer.

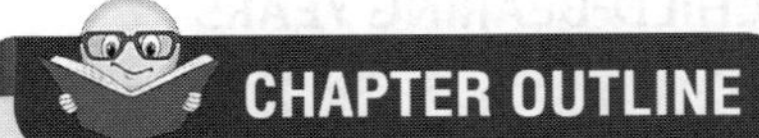

- Introduction
- Physiotherapy assessment of menstrual disorders
  - Obesity assessment
  - Quality of life
  - Pain assessment
- Assessment in child-bearing years
  - Antenatal period
  - Assessment in postnatal period
  - Assessment of diastasis recti
- Assessment following gynecological and obstetrical surgeries
  - Assessment following cesarean section
  - Assessment following hysterectomy
- Assessment of pelvic floor muscles
  - Manual muscle testing of pelvic floor muscles
  - Transvaginal pelvic floor muscle examination
  - Pelvic floor manometry
  - Electromyography
  - Ultrasound examination
  - Transrectal pelvic floor muscle examination
- Assessment for urinary incontinence
- Assessment of females in the transition period and menopause
- Assessment of elderly women
  - Health screening for elderly women
  - Physical therapy assessment for senior citizen women
- Assessment of women with breast cancer

INTRODUCTION

Women's reproductive and sexual health has a distinct difference compared to men's health. Even in developed countries pregnancy and childbirth are associated with substantial risks to women with maternal mortality. Comorbidity from other non-reproductive diseases such as cardiovascular disease contributes to both the mortality and morbidity of pregnancy, including preeclampsia. Sexually transmitted infections have serious consequences for women and infants, with mother-to-child transmission leading to outcomes such as stillbirths and neonatal deaths, and pelvic inflammatory disease leading to infertility. In addition infertility from many other causes, birth control, unplanned pregnancy, unconsensual sexual activity and the struggle for access to abortion create other burdens for women.

As women age, they face challenging health issues. Their average life expectancy is longer than their male counterparts, yet they often have multiple chronic, ongoing health problems that complicate their care, accentuate their

Box 4.1: Assessment common to all women.

- Age
- Occupation/lifestyle
- Address
- Marital status—duration of marriage and consanguinity

Medical and surgical history—if present

- Medical history: DM-II, respiratory, back pain, GI dysfunction, neurological condition, dietary issues and difficulty in ADL.
- Obstetrical history:
  - Number of pregnancies and deliveries (gravida and parity)
  - Type of deliveries, vaginal or C-section—full-term normal, LSCS, episiotomy
  - Birth weight of babies, any congenital abnormalities in previous babies
  - Birth trauma (episiotomy, lacerations, forceps)
  - Postpartum problems
  - Back pain prenatal or postpartum
  - Previous abortions if any
  - Menstruation details
  - Other diseases like PID, rubella, toxoplasmosis, etc.
  - Postural hypotension
  - Any trauma during pregnancy
- Gynecological history—surgeries like hysterectomy, laparoscopic surgery, prolapse repair, etc., hormonal status, fibroids, cysts, etc.
- Sexual activity—sexual health or pelvic pain
- Menstrual history—including menopause

Personal history: Sleeping habits, lifestyle, any addiction—smoking, alcohol

Drug history: Drugs taken during pregnancy, oral contraceptives, intrauterine devices

Family history: History of twin pregnancy in family, congenital defects

Psychological history: Anxiety, depression, emotional disturbances, stress related to pregnancy

infirmity, and reduce their quality of life. An understanding of the differences in disease frequencies, presentations, and response to treatments is necessary to provide older adult women with optimal health care.

Box 4.1 shows points of assessment common to all women as applicable.

PHYSIOTHERAPY ASSESSMENT FOR MENSTRUAL DISORDERS

Demographic details are integral part of the assessment in menstrual disorders like dysmenorrhea, polycystic ovary syndrome (PCOS). This is followed by the history of commencing of the menstrual problems including the chief complaints of the female. Various menstrual disorders need a baseline assessment of obesity as it is one of the major causes for the same. Body mass index (BMI), waist hip ratio and polycystic ovary syndrome questionnaire (PCOSQ) scale are a few measures that can be assessed before managing PCOS.

Obesity Assessment

Body mass index is defined as the body mass divided by the square of the body height, and is expressed in units of kg/m^2, resulting from mass in kilograms and height in meters **(Table 30.1)**.

The ***waist-hip ratio*** or waist-to-hip ratio (***WHR***) is the dimensionless ratio of the circumference of the waist to that of the hips **(Table 30.1,** also *see* Chapter 30: Obesity in Women).

Quality of Life

Polycystic ovary syndrome questionnaire (PCOSQ) is a questionnaire developed to measure the health-related quality of life (HRQoL) of women with PCOS. It contains 26 items, measuring 5 areas of HRQoL:

- Emotional (8 items)
- Body hair (5 items)
- Weight (5 items)
- Infertility (4 items)
- Menstrual problems (4 items)

Pain Assessment

Pain is a subjective symptom, which is not easily 'observed' or 'detected' by anyone other than the afflicted person. There is also no way to precisely 'measure' pain, e.g., through the use of a clinical test. Instead, it is up to the patient to try to accurately describe the severity and type of pain experienced. The best way to do this for period pain is to track symptoms. The Universal pain assessment tool can be used to 'score' period pain levels.

ASSESSMENT IN CHILD-BEARING YEARS

Antenatal Period

During pregnancy there are progressive anatomical, physiological, hormonal and biochemical changes not only confined to the genital organs but also to all systems of the body. It is the process of maternal adaptation to the increasing demands of the growing fetus. The significant physical and physiological changes occurring during the child-bearing year require musculoskeletal adaptations. Before planning a rehabilitation program for the same, a detailed assessment helps to specifically work on the areas of need.

Subjective Examination

Demographic details as described in **Box 4.1**.

- Age (<17 years and >35 years is considered as 'high risk')

Chief complaints

- Musculoskeletal problems including cramps, radiating pains, low back pain, SI joint pain, numbness or tingling, etc.
- Frequency of micturition
- Period of amenorrhea
- General weakness
- Blood pressure changes
- Headache
- Trimester wise complaints
- Swelling in limbs

Obstetric history is described in **Box 4.1**

Other system history

- ❖ Incontinence history
- ❖ Prolapse history
- ❖ Burning micturition
- ❖ Loss of appetite
- ❖ Loss of weight or abnormal weight gain
- ❖ Constipation, piles, etc.
- ❖ Heartburns

Pain history

- ❖ Onset of symptoms
- ❖ Duration of symptoms
- ❖ Type and location of pain
- ❖ Aggravating and relieving factors

Objective Examination

- ❖ General condition
- ❖ Vital signs—blood pressure, heart rate, pulse, respiratory rate, SpO_2
- ❖ Trophic changes related to pregnancy—e.g., chloasma gravidarum, linea nigra, striae gravidarum, etc.
- ❖ Scar from previous surgery in case of multipara, edema over hands and legs—girth measurement, volumetric measurement
- ❖ Posture in standing, sitting and lying—look for cervical or lumbar lordosis, rounded shoulders, hyperextended knees, etc.
- ❖ Gait:
  - ◆ Identify deviation from normal gait pattern, spatial and temporal measures, wider base of support, etc.
  - ◆ Kinematic analysis of gait during pregnancy provides information about the anatomical changes with advancement of pregnancy
- ❖ Range of motion—there may be hypermobility of joints due to ligament laxity, restricted range due to edema, back pain or postural problems.
- ❖ Manual muscle testing:
  - ◆ Abdominal muscles (Oxford method)
  - ◆ Gluteal muscles (Oxford method)
  - ◆ Perineal muscles (*refer* PFM assessment)
- ❖ Diastasis recti

Assessment of Psychological State

Any of the following scales can be used:

- ❖ Edinburgh postnatal depression scale
- ❖ Pregnancy-related anxiety scale
- ❖ Development of antenatal psychological stress scale
- ❖ Pregnancy experience scale

Exercise Testing

Maximal exercise testing should not be performed on pregnant women unless medically necessary. If a maximal exercise test is to be done, then it should be carried out with physician supervision after the woman has been medically evaluated for contraindications to exercises. (ACSM guidelines for exercise testing and prescription)

The Canadian Society for Exercise Physiologists Physical Activity Readiness Medical Examination for Pregnancy (PARmed-X for pregnancy) or the Electronic Physical Activity Readiness Medical Examination (ePARmed-X+) should be used for the health screening of pregnant women before their participation in exercise programs.

Assessment in Postnatal Period

The postpartum period, also known as the puerperium and the "fourth trimester," refers to the time after birth when maternal physiologic changes related to pregnancy return to the nonpregnant state. In addition to physiologic changes and medical issues that may arise during this period, healthcare providers should be aware of the psychological needs of the postpartum mother and be sensitive to cultural differences that surround childbirth, which may involve eating particular foods and restricting certain activities.

The assessment during postnatal period along with antenatal assessment, includes:

Postnatal History/Assessment (Also see Chapter 22: Postnatal care)

- ❖ Place of delivery
- ❖ Type of labor (induced or spontaneous)
- ❖ History of breastfeeding
- ❖ Mother's blood pressure
- ❖ Breast examination—engorgement, sore and cracked nipples
- ❖ Abdominal status
- ❖ Uterine involution and cervix status
- ❖ Smear test (if needed)
- ❖ Discussing contraception
- ❖ For primiparas—check for perineal pain and sexual problems
- ❖ Scar (of episiotomy or LSCS)—the length of scar, type, condition whether infected, healed, redness, adherence, etc., should be evaluated.
- ❖ Genitourinary dysfunction/pain:
  - ◆ Fecal incontinence
  - ◆ Stress incontinence
  - ◆ Constipation
  - ◆ Urinary retention
  - ◆ Urgency
- ❖ Musculoskeletal dysfunction/pain:
  - ◆ Diastasis recti abdominis
  - ◆ Low back pain
  - ◆ Pain in epidural site
  - ◆ Thoracic pain
  - ◆ Coccydynia
  - ◆ Symphysis pubis pain
  - ◆ After pain (postpartum lower abdominal pain)
- ❖ Circulatory dysfunction/pain:
  - ◆ Varicose veins
  - ◆ Edema
  - ◆ Superficial/deep vein thrombosis
  - ◆ Pulmonary embolism
  - ◆ Hemorrhoids
- ❖ Fatigue

- Psychological symptoms—baby/maternity blues, puerperal psychosis, postnatal depression
- Sexual problems (also *see* Chapter 16: Psychosexual Dimensions of Women's Health).

Assessment of Diastasis Recti

Diastasis recti is separation of the rectus abdominis muscles in the midline at linea alba. The integrity and continuity of the abdominal musculature are disrupted. Any separation larger than two finger width is considered significant. It may occur in pregnancy as a result of hormonal effects on the connective tissue and the biomechanical changes of pregnancy, it may also develop during labor, especially with excessive breath-holding during the second stage. It appears to be less common in women with good abdominal tone before pregnancy.

Examination

- The test can be performed during pregnancy and after third postpartum day for optimal accuracy. The patient is in hook lying position. Ask the patient to slowly raise her head and shoulders off the floor, reaching her hands toward the knees, until the spines of scapulae leave the floor.
- Place the fingers of one hand horizontally across the midline of the abdomen at the umbilicus **(Fig. 4.1)**. If a separation exists, the fingers sink into the gap between the rectus muscles, or a visible bulge between the rectus bellies may be appreciated. The number of fingers that can be placed between the muscles bellies is noted. Also *see* Chapter 22: Postnatal Care.

ASSESSMENT FOLLOWING GYNECOLOGICAL AND OBSTETRICAL SURGERIES

Assessment Following Cesarean Section

Cesarean section (C-section) is a major abdominal surgery involving delivery of infant by incisions in the abdominal and uterine wall rather than pelvis and vagina. It may be carried out under either epidural or general anesthesia.

Assessment includes:

- Demographic details
- Gynecological and obstetric history **(Box 4.1)**
- Pain examination at incision site
- Vitals assessment
- Chest examination—auscultation, chest expansion (post anesthesia and surgery)
- Wound/scar examination including:
  - State of healing
  - Size of the wound/scar
  - Adherence
  - Signs of infection
- Motor examination:
  - Range of motion of limbs
  - Strength of abdominals
  - Endurance
  - Tightness of muscles of limbs
- Pelvic floor muscle examination (*refer* PF examination described later)
- Assessment of diastasis recti (described earlier)
- Gait examination
- Functional assessment (Also *see* Chapter 23: Cesarean Section).

Clinical Pointer

Assessment of abdominals and pelvic floor muscles should be avoided till after the surgical wound heals/ 4–6 weeks post-surgery.

Assessment Following Hysterectomy

Hysterectomy is surgical removal of uterus.

Assessment can be same as C-section. Pelvic floor muscle examination can be done approximately 4-6 weeks after

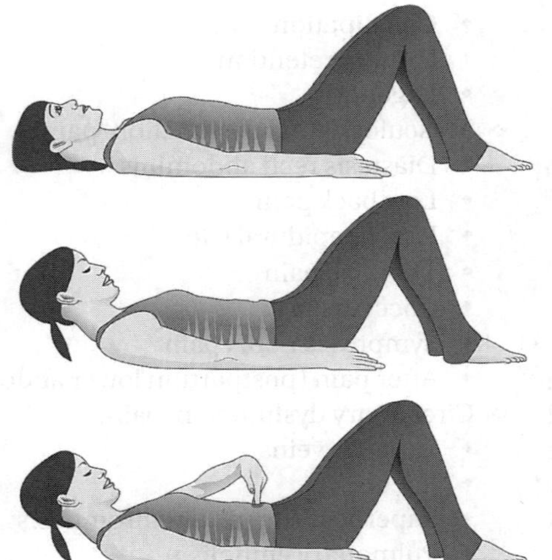

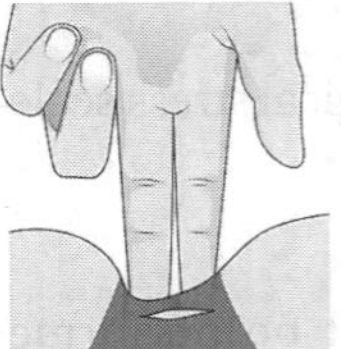

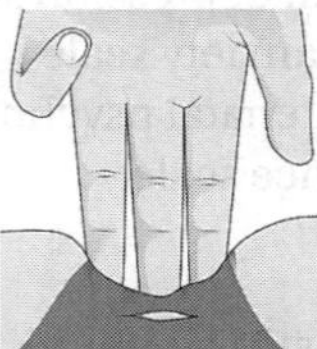

Fig. 4.1: Examination of diastasis recti.

hysterectomy (Also *see* Chapter 13: Gynecological Conditions: Clinical and Physiotherapy— Part II).

ASSESSMENT OF PELVIC FLOOR MUSCLES

The pelvic floor muscles (PFM) consist of approximately 70% slow-twitch (type 1) and 30% fast-twitch (type 2) muscle fibers. Although the PFM are thought to work tonically and reflexly during routine daily activities, voluntary contractions are required for training. Knowledge of the female pelvic musculature is essential to understanding the pathophysiology of conditions such as urinary incontinence (UI) and stages of pelvic organ prolapse (POP) **(Table 4.1)**. In addition, this knowledge helps examiners more accurately interpret findings from a digital pelvic examination. Conditions such as UI usually occur as result of a dysfunction of the bladder and/or the urethra along with, in most cases, weakness of the pelvic floor muscles (PFMs).

PFM weakness is recognized as one of the problems encountered in patients with urinary and fecal incontinence, and re-education should address the perceived deficit, be it in the slower/and fast-twitch muscle fibers. **Box 4.2** shows the risk factors for development of weak PFM. The Minute Quiz for Urinary Incontinence is a short questionnaire which can be used as an assessment tool. There are several ways to assess the PFM, including:

- Digital palpation
- Pressure perineometer
- Electromyography (EMG)
- Ultrasound scanning
- Magnetic resonance imaging (MRI)

Evaluation of muscle strength and endurance provides information on the severity of muscle weakness and forms the basis of patient-specific exercise programs.

Table 4.1: Stages of pelvic organ prolapse.

Stage 0 (not often used)	No prolapse
Stage 1	Descent to any point 1 cm above the hymen
Stage 2	Descent to the hymen
Stage 3	Descent 1 cm or more distal to the hymen

Box 4.2: Risk factors for pelvic floor muscle weakness.

- Multiple vaginal deliveries, high infant birth weights: can cause neuromuscular injury and stretching
- Chronic elevations in abdominal pressure related to:
  - Constipation (chronic straining with defecation)
  - Chronic cough (from conditions such as chronic lung disease, long-term smoking)
  - Heavy or improper lifting
- Obesity: Places chronic strain on pelvic floor
- Advancing age: Results in decreased collagen strength
- Lack of estrogen in pelvic tissue: Leads to loss of elasticity in vaginal wall, loss of pelvic muscle tone, thinning of vaginal wall, and devascularization of tissues

Subjective assessment:

- Demographics and history as described in **Box 4.1**
- Obstetric and gynecological history as described in **Box 4.1**
- Chief complaints (pain, discomfort, heaviness): Chief complaints in words of patients would easily be able to take towards type of pelvic floor dysfunction.
- Urinary leakage
- Pelvic organ prolapse **(Table 4.1)**

Postural and gait observation: Changes in frequent static and dynamic biomechanics of lumbopelvic junction can lead to overstretched or over compressed PFM dysfunctions. Prolonged sitting can lead to over flexion of the coccyx which can create disturbance in PFM alignments. It fails to maintain normal tone of pelvic floor muscles which can lead to trigger point formation and hypertonus dysfunction.

Objective assessment:

- Vulvar or perineal observation
- Vaginal and rectal examination
- External palpation (urogenital triangle–urorectal triangle)
- Internal palpation (deep pelvic floor muscle)
- Perineometer
- Pelvic ultrasonography
- Electromyography

Manual Muscle Testing of Pelvic Floor Muscles

- Oxford scale or Harvard Scale **(Table 4.2)**
- Laycock quantitative assessment scale (PERFECT)

PERFECT is an acronym with:
P = representing power (or pressure, a measure of strength using a manometric perineometer)
E = endurance
R = repetitions
F = fast contractions, and finally
ECT = every contraction timed

The scheme was developed to simplify and clarify PFM assessment.

Transvaginal Pelvic Floor Muscle Examination

Indications

- Pelvic pain
- Pelvic organ prolapse
- PF dysfunctions
- Incontinence
- History of sexual dysfunction
- Vaginal laxity

Table 4.2: Oxford scale/Harvard scale.

Modified Oxford grading scale for pelvic floor muscles	
0	No muscle activity
1	Minor muscle "flicker"
2	Weak muscle activity without a circular contraction
3	Moderate muscle contraction
4	Good muscle contraction
5	Strong muscle contraction

Contraindications

- Lack of consent
- Six-week postpartum and post-surgery
- Severe vaginitis and infection
- During menstruation and pregnancy
- Sexual abuse
- Severe pelvic pain
- Age less than 18 and pediatric patients
- Physician's restrictions and surgery, recent radiotherapy

Procedure (for Digital Assessment)

- Patient is positioned in crook-lying position with a neutral lumbar spine, hips abducted and feet apart, on a waterproof underpad covering sheet bed. Other materials required would be vinyl or latex gloves and a bin.
- Thorough handwashing must be done and open wounds should be covered.
- Ideally one should start with one finger examination rather than two, as two fingers can create a mild stretch to muscle spindle and reflex facilitation of muscle can misguide reading or palpation. However, if there is muscle laxity then two fingers, index and middle can be used **(Fig. 4.2)**.
- It is important that the therapist pays attention to patient's body language and leg position which can anticipate pain due to PFM examination. A pain free and extremely gentle examination should be ensured to the patient while inserting gloved and lubricated single finger.
- Palpate for painful spots, trigger points, muscle spasms, myofascial adhesions, etc.
- Ask the patient to contract her PFM as hard as possible and ask her to try to squeeze examiner's finger together and lift it inward and in upward direction. Strong muscles will be felt as thick and firm band of muscles, compared to weak or loose muscles which can feel thin and flabby. Pubococcygeus (PC) muscle is felt as 1-2 cm band at lateral vaginal wall, while puborectalis (PR) can be palpated posteriorly when the examiner presses posteriorly and over the rectal contents.
- Ask the patient to cough (KNACK technique) while trying to hold PFM without losing grip on examiner's finger and observe any descent, bulging or urine loss. Ask patient to create submaximal contraction to access control, later eccentric strength and control of muscles can be examined by slowly releasing the fully contracted muscles by 10% progressively.
- Pelvic floor muscle coordination can be assessed by asking patient to contract and relax quickly and slowly, checking ability to relax quickly and completely, checking time taken to reach maximum firm contraction which will provide information about timing for fast twitch muscle fibers to respond. Progressive reduction of these timings on coughing like activities can help to gain better continence.
- Make sure to maintain eye contact and assess body language to figure out patient's cooperation and comfort level while doing transvaginal examination.

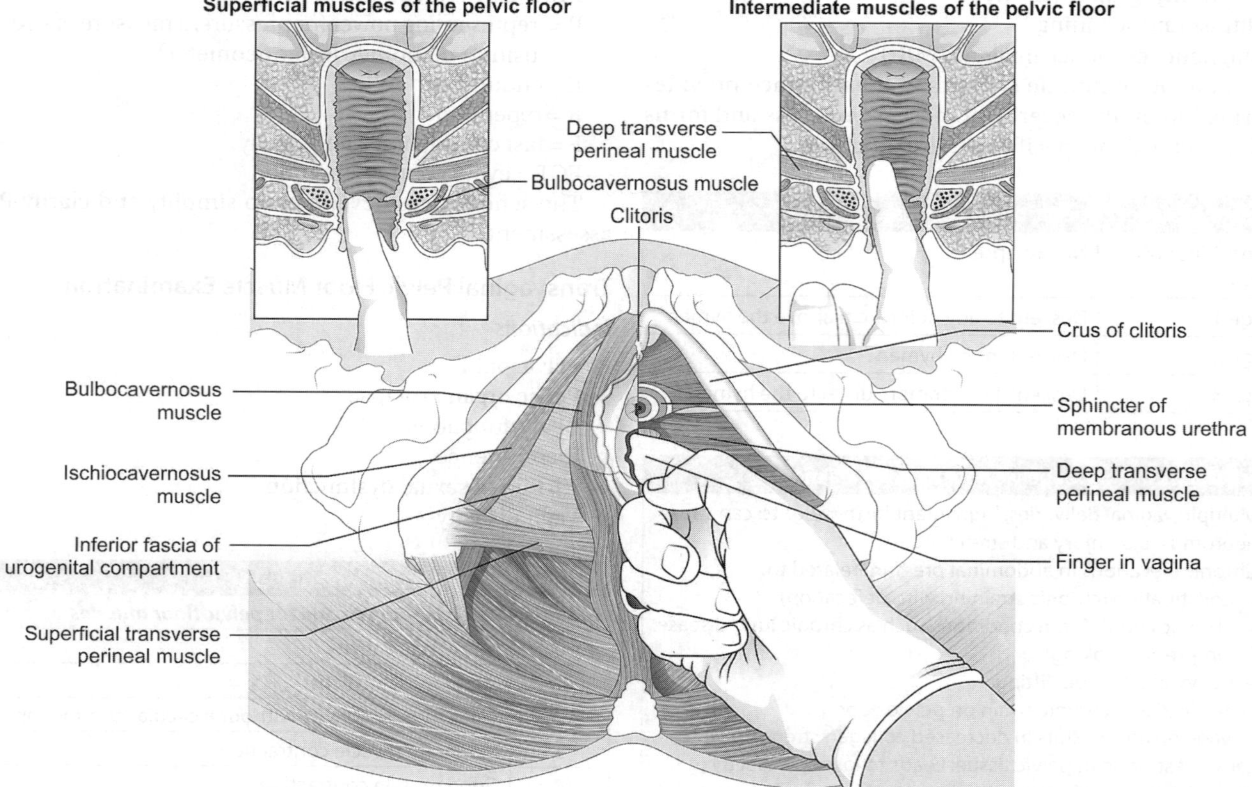

Fig. 4.2: Digital examination of pelvic floor muscles *(For color version, see Plate 1)*.

With perineometers—air filled pressure probe is used to register vaginal pressure as an indication of pelvic floor strength.

With vaginal weights—weights such as cones of increasing mass are developed as a method of providing biofeedback and resistance for pelvic floor musculature.

Pelvic Floor Manometry

Measurement of resting pressure or pressure rise generated during contraction of the PFM using a manometer connected to a sensor, which is inserted into the urethra, vagina or rectum. Pelvic floor manometric tools measure pressure in mmHg, hPa or cmH_2O. **Table 4.3** shows the classification using manometry.

Electromyography

It is the most effective method of objectively recording the muscle activity. Fine wire or needle electrodes are placed on the perineum and records are taken for superficial muscle activity. Surface electrodes are used intravaginally or intra anally in some rehabilitation centers as biofeedback mechanism.

Ultrasound Examination

Patients PFM can be assessed with ultrasound machine through abdominal sonography.

Transrectal Pelvic Floor Muscle Examination

Procedure

- Position the patient in left-lateral position as it enables examiners to perform transrectal examination and easily palpate puborectalis and external anal sphincter at rest and during PFM contraction.
- Examiner's properly lubricated index finger is introduced through the anus to the rectum up to 3–4 cm.
- Instruct the patient to squeeze the finger as if to stop passing of gas. Sling like puborectalis muscle pulls the examiner's finger anteriorly.
- For relaxation, at the time patient relaxes pelvic floor muscles (instruct as if emptying the bowel) examiner should feel opening of anal sphincter along with release of puborectalis posteriorly towards coccyx.

ASSESSMENT FOR URINARY INCONTINENCE

Urinary incontinence (UI) is the loss of bladder control. Incontinence affects twice as many women as men. This may be because pregnancy, childbirth, and menopause may make urinary incontinence more likely. Unfortunately, problems like UI which are silently existing and affecting the quality of life of women are not noticed much.

Less than 50% of females with UI consult the doctor, but screening at primary level is mandatory to provide early intervention and prevention. International Continence Society women guidelines 2013 has recommended asking the following question to all women aged >22 years at every visit:

'Is voiding the bladder or leakage of urine a problem for you?'. If the answer is positive then further evaluation of the women will give an appropriate diagnosis.

Table 4.3: Classification of pelvic floor function according to manometry pressure in women.

Classification	*Manometry values (cm H_2O)*
Very weak	7.5–14.5 mm Hg
Weak	14.6–26.5 mm Hg
Moderate	26.6–41.5 mm Hg
Good	41.6–60.5 mm Hg
Strong	> 60.6 mm Hg

History and Clinical Examination

A proper history along with perineal area observation, palpation and examination are included here. Perineum should be observed for skin infection, vaginal discharge, prolapse, episiotomy scar, perineal surgery or any hemorrhoids. A simple bedside clinical test to diagnose stress incontinence is cough test performed with full bladder. A sign of prolapse or leakage should be noted.

Frequency Volume Chart

Frequency volume charts are an essential adjunct to both the assessment of patients at presentation and the evaluation of new treatments for filling and voiding dysfunction. The time of voiding and quantity of urine passed per micturition episode has to be recorded. The patient should be provided with a jug to void the urine.

The normal frequency of micturition is 6–8 times per 24 hours. Normal volume of urine in day time is 250–450 mL. A normal healthy woman wakes up not more than once in the night to void urine.

Details obtained from the chart are:

- Number of times the subject visits the toilet
- Accurate extent of nocturia
- Difference between voiding episodes in day and night
- Total and individual volume voided during day
- Incidence of leakage with probable reason
- Drinks intake with amount during day
- Total amount of caffeine consumed

Pad Test

The pad test is a noninvasive diagnostic tool for urinary incontinence. It is an easy to perform, inexpensive test with utilization in both the daily patient care and clinical research. One-hour pad tests are most suitable in establishing initial diagnosis, the 24-hr test serves most often for evaluation of treatment outcomes, and longer pad tests are used in clinical studies.

Procedure:

- The test is started without the patient voiding.
- Preweigh the perineal pad and ask patient to place it in panty.
- The patient is asked to drink around 500 mL of sodium-free liquid (e.g., distilled water) within 15 minutes and asked to sit or rest until initial half an hour.

- Then the patient is asked to stroll around for next 30 minutes, ascend and descend stairs and perform following exercises; sit to stand (x10), coughing vigorously (x10), running on spot for 1 minute, bending down to pick up a small object (x5), wash hands under cold water for 1 minute.

At the end of 1 hour of the test, the pad is weighed and the difference is observed. An increase of up to 1 g is considered normal which could be due to sweating and vaginal discharge. More increase in weight of the pad can suggest urine leakage, but because of its artificiality and stressfulness it was shown to be an unsatisfactory screening test.

Voiding Diaries

A bladder diary, also known as a voiding diary **(Table 4.4)**, is indispensable to urologists for the evaluation of symptoms and causes associated with overactive bladder. A bladder diary is kept by the patient over the course of three to seven days, and allows the healthcare provider to evaluate the

Table 4.4: 3 Days bladder diary.

Day 1	*Fluids*		*Urination*				*Accidents*		
Date *dd/mm/yy*	*What kind?*	*How much?*	*How many times?*	*How much?*	*Did you feel a strong urge to urinate?*	*What activity did this interrupt?*	*Did you have an accident?*	*How much did you leak?*	*What were you doing at the time?*
6 AM–9 AM				S M L	Yes No		Yes No	S M L	
9 AM–12 PM				S M L	Yes No		Yes No	S M L	
12 PM–3 PM				S M L	Yes No		Yes No	S M L	
3 PM–6 PM				S M L	Yes No		Yes No	S M L	
6 PM–9 PM				S M L	Yes No		Yes No	S M L	
9 PM–12 AM				S M L	Yes No		Yes No	S M L	
12 AM–3 AM				S M L	Yes No		Yes No	S M L	
3 AM–6 AM				S M L	Yes No		Yes No	S M L	

Day 2	*Fluids*		*Urination*				*Accidents*		
Date *dd/mm/yy*	*What kind?*	*How much?*	*How many times?*	*How much?*	*Did you feel a strong urge to urinate?*	*What activity did this interrupt?*	*Did you have an accident?*	*How much did you leak?*	*What were you doing at the time?*
6 AM–9 AM				S M L	Yes No		Yes No	S M L	
9 AM–12 PM				S M L	Yes No		Yes No	S M L	
12 PM–3 PM				S M L	Yes No		Yes No	S M L	
3 PM–6 PM				S M L	Yes No		Yes No	S M L	
6 PM–9 PM				S M L	Yes No		Yes No	S M L	
9 PM–12 AM				S M L	Yes No		Yes No	S M L	
12 AM–3 AM				S M L	Yes No		Yes No	S M L	
3 AM–6 AM				S M L	Yes No		Yes No	S M L	

Day 3	*Fluids*		*Urination*				*Accidents*		
Date *dd/mm/yy*	*What kind?*	*How much?*	*How many times?*	*How much?*	*Did you feel a strong urge to urinate?*	*What activity did this interrupt?*	*Did you have an accident?*	*How much did you leak?*	*What were you doing at the time?*
6 AM–9 AM				S M L	Yes No		Yes No	S M L	
9 AM–12 PM				S M L	Yes No		Yes No	S M L	
12 PM–3 PM				S M L	Yes No		Yes No	S M L	
3 PM–6 PM				S M L	Yes No		Yes No	S M L	
6 PM–9 PM				S M L	Yes No		Yes No	S M L	
9 PM–12 AM				S M L	Yes No		Yes No	S M L	
12 AM–3 AM				S M L	Yes No		Yes No	S M L	
3 AM–6 AM				S M L	Yes No		Yes No	S M L	

(S: small, M: medium, L: large)

patient's bladder function based on fluid intake and output. The diary captures how much fluid the patient is taking in during the day, how frequently the patient is urinating both day and night, if there are leaking accidents, and how much urine was lost. The diary consists of three sections:

1. Fluids
2. Urination
3. Accidents

Completing a bladder diary is a simple process. The patient begins their diary when they wake up each morning and continues making notes throughout the day.

The International Continence Society recommends that voiding diaries should be included in clinical evaluation of subjects with lower urinary tract syndrome.

Paper Towel Test

This test is performed in standing position. The patient holds a colored paper towel against the perineum and coughs strongly three times. Any leakage absorbed by the paper towel will change the color.

Alternatively, the test can be performed in stride standing after removing the underwear. The patient is asked to cough 3 times and leakage falls on the towel. Assessment of leakage can be measured by weighing or measuring the area of dampness.

Muscle Testing of Pelvic Floor

See PFM assessment

QOL Assessment

This includes following questionnaires and analogue scales:

- Incontinence severity index (ISI)
- International Consultation on Incontinence Questionnaire (ICIQ)
- Incontinence Impact Questionnaire (IIQ)
- Pelvic Floor Impact Questionnaire (PFIQ)
- Urogenital Distress Inventory (UDI)
- Pelvic Floor Distress Inventory (PFDI)
- Short form 36 (SF-36)

ASSESSMENT OF FEMALES IN THE TRANSITION PERIOD AND MENOPAUSE

The core symptoms of menopause include vasomotor and vaginal symptoms, insomnia, and mood changes. Assessment of females in this period can be focused upon points shown in **Box 4.3**. For detailed assessment of women during menopause *refer* Chapter 9: Menopause.

Box 4.3: Assessment of women during menopause.

- Biochemical Investigations in the form of hormonal profile (LH, FSH, estrogen)
- Vasomotor symptoms
- QoL assessment
- Menopausal symptoms assessment
- Sleep assessment: Polysomnography, sleep questionnaires [e.g., Functional Outcomes of Sleep Questionnaire (FOSQ), Pittsburgh Sleep Quality Index (PSQI)]

ASSESSMENT OF ELDERLY WOMEN

Senior women are at greater risk than men for many conditions and are affected differently by many diseases that impact both sexes. However, women more often face multiple chronic conditions that affect their daily lives, such as diabetes, hypertension, or arthritis. Common health conditions for elderly women include heart diseases, cancer, stroke, diabetes, obesity, arthritis, Alzheimer's disease, etc., out of which musculoskeletal problems being the commonest.

Health Screening for Elderly Women

Screening for following conditions should be performed on a regular basis:

- Blood pressure screening
- Cervical and breast cancer screening
- Colorectal cancer screening
- Lung cancer screening
- Cholesterol and heart disease screening
- Diabetes screening
- Dental examination
- Eye examination
- Hearing test
- Infectious diseases screening
- Skin examination
- Immunization
- Osteoporosis screening
- Obesity assessment
- Physical examination

Physical Therapy Assessment for Senior Citizen Women

There is a set of physical therapy assessment for the senior citizen women. Senior citizen fitness tests are practical and straightforward assessments of cardiovascular fitness, strength, and flexibility that require little or no equipment. The tests are as follows:

- Test of the chair stand—testing lower body strength
- The arm curl test—testing upper body strength
- Sit and reach test in a chair—lower body flexibility test
- Scratch test on the back—upper body flexibility test
- The 8-foot-up-and-go test—agility test
- 6-minute walk test—assess aerobic endurance

ASSESSMENT OF WOMEN WITH BREAST CANCER

Breast cancer can occur in both men and women, but it is far more common in women.

Assessment includes:

- Demographic details **(Box 4.1)**
- Surgical and medical history—pertinent history and pain history:
  - Date of surgery
  - Diagnosis and type of surgery/mastectomy

- Affected side
- Number of radiations
- Chemotherapy

❖ Chief complaints
❖ Compression bandages duration
❖ Investigations
❖ Observation
- Posture
- Skin color
- Muscle atrophy
- Scar
- Edema

❖ Examination
- Temperature
- Sensory examination
- Range of motion of limbs
- Muscle strength
- Swelling or edema—details described in Chapter 29: Cancer and Lymphedema.

Summary

This chapter provides details about physical therapy assessment of women in different conditions like pelvic floor dysfunction, childbearing years, gynecological and obstetric surgeries, menstrual disorders, elderly women and conditions like breast cancer. Explanation about its subjective, objective and quality of life assessment is described in detail for various conditions.

CLINICAL EXAMPLE

A 27-year-old female presented with 5 months of amenorrhea and was diagnosed as being 20 weeks pregnant by her obstetrician.

❖ Name: Ms. A
❖ Age: 27 years
❖ Occupation: Homemaker
❖ Address: XYZ
❖ Chief complaint: Occasional low back pain
❖ Marital status: Married since 2.5 years with no history of consanguinity
❖ History of presenting illness: The subject has developed low back pain since past 2 weeks which is occasional and occurs only after standing for more than 1 hour.
❖ Medical history: Polycystic ovarian syndrome since several years
❖ Obstetrical history: $G_1P_0L_0A_0$
❖ Gynecological history: Subject had history of irregular menses due to polycystic ovarian syndrome which was managed by hormonal medications
❖ Sexual activity: Normal
❖ Personal history: NAD
❖ Drug history: Subject is on iron, folic acid and calcium supplements
❖ Family history: NAD
❖ Psychological history: NAD
❖ Pain examination:
- Onset: Since 2 weeks
- Location: Lower lumbar and sacral areas
- Type: Dull aching
- Aggravating factor: Standing for more than an hour
- Relieving factor: Rest
- Intensity: 0 on rest; 4/10 on activity (standing)

❖ Objective examination:
- General condition: Good
- Vitals: NAD
- Trophic changes due to pregnancy: Linea Nigra, hyperpigmentation of areola present
- Edema: Absent
- Scar: Absent
- Range of motion: Normal for all joints
- Manual muscle testing: Normal for major muscle groups
- Pelvic floor muscle assessment: Since there was no complaint or risk factor noted, internal examination was omitted
- Posture assessment: Wide base of support with increased lumbar lordosis and anterior pelvic tilt seen in standing
- Gait assessment: NAD

❖ Psychological state: Normal (evaluated using Pregnancy-related anxiety scale)
❖ Exercise testing: NAD (evaluated using 6 minute walk test)
❖ Investigations: All blood investigations were within normal range; all ultrasound scans suggested no abnormalities
❖ Functional assessment: NAD (evaluated using Functional Independence Measure)
❖ Impairments:
- Low back pain
- Increased lumbar lordosis and anterior pelvic tilt

❖ Physical and functional diagnosis: A 27-year-old female presented with low back pain on standing for more than an hour and amenorrhea since 5 months. She has increased lumbar lordosis and anterior pelvic tilt and was diagnosed as being 20 weeks pregnant by her obstetrician.

Review Questions

1. Explain in detail about the transvaginal and transrectal assessment of pelvic floor muscles.
2. When and how will you assess the women for diastasis recti?
3. What are the important points of consideration during assessment of women having menstrual disorders?
4. What are the different methods of assessment of urinary incontinence?
5. Write in detail about health screening and physical therapy assessment for elderly women.
6. Explain in detail about points of assessment for a woman suffering from breast cancer.

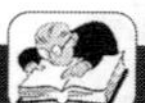

Bibliography

1. American College of Sports Medicine. ACSM's guidelines for exercise testing and prescription, 10th edition. Philadelphia: Wolters Kluwer; 2018. P.197-8.
2. Bryan NP, Chapple CR. Frequency volume charts in the assessment and evaluation of treatment: How should we use them? Eur Urol. 2004;46(5):636-40.
3. Bø K, Frawley HC, Haylen BT, Abramov Y, Almeida FG, Berghmans B, et al. An International Urogynecological Association (IUGA)/International Continence Society (ICS) joint report on the terminology for the conservative and nonpharmacological management of female pelvic floor dysfunction. Neurourol Urodyn. 2017;36(2):221-44. doi:10.1002/nau.23107. PMID: 27918122.
4. Carcio HA. Digital assessment of the pelvic floor muscles: A neglected technique. Womens Healthcare. 2018;6(1):34-7.
5. Dugdale DC III, Zieve D, Conaway B, ADAM Editorial team. MedlinePlus [Internet]. Bethesda (MD): US National Library of Medicine; 2021 Aug 17 [updated 2021 Aug 17; cited 2022 Oct 17]. Available from: https://medlineplus.gov/
6. Het's Manual of Pelvic Floor Rehabilitation—WOW IIPRE, 1st edition. New Delhi: Jaypee Brothers Medical Publishers; 2020.
7. King S. Period pain—What's normal? [Internet]. Menstrual Matters; 2018 [cited 2022 Oct 17]. Available from: https://menstrual-matters.com/blog/period-pain-norm/
8. Krhut J, Zachoval R, Smith PP, Rosier PF, Valansky L, Martan A, et al. Pad weight testing in the evaluation of urinary incontinence. Neurourol Urodyn. 2014;33(5):507-10. doi:10.1002/nau.22436. PMID: 23797972.
9. Laycock J, Jerwood D. Pelvic floor muscle assessment: The PERFECT scheme. Physiotherapy. 2001;87(12):631-42.
10. Mantle J, Haslam J, Barton S. Physiotherapy in obstetrics and gynaecology, 2nd edition. London: Butterworth-Heinemann; 2005.
11. National Library of Medicine; National Center for Biotechnology Information. PLoS One. 2017;12(10):e0187045. doi:10.1371/journal.pone.0187045.
12. Office on Women's Health. Urinary incontinence [Internet]. Washington (DC): US Department of Health and Human Services; 2021 [cited 2022 Oct 17]. Available from: https://www.womenshealth.gov/a-z-topics/urinary-incontinence
13. Physiopedia. Cesarean Section. 2022 Aug 6 [cited 2022 Oct 17]. Available from: https://www.physio-pedia.com/Cesarean_Section
14. Rikli RE, Jones CJ. Measuring functional fitness of older adults. J Active Aging. 2002;1(1):24-30.
15. Sheth M, Rangey PS, Vyas LJ, Sharma S. Physiotherapy in general medical and surgical conditions, 1st edition. New Delhi: Jaypee Brothers Medical Publishers; 2022.
16. Urology Austin. Bladder diary [Internet]. 2022 [cited 2022 Oct 17]. Available from: https://urologyaustin.com/general-urology/bladder-diary/
17. Weir CB, Jan A. BMI classification percentile and cut off points. In: StatPearls [Internet]. Treasure Island (FL): StatPearls Publishing; 2022 [updated 2022 Jun 27; cited 2022 Oct 17]. Available from: https://www.ncbi.nlm.nih.gov/books/NBK541070/

Multiple Choice Questions (MCQs)

To test your understanding and recall of key concepts.

1. **The polycystic ovary syndrome questionnaire (PCOSQ) is used to assess__________.**
   A. Pelvic floor muscle strength
   B. Health-related quality of life (HRQoL)
   C. Intensity of pain
   D. Urinary incontinence
2. **Assessment of diastasis recti in a postnatal female can detect__________.**
   A. Pelvic organ prolapse
   B. Separation of rectus abdominis muscles
   C. Hormonal dysfunction
   D. Postpartum depression
3. **Waist-to-hip ratio of 0.88 in a female subject is indicative of__________.**
   A. Excellent level of fitness
   B. Good level of fitness
   C. No risk for health complications
   D. Risk for health complications
4. **A 30-year-old postnatal woman reports difficulty holding urine while sneezing. Which muscle group should be evaluated?**
   A. Rectus abdominis muscles
   B. Pelvic floor muscles
   C. Gluteal muscles
   D. Quadriceps muscles
5. **During a physical therapy session, a pregnant woman presents with low back pain and an anterior pelvic tilt. Which exercise would be most effective?**
   A. Pelvic tilt exercises
   B. Abdominal crunches
   C. Deep squats
   D. High-intensity interval training
6. **Which assessment method would be most appropriate to identify pelvic floor dysfunction in a patient with urinary incontinence?**
   A. Electromyography
   B. Blood pressure monitoring
   C. Treadmill stress test
   D. Reflex testing
7. **A multiparous patient demonstrates weak pelvic floor muscles during digital palpation. Which of the following could be a contributing factor?**
   A. Increased estrogen levels
   B. Chronic constipation
   C. Low body weight
   D. High blood pressure

ANSWERS

1. B	2. B	3. D	4. B	5. A
6. A	7. B			

Chapter 5

Laboratory and Molecular Investigations in Women's Health

Ajay Junnarkar

LEARNING OBJECTIVES

At the end of the chapter, the reader will be able to:

- Know the investigations carried out in conditions seen in women like anemia, infertility, polycystic ovary syndrome.
- Learn about the investigations carried out for diagnosis in infections.
- Know the protocols in testing during pregnancy.
- Know the investigations for osteoporosis.
- Gain knowledge for screening and testing for cancer in women.

CHAPTER OUTLINE

- Introduction
  - Role of pathology
- Anemia
- Thyroid disorders
- Infections and sexually transmitted infections
  - Acute phase reactants
- Infertility
- Polycystic ovary syndrome
- Pregnancy
  - Maternal prenatal screening
  - Gestational diabetes
- Osteoporosis
- Cancer in women
  - Breast cancer
  - BRCA1 and BRCA2 tests
  - Cervical cancer
  - Lynch syndrome

INTRODUCTION

The National Health Policy (NHP) quotes "Women's health refers to the branch of medicine that focuses on the treatment and diagnosis of diseases and conditions that affect a woman's physical and emotional well-being."

The WHO states that "....A woman's right to the enjoyment of the highest standard of health must be guaranteed throughout her lifetime, equal to that of men. Women are affected by many of the same health conditions as men, but women experience them differently due to both genetics and the social construction of gender."

Sustainable Development Goal 3 includes an ambitious target: "reducing the global maternal mortality rate (MMR) to less than 70 per 100,000 births, with no country having a maternal mortality rate of more than twice the global average".

Some of the health issues faced by women in their lifetime include:

- Anemia
- Infections and sexually transmitted infections
- Infertility
- Polycystic ovarian syndrome (PCOS)
- Diabetes
- Hypertension
- Pregnancy-related health issues
- Lifestyle disorders
- Cancer

Role of Pathology

The modern pathology lab is no more simply a diagnostic tool. With the advent of advanced technology and newer methodologies the laboratory can help not only in diagnosis of medical disorders but can also aid in prognostication, prediction and treatment.

ANEMIA

Anemia is defined as a decrease in the red cell mass—depicted by low hemoglobin and/or a low hematocrit [packed cell volume (PCV)] in a routine complete blood count (CBC) report. It manifests with symptoms of tiredness, dizziness, shortness of breath, amongst others.

In women, the common causes are:
- Increased blood loss (menstrual, postpartum, post-menopausal)
- Malnutrition (in children, during pregnancy, dietary deficiency)
- Chronic disease/inflammation (hypothyroidism, diabetes, rheumatoid arthritis, Crohn's disease).

The following lab tests may be done to determine the cause of anemia:
- CBC with peripheral blood film examination
- Serum iron/total iron binding capacity (TIBC)/Ferritin
- Serum vitamin B_{12}, serum folate
- Liver function tests
- Renal function tests
- Tests for autoimmune disorders
- Thyroid function tests

Complete Blood Count

A complete blood count (CBC) complemented with a peripheral blood film examination generally indicates the severity and type of anemia [hemoglobin (Hb), red blood cell (RBC) count, PCV].

The red blood cell indices provide an average numeric value of the red cell hemoglobin content:
- Mean corpuscular hemoglobin (MCH)
- Mean corpuscular hemoglobin concentration (MCHC)
- Mean corpuscular volume (MCV)
- Red-cell distribution width (RDW) is the degree of variation of red-cell size.

Coupled with peripheral blood examination, a morphological diagnosis of the type of anemia can be made:
- Microcytic
- Macrocytic
- Normocytic

This helps to narrow down the etiology, and with the aid of other appropriate biochemical tests, can lead to a conclusive diagnosis.

The white blood cell (WBC) counts and morphology along with platelets are indicative of infections (acute and chronic), leukemias (acute and chronic) and various bone marrow related disorders.

Serum Iron/TIBC/Ferritin

Box 5.1 shows the normal range for iron.

In iron-deficiency state:
- The total iron binding capacity (TIBC) increases
- Ferritin decreases
- Serum iron levels are maintained.

The presence of concomitant infections can raise serum ferritin to normal levels in spite of iron deficiency, as ferritin is also an acute phase reactant.

Box 5.1: Normal range for iron.

The normal range in adults is:
- Iron: 50–160 μg/dL
- TIBC: 250–400 mg/dL
- Ferritin: 12–300 μg/L

Box 5.2: Normal range for vitamin B_{12}.

Normal range of Vitamin B_{12}: 200–900 pg/mL

Box 5.3: Normal range for folic acid.

- Serum: 5–16 ng/mL
- Red cell folate: >150 ng/mL

Vitamin B_{12}

Box 5.2 shows the normal range for vitamin B_{12}.
- Strict vegetarians show a higher prevalence of vitamin B_{12} deficiency. Menopausal and perimenopausal women are more susceptible to deficiency due to hormonal changes.
- Demands for vitamin B_{12} increase during times of physical stress.
- Exogenous sources of B_{12} are meat and dairy products, which provide the B_{12} that is absorbed on a daily basis in the presence of an acidic stomach and intrinsic factor.
- Vitamin B_{12} deficiency is one of the major causes of macrocytic anemia but may also be present in normocytic patients. A deficiency of vitamin B_{12} promotes neurologic deficits, such as bilateral paresthesias of the lower extremities, loss of vibratory sensation, and disequilibrium-neurologic deficits that significantly affect quality of life, making this nutritional deficit worthy of recognition and treatment.

Folic Acid

Box 5.3 shows the normal range for folic acid. Dietary insufficiency is commonly seen in pregnant women, especially in tropical countries like India. Folate deficiency results in megaloblastic anemia. Studies indicate that adequate supplementation in pregnancy prevents the birth of babies with neural tube defects.

In addition renal, hepatic, thyroidal and several systemic disorders can cause concomitant anemia. Renal function tests, liver function tests, thyroid function tests and tests for autoimmune conditions are useful in determining the exact etiology.

THYROID DISORDERS

The thyroid gland secretes the two hormones:
1. Thyroxine/T4 (3,5,3'5'-tetraiodothyronine)
2. Small amounts of T3 (3,5,3'-triiodothyronine)

Both exist as bound (total T3 and T4) and as free forms (free T3 and free T4) in the serum. The thyroid hormone syntheses are regulated by TSH (thyrotropin or thyroid stimulating hormone), secreted by the pituitary gland.

Thyroid disorders have a higher prevalence in women compared to men. The functional disorders—hypothyroidism and hyperthyroidism, can be diagnosed by evaluating serum levels of T3, T4, free T3, free T4 and TSH in most of the cases.

Clinical Pointer

In general, hypothyroidism is characterized by high TSH, low T3/free T3 and low T4/free T4, while hyperthyroidism results from low TSH and high T3/free T3 and high T4/free T4. Goiter refers to enlargement of the thyroid gland and is endemic in areas of iodine deficiency.

Three thyroid autoantigens responsible for autoimmune disorders of the thyroid gland are:
1. Anti-TPO (Thyroid peroxidase antibody)
2. Anti-Tg (Anti-thyroglobulin antibody)
3. TRAb (TSH receptor antibodies)

INFECTIONS AND SEXUALLY TRANSMITTED INFECTIONS

The evaluation of infections requires a basic work-up which includes:
- ❖ CBC with ESR
- ❖ Urine examination
- ❖ Appropriate organ function tests

Acute-phase reactants help to diagnose and monitor inflammation in general.

Acute Phase Reactants

Box 5.4 shows some of the biochemical markers used to monitor inflammation.

C-reactive Protein

C-reactive protein (CRP) is a valuable marker and highly sensitive in acute inflammation (especially bacterial infections) and tissue necrosis.
- ❖ Blood levels are typically elevated 4–8 hours after tissue injury.
- ❖ Blood levels return to normal 48–72 hours after cessation of inflammation.
- ❖ Persistent elevation usually indicates ongoing inflammation or chronic infection.
- ❖ Of late, it has been used to predict risk of cardiovascular disease, given the role of proinflammatory factors in atherogenesis and vascular endothelial damage.

Box 5.5 shows normal ranges for CRP and transferrin.

Fibrinogen

Normal plasma levels are 150–400 mg/dL and these may be elevated 10–15 fold during infection. The ESR also increases as a result.

Box 5.4: Biochemical markers to monitor inflammation.
- C-reactive protein (CRP)
- Fibrinogen
- Transferrin
- Ferritin
- Alpha-1 antitrypsin
- Lactoferrin
- Albumins

Box 5.5: Normal ranges for CRP.
- Normal reference range for C-reactive protein (CRP) is <6 mg/L
- Normal range for transferrin is 200–400 mg/dL

Transferrin and Ferritin (See Box 5.1)

- ❖ Transferrin is measured as total iron binding capacity (TIBC) in the serum.
- ❖ Low transferrin levels are seen in infection, liver and kidney damage and malignancies.
- ❖ It is usually assayed with serum ferritin which rises in infective and inflammatory conditions.

INFERTILITY

The evaluation of the female reproductive system requires a step-wise approach employing proper clinical data, radiological workup and also appropriate hormone assays. Disturbances of the normal menstrual pattern are an indication of ovarian dysfunction. Following a proper clinical history the hormones shown in **Box 5.6** may be measured to assess endocrine function.

POLYCYSTIC OVARY SYNDROME

Polycystic ovary syndrome (PCOS) is one of the common endocrinopathies seen in women, and also an important cause of infertility. Its diagnosis encompasses several criteria—clinical, radiologic, biochemical and exclusionary. The laboratory evaluation entails assays of:
- ❖ Testosterone/free testosterone
- ❖ Dehydroepiandrosterone sulfate (DHEAS)
- ❖ Follicle-stimulating hormone (FSH)
- ❖ Luteinizing hormone (LH)
- ❖ Prolactin
- ❖ 17-OH progesterone

An oral glucose tolerance test with insulin levels is also advised since insulin resistance is one of the features of this disorder.

PREGNANCY

Screening for anemia, thyroid disorders and STIs are essential during pregnancy. Fetal health monitoring especially for congenital defects are now mandatory.

Box 5.6: Hormones studied in infertility.
- Beta-hCG (Beta–human chorionic gonadotropin)
- Prolactin
- Follicle-stimulating hormone (FSH)
- Luteinizing hormone (LH)
- Thyroid-stimulating hormone (TSH)
- Free T4
- Testosterone
- Dehydroepiandrosterone sulfate (DHEAS)
- 17-OH Progesterone

Maternal Prenatal Screening

Second-trimester screening of a pregnant woman's serum for markers of congenital abnormalities such as fetal trisomy 21 (Down syndrome) and neural tube defects has become an important part of antenatal care. The protocol most commonly used is the triple marker screen, which measures:

- Serum levels of alpha-fetoprotein (MSAFP)
- Unconjugated estriol (uE3)
- Beta-human chorionic gonadotropin (beta-hCG)

The results of these tests are used to derive a value known as a ***multiple of the median*** (MoM). An algorithm that combines maternal age with MoMs can be used to calculate the risk for chromosomal disorders such as trisomy 21 and 18.

- ***Alpha fetoprotein (AFP)*** alone-corrected for weight, race, insulin-dependent diabetes, and multiple pregnancies can be used to predict the risk of fetal neural tube defect.
- ***Triple marker screening*** identifies trisomic pregnancies and neural tube defects.
- A "***quadruple test***" screen is also used in the second trimester, combining inhibin assay with the triple marker test.
- Early assessment for trisomy 21 can also be done between 9 and 12 weeks by measuring maternal serum ***pregnancy associated plasma protein*** (PAPP-A) and ***serum beta-human chorionic gonadotrophin (beta-hCG)***. Low PAPP-A in the first trimester has been associated with fetal loss, abruption, preeclampsia, and fetal growth restriction. In contrast, beta-hCG levels on average will double in pregnancies at risk for trisomy 21.

Table 5.1 shows the patterns of triple screen test results and their interpretations.

Gestational Diabetes

Gestational diabetes mellitus (GDM) is defined as any degree of glucose intolerance with onset or first recognition during pregnancy.

Women with obesity, previous history of diabetes/GDM, history of abnormal glucose tolerance, history of poor obstetric outcome and family history of diabetes are at a higher risk of developing GDM. Women with GDM have a higher risk for preeclampsia, spontaneous abortions and fetal anomalies.

The WHO criteria for diagnosis of GDM and diabetes in pregnancy are shown in **Table 5.2**.

Once diagnosed with GDM or diabetes, it is essential to self-monitor blood glucose levels in order to achieve optimal control. Glucose targets are:

Table 5.1: Patterns of triple screen test results and their interpretations.

Condition	*MSAFP level*	*uE3 level*	*hCG level*
NTD	Increased	Normal	Normal
Trisomy 21	Low	Low	Increased
Trisomy 18	Low	Low	Low
Molar pregnancy	Low	Low	Very high
Multiple gestation	Increased	Normal	Increased
Fetal death (stillbirth)	Increased	Low	Low

(NTD: neural tube defect)

Table 5.2: The WHO criteria for the diagnosis of GDM and diabetes in pregnancy.

	GDM	*Diabetes*
Fasting plasma glucose	92–126 mg/dL	>126 mg/dL
75 g oral glucose tolerance test		
1-hour postprandial-glucose	≥180 mg/dL	–
2-hour postprandial-glucose	153–199 mg/dL	≥200 mg/dL
		RBS >200 mg/dL with symptoms
		HbA1C >6.5%

- Fasting plasma glucose <95 mg/dL and
- Either 1-hour postprandial glucose <140 mg/dL or 2-hour postprandial glucose <120 mg/dL.

OSTEOPOROSIS

Osteoporosis is common in women in the postmenopausal period. The diagnosis of primary osteoporosis rests on radiological findings combined with exclusion of secondary causes. This may require biochemical assays of various metabolites involved in bone formation and remodeling.

Serum Calcium

Box 5.7 shows the normal serum levels of calcium.

In the blood, calcium exists as:

1. Free or ionized calcium
2. Plasma protein-bound calcium
3. Anion bound complexes.

The blood levels are mainly regulated by parathyroid hormone (PTH) and active vitamin D_3. Hypocalcemia can be caused by:

1. Deficiency of PTH production or secretion
2. Deficiency of vitamin D
3. Defective bone mineralization with normal PTH and vitamin D.

Chronic renal failure is a significant cause of osteomalacia and must be evaluated with appropriate renal function tests.

Vitamin D

Vitamin D (cholecalciferol) plays an essential role as a hormone in the control of calcium and phosphorus.

UV light exposure of the skin converts naturally occurring 7-dehydrocholesterol to cholecalciferol or vitamin D_3. Diet-derived cholecalciferol from animal sources is called ergocalciferol or vitamin D_2. Both vitamin D_3 and vitamin D_2, require two hydroxylations to convert to its active form—1, 25 dihydroxycholecalciferol. Most of the laboratory instruments assay 25-hydroxyvitamin D as it is more stable in serum and has a longer half-life.

Vitamin D deficiency and insufficiency have been defined as a 25-hydroxyvitamin D <20 ng/mL and 21–29 ng/mL, respectively.

Box 5.7: Normal serum levels of calcium.

The normal serum levels of calcium range from 8.5–11 mg/dL.

Parathyroid Hormone

Parathyroid hormone (PTH) maintains physiological levels of ionized calcium. Calcitonin, phosphorus and magnesium also play an important role in mineral and bone metabolism. Their assays are used in conjunction with the other metabolites for determining the etiology of metabolic bone disorders.

CANCER IN WOMEN

Breast and cervical cancer are the two most common causes of cancer in women in India. Some of the important screening techniques for early detection and diagnosis are:

- Self-examination
- Mammography
- Genetic testing
- PAP smear examination

These can be supplemented with the following when indicated, for more precise diagnosis

- Tissue biopsies
- FNACs

Breast Cancer

Regular screening is the best way to detect early breast cancer. The American Cancer Society recommendations for women who are at average risk for developing breast cancer are shown in **Box 5.8**.

Suspicious lesions are stratified according to BI-RADS (*See* **Chapter 6:** Radiological Investigations in Women's Health) score based on the mammogram and USG. This is frequently followed by a needle biopsy of the lesion, which is then examined under the microscope for presence of carcinoma. If present, the invasive carcinoma is classified using the Nottingham-Bloom-Richardson system into one of three grades.

Hormone Receptor (ER, PR) and HER-2 Status

- It has long been known that the growth of breast cancer cells is (at least partly) driven by the hormones-estrogen and progesterone. In normal breast tissue these receptors subserve physiological functions. Roughly two-thirds of breast cancer patients carry these (either or both) receptors in their cells, which can be detected in the biopsied tissue sample by the pathologist using the technique of immunohistochemistry (IHC). Employing a scoring system the cancerous tissue is labeled either *"ER, PR positive" or "ER, PR negative"*. The purpose is to identify ER/PR (estrogen receptor/progesterone receptor) positive patients who will benefit from hormonal therapy (e.g., Tamoxifen) to treat their cancers.
- About one fifth of breast cancers also overexpress a protein, Human epidermal growth factor receptor 2 (HER-2), on the cell surface. Though *HER-2 positive* breast cancers have a more aggressive clinical course, these cancers can be effectively treated by targeting the HER-2 receptors (targeted therapy, e.g., Herceptin). The biopsy samples are used to detect the presence of HER-2 receptors employing the techniques of IHC and/or FISH (Fluorescent In-Situ Hybridization).

Box 5.8: Screening for breast cancer.

- **Women aged 40 to 44** years should have the choice to start annual breast cancer screening with a mammogram (X-ray of the breast) if they wish to do so.
- **Women aged 45 to 54** should get a mammogram every year.
- **Women 55 and older** can switch to a mammogram every 2 years, or can continue yearly screening.
- **Women at high-risk for breast cancer**– because of their family history, a genetic mutation, or other risk factors—should be screened with MRI along with a mammogram.

Clinical Pointer

Testing for ER, PR and HER-2 status is now an essential part of the standard protocol worldwide to evaluate breast carcinoma.

BRCA1 and BRCA2 Tests

BRCA1 and BRCA2 are genes in the human body whose normal function is to repair DNA damage in the cells. Mutation in either or both of the genes is associated with an increased risk for developing cancer, especially breast and ovarian cancer, along with a few other types of cancer. Hence, testing for these mutations, along with other cancer predisposing genes, has become advisable in women who have a family history of breast cancer, especially cancer developing at an early age. The tests are performed using blood samples.

Cervical Cancer

The Papanicolaou test (Pap Test) and HPV DNA test are the two screening methods for cervical cancer.

The Pap Test

- The Pap test involves collection of cells from the transformation zone of the cervix and either spreading them directly on glass slides or preserving them in specialized liquid media for subsequent processing.
- The latter method [(liquid-based cytology (LBC)] has the advantage of providing adequate material for both Pap tests and human papillomavirus (HPV) DNA tests, from the same sample.
- The collected samples are processed in the labs and reported by pathologists using a standard set of terms as outlined in the Bethesda System. The Bethesda system consists of several morphologic categories for reporting the squamous and glandular cells in the smears, ranging from "negative for intraepithelial lesion or malignancy (NILM)" to "squamous cell carcinoma/adenocarcinoma". Each category is associated with definite clinical connotations, prognostication and follow-up/treatment protocols.
- The primary aim of the Pap test is to detect precancerous lesions before they develop into invasive cancers. Concomitant testing for HPV DNA increases the sensitivity of the test and also lengthens the period to repeat testing (5 years vs. 3 years) when compared to Pap test alone.

Lynch Syndrome

- Lynch syndrome is an autosomal dominant condition closely associated with colorectal, endometrial and ovarian cancer.
- It is the most common inherited cancer predisposition syndrome.
- Lynch syndrome arises from inherited mutations, known as pathogenic variants, in the genes encoding the proteins of the highly conserved DNA mismatch repair (MMR) system.
- Women with Lynch syndrome are at increased risk of both endometrial and ovarian cancer and should be offered personalized counseling regarding family planning, red flag symptoms and risk-reducing strategies.

Summary

Biochemical investigations aid in diagnosis, prognostication, prediction and treatment of medical disorders. They are especially important in women as they can help in early diagnosis of many disorders like cancer, anemia, infertility, etc. and reduce morbidity and mortality to a great extent. Investigations during pregnancy aid in knowing the nutritional status of the mother and fetus and also the developmental status of the fetus. In lieu of biochemical investigations, the diagnostic procedure is delayed and can result in poor treatment outcomes.

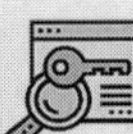

Review Questions

1. Which tests help to diagnose anemia?
2. What are the screening protocols in pregnancy?
3. What are the tests done to help diagnose cancer?
4. Write short notes on:
   a. Importance of biochemical investigations for women
   b. Biochemical investigations for osteoporosis
   c. Biochemical investigations for infertility

Bibliography

1. Henry's Clinical Diagnosis and Management by Laboratory Methods. 22nd edition.
2. Holick MF, Binkley NC, Bischoff-Ferrari HA, Gordon CM, Hanley DA, Heaney RP, Murad MH, Weaver CM; Endocrine Society. Evaluation, treatment, and prevention of vitamin D deficiency: an Endocrine Society clinical practice guideline. J Clin Endocrinol Metab. 2011;96(7):1911-30. doi: 10.1210/jc.2011-0385. Epub 2011 Jun 6. Erratum in: J Clin Endocrinol Metab. 2011 Dec;96(12):3908. PMID: 21646368.
3. https://emedicine.medscape.com/article/1172273-clinical#b5.
4. https://www.cancer.org/healthy/cancer-facts/cancer-facts-forwomen.html.
5. Metzger BE, Coustan DR (Eds.): Proceedings of the Fourth International Workshop—Conference on Gestational Diabetes Mellitus. Diabetes Care 21. 1998;(Suppl. 2):B1–B167.
6. WHO. Fact sheet: Maternal Mortality.

Multiple Choice Questions (MCQs)

To test your understanding and recall of key concepts.

1. **What is the main function of parathyroid hormone (PTH)?**
   A. Regulate sodium levels
   B. Control blood glucose levels
   C. Maintain physiological calcium levels
   D. Enhance vitamin B_{12} absorption
2. **Which of the following is *true* for folic acid?**
   A. Dietary insufficiency is commonly seen in tropical regions
   B. Folate deficiency results in megaloblastic anemia
   C. Folate deficiency in pregnancy can prevent neural tube defects in fetus
   D. All of the above
3. **Which of the following biochemical markers are used to monitor inflammation?**
   A. C-reactive protein (CRP)
   B. Thyroxine/T4
   C. Mean corpuscular hemoglobin concentration (MCHC)
   D. Serum iron
4. **Which test is used to evaluate neural tube defects in pregnancy?**
   A. Serum beta-hCG
   B. Alpha-fetoprotein (AFP)
   C. PAPP-A (pregnancy associated plasma protein)
   D. Transferrin levels
5. **A pregnant woman is diagnosed with gestational diabetes mellitus (GDM). Which of the following test results supports this diagnosis?**
   A. Fasting glucose >80 mg/dL; 1-hour postprandial glucose >120 mg/dL
   B. Fasting glucose >92 mg/dL; 1-hour postprandial glucose >180 mg/dL
   C. Fasting glucose >75 mg/dL; 2-hour postprandial glucose >140 mg/dL
   D. Random glucose >150 mg/dL with no symptoms
6. **A 65-year-old postmenopausal woman presents with severe bone pain and fractures. What should be the key elements of her assessment?**
   A. Serum calcium, vitamin D levels, DEXA scan
   B. Full thyroid panel, blood glucose, lipid profile
   C. CBC, CRP, hormone receptor testing
   D. Mammogram, MRI, tumor marker assay

ANSWERS

1. C	2. D	3. A	4. B	5. B
6. A				

Chapter 6

Radiological Investigations in Women's Health

Hiran Pandya

LEARNING OBJECTIVES

At the end of the chapter, the reader will be able to:
- Have a brief understanding of various radiological modalities.
- Know the pros and cons of the imaging techniques.
- Gain knowledge about different imaging techniques used for various conditions in females.

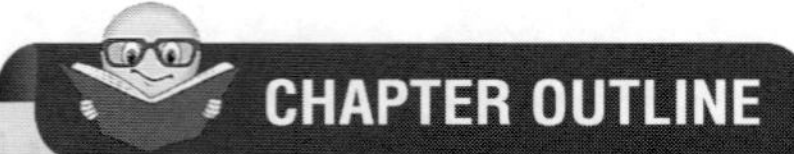

INTRODUCTION

National Institute of Health and Family Welfare of India define women's health as the branch of medicine that focuses on the treatment and diagnosis of diseases and conditions that affect a woman's physical and emotional well-being. Because they are often discriminated against due to sociocultural issues in many nations, the health of women and girls is a topic of particular concern. Radiology plays a significant part in guiding therapy and assessing the prognosis of the conditions. There are various conditions which are only seen in women due to the different anatomical and physiological working of the bodies. Issues like pregnancy, radiosensitive breast tissue, lactation, etc., pose a significant challenge to medical imaging. Due to these issues, it is crucial to pay close attention to gynecologic imaging radiation exposure over the course of a person's lifetime. In this chapter, we will look at various radiological modalities and their uses in female-specific conditions.

MAGNETIC RESONANCE IMAGING

Magnetic resonance imaging (MRI) is a technique which uses non-ionizing radiations to create images. There are two types of imaging signals in an MRI namely, T1 and T2 as shown in **Table 6.1**. To prevent significant injury to patients and personnel, safety precautions must be carefully observed, which calls for specialized MRI compatible equipment and strict adherence to safety regulations.

Table 6.1: Difference between T1 and T2 MRI.

T1 MRI	*T2 MRI*
• Also referred to as the anatomy sequence as the anatomy of structures is clearer and the water is not visible • The water does not show any signal and hence is black	• Also called the pathological sequence as the high signal of water shows effusion and fluid collection easily • The water has high signal so it appears white

Breast MRI

Even though mammograms are the most commonly used modality for evaluating the breast tissue, there are a certain percentage of breast cancer which go undiagnosed. That is when contrast-enhanced magnetic resonance (ce-MR) imaging **(Figs. 6.1 and 6.2)** of the breast comes into play.

American College of Radiology (ACR) appropriateness criteria states that ce-MR is to be used for women considered high-risk which includes:

- Women having *BRCA1* and *BRCA2* gene mutation and their untested first-degree relatives
- Having history of chest irradiation between 10 to 30 years of age
- Women with 20% or greater lifetime risk of breast cancer
- Have Li-Fraumeni syndrome, Cowden syndrome, or Bannayan-Riley-Ruvalcaba syndrome, or have first-degree relatives with one of these syndromes.

Indications

Indications for breast MRI are:

- High-risk patients
- Personal or family history

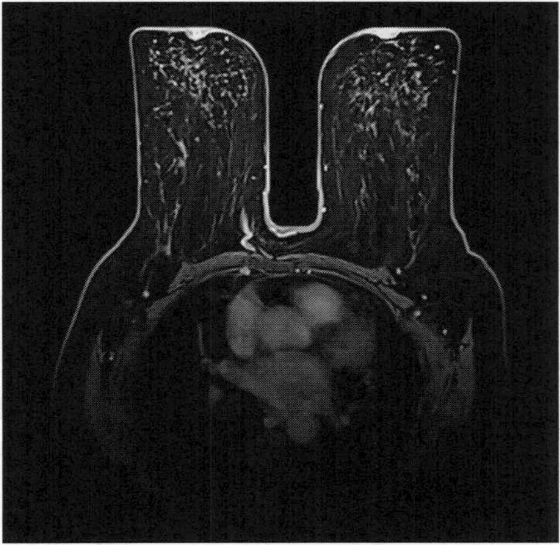

Fig. 6.1: Normal breast in post contrast T2.

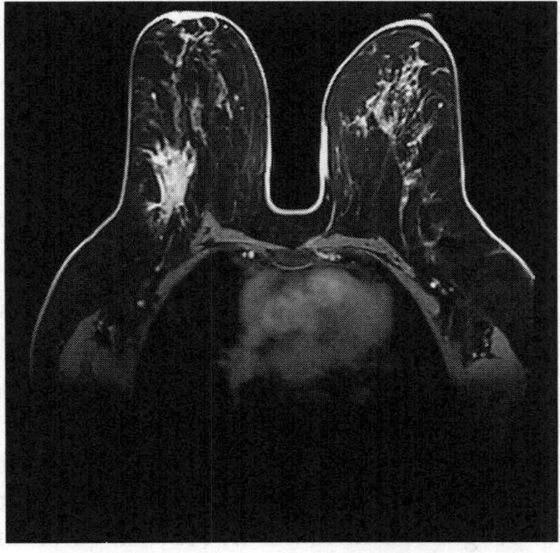

Fig. 6.2: Right breast carcinoma (BI-RADS V) in post contrast T2.

- Assessment of unknown primary, local magnitude of disease, multicentricity and bilaterally especially in dense breasts
- Pre and postoperative assessment of patients
- Seeing the result of the neoadjuvant chemotherapy
- Checking silicon implants

Abdomen and Pelvis MRI

MRI has become the primary modality for making diagnoses and directing treatment for individuals with gynecological illnesses. MRI is helpful in detecting endometriosis as well as pelvic adhesions due to obstructive anomalies.

A survey performed by The European Society of Urogenital Radiology (ESUR) showed that MRI was most commonly advised for detection and staging of gynecologic neoplasms, followed by assessing suspected or confirmed recurrent pelvic tumor (78.45%) and sonographically indeterminate adnexal mass.

MRI is also the choice of investigation over ultrasound and CT scan to check the staging of cervical cancer. Some of the other indications they found were:

- Evaluation of pelvic pain
- Endometriosis
- Assessment of fibroids
- Identification of congenital anomalies
- Checking for complications post pelvic surgery
- Also used in assessing abdominal pain in pregnant women

Fetal MRI

An essential diagnostic imaging supplement to ultrasonography is fetal magnetic resonance imaging (MRI), especially for monitoring fetal brain development.

It helps in either confirming the findings of the ultrasound or helps in gaining additional information. However, it is not currently employed as the primary screening technique in prenatal treatment.

American Congress of Obstetricians and Gynaecologists (ACOG), proposed the guidelines which also suggested the use of MRI when the ultrasound does not show clear results. This is done to improve the precision of diagnosis, especially in cases of posterior localization of the placenta or abnormally invasive placenta (AIP).

Additionally, it has been discovered that fetal MRI is useful in monochorionic twin pregnancies following the iatrogenic or natural death of a co-twin to detect pathological abnormalities in the surviving twin.

The indications of fetal magnetic resonance imaging according to the recommendations of the American College of Radiology (ACR), and Society for Pediatric Radiology (SPR) are:

- **Brain:**
  - Congenital anomalies
  - Screening fetuses with a family risk for brain anomalies-tuberous sclerosis malformations of cerebral cortical development
  - Vascular abnormalities: Vascular malformations
- **Spine:** Such as neural tube defects; vertebral anomalies

- **Skull, face and neck:** Masses of the face and neck like venolymphatic malformations; teratomas; facial clefts
- **Thorax:**
  - Congenital pulmonary airway malformations
  - Congenital diaphragmatic hernia
  - Effusion
  - In cases with the risk of pulmonary hypoplasia secondary to oligohydramnios, chest mass, or skeletal dysplasias for volumetric assessment of lung
- **Abdomen, retroperitoneal and pelvis:**
  - Location of tumors, such as hemangiomas, neuroblastomas
  - Suprarenal or renal masses, genitourinary anomalies
  - Complex lower urinary tract obstruction
- **Fetal surgery assessment:**
  - Meningomyelocele; sacrococcygeal teratomas.
  - Processes obstructing the airway (e.g., neck mass or congenital high airway obstruction)
  - Complications of monochorionic twins needing surgery

COMPUTERIZED TOMOGRAPHY

Computerized tomography (CT) gives us cross sectional images of the body parts with the help of X-rays.

Contrast CT uses iodine containing liquid which is injected intravenously and is commonly used in scanning the pelvic, chest or abdomen. The anatomy, physiology, as well as the pathophysiology of the specific organs are taken into consideration when intravenous contrast is used. It can be helpful in identification of vascular structure malformations as well as infection-related pathologies.

Another method is the ***Computerized Tomography Angiography*** (CTA) which also uses iodine contrast and helps in evaluation of the vascular structure in detail.

Advantages

- Fast, noninvasive and painless diagnosis
- Can be used in emergency for quick diagnosis of internal injury
- Patients body has no radiations after performing CT scan
- Less sensitive than MRI to patient movement
- Less expensive and more readily available than MRI
- Images of bone, soft tissue, and blood vessels can be obtained at the same time.
- Implanted medical device is not an issue when getting a CT scan
- As it has Real-time imaging, it can be a useful tool for directing needle aspirations and needle biopsies, especially for lungs, abdomen, bones and pelvis.

Disadvantages

- Cannot distinguish soft structures like ligaments as well as MRI
- Less sensitive in identifying white matter affection of the brain as compared to MRI
- Limited use in diagnosis of posterior fossa or brainstem pathology
- Pregnant women are only advised CT scan when absolutely necessary.

Fetal CT

This investigation is only performed when there is a doubt in the diagnosis after ultrasound. Additionally, only a low dose is used so that the fetal skeleton is clearly seen but the body is not. The radiation dose is the main danger of this procedure. It should be kept as low as is practically possible.

It is used when the fetus has severe bone abnormalities, during the second and third trimesters of gestation.

Abdominal and Female Genital Tract CT

Normally, ultrasound is the modality of choice for the diagnosis of any condition related to the genital tract. However, CT scan can be performed to confirm the diagnosis of malignancy, in follow-up and provide more information about the characteristic of the lesion.

Due to its excellent morphological resolution and capacity to show a variety of structures, including bones, lungs, abdominal viscera, and pelvic organs, CT is recommended in many abdominal disorders. The use of CT is constrained by the presence of ionizing radiation.

Indications

Some of the indications for abdominal and pelvic CT suggested by the American College of Radiologists (ACR) are:

- Assessing abdomen or pelvic trauma
- Renal, adrenal, and urinary tract disorders.
- Fluid collections or known or suspected abdominal or pelvic masses, including gynecological masses
- Evaluation of inflammatory processes in the abdomen or pelvis, such as inflammatory bowel disease and infectious bowel disease
- Finding issues after abdominal and pelvic surgery, such as an abscess, a radiation change, and the development of a fistula
- Primary or metastatic malignancies, including lesion characterization (e.g., focal liver lesion), staging, and treatment monitoring
- Evaluating the effectiveness of treatment for tumors, including perfusion research
- Assessment of bowel blockage or gastrointestinal hemorrhage
- Guidance for abdominal or pelvic interventional or therapeutic operations
- Follow-up examination after interventional or therapeutic operations in the belly or pelvis, including abscess drainage
- Planning radiation and chemotherapy treatments
- Assessment of the recipient before and after the transplant

CT is helpful in assessing lymph node status, tumor size, parametrial invasion, and distant metastasis, all of which are crucial prognostic variables in cervical carcinoma. This makes its use widespread in cervical cancer clinical staging.

ULTRASONOGRAPHY

Ultrasonography (USG) is an eminent imaging technology, also known as Ultrasound which has many applications in women's health. Three-dimensional (3D) and four-dimensional (4D) ultrasound has become rapidly popular. There are two major techniques of performing ultrasound, namely, transabdominal (TAS) and transvaginal (TVS).

1. The *transabdominal* (TAS) is performed by using the transducer head over the abdomen with full bladder and is commonly used to see the organs like kidney, liver, gallbladder, etc. In Obstetrics, it is used to check on the intrauterine pregnancy, intra-abdominal free fluid, abdominal aortic aneurysm, and hydronephrosis.
2. *Transvaginal (TVS)* ultrasound uses a high-frequency transducer which gives better resolution of both the uterus and ovaries. It should be performed with an empty bladder, where the transducer head is inserted into the vagina.

Even though TVS has better quality of images, it has its own limitations, as it cannot be performed in younger females, comparatively causes more discomfort in older women, and in some regions, it may not be culturally accepted.

Doppler Ultrasound is another technique which can assess the blood flowing through the vessels. It is a type of transvaginal technique which includes color-coded Doppler, two-dimensional (2D) and three-dimensional (3D) power Doppler ultrasonography.

Advantages

- Non-ionizing sound waves used, have no carcinogenesis which makes it safer for evaluating fetal and gonadal tissue.
- It is a machine which is more readily available than MRI and CT scan.
- Less expensive than CT scan or MRI.
- Easily portable as compared to CT scan and MRI.
- Lesser contraindications as compared with MRI or contrast-enhanced CT.
- Helps in examination of anatomy as well as physiology (such as fetal heart rate) as it gives real-time image.
- Images may not be as adversely affected by metallic objects, unlike CT or MRI.

Disadvantages

- Proper training required for accurate and effective usage of the device.
- Not capable of evaluating the internal structure of tissue types with high acoustical impedance (e.g., bone, air).
- One of the side effects is the thermal heating or mechanical injury which can occur at tissue level which may harm the fetus.
- It has its own distinct artifacts (US artifacts), which can lead to chances of low-quality image or misinterpretation.

Obstetrics Ultrasound

USG is used throughout the gestational period to monitor the pregnancy as it gives a high definition 2-dimensional real time image in various planes **(Figs. 6.3A and B)**. Nowadays, 3D ultrasound **(Figs. 6.4 and 6.5)** is also used to give a proper picture in the form of face and behaviors like yawning of the fetus development. USG is performed to find out the following:

- Find the presence of a living fetus
- Determine the age of pregnancy
- Check for ectopic pregnancy
- Check for congenital abnormalities in the embryo
- Check the fetal heart rate
- Determine position of the fetus and the placenta
- Check for premature rupture of the membranes
- Check for multiple pregnancies
- Determine the amount of amniotic fluid around the fetus
- Examine to see the opening or shortening of the cervix
- Examine the growth and the health of the fetus

Breast Ultrasound

Ultrasound of breast is used normally as a secondary form of investigation after mammogram. It is preferred in younger women.

- It can be an alternate to mammogram as it is cheaper, portable and can effectively find out palpable abnormalities in the breast.
- It can differentiate cystic from solid masses and demonstrate those features of solid masses that would denote the mass as suspicious and warranting biopsy.

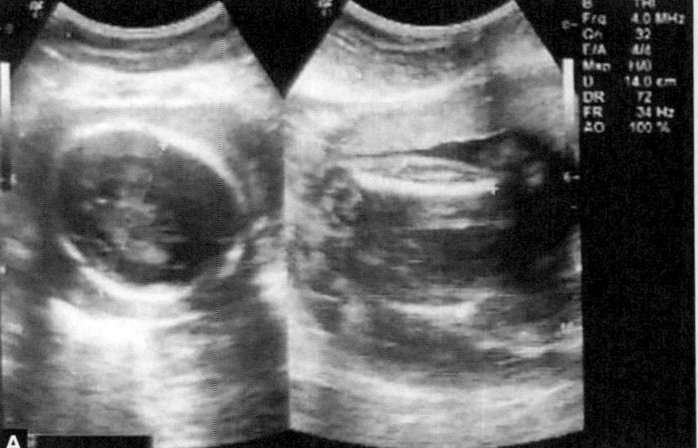

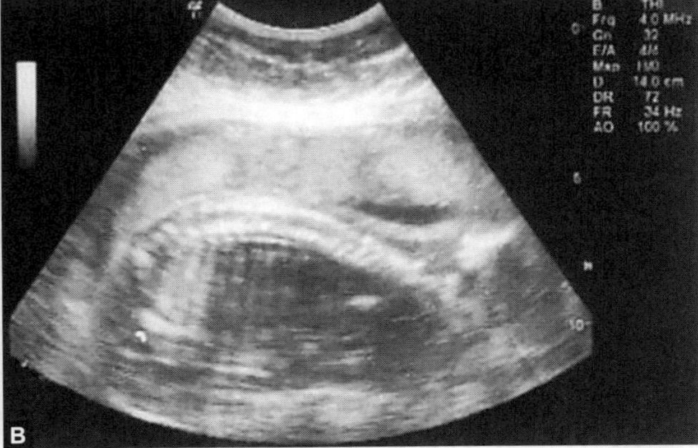

Figs. 6.3A and B: Monitoring fetal growth in the uterus by USG.

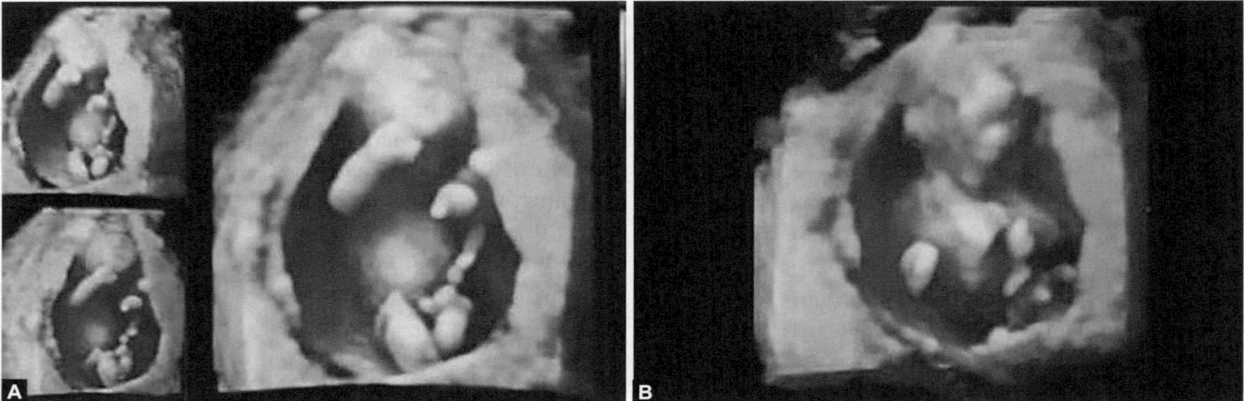

Figs. 6.4A and B: A 3D ultrasound image of the fetus during the first trimester of pregnancy.

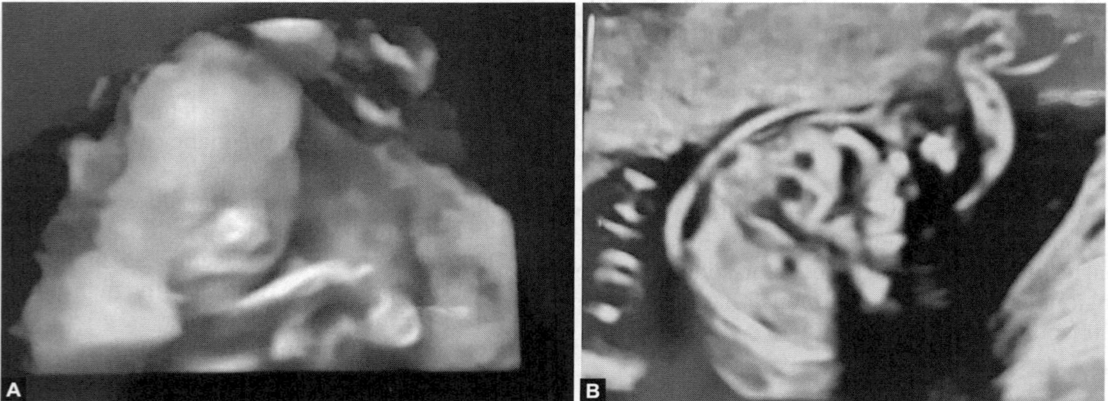

Figs. 6.5A and B: A 4D ultrasound of the fetus growth during the second trimester of pregnancy.

- Ultrasound is a particularly useful diagnostic modality in dense breast tissue, often detecting breast cancers obscured on mammography.
- In cases where biopsy is needed, ultrasound helps in guiding the subsequent procedures, further improves its utility in the diagnosis of breast cancer.

Abdomen and Pelvis Ultrasound

In most cases, ultrasound is the first imaging technique used in abdominal pathology. It is used to study the peritoneal cavity and organs in the abdomen and the pelvis like the gallbladder, spleen, uterus, kidney, liver, etc. It is also used for guiding diagnostic procedures in abdominal pathology.

Indications for Abdominal US

- Abdominal pain
- Vaginal bleeding
- Hydronephrosis
- Free fluid in the abdominal cavity due to blunt trauma
- Cirrhosis and portal hypertension
- Suspected hypertrophic pyloric stenosis
- Search for metastatic disease
- Evaluation of uncontrolled hypertension
- Suspected renal artery stenosis
- Urinary tract infection, etc.

The pelvic ultrasound is used alongside physical examination to confirm the presence of pelvic mass, and to evaluate its size, contour, and character, to determine the organ of origin, evaluate for involvement of other organs.

Indications of USG of Pelvis

- Infertility
- Pelvic pain
- Abnormal vaginal bleeding
- Endometriosis
- Disorders of menstruation
- Uterine fibroids **(Figs. 6.6A and B)**
- Polycystic ovary syndrome
- Abnormal or limited physical examination
- Suspicion of mass or infection
- Localization of intrauterine contraceptive device (IUD)
- Guidance for interventional procedures

Diagnostic Criteria for Polycystic Ovary Syndrome

- One of the diagnostic criteria for polycystic ovary syndrome (PCOS) according to the Rotterdam consensus is the presence of the polycystic ovary (PCO) seen during an ultrasound examination.
- The other two criteria being, clinical and/or biochemical symptoms of hyperandrogenism as well as oligo- and

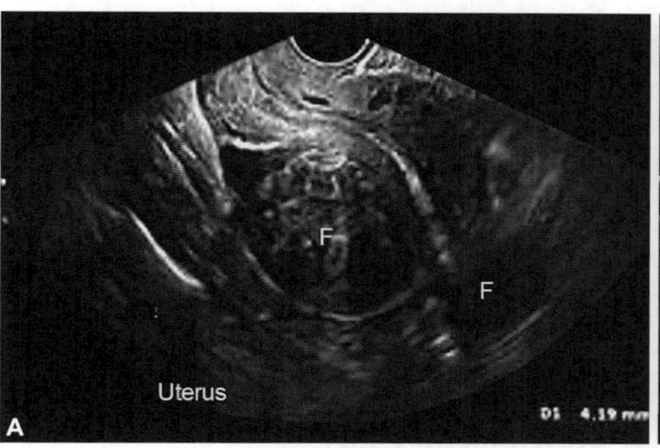

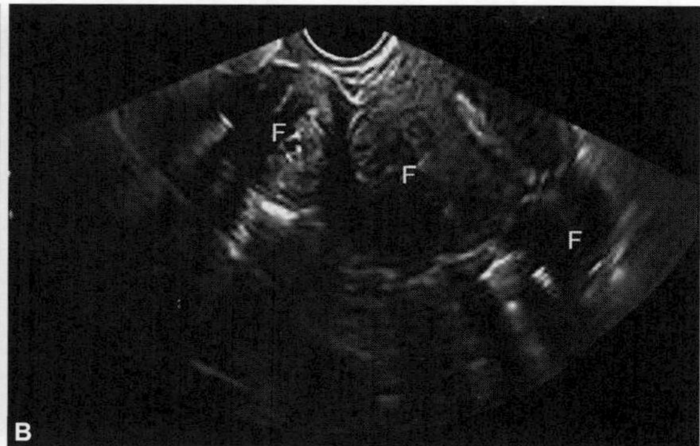

Figs. 6.6A and B: Enlarged uterus and multiple fibroids on USG.

anovulation. When any two out of the three criteria are present, the diagnosis of PCOS can be confirmed.

In conditions such as dysmenorrhea, where there is presence of pelvic pain, USG can be used to check the organs of the pelvis.

- The preferred technique for doing the initial assessment is by transvaginal ultrasonography.
- Transabdominal pelvic ultrasonography is preferred in non-sexually active adolescents and young women to ensure patient comfort.
- Ultrasound can be used to identify dysmenorrhea linked to adnexal pathology or uterine anomalies.

SONOHYSTEROGRAPHY

Sonohysterography (SHG) supplements transvaginal ultrasound as a way of better evaluating the endometrium since it improves the endometrial visibility than is possible with conventional transvaginal ultrasonography. It involves injecting a tiny amount of sterile saline into the uterine cavity and using an ultrasound transducer to examine the uterine lining.

Indications for SHG

- Abnormal uterine bleeding
- Infertility and repeated abortion
- Congenital abnormality of the uterine cavity
- Pre or postoperative assessment of uterine myomas, polyps or cysts
- Additional investigation of suspected endometrial abnormalities detected by transvaginal sonogram
- Insufficient transvaginal sonographic imaging

Contraindications of SHG

The main contraindications of SHG include:

- Pregnancy
- Pelvic infection
- Excessive vaginal bleeding

MAMMOGRAPHY

Breast cancer is one of the major conditions which affects the women around the world.

Mammography is a special examination method to examine the breast using low-level of X-rays. A mammography examination is called a mammogram. It is considered the gold standard in early detection and identification of the carcinoma of the breast. A normal mammogram is two-dimensional in shape where images of breast are taken from side to side and top to bottom **(Fig. 6.7)**.

Clinical Pointer

The American College of Radiology (ACR) and Society of Breast Imaging (SBI) recommends annual mammograms for women after 40 years of age.

There are two types of mammography which are performed namely, diagnostic mammography and screening mammography.

- The *diagnostic mammography* is done for patients who have abnormal findings like lump in the breast or discharge from the nipples which the patient or her doctor may have found.
- On the other hand, *screening mammography* is done for early diagnosis of asymptomatic women.
- Another type of mammography is called the *digital breast tomosynthesis* (DBT), which is a three-dimensional (3D) mammography. It allows the view of the breast in 3 dimensions in the multiple thin slides of the whole breast. However, the dosage of exposure is slightly higher than the normal mammogram.
- *Galactography*, also known as *Ductography*, uses mammography to evaluate the nipple discharge. It utilizes contrast dye which is injected into the breast before the X-ray, to give a more detailed picture of the milk ducts.

Among other techniques we have is the *magnetic resonance (MR) mammogram* which is emerging in use nowadays. It has received clinical approval for a number of indications.

Indications of Magnetic Resonance (MR) Mammogram

- Diagnosis of cancer with an unknown source
- Screening of high-risk women for breast cancer
- Diagnosis of recurrent breast cancer
- Evaluation of the breast with implants
- Staging of local breast cancer

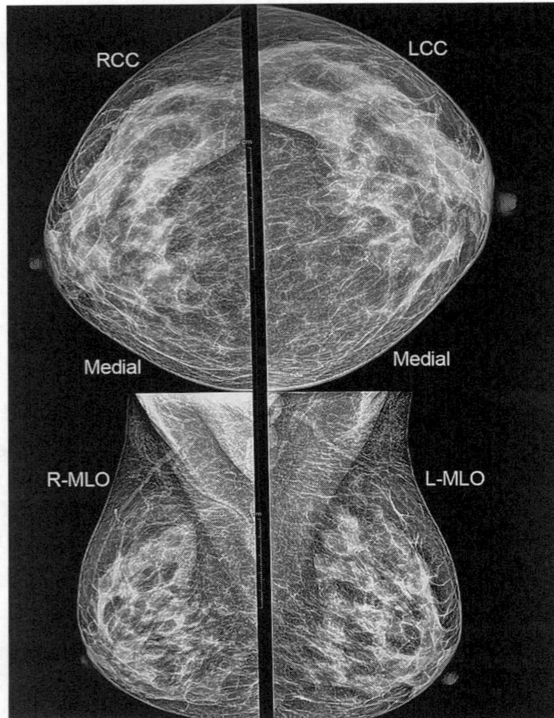

Fig. 6.7: Mammogram with BI-RADS 2.

Advantages of Mammography

- Helps in reducing the mortality rates due to carcinoma of the breast
- Detection of all types of cancer can be done including invasive ductal and invasive lobular cancer
- Screening mammography identifies even small tumors, this gives the patient more treatment options
- The use of screening mammography increases the detection of small abnormal tissue growths confined to the milk ducts in the breast, called ductal carcinoma in situ (DCIS).

Disadvantages of Mammography

- Overdiagnosis of tumors, that is identifying tumors that may never become symptomatic in the patients.
- Getting false positive results which make further investigations necessary.

BREAST IMAGING-REPORTING AND DATA SYSTEM

Breast imaging-reporting and data system (BI-RADS) is a system created by the American College of Radiology which is used as a risk analysis system in breast imaging such as mammography, MRI and ultrasound. It aims to standardize management guidelines for breast lesions and enhance communication through breast imaging reports.

It helps radiologists interpret findings, use the proper assessment and recommendations, audit their breast imaging practice to verify that quality standards are maintained, and improve patient care. It consists of the following categories as shown in **Table 6.2** as published in 2013.

Table 6.2: Category of BI-RADS assessment.

BI-RADS 0	Incomplete
BI-RADS 1	Negative
BI-RADS 2	Benign
BI-RADS 3	Probably benign
BI-RADS 4	Suspicious
BI-RADS 5	Highly suggestive of malignancy
BI-RADS 6	Known biopsy proven malignancy

ABDOMINAL X-RAY

X-rays are a type of electromagnetic energy.

Indications

It can be used for various abdominal conditions such as:
- Intestinal blockages
- Ingestion of external foreign items
- Kidney and urinary bladder stones and gallstones
- Perforations of the stomach or intestine, etc.

Advantages

- Minimally invasive procedure with very few risks
- Painless
- Equipment is widely used and reasonably priced and easily available as compared to MRI
- Helpful in emergency diagnosis and treatment

Disadvantages

- Images are not as detailed as those of other approaches such as CT of the abdomen and pelvis or MRI.
- To better understand the findings of an abdomen X-ray or to search for abnormalities that the abdominal X-ray missed, other imaging studies may be required.
- Not advisable for pregnant women.

DUAL-ENERGY X-RAY ABSORPTIOMETRY

Osteoporosis is a condition which leads to low bone mass, degeneration of bone tissue, and disruption of bone microarchitecture. This leads to decreased bone strength and increases the risk of fractures. The diagnosis of osteoporosis is done by measuring the bone mineral density (BMD) and most common method of measuring the BMD is the Dual-energy X-ray absorptiometry (DEXA). It is normally performed over the lumbar spine as well as both the femoral neck of the patient **(Fig. 6.8)**. A Z score is generated by comparing the measured bone mineral density to a database of patients with normal bone mineral density for their age and sex. The difference between the patient's measurement and that of a young healthy adult is known as a T score. The WHO diagnostic criteria of osteoporosis are shown in **Table 6.3**.

Advantages

- It is fast, quick and a simple procedure
- Noninvasive procedure

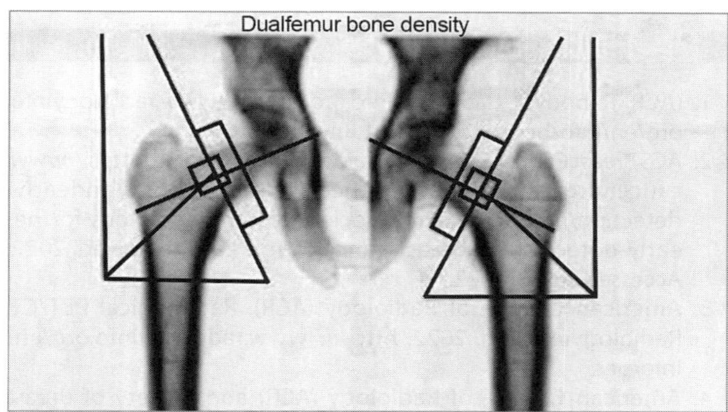

Fig. 6.8: DEXA scan of bilateral femur of a patient with a T score of −0.7 which indicates normal bone mineral density.

Table 6.3: WHO diagnosis criteria of osteoporosis based on BMD.

T score	*Classification*
T ≥ -1 and above	Normal
−2.5 < T<-1	Osteopenia
T≤−2.5	Osteoporosis
T≤−2.5 along with one or more fragility fracture	Severe osteoporosis

- Used to make a decision on whether treatment is required
- Checking and monitoring the effect of the treatment
- No radiation remains in the body

Disadvantages

- Expensive equipment
- Non-portable machine
- The measurements of bone density made using various DEXA systems cannot be directly compared. Hence, the follow-up examinations should be ideally performed using the same machine.

POSITRON EMISSION TOMOGRAPHY

Positron emission tomography (PET) is a part of nuclear imaging which combines molecular and anatomical imaging using radioactive material. The process entails injecting a radiopharmaceutical that emits positrons intravenously, waiting for systemic absorption, and then scanning for patterns of radiopharmaceutical buildup in the body. Fluorodeoxyglucose (FDG) called F-18 is a commonly used radio-pharmaceutical agent which is similar to glucose.

PET scan can also be combined with the CT scan or MRI. PET/CT is more common than PET/MRI. The advantage of PET/CT is that it allows the view of both anatomical and physiological structure of the body.

PET scan has better sensitivity to the growing cancer cell **(Fig. 6.9)** but is not a very good tool to show the anatomy. Whereas CT scan has a greater advantage of showing the anatomy, size as well as the anatomical location of the tumor but not the metabolic activity of the tumor. Hence, this combination gives more precise information and a confirmed diagnosis.

Indications

It is commonly used for the following procedures:

- Detecting or diagnosing cancer
- Checking the spread of cancer
- Checking the prognosis of the condition
- Assessing the viability and metabolism of the tissue
- Detecting cause of fever of unknown origin
- Examining any abnormalities of the brain, such as tumors, memory problems, convulsions, and other conditions of the central nervous system, the heart and brain in a healthy person
- Assessing myocardial viability to see which parts of the heart are affected by a myocardial infarction.
- Restaging of breast cancer.

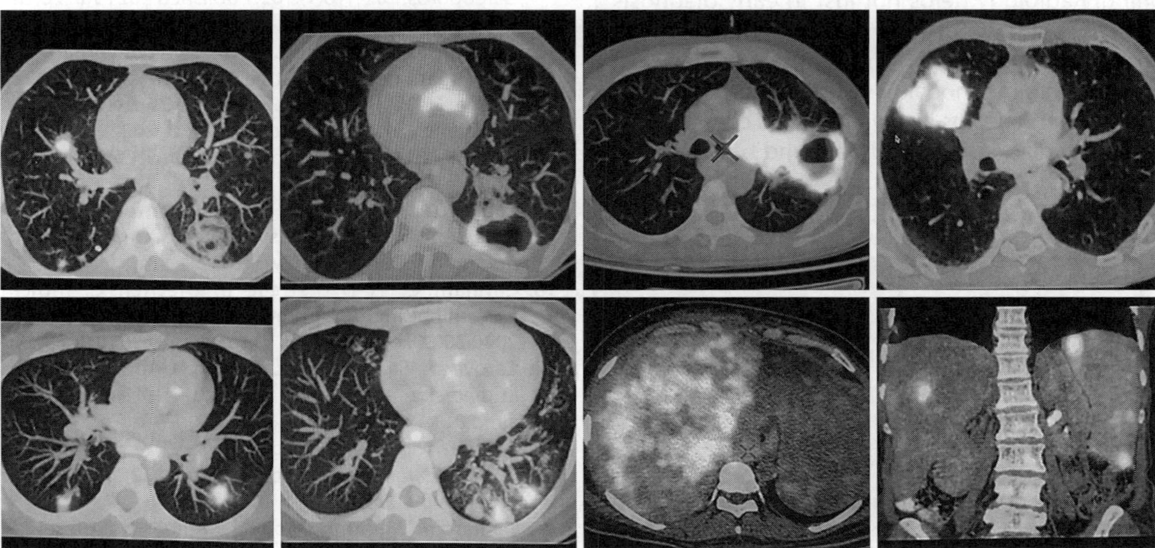

Fig. 6.9: PET scan showing lung cancer.

Advantages

- Both anatomical and functional information can be sought which is not the case in MRI and CT scan.
- Better at assessing locoregional lymph nodes as compared to CT.
- Cost effective and may provide more precise information than exploratory surgery.
- When CT and PET are performed together rather than separately, the patient benefits from improved convenience.

Disadvantages

- Requires intravenous injection.
- Time consuming as the radioactive drug takes time to accumulate in the area of interest.
- Image resolution is not as high as CT or MRI.
- Not advisable for pregnant women.

PET has shown to be effective in staging advanced disease, monitoring therapy, restaging, and finding recurring disease.

- However, it is typically not advisable in the initial diagnosis and screening of majority of the patients. It has been found that it can offer more information than a CT, MRI, or bone scan in 29% of the cases.
- However, in case the initial lesions are small, well-defined, and slow-growing, like lobular carcinoma and ductal carcinoma in situ, PET may not be able to identify them.
- False negatives may result from PET's inability to detect tiny metastases in normally sized axillary nodes.
- Therefore, additional testing is still necessary if a PET scan for axillary nodes in a breast cancer patient is negative.
- ***FDG-PET*** has also demonstrated good sensitivity in the identification of cervical malignancies and can consistently show the degree of nodal involvement, assisting in proper therapy planning.

Summary

Women face various unique challenges in the health domain due to their different anatomical and physiological functioning. Radiology helps not just in early diagnosis but also in keeping a track of the condition and the effectiveness of the treatment. This chapter gives an idea about various imaging modalities pertaining to women's health. Each technique has its own pros and cons and the best method of diagnosis should be found based on the what is best suited for the patient.

Review Questions

1. What are the various imaging techniques used for diagnosing carcinoma of the breast?
2. What are the advantages and disadvantages of Computerized Tomography?
3. What is BI-RADS? Write the various categories of BI-RADS assessment.
4. What are the various techniques of ultrasound used in women's health?
5. State the indications of sonohysterography.

Bibliography

1. (ACR) R. bodyct. Radiologyinfo.org. https://www.radiologyinfo.org/en/info/bodyct. Accessed July 8, 2022.
2. ACS Breast Cancer Screening Guidelines. Cancer.org. https://www.cancer.org/cancer/breast-cancer/screening-tests-andearly-detection/american-cancer-society-recommendations-forthe-early-detection-of-breast-cancer.html. Last reviewed 2022. Accessed July 8, 2022.
3. American College of Radiology (ACR). Radiological PET/CT. Radiologyinfo.Org, 2022, https:// www.radiologyinfo.org/en/info/pet.
4. American College of Radiology (ACR) and Society of Breast Imaging (SBI) Breast Cancer Screening Guidelines for Women at High Risk for the Disease.
5. American College of Radiology--SPR Practice parameter for the safe and optimal performance of fetal magnetic resonance imaging (MRI). 2022.
6. American College of Radiology. X-ray (Radiography)--Abdomen. Radiologyinfo.org. https://www.radiologyinfo.org/en/info/abdominrad. Accessed July 6, 2022.
7. Anand SS, Singh H, Dash AK. Clinical Applications of PET and PETCT. Med J Armed Forces India. 2009;65(4):353-58. doi:10.1016/S0377-1237(09)80099-3.
8. Aoki TT, Grecu EO, Srinivas PR, Prescott P, Benbarka M, Arcangeli MM. Prevalence of osteoporosis in women: variation with skeletal site of measurement of bone mineral density. Endocr Pract. 2000;6(2):127-31. doi:10.4158/EP.6.2.127.
9. Bachanek M, Abdalla N, Cendrowski K, Sawicki W. Value of ultrasonography in the diagnosis of polycystic ovary syndrome--literature review. J Ultrason. 2015;15(63):410-22. doi:10.15557/JoU.2015.0038.
10. Balasubramanian P, Murugesan VK, Boopathy V. The role of MR mammography in differentiating benign from malignant in suspicious breast masses. J Clin Diagn Res. 2016;10(9):TC05-TC08. doi:10.7860/JCDR/2016/21820.8456.
11. Benseler J. The Radiology Handbook: A Pocket Guide To Medical Imagining.
12. Bhadada SK, Chadha M, Sriram U, et al. The Indian Society for Bone and Mineral Research (ISBMR) position statement for the diagnosis and treatment of osteoporosis in adults. Arch Osteoporos. 2021;16(1):102. Published 2021 Jun 26. doi:10.1007/s11657-021-00954-1.
13. Breast cancer. Who.int. https://www.who.int/news-room/fact-sheets/detail/breast-cancer#:~:text=In%202020%2C%20there%20were%202.3,the%20world's%20most%20prevalent%20cancer. Accessed July 8, 2022.
14. Butler P. Applied Radiological Anatomy. Cambridge: Cambridge University Press; 2012.
15. Cancer Treatment centres of America. https://www.cancercenter.com/cancer-types/breast-cancer/diagnosis-and-detection/ductogram. Accessed July 6, 2022.
16. Caraiani C, Yi D, Petresc B, Dietrich C. Indications for abdominal imaging: When and what to choose? J Ultrason. 2020;20(80):e43-e54. doi:10.15557/JoU.2020.0008.
17. Carovac A, Smajlovic F, Junuzovic D. Application of ultrasound in medicine. Acta Inform Med. 2011;19(3):168-71. doi:10.5455/aim.2011.19.168-171.
18. European Society of Radiology 2009. The future role of radiology in healthcare. Insights into imaging. 2010;1(1):2-11. doi:10.1007/s13244-009-0007-x
19. Gaillard F. Mammography | Radiology Reference Article | Radiopaedia.org. Doi.org. https://doi.org/10.53347/rID-1644. Accessed July 8, 2022.

20. Gatta G, Di Grezia G, Cuccurullo V, et al. MRI in pregnancy and precision medicine: A review from literature. J Pers Med. 2021;12(1):9. Published 2021 Dec 23. doi:10.3390/jpm12010009.
21. Goodman TR, Amurao M. Medical imaging radiation safety for the female patient: rationale and implementation. Radiographics. 2012;32(6):1829-37. doi:10.1148/rg.326125508.
22. International Commission on Radiological Protection. Information for patients, family members, carers and the public--ICRPaedia.Icrpaedia.org. http://icrpaedia.org/Information_for_patients,_ family_members,_carers_and_the_public. Accessed July 27, 2022.
23. International evidence-based guideline for the assessment and management of polycystic ovary syndrome. Copyright Monash University, Melbourne, Australia 2018.
24. Kho K, Shields J. Diagnosis and Management of Primary Dysmenorrhea. JAMA. 2020;323(3):268. doi:10.1001/jama.2019.16921.
25. Kurzweil A, Martin J. Transabdominal Ultrasound. [Updated 2021 Aug 13]. In: StatPearls [Internet]. Treasure Island (FL): StatPearls Publishing; 2022. Available from: https://www.ncbi.nlm.nih.gov/books/NBK534813/
26. Lecchi M, Fossati P, Elisei F, Orecchia R, Lucignani G. Current concepts on imaging in radiotherapy. Eur J Nucl Med Mol Imaging. 2008;35(4):821-37. doi:10.1007/s00259-007-0631-y
27. Loberg M, Lousdal ML, Bretthauer M, Kalager M. Benefits and harms of mammography screening. Breast Cancer Res.2015;17(1):63. doi:10.1186/s13058-015-0525-z
28. Mittal M, Deolia S, Agrawal A, Chaturvedi H, Agrawal G, Chhabra KG. Prevalence of breast imaging reporting and data system (BIRADS) categories and breast consistencies in Central India—A cross-sectional survey. J Family Med Prim Care. 2021;10(9):3219-22. doi: 10.4103/jfmpc.jfmpc_2494_20. Epub 2021 Sep 30. PMID: 34760733; PMCID: PMC8565158.
29. Nana A, Slater GJ, Stewart AD, Burke LM. Methodology review: using dual-energy X-ray absorptiometry (DXA) for the assessment of body composition in athletes and active people. Int J Sport Nutr Exerc Metab. 2015;25(2):198-215. doi:10.1123/ijsnem.2013-0228.
30. National Health Portal. https://www.nhp.gov.in/healthlyliving/women-s-health. Published 2022. Accessed July 6, 2022.
31. Niazi, M. Transabdominal vs Transvaginal Sonography—Comparison in Pelvic Pathologies. Journal of Rawalpindi Medical College. 2015;19(3):223-6. https://www.journalrmc.com/index.php/JRMC/article/view/242.
32. Nougaret S, Lakhman Y, Gourgou S, et al. MRI in female pelvis: an ESUR/ESR survey. Insights into Imaging. 2022;13(1):60. https://doi.org/10.1186/s13244-021-01152-w
33. Obstetric Ultrasound.Radiologyinfo.org. https://www.radiologyinfo.org/en/info/obstetricus. Accessed July 8, 2022.
34. Piessens S, Edwards A. Sonographic evaluation for endometriosis in routine pelvic ultrasound. J Minim Invasive Gynecol. 2020;27(2):265-66. doi:10.1016/j.jmig.2019.08.027.
35. Prasad TV, Thulkar S, Hari S, Sharma DN, Kumar S. Role of computed tomography (CT) scan in staging of cervical carcinoma. Indian J Med Res. 2014;139(5):714-19.
36. Prayer D, Malinger G, Brugger PC, et al. ISUOG Practice Guidelines: performance of fetal magnetic resonance imaging. Ultrasound Obstet Gynecol. 2017;49(5):671-80. doi:10.1002/uog.17412.
37. Radhakrishna S, Agarwal S, Parikh PM, et al. Role of magnetic resonance imaging in breast cancer management. South Asian J Cancer. 2018;7(2):69-71. doi:10.4103/sajc.sajc_104_18.
38. RI|Changeset|Radiopaedia.org.Images.radiopaedia.org.https://images.radiopaedia.org/articles/6317/changesets/179909/edits. 2022. Accessed July 8, 2022.
39. Rotterdam ESHRE/ASRM-Sponsored PCOS consensus workshop group. Revised 2003 consensus on diagnostic criteria and long-term health risks related to polycystic ovary syndrome (PCOS). Hum Reprod. 2004;19(1):41–7. [PubMed] [Google Scholar].
40. Salari N, Ghasemi H, Mohammadi L, et al. The global prevalence of osteoporosis in the world: a comprehensive systematic review and meta-analysis. J Orthop Surg Res. 2021;16(1):609. doi:10.1186/s13018-021-02772-0.
41. Saleem SN. Fetal MRI: An approach to practice: A review. J Adv Res. 2014;5(5):507-23. doi:10.1016/j.jare.2013.06.001.
42. Saul T, Siadecki SD, Berkowitz R, Rose G, Matilsky D, Sauler A. M-Mode ultrasound applications for the emergency medicine physician. J Emerg Med. 2015;49(5):686-92. doi:10.1016/j.jemermed.2015.06.059.
43. Shaw P, Robinson S, Abai B. Radiation safety for women: What physicians and patients need to know. Vascular Disease in Women. 2021:415-36. doi:10.1016/b978-0-12-822959-0.00011-0.
44. Sood R, Rositch AF, Shakoor D, Ambinder E, Pool KL, Pollack, et al. Ultrasound for breast cancer detection globally: A systematic review and meta-analysis. Journal of Global Oncology, 2019;2019(5):1-17. https://doi.org/10.1200/JGO.19.00127.
45. Sozen T, Ozışık L, Başaran NC. An overview and management of osteoporosis. Eur J Rheumatol. 2017;4(1):46-56. doi:10.5152/eurjrheum.2016.048.
46. The Society for Pediatric Radiology. Fetal CT: General Information. Pedrad.org. https://www.pedrad.org/Specialties/Fetal-Imaging/Fetal-CT-General-Information. Accessed July 8, 2022.
47. Tollens F, Baltzer PAT, Dietzel M, et al. Cost-Effectiveness of MR Mammography in Breast Cancer Screening of Women With Extremely Dense Breasts After Two Rounds of Screening. Front Oncol. 2021;11:724543. Published 2021 Sep 9. doi:10.3389/fonc.2021.724543.
48. Wladimiroff J, Eik-Nes S. Ultrasound in Obstetric and Gynaecology. Elsevier Limited; 2009.
49. Yang T, Pandya A, Marcal L, et al. Sonohysterography: Principles, technique and role in diagnosis of endometrial pathology. World J Radiol. 2013;5(3):81-7. doi:10.4329/wjr.v5.i3.81.

Multiple Choice Questions (MCQs)

To test your understanding and recall of key concepts.

1. **What is the primary imaging modality for detecting fetal abnormalities?**
   A. Mammography
   B. Ultrasound
   C. MRI
   D. PET scan

2. **What does the T1 signal in MRI primarily highlight?**
   A. Pathological sequences
   B. Water and fluid collections
   C. Anatomical structures
   D. Air-filled spaces

3. **Which of the following imaging modalities is considered the investigation of choice for local staging of cervical cancer due to its superior soft-tissue resolution?**
   A. Ultrasound B. CT scan
   C. MRI D. X-rays

4. Why is MRI preferred over CT for imaging pelvic soft tissues?
A. It is less expensive.
B. It provides better soft-tissue contrast.
C. It requires less time to complete.
D. Minimal contraindications.

5. What is the role of BI-RADS in breast imaging?
A. It categorizes imaging modalities based on cost.
B. It standardizes breast lesion assessment and recommendations.
C. It identifies contraindications for mammography.
D. It evaluates radiation exposure risks.

6. A 35-year-old woman with dense breast tissue requires breast imaging. Which modality is most appropriate?
A. Mammography
B. Breast ultrasound
C. PET scan
D. Dual-energy X-ray absorptiometry (DEXA)

7. A patient presents with suspected pelvic adhesions. Which imaging modality would be most useful?
A. Transabdominal ultrasound
B. Pelvic MRI
C. Abdominal X-ray
D. CT scan of the pelvis

8. How can dual-energy X-ray absorptiometry (DEXA) contribute to patient management in osteoporosis?
A. By assessing the bone mineral density
B. By identifying soft tissue masses
C. By evaluating the effectiveness of chemotherapy
D. By detecting pathological fractures in real-time

ANSWERS

1. B	2. C	3. C	4. B
5. B	6. B	7. B	8. A

Chapter 7

International Classification of Functioning in Women's Health

Suvarna Ganvir, Shyam Ganvir

LEARNING OBJECTIVES

At the end of the chapter, the reader will be able to:

- Define International Classification of Functioning (ICF).
- Describe the terminologies used in describing the ICF for a particular condition.
- Describe the relevance of using ICF in different conditions related to women.
- Understand the concept of ICF for a particular disease condition related to women's health.
- Describe the clinical and research related use of ICF for a physiotherapist.

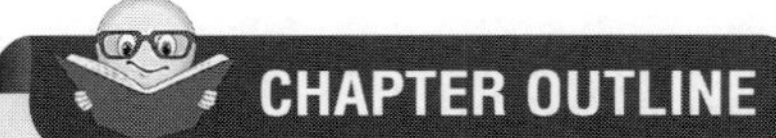

- Introduction
- International classification of functioning
- Terminologies used in ICF
  - Body structure
  - Body function
  - Activities and participation
  - Environmental factors
  - The qualifiers
  - Contextual factors
- Applications of ICF
- ICF core sets
  - Postpartum period
  - Fall risk
- Breast cancer
- Urinary incontinence

INTRODUCTION

Patient-Centered Care (PCC) has been defined as "care that is respectful of and responsive to individual patient preferences, needs and values". ***Patient-Reported Outcomes*** (PROs) and shared decision-making are key components of PCC because they encourage and empower patients to play an active role in their own care. These PROs are described by patients in their own words which are focused towards the patient's life experiences. Thus, it helps to note the information which otherwise may get overlooked in a busy clinical setting. This also facilitates clinician—patient communication and shared decision-making. This may provide right direction to the treatment goals and thus overall quality of treatment may improve.

International Classification of Functioning (ICF) serves the purpose of providing a comprehensive list of patient-related outcomes in terms of Activities and Participation. Thus, shared decision-making using ICF can be facilitated.

For a clinician it is equally important to know the body structures and functions affected in a patient which has a direct impact on activities and participation. The International Classification of Functioning, Disability and Health (ICF) provides a useful framework for achieving this understanding, and constitutes a common language among the different health professionals. According to the ICF, the problems associated with a disease may concern body functions and body structures, activities and participation in life situations. Health states and the development of disability are modified by contextual factors such as environmental and personal factors.

Literature has identified Women's Health as a domain founded from the clinical area of Obstetrics and Gynecology that is involved in the care of women in relation to childbirth, both antenatally and postnatally, including the teaching of

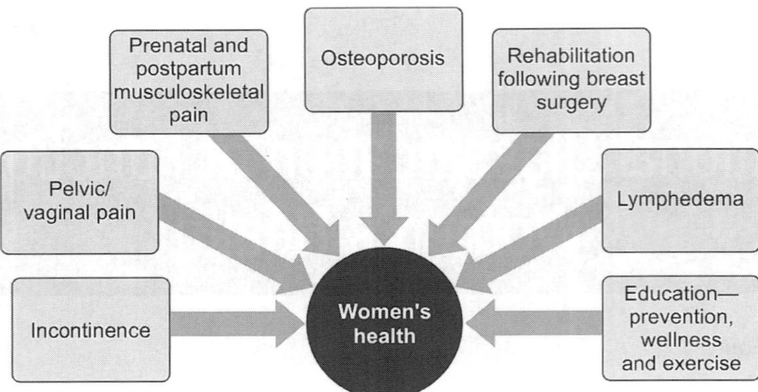

Fig. 7.1: Scope of women's health.

antenatal classes, in the treatment of incontinence, and in the care of women undergoing gynecological surgery. The scope of practice has now increased to include all health concerns of women **(Fig. 7.1)**.

INTERNATIONAL CLASSIFICATION OF FUNCTIONING

The International Classification of Functioning, Disability, and Health (ICF) provides a useful framework for classifying patients' problems and describing them in a standardized language for professionals worldwide. The second part of the ICF covers contextual factors, including environmental, and personal issues. In the ICF, having a problem may mean an impairment, limitation, restriction, or barrier, depending on the component.

The ICF focuses on three components **(Fig. 7.2)**, which underscores the importance of the interplay and influence of both internal and external factors to each individual's health status:

- **Body functions and structures**
- **Activities and participation** (at individual and societal levels)
- **Personal and environmental factors** (at a contextual level).

TERMINOLOGIES USED IN ICF

Box 7.1 describes some of the terms related to ICF.

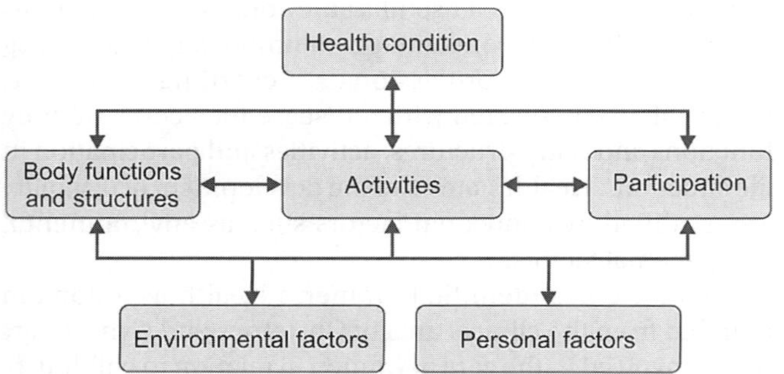

Fig. 7.2: Components of ICF.

Box 7.1: Terms related to ICF.

- **Body functions:** The physiological functions of body systems (including psychological functions).
- **Body structures:** Anatomical parts of the body such as organs, limbs and their components.
- **Impairments:** Problems in body function and structure such as significant deviation or loss.
- **Activity:** The execution of a task or action by an individual.
- **Participation:** Involvement in life situation.
- **Activity limitations:** Difficulties an individual may have in executing activities.
- **Participation restrictions:** Problems an individual may experience in involvement in life situations.
- **Environmental factors:** The physical, social, and attitudinal environment, in which people live and conduct their lives.

Body Structure

- Structure of the nervous system
- The eye, ear and related structures
- Structures involved in voice and speech
- Structure of the cardiovascular, immunological and respiratory systems
- Structures related to the digestive, metabolic and endocrine systems
- Structure related to genitourinary and reproductive systems
- Structures related to movement, skin, and related systems.

Body Function

The ICF has a separate chapter for each of the domains:

- Mental functions
- Sensory functions and pain
- Voice and speech functions
- Functions of the cardiovascular, hematological, immunological and respiratory systems
- Functions of the digestive, metabolic, endocrine systems, genitourinary and reproductive functions
- Neuromusculoskeletal and movement-related functions
- Functions of the skin and related structures.

Activities and Participation

- Learning and applying knowledge
- General tasks and demands
- Communication
- Mobility
- Self-care
- Domestic life
- Interpersonal interactions and relationships
- Major life areas—community, social and civic life.

Environmental Factors

- Products and technology
- Natural environment and human-made changes to environment
- Support and relationships
- Attitudes, Services, systems and policies.

Depending on which body part is affected or which system of the body is diseased, the healthcare professional can refer the concerned chapter and can decide the codes and its qualifiers.

For example:

Body structure is denoted as s and the corresponding item in each chapter is given the coding such as, e.g.:

- s720: Structure of shoulder region
- s810: Structures of areas of skin

Similarly, body function is denoted as b, e.g.:

b28010: Pain in head and neck

Activities and participation are denoted as d and classified as, e.g.:

- d230: Carrying out daily routine
- d420: Transferring oneself
- d475: Driving
- d920: Recreation and leisure

Environmental factors are coded as e and classified as e.g:

- e115: Products and technology for personal use in daily living
- e155: Design, construction and building products and technology of buildings for private use
- e355: Health professionals

The Qualifiers

The list of domains in ICF becomes a classification when qualifiers are used. Qualifiers record the presence and severity of a problem in functioning at the body, person and societal levels.

For the classifications of body function and structure, the ***primary qualifier*** indicates the presence of an impairment and, on a five-point scale, the degree of the impairment of function or structure:

- No impairment
- Mild
- Moderate
- Severe
- Complete

In the case of the Activity and Participation list of domains, two important qualifiers are provided. Together, these qualifiers enable the user to code essential information about disability and health. The ***Performance qualifier*** describes what an individual does in his or her *current environment.* Since the current environment always includes the overall societal context, performance can also be understood as "involvement in a life situation" or "the lived experience" of people in their actual context. (The 'current environment' will be understood to include assistive devices or personal assistance, whenever the individual actually uses them to perform actions or tasks.)

Qualifiers are as follows:

1. No problem
2. Mild problem
3. Moderate problem
4. Severe problem
5. Complete problem
6. Not specified
7. Not applicable

The ***Capacity qualifier*** describes an individual's ability to execute a task or an action. This construct indicates the highest probable level of functioning of a person in a given domain at a given moment. When a person has a capacity problem associated with a health condition, therefore, that incapacity is a part of their state of health. To assess the full ability of the individual, one would need to have a "standardized environment" to neutralize the varying impact of different environments on the ability of the individual. In practice, there are many possible environments that we could use for this purpose. That is, a standardized environment might be:

- An actual environment commonly used for capacity assessment in test settings; or
- An assumed environment thought to have a uniform impact; or
- An environment with precisely defined parameters based on extensive scientific research.

Whatever it is in practice, this environment can be called 'uniform' or 'standard' environment. The capacity construct therefore reflects the environmentally-adjusted ability of the individual in a specified domain. The Capacity qualifier assumes a 'naked person' assessment, that is, the person's capacity without personal assistance or the use of assistive devices. For assessment purposes, this environmental adjustment has to be the same for all persons in all countries to allow for international comparisons.

Clinical Pointer

The gap between capacity and performance reflects the difference between the impacts of current and uniform environments, and thus provides a useful guide as to what can be done to the environment of the individual to improve performance.

Contextual Factors

"***Environmental factors***" can be subdivided into:
- *Individual factors* (the features and interactions present in a person's immediate living, working, and socializing environment) and
- *Societal factors* (the formal and informal rules or laws, social structures, and available services and support in the person's living or working environments, community, or society).

Environmental factors greatly influence the extent to which a health condition affects the person's ability to perform activities or to participate in life.

Personal factors constitute the second contextual factor type in the ICF model. These individual background characteristics are not considered to be a part of the health condition of interest. Examples of these characteristics include:
- Sex
- Race
- Age
- Socioeconomic status
- Fitness
- Habits
- Coping styles
- Education
- Comorbidities
- Social background
- Past and current events
- Behavior patterns

These important contextual factors are included in the ICF model because of the potential effects that some or all of them have on various outcomes. For example, socioeconomic status is known to be an important factor in health outcomes, habits related to physical activity influence many aspects of health and functional ability, and depression presents a challenging barrier to participation for many people. **Table 7.1** shows the qualifiers for environmental barriers and facilitators.

APPLICATIONS OF ICF

The ICF can be useful as a clinical tool for:
- Health needs assessment and matching treatments with specific conditions
- As a statistical tool for comparing services
- As a research tool for measuring outcomes, environmental factors, or quality of life.

Despite its potential, the length and time required to use the ICF in the clinical context represent important obstacles, and the development of ICF-based instruments is encouraged.

Table 7.1: The qualifiers for environmental barriers and facilitators.

	Qualifier for environmental barriers		***Qualifier for environmental facilitators***
(-0)	No barrier	(+0)	No facilitator
(-1)	Mild barrier	(+1)	Mild facilitator
(-2)	Moderate barrier	(+2)	Moderate facilitator
(-3)	Severe barrier	(+3)	Substantial facilitator
(-4)	Complete barrier	(+4)	Complete facilitator
(-8)	Barrier, not specified	(+8)	Facilitator, not specified
(-9)	Not applicable	(+9)	Not applicable

ICF CORE SETS

For the ease of application, WHO has developed Core sets for different conditions incorporating the relevant domains and the chapters along with codes. These are called as Core sets. Core sets facilitate a systematic and comprehensive description of functioning which can be utilized in clinical practice as well as for research. The core sets make the ICF more applicable for everyday use. These condition specific core sets include composite information about specific health conditions, condition groups and settings. In clinical practice, ICF core sets, together with ICF qualifiers can be employed to identify the level of impairment in body functions and structures, limitations in activities, restrictions in participation, and the extent of influence environmental factors have on the functioning of a specific patient.

Detailed information on individual ICF core sets is available at www.icf-research-branch.org or www.icf-core-sets.org. ICF core sets for musculoskeletal, neurological, cardiopulmonary conditions and few general conditions are available.

However, there are none related to conditions related to Women's health. Hence there is a lot of scope for research in this aspect of ICF and women's health.

In a recent research study, following components of ICF have been used to understand the issues associated with this population as shown in **Table 7.2**.

Postpartum Period (PNC)

Mothers often have physical complaints such as problems of:
- Functions of sleep and pain sensation
- Urinary or fecal incontinence
- Sexual dysfunction
- Pelvic organ prolapse

These complaints vary according to:
- Biological factors
- The dependence level of the baby for care
- The level of social support received

Moreover, the impairment of pelvic floor muscle function **(Fig. 7.3)** is also widespread and occurs as a result of:
- Reduced tonus
- An overload of pelvic region structures
- Multiparity
- Traumas resulting from childbirth

Women in the immediate postpartum period usually have difficulties regarding their mobility and transfers. Many mothers face difficulties in performing their daily routine and taking care of their health, which can generate stress, frustration, and mental illness. These problems consequently

Table 7.2: Components of ICF associated with women's health.

Personal factors	*Body function*	*Body structure*	*Activities*	*Environmental factors*
i110 Age	b134 Sleep functions	s410 Structure of cardiovascular system	d230 Carrying out daily routine	e115 Products and technology for personal use in daily living
i150 Educational background	b152 Emotional functions	s430 Structure of respiratory system	d450 Walking	e120 Products and technology for personal indoor and outdoor mobility and transportation
i160 Occupational background	b280 Sensation of pain	s610 Structure of urinary system	d570 Looking after one's health	e155 Design, construction, and building products and technology of buildings for private use
i170 Economical background	b415 Blood vessel functions	s620 Structure of pelvic floor	d5700 Ensuring one's physical comfort	e310 Immediate family
i210 Position in the family	b440 Respiration functions	s630 Structure of reproductive system	d640 Doing housework	e315 Extended family
i220 Position in partnership and marriage	b515 Digestive functions	s6302 Breast and nipple	d6600 Assisting others with self-care	e320 Friends
i530 Personal attitudes	b525 Defecation functions	s730 Structure of upper extremity	d760 Family relationships	
i74012 Habits	b620 Urinary functions	s740 Structure of pelvic region	d770 Intimate relationships	
i74015 Lifestyle	b6202 Urinary continence	s750 Structure of lower extremity	d7702 Sexual relationships	e325 Acquaintances, peers, colleagues, neighbors and community members
	b640 Sexual functions		d850 Remunerative employment	e355 Health professionals
	b6603 Lactation	s760 Structure of trunk	d920 Recreation and leisure	e360 Other professionals
	b730 Muscle power functions	s7601 Muscles of trunk	d9205 Socializing	e460 Societal attitudes
	b7305 Power of muscles of the trunk			e540 Transportation services, systems, and policies
	b760 Control of voluntary movement functions			e575 General social support services, systems and policies
	b820 Repair functions of the skin			e580 Health services, systems, and policies
				e590 Labor and employment services, systems and policies

lead to negative changes in performance of activities and participation. According to the current perinatal health promotion model, the attitudes of family members, friends, and health professionals play an essential role as a support network for women and must be considered from a biopsychosocial perspective.

Fall Risk

The ICF allows a comprehensive study of fall risk that includes medical, social and psychological risk factors. As fall risk is multidimensional, the ICF is appropriate to systematically investigate falls in the clinical practice. Further, the ICF has already been embraced across a number

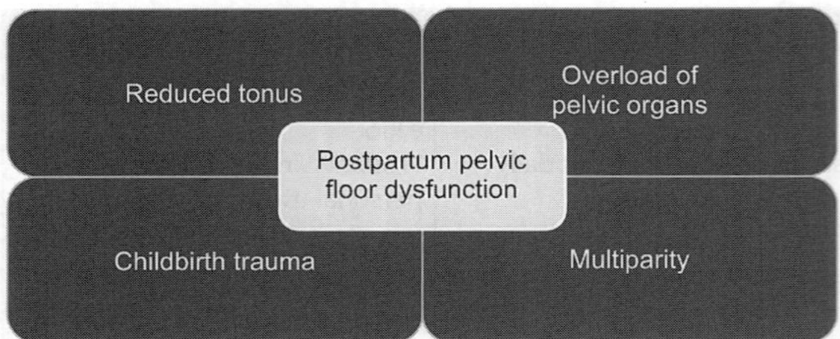

Fig. 7.3: Common causes of pelvic floor dysfunction in postpartum women.

of falls-related disciplines, such as occupational therapy and rehabilitation, but has not been specifically related to fall risk. The interactions between the ICF components are reciprocal. Therefore, the ICF accommodates the dynamic interactions underpinning fall risk, so that any change in one of the ICF components can influence other interactions within the framework. In a study of the ICF and clinical assessment measures in relation to falls following stroke, the ICF was found to match the multidimensional nature of fall risk. However, this relationship was not empirically tested. Furthermore, little evidence exists on how to reliably map the ICF to fall risk, or whether an analysis of fall risk using the ICF components is able to confirm the theoretical assumptions underpinning the ICF.

BREAST CANCER

Due to advances in the treatment of breast cancer, including the combined use of surgical intervention, radiation therapy and chemotherapy, cancer survival rates have increased to 50%. However, breast cancer is associated with a wide range of functional impairments.

- Pain, limited range of motion and lymphedema of the affected arm can result from primary surgical treatment. Untreated lymphedema gradually worsens with time.
- Anxiety, depression, loss of energy or fatigue, and sleeping problems are common responses to stressors.
- A significant proportion of women also suffer from disturbances in body image and self-concept.
- Moreover, social isolation and disruptions in family and sexual relationships are related to fears of recurrence and death.
- Finally, the side-effects of treatment, as well as inactivity secondary to treatment, can impair activity and participation, decrease independence and affect quality of life.

Taking the diversity of consequences of breast cancer into account, a multidisciplinary approach seems appropriate. Rehabilitation after breast cancer requires a multiprofessional team including physicians, psychologists, nurses, social workers and particularly physiotherapists **(Fig. 7.4)**. Physiotherapists are part of the multiprofessional team to prevent and restrict physical sequelae. In order to reach these rehabilitation goals, physiotherapists use different systemic treatment approaches and advise patients regarding

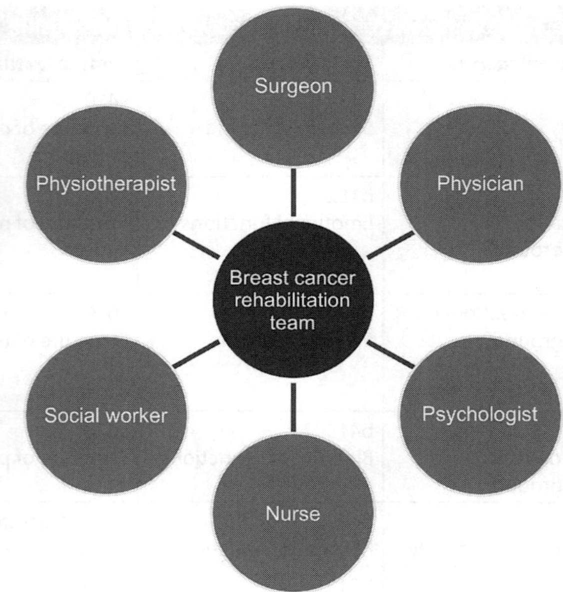

Fig. 7.4: Rehabilitation team for breast cancer.

prevention or how to apply compensation strategies. To optimize interventions aimed at maintaining functioning and minimizing disability, a proper understanding of the patient's functioning and health status is needed.

The International Classification of Functioning, Disability and Health (ICF) Core set for Breast Cancer represents an attempt of the ICF to present the typical gamut of issues commonly seen in the functioning and contextual factors of the affected subjects that may influence the patient's overall functioning. ICF core set is available for Breast Cancer in comprehensive and brief form which includes all the related domains under the categories of ICF. The content validity of these core sets from the perspective of physiotherapists was examined by Andrea Glaessel in 2011. Based on the discussion of the results of this study, a revised version of the ICF Core set for Breast Cancer could be created. Finally, as the Comprehensive ICF Core Set for Breast Cancer defines 'what to measure' but not 'how to measure', future studies could focus on the operationalization of the ICF categories.

URINARY INCONTINENCE

The American Physiotherapy Association defines Urinary Incontinence as involuntary loss of urine. Though this constitutes an impairment of body functions denoted by ICF code b6202 but has far more consequences which can be more efficiently described by ICF. Urinary incontinence may lead to activity limitations like inability to reach toilet in time, frequent urination, etc. In addition, it may also affect the patient's lived experiences thus leading to participation restrictions like avoidance of social activities, travel, etc. The above mentioned impairments and restrictions can be influenced by environmental and personal factors such as access to sanitation, mobility, attitudes, support, etc.

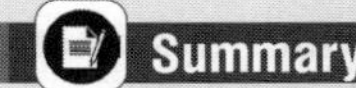

Summary

ICF is an umbrella term describing the effect of a disease on functioning of an individual. For a physiotherapist who is concerned primarily with functional independence, it is important to understand this impact in a greater detail so that remedial measures can be taken to reduce the impact and improve functional recovery. Though the literature related to the use of ICF in different women related conditions is scanty, it can be viewed as an opportunity to develop core sets for these commonly seen conditions and hence the responsibility on the shoulders of physiotherapists is big.

CLINICAL EXAMPLE

A 20-year-old female with 6 months of pregnancy is complaining of back pain in thoracolumbar region and referred for physiotherapy. Pain is localized to back and is more during rest. She is a teacher by occupation and plans to continuing to work till 8th month of pregnancy. On NPRS pain is 5/10 at rest and 3/10 during movements and no abnormal restriction of movements is present.

ICF description will include structural impairments related to pregnancy whereas structural integrity will be in terms of neurological, cardiothoracic system. Movements should be carefully analyzed in terms of quantity and quality. Pain at rest indicates more of muscle fatigue or early spasm. And hence should be carefully noted. All system descriptions should be elaborated and mention that other systems have intact structural integrity.

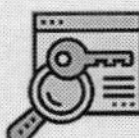

Review Questions

1. What are the components of ICF?
2. What are qualifiers? How are these classifiers applicable in women-related conditions?

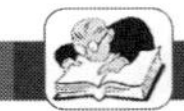

Bibliography

1. Bulhões É, Dantas T, Dantas JH, Souza ÍN, Castaneda L, Dantas DS. Functioning of women in the postpartum period: an International Classification of Functioning, Disability and Health-based consensus of physical therapists. Braz J Phys Ther. 2021;25(4):450-9.
2. Gass S, Kuhn M, Koenig I, Radlinger L, Koehler B. Development of an ICF-based questionnaire for urinary and/or fecal incontinence (ICF-IAF): the female patients' perspective using focus groups (subproject). Neurourol Urodyn. 2019;38(6):1657-62.
3. Glaessel A, Kirchberger I, Stucki G, Cieza A. Does the Comprehensive International Classification of Functioning, Disability and Health (ICF) Core Set for breast cancer capture the problems in functioning treated by physiotherapists in women with breast cancer? Physiotherapy. 2011;97(1):33-46.
4. ICF Case Studies. Bowel and bladder management: evaluation [Internet]. 2022 [cited 2025 Sep 21]. Available from: https://www.icf-casestudies.org/case-studies/bowel-andbladder-management/evaluation
5. ICF Core Sets [Internet]. 2022 [cited 2025 Sep 21]. Available from: https://www.icf-core-sets.org/en/page0.php
6. Ibsen C, Maribo T, Nielsen CV, Hørder M, Schiøttz-Christensen B. ICF-based assessment of functioning in daily clinical practice: a promising direction toward patient-centred care in patients with low back pain. Front Rehabil Sci. 2021;2:732594.
7. Mehraban A, Mackenzie L, Byles J, Gibson R, Curryer C. Can the International Classification of Functioning, Disability and Health (ICF) be used to understand risk factors for falls in older Australian women? Health (Irvine Calif). 2013;5(1):39-48.

Multiple Choice Questions (MCQs)

To test your understanding and recall of key concepts.

1. **What is the primary focus of the International Classification of Functioning (ICF)?**
   A. Diagnosis of disease
   B. Patient's abilities and contextual factors
   C. Clinical imaging techniques
   D. Pharmaceutical interventions
2. **In ICF, which term refers to anatomical parts of the body such as organs and limbs?**
   A. Body functions
   B. Activities
   C. Body structures
   D. Environmental factors
3. **Why are contextual factors important in ICF?**
   A. They put emphasis on the disease pathology
   B. They define the environmental and personal influences on an individual's health
   C. They categorize diseases into different chapters
   D. They identify treatment protocols for specific conditions
4. **What role does the Performance qualifier play in ICF?**
   A. Measures an individual's potential capabilities
   B. Assesses the impact of societal attitudes on participation
   C. Describes what an individual does in their current environment
   D. Evaluates anatomical abnormalities in body structures
5. **A woman with breast cancer reports difficulty lifting her arm after surgery. Which ICF code could best describe this limitation?**
   A. d475: Driving
   B. d450: Walking
   C. d430: Lifting and carrying objects
   D. d530: Toileting

6. How can the gap between capacity and performance qualifiers guide intervention planning?

A. It highlights the need for additional medical imaging
B. It identifies environmental modifications to improve functional performance
C. It suggests the best pharmacological treatment for the condition
D. It determines the severity of anatomical impairments

7. A 20-year-old pregnant woman reports back pain during rest. Which factors should be analyzed using ICF?

A. Structural impairments related to pregnancy
B. Quality and quantity of movement patterns
C. Contextual factors impacting health
D. All of the above

8. While designing an ICF-based assessment plan for a woman with postpartum pelvic floor dysfunction, which of the following should be included?

A. Body function evaluations (e.g., urinary continence)
B. Activity assessments (e.g., self-care)
C. Environmental and personal factors (e.g., family support)
D. All of the above

ANSWERS

1. B	2. C	3. B	4. C
5. C	6. B	7. D	8. D

Section 3

Management Strategies in Women's Health

Section Outline

Chapter 8

Adolescence, Puberty and Menarche

Pothiraj Pitchai, Mayur Revadkar

LEARNING OBJECTIVES

At the end of the chapter, the reader will be able to:

- Define adolescence, puberty and menarche.
- Identify the physiological changes happening during puberty and at menarche.
- Discuss the disorders of puberty and menstruation.
- Describe the physiotherapy management for health issues encountered by adolescent girls at pubertal age.

CHAPTER OUTLINE

INTRODUCTION

'Adolescence' is the transition period between childhood and adulthood. It includes physical, psychological and social changes. 'Puberty' is the term used to describe biological changes which occur as a child develops and becomes capable of reproduction. During puberty in females, one of the most important events is 'Menarche', which means onset of menstruation. This phase of woman's life is predominantly guided by the 'hypothalamic pituitary-ovarian axis'.

ADOLESCENCE

Adolescence is the phase of life between childhood and adulthood, from ages 10 to 19 years. It is a unique stage of human development and an important time for laying the foundations of good health. Adolescents experience rapid physical, cognitive and psychosocial growth. This affects how they feel, think, make decisions, and interact with the world around them.

- For 10–14-year-old the leading risks for health are related to water, hygiene and sanitation.
- Risks for 15–19-year-old are more often related to behaviors, such as alcohol use and unsafe sex.

Poor diet and low physical activity are additional challenges which begin in childhood and adolescence, as does sexual abuse. Older adolescent girls are disproportionately affected by intimate partner violence. Pregnancy complications and unsafe abortions are the leading causes of death among 15–19-year-old girls. Most adolescent mortality and morbidity are preventable or treatable, but adolescents face specific barriers in accessing health information and services.

PUBERTY

Definition

Puberty in girls is the period, which links childhood to adulthood. It is the period of gradual development of secondary sexual characters.

Physiological Changes of Puberty

Breast Budding

- When ovaries start to produce and release estrogen, fat in the connective tissue starts to build up **(Fig. 8.1)**. The duct system also starts to grow, the glands vascularize, and the areolae enlarge and become more pigmented.
- Estradiol and progesterone are the principal stimulators of the mammary glands during adulthood; progesterone alone has little effect. In addition, growth hormone (GH), thyroid hormone, and adrenal glucocorticosteroids have permissive effects.
- The ductal cells alternately proliferate and regress in response to changing levels of estradiol and progesterone during each menstrual cycle, with proliferation being maximal in the late luteal phase after sustained exposure to high levels of progesterone. Breast growth is also referred to as *thelarche.*

Pubic and Axillary Hair Growth

- Pubic hair growth generally occurs after breast development and followed by this, there is axillary hair growth. Approximately six months after thelarche begins, *pubarche*, or growth of pubic hair, typically occurs.
- Pubic hair initially appears light, sparse and straight but will become coarse, thick, and dark throughout the course of puberty.
- Approximately two years after pubarche, axillary hair begins to grow, a secondary sexual characteristic mediated by testosterone.

Growth in Height

- With puberty, there is sudden spurt in height.
- Before puberty, boys and girls grow at similar speeds, but during puberty boys grow more than girls.
- Normal growth is controlled by a number of hormones such as:
    - Growth hormone, made in the pituitary gland, which is the most important factor
    - Thyroid hormone
    - Sex hormones—testosterone or estrogen.

Menstruation

- The onset of menstruation is the hallmark sign of puberty.
- Menarche occurs near the end of Tanner stage IV **(Box 8.1 and Fig. 8.2)** after a year-long rise in daily estradiol output. High estradiol levels at this time exert negative feedback on the gonadotropic axis to suppress it, leading to cyclic estrogen levels and uterine bleeding.
- At the time of menarche, positive estradiol feedback on the axis is not yet established; therefore, ovulation rarely occurs. Uterine bleeding occurs with varying cyclicity until the mechanism of estrogen-induced LH surge is mature and ovulatory cycles occur. This process generally takes a year or more after menarche to become fully established.

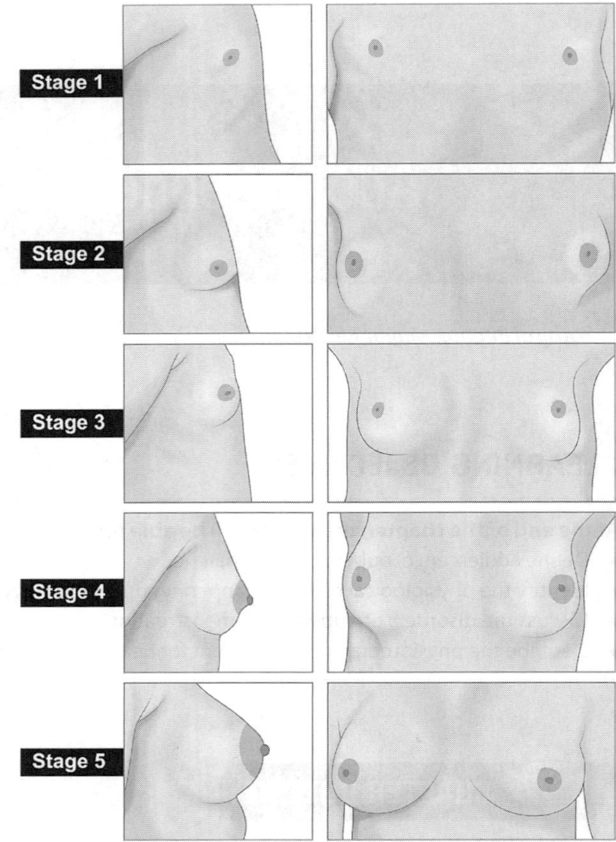

Fig. 8.1: Breast changes during puberty.

Box 8.1: Tanner scale.

The Tanner scale [also known as the Tanner stages or Sexual Maturity Rating (SMR)] is a scale of physical development in children, adolescents and adults. The scale defines physical measurements of development based on external primary and secondary sex characteristics, such as the size of the breasts, genitals, testicular volume and development of pubic hair.

Onset of Puberty

Onset of puberty is usually around 10 to 16 years.

External confounding factors, among others, which can affect the onset of puberty, are:

- **Genetic:** The cause of central precocious puberty (early onset) is often unknown.
- **Nutrition and body weight:** Girls begin puberty at an earlier age as compared to past decades. Overweight or obese children are more likely to enter puberty early. The progression of puberty is affected by nutrition. Severe primary or secondary malnutrition can also delay the onset and progression of puberty. The higher incidence of anorexia nervosa and bulimia in adolescents imposes a nutritional risk on pubertal development.

Staging pubic hair development

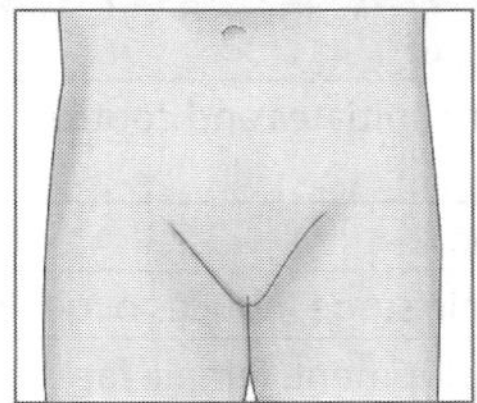

Pubic hair stage 1
Prepubertal. The vellus over the pubis is no further developed than that over the abdominal wall, i.e., no pubic hair

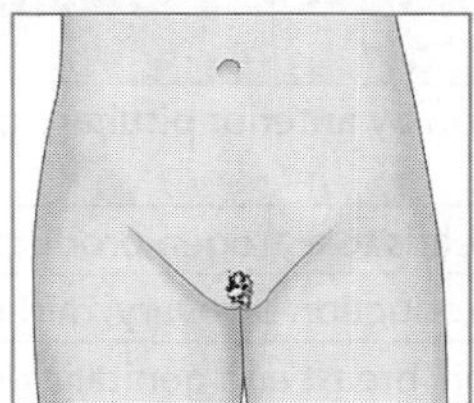

Pubic hair stage 2
Sparse growth of slightly pigmented, longer but still downy hair, straight or only slightly curled, appearing chiefly along the labia

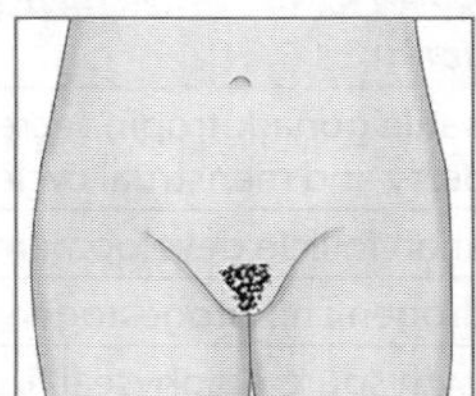

Pubic hair stage 3
The hair is considerably darker, coarser, and more curled. The hair spreads sparsely over the mons

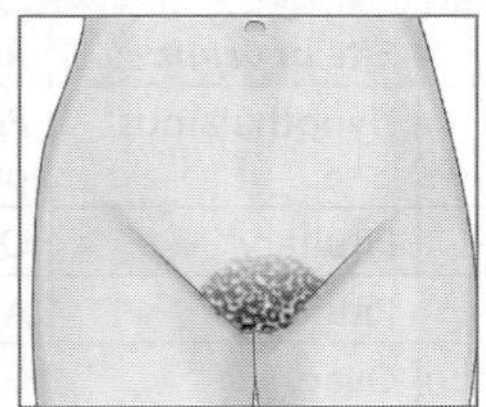

Pubic hair stage 4
The hair now resembles adult type. The area covered is still smaller than that in the adult, but the hair is beginning to spread across the mons. There is no hair spread to the medial thighs

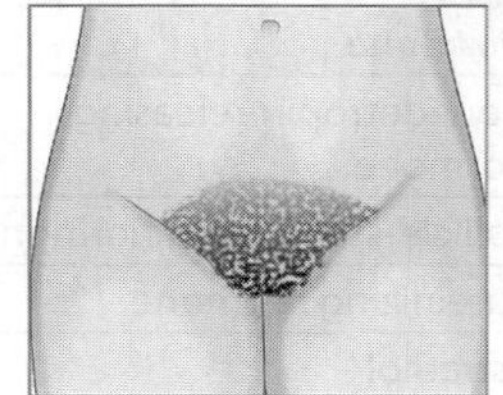

Pubic hair stage 5
The hair is adult in type and quantity, darker, coarse, and curled, and distributed in the classic female triangle. Some individuals may have hair spread to the medial thighs

Staging breast development

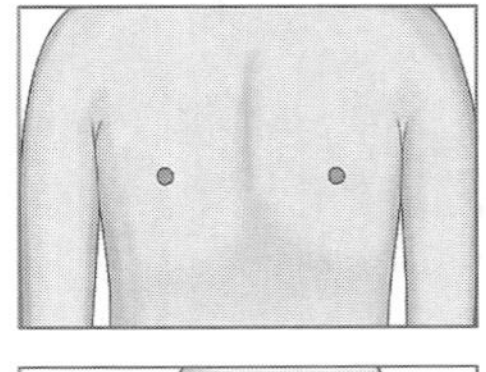
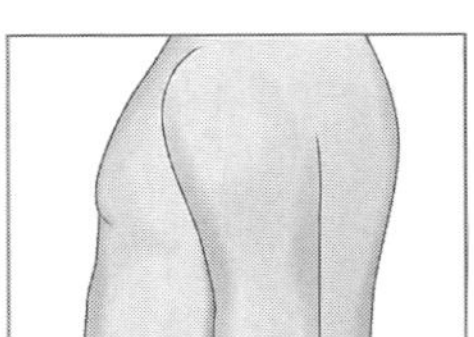

Breast stage 1
There is no development. Only the papilla is elevated

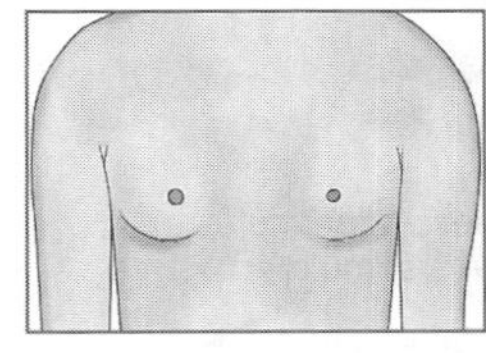
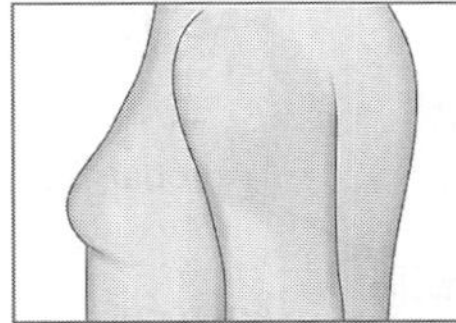

Breast stage 2
The "breast bud" stage. The areola widens, darkens slightly, and elevates from the rest of the breast as a small mound. A bud of breast tissue is palpable below the nipple

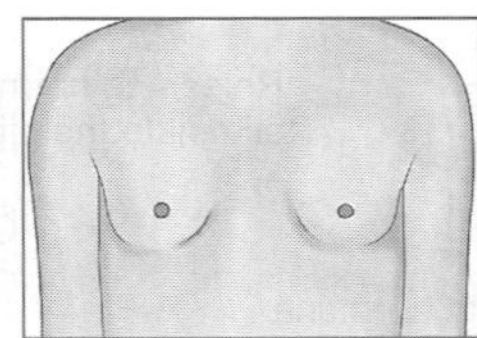
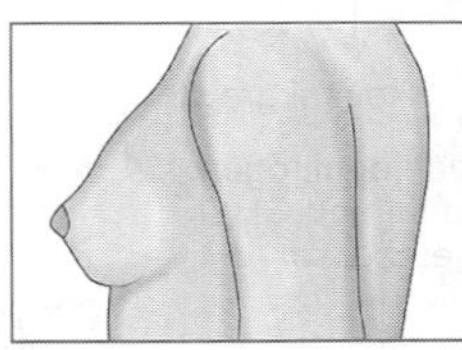

Breast stage 3
The breast and areola further enlarge and present a rounded contour. There is no separation of contour between the nipple and areola and the rest of the breast. The breast tissue creates a small cone

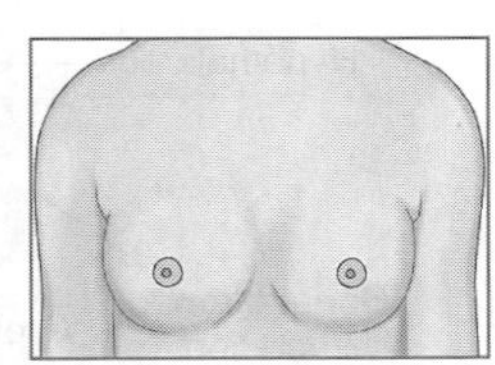
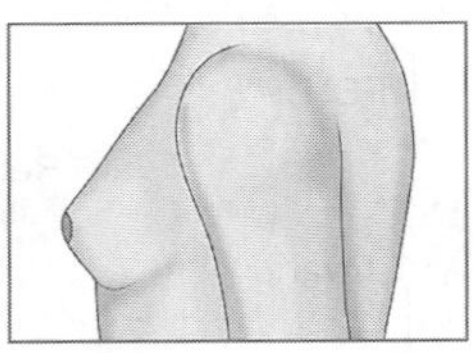

Breast stage 4
The breast continues to expand. The papilla and areola project to form a secondary mound above the rest of the breast tissue

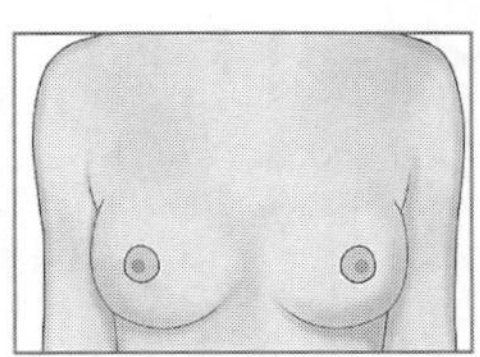
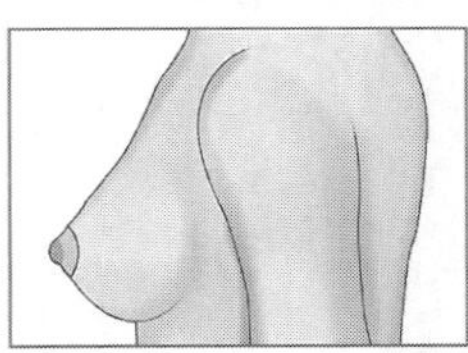

Breast stage 5
The mature adult stage. The secondary mound made by the areola and nipple, present in stage 4, disappears. Only the papilla projects. The diameter of the breast tissue (as opposed to the height) has extended to cover most of the area between the sternum and lateral chest wall

Fig. 8.2: Tanner staging.

- **Psychological state:** Environmental factors have been related to pubertal development. Stress is the environmental factor of interest and has typically been divided into two categories of predictors: physical stressors and psychosocial stressors. Increased physical stressors (e.g., decreased nutritional intake or increased exercise) are more often associated with delayed pubertal timing. Psychosocial stressors (e.g., family conflict or depressed mood) are often associated with accelerated pubertal timing.
- **Social and cultural background:** The influence of parental and peer relationships, as well as the broader culture, shapes many aspects of adolescent development. Adolescents can be easily swayed by their close relationships. Culture is learned and socially shared, and it affects all aspects of an individual's life. Social responsibilities, sexual expression, and belief-system development, for instance, are all likely to vary based on culture.
- **Exposure to light:** Researchers have found exposure to blue light to be associated with decreased levels of melatonin, increased levels of two major reproductive hormones (estradiol and luteinizing hormone), and changes in ovarian tissue that may be indicative of early onset of puberty in females. Studies have found use of blue-light emitting mobile devices to be correlated with disruptions in sleep patterns potentially due at least in part to changes in melatonin levels. Melatonin levels on average tend to be higher right before one enters puberty.

Endocrinology in Puberty

The specific mechanism controlling the time of onset of puberty is complex and is still not understood completely. It is believed, there is activation of 'Hypothalamic-Pituitary-Ovarian Axis' at the time of puberty due to GnRH. Multiple hormones control this orchestra as explained in **Table 8.1** and **Figure 8.3**.

Changes in Genital Organs

- **Ovaries:** Ovaries become more oval and bulkier due to follicular enlargement.
- **Uterine body:** The size of uterus increases rapidly in comparison to cervix.

Table 8.1: Hormones associated with puberty.

Hormone	*Site of origin*	*Action*
Gonadotropin-releasing hormone	Hypothalamus	Pulsatile gonadotropin secretion by anterior pituitary gland initiates and controls puberty and menstrual cycle
Follicle-stimulating hormone	Pituitary	Ovarian follicle development leads to estrogen production
Luteinizing hormone	Pituitary	Androgen and progestogen production by ovary; mid-cycle surge induces ovulation
Estradiol	Ovary	Growth spurt; epiphyseal fusion; breast and genitalia development; female fat distribution; production of proliferative endometrium. Triggers mid-cycle surge of luteinizing hormone
Progesterone	Ovary	Breast development; production of secretory endometrium
Androgens	Adrenal gland and ovary	Pubic, axillary and other body hair growth; muscle mass increase; skin thickening and increased sebum production by sebaceous glands

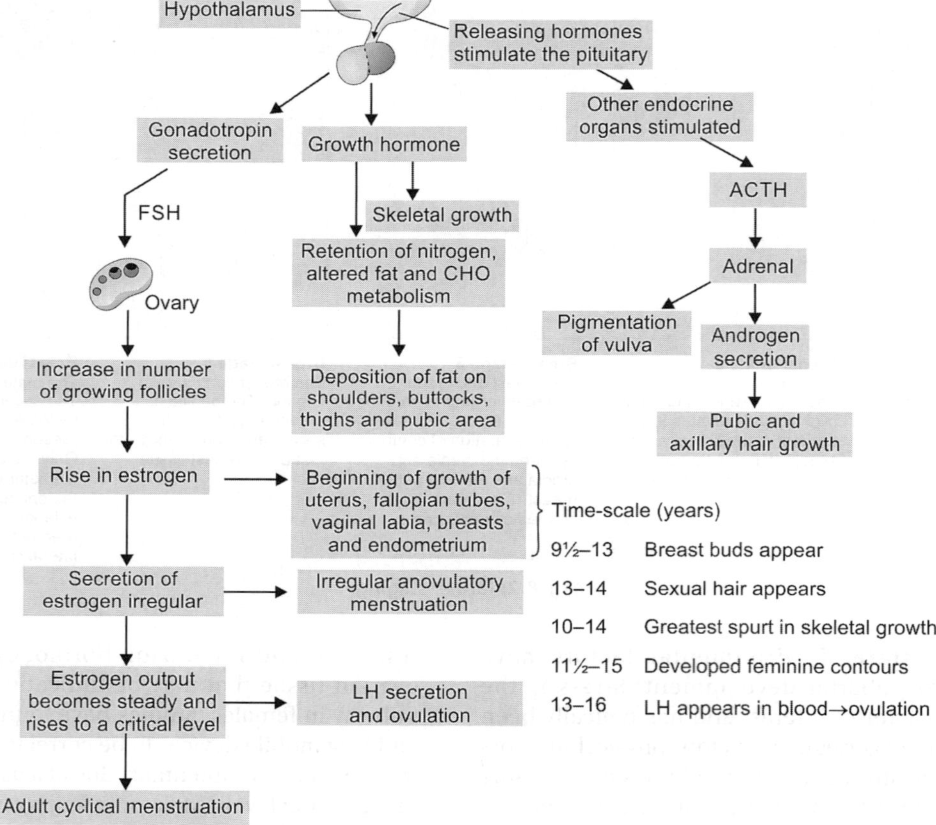

Fig. 8.3: Endocrinology of puberty.

- **Vagina:** Vagina is covered with many layers of stratified epithelium. The vaginal pH becomes more acidic ranging between 4-5.
- **Vulva:** There is increase in size of mon pubis and labia minora.
- **Breast:** There is proliferation of duct systems and deposition of fat in breast tissue.

Common Disorders of Puberty

Precocious Puberty

When signs of puberty are evident before the age of 8 years or menstruation starts before age of 10 years, it is called precocious puberty. It is due to premature activation of the hypothalamic-pituitary-ovarian axis.

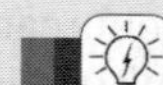

Clinical Pointer

Children who are significantly overweight have a higher risk of developing precocious puberty.

Delayed Puberty

When signs of puberty are not evident by 13–14 years of age or menarche appears as late as 16 years of age.

- Several factors can cause delayed puberty, such as:
  - Chronic illnesses like diabetes, anorexia or bulimia
  - Excessive exercise
  - Trauma to the head
  - Chemotherapy or radiation treatments for cancer
  - Hypothyroidism

Puberty Menorrhagia

- When periods are heavy, irregular or scanty.
- The commonest cause is immaturity of the hypothalamic-pituitary-ovarian axis, leading to inadequate positive feedback and sustained high estrogen levels.
- Many girls suffer from anemia due to excessive blood loss.

MENARCHE

The word Menarche is derived from Ancient Greek, *mēn*-'month', and *arkhē*—'beginning', which means—the first menstrual cycle. Menarche is defined as onset of first menstruation in an adolescent girl's life. It is one of the markers of puberty. It is considered as an important event in adolescent girls as it indicates the possibilities of reproductive capacity. However, among postmenarcheal girls, 80% of the cycles are anovulatory during the first-year postmenarche, 50% and 10% in third year and 6th year respectively. Menarche generally occurs without any warning sign and often it is painless. The onset of menarche varies across the globe. In developing countries like India, it occurs between the ages of 9–16 years with the mean age of 12.52 to 13.76 years.

Determinants

The onset of menarche differs significantly and the determinants are as follows:

- **Genetics:** Mother's age at menarche determines the girl's pubertal maturation and their age at menarche.
- **Ethnicity and race:** Black girls tend to reach puberty and menarche at an early age as compared to white girls.
- **Nutritional factors:** Increased energy-adjusted intake, high intake of animal protein, iron, polyunsaturated fatty acid rich food diet and high calories food increase chances of early menarche.
- **Anthropometric factors:** Increased body mass index, waist circumference and higher subcutaneous fat at prepubertal age influence the early onset of menarche.
- **Physical activity:** Increased physical activity delays the onset of menarche.
- **Environmental factors:** Families with higher socioeconomic status, urban families, higher parental education and small family size, all lead to an early onset of menarche.

Physiology

The so-called "Mini-Puberty" occurs during early fetal life and early infancy, where the hypothalamic GnRH is released and activates the hypothalamic-pituitary-gonadal (HPG) axis for the production of sex hormones. This axis controls puberty and reproduction, and is regulated by complex inhibitory and excitatory neurons. Later in childhood, this axis becomes inactive. However, the onset of puberty, in females, begins only after the reactivation of the hypothalamic gonadotropin-releasing hormone secretory system in hypothalamus and setting of a maturing hypothalamic-pituitary-ovarian (HPO) axis. This axis controls and regulates the gonadal development and function. The function of the HPO axis is shown in **Figure 8.4**.

However, the exact mechanism of reactivation of GnRH. Menarche usually occurs 2 to 3 years after thelarche and 6 months after the peak height velocity during the pubertal growth height. Once the adolescent enters Tanner stage 4, the first menstruation begins. Generally, the HPO axis is immature during the early years after the menarche, therefore menstrual cycles are anovulatory and irregular. The range of menstrual cycles in these years becomes either short cycle, i.e., less than 20 days, or long cycle, i.e., more than 45 days. However, by the end of three years after the menarche, the menstrual cycle becomes typically like an adult cycle with an average range of 21 to 34 days long duration.

Timing

- The menarche that occurs in 11 years or less is called early menarche
- Late menarche is defined as menarche occurring at or later than 15 years of age.
- Anomalies in timing of menarche invite various physical and psychosocial problems in adolescent girls.

Early Menarche

Menarche at an early age can lead to the development of:

- Premature fusion of epiphyseal growth plates leading to shorter stature
- Increased cardiovascular risk
- Obesity
- Metabolic syndrome
- Type II diabetes
- High-risk of developing breast cancer

Numerous studies across the globe also identified that early menarche is highly associated with early pregnancy, sexual intercourse, sexually transmitted disease, anxiety and depression. The causes for early menarche are as follows:

- Stressful family environment
- Families of high socioeconomic status
- Consumption of more animal protein
- Consumption of less vegetable protein
- Overweight or obese BMI
- Formula feeding during early infancy

Late Menarche

The adolescent girl who has not reached their menarche by the age of 15 or three years after the onset of thelarche is called one with late menarche. Delayed menarche has been reported to lead to osteoporosis as well as increased risk for Alzheimer's. The causes for late menarche are as follows:

- Low body mass index
- Eating disorder: Anorexia nervosa

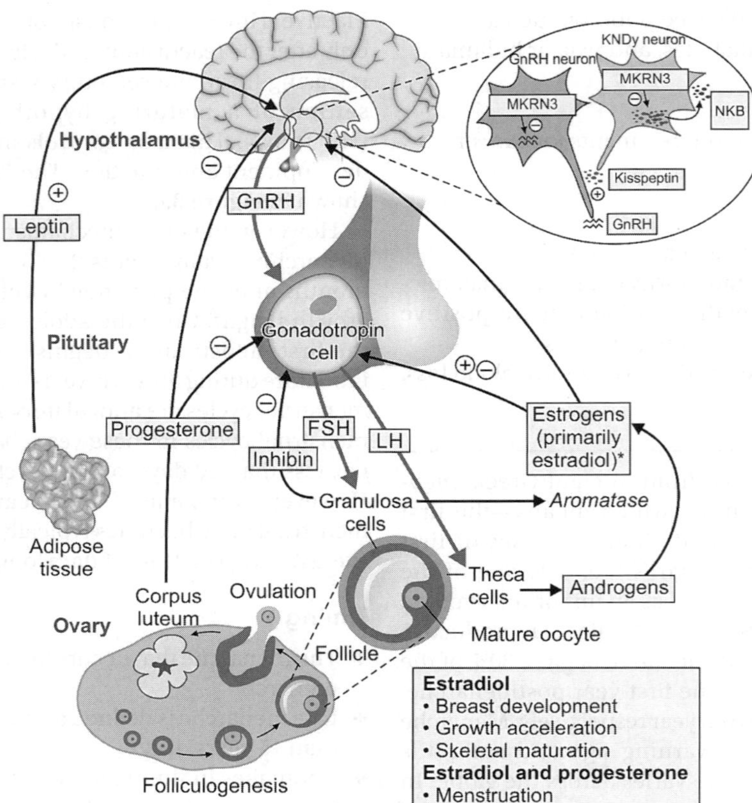

Fig. 8.4: Hypothalamic-pituitary-ovarian axis.

- Intense exercise (athletes) for more than 3 hours per day
- Abnormalities of female genitourinary tract

MENSTRUAL CYCLE

Menstrual cycle or menstruation **(Box 8.2)** is a series of changes that take place in childbearing phase, between menarche and menopause. It includes regular cyclic changes that take place every 28 days. The normal menstrual cycle in adolescent girls is shown in **Table 8.2**. It is regulated by the hypothalamic-pituitary-ovarian (HPO) axis where there is a constant interaction between, hypothalamus, pituitary, ovaries, uterine lining and cyclic production of gonadotropic and steroid hormones. Menstrual cycle leads to vaginal bleeding due to shedding of uterine mucosa. Menstrual cycle is considered as periodic preparation for pregnancy and therefore, it is an important factor which not only influences the reproductive health, but also the overall well-being in woman's life.

Box 8.2: Menstruation.

Menstruation is the visible manifestation of cyclic physiologic uterine bleeding that occurs due to shedding of the endometrium resulting from invisible physiologic interplay of hormones mainly through the hypothalamo-pituitary-ovarian axis.

Table 8.2: Normal menstrual cycles in adolescent girls.

Menarche (mean age)	13 ± 1.1 years
Menstrual cycle duration	21–35 days
Menstrual flow duration	5–6 days
Menstrual product use	Three to six pads per day

Cycle and Phases of Menstrual Cycle

The menstrual cycle consists of:

- **Ovarian cycle:** The ovarian cycle describes the changes that take place in ovarian follicles. It constitutes of the development and maturation of a follicle, ovulation and formation of corpus luteum and its degeneration. All these events occur within 4 weeks.
- **Uterine cycle:** The uterine cycle describes the changes that occur in endometrial lining of the uterus. This lining consists of basal layer and superficial functional layer. The superficial functional layer, is under the influence of fluctuating cyclic ovarian hormones such as estrogen and progesterone, and is shed during menstruation.

These cycles can be further divided into phases as shown in **Table 8.3**.

In menstruation cycle, the ovarian and uterine events take place simultaneously. When the follicular phase begins in the ovaries, the uterus undergoes proliferative phase concurrently whereas, the luteal phase in ovaries corresponds to the secretory phase in uterus.

Table 8.3: Phases of menstrual cycle.

Ovarian cycle	• Follicular phase • Ovulation • Luteal phase
Uterine cycle	• Proliferative phase • Secretory phase • Menstruation

Mechanism of Menstruation

The span of the menstrual cycle is between the first day of menstrual bleeding of one cycle to the first day of menstrual bleeding of the next cycle.

- It is regulated by the hormones that are secreted by negative feedback and positive feedback mechanism through hypothalamo-pituitary-ovarian axis.
- After the onset of puberty, the hypothalamus secretes GnRH in a pulsatile manner. This in turn stimulates the anterior lobe of the pituitary gland to secrete FSH and LH, which target the ovaries **(Fig. 8.5)**.

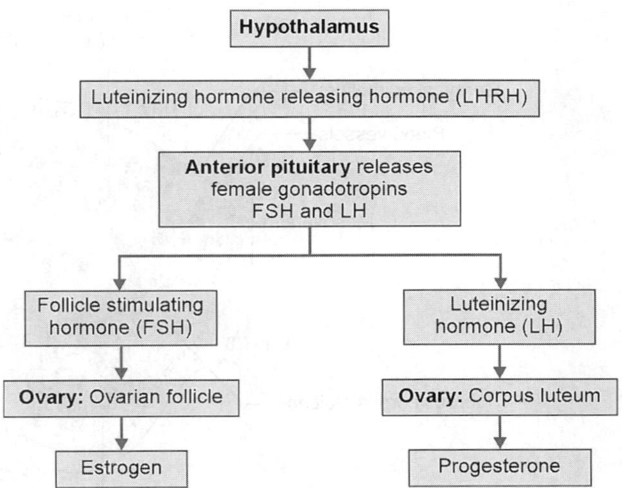

Fig. 8.5: Hypothalamus and its role in menstruation.

Follicular Phase

- The follicular phase of the menstrual cycle begins from day 5 and extends up to day 14 of cycle, till the ovulation, for the average 28 days duration of the menstrual cycle. During this phase, the primordial follicle goes through the developmental and growth changes to become a matured follicle **(Fig. 8.6)**.
- In ovary, the primordial follicle consists of immature ovum and is surrounded by an incomplete granulosa cell. Under the influence of FSH, the primordial follicle undergoes many changes and eventually becomes a primary follicle. During this stage, the ovum is completely surrounded by granulosa cell, the size of the ovum and follicle gradually increase.
- About 6 to 8 primary follicles further undergo developmental changes, but only the dominant follicle becomes vesicular follicle. The granulosa cell is now covered by theca cell/follicular sheet and finally develops into a matured follicle, called Graafian follicle, by 14th day of cycle **(Fig. 8.7)**.

The FSH acts on the granulosa cells and produces estrogen. Estrogen has three functions:

1. To provide negative feedback to FSH to reduce the production of FSH, thereby leading to atresia of the non-dominant follicles
2. Transportation of estrogen to the uterus brings about proliferatory changes in uterine endometrium
3. To provide positive feedback to FSH for the release of LH and this event is called LH surge.

The release of the LH too has three functions:

1. It acts on the granulosa cells and produces a small quantity of progesterone before the ovulation. This progesterone provides positive feedback for the release of FSH and LH, called FSH surge and LH surge, respectively.
2. LH acts on the theca interna cells and produces androgens. These androgens get converted as estrogen at the granulosa cell by the enzyme called aromatase.

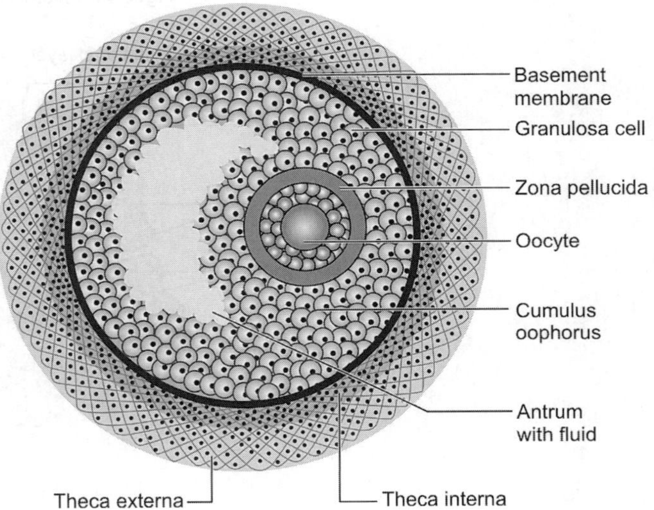

Fig. 8.6: Mature follicle.

3. LH acts on the matured follicle called Graafian follicle where the primary oocyte is converted into secondary oocyte. It ruptures the Graafian follicle, releases the secondary oocyte and results in ovulation, marking the end of proliferative phase.

Proliferative Phase

- Along with changes in the ovarian follicle, the endometrial layer of the uterus also undergoes changes which extend from day 5 or 6 to till ovulation (day 14). This phase is called as proliferative phase.
- As the ovarian estrogen concentration increases, it helps to regenerate the surface of the endometrium followed by increase in the growth and thickness of the endometrial layer including the stroma cell, gland, epithelium and the spiral arteries **(Fig. 8.8)**.
- Additionally, the estrogen also brings about changes in the cervix. The channel in the cervix produces a watery

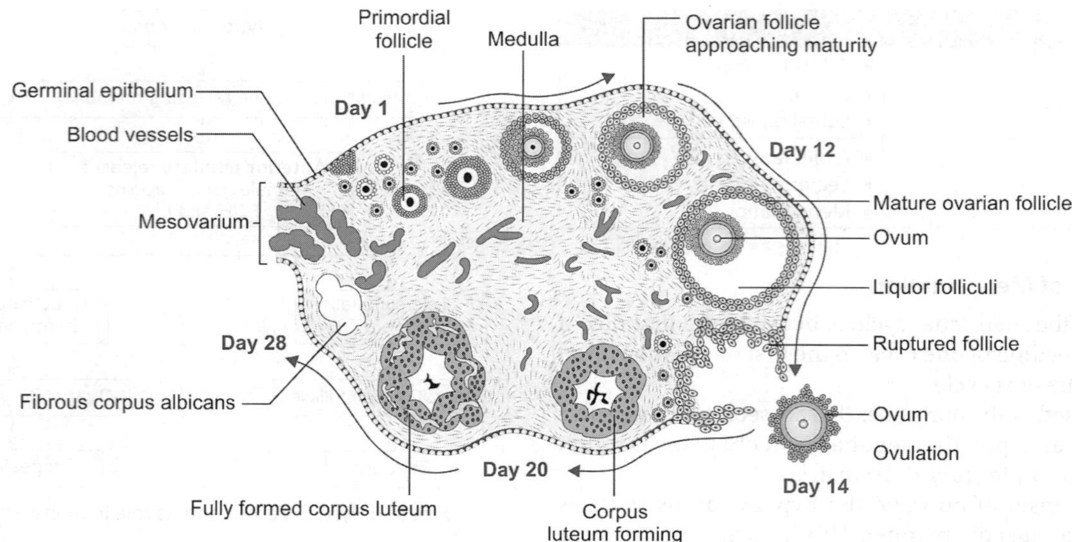

Fig. 8.7: Development of ovarian follicle.

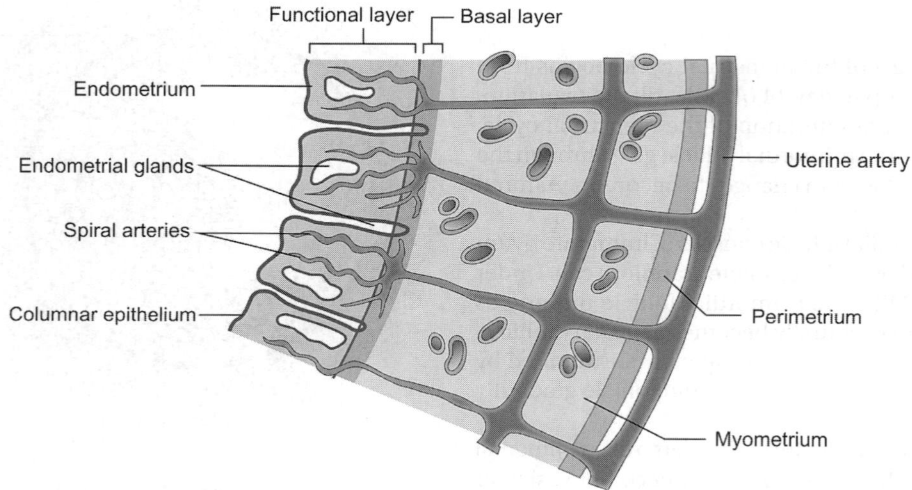

Fig. 8.8: Layers of uterine wall.

mucoid discharge to make the vagina less acidic and create a healthy environment for the incoming sperm. Around this phase, the primordial ovarian follicle begins to mature into a Graafian follicle.

Luteal Phase

- Luteal phase occurs in the second phase of menstrual cycle that extends between day 15 to day 28 of menstrual cycle.
- After ovulation, the ruptured Graafian follicle develops into corpus luteum and therefore it is called luteal phase.
- Corpus luteum is a granular yellow body. Under the influence of LH, the corpus luteum produces progesterone, estrogen and inhibin. The granulosa cell of the corpus luteum secretes large quantity of progesterone and theca cells produce small amount of estrogen. Thus, it acts as a temporary endocrine gland.
- The small amount of estrogen causes further proliferation of the endometrium for more thickness of the endometrial layer. Whereas, progesterone is transported to the uterus and it causes further enlargement of the stroma, further growth of the glands and brings about secretory changes in the uterine endometrium.
- If the ovum is fertilized, the size of the corpus luteum increases and it becomes active until the development of placenta which is capable enough to produce these hormones and then it degenerates. Thus, it helps to maintain pregnancy.
- If the ovum is not fertilized, the increased level of progesterone postovulation, gives rise to negative feedback for FSH and LH release. Reduction of LH causes degeneration of corpus luteum.

Secretory Phase

- During this phase, along with corpus luteum, the uterus also prepares for the possible fertilized ovum implantation. Under the influence of progesterone, the blood supply to the endometrium increases, the secretory gland produces more watery mucus in endometrium, uterine tube and in the cervix for assisting incoming spermatozoa.

- The secreted amount of progesterone reaches its maximum production on day 8 of the menstrual cycle. This increased level of progesterone, post ovulation, gives rise to negative feedback for FSH and LH release. Low level of FSH prevents development and growth of follicles from the current cycle. Due to decreased level of LH, the corpus luteum undergoes degeneration and the production of progesterone is reduced.
- In the absence of progesterone, the secretory function of the endometrium cannot survive; this brings about shedding of uterine endometrium. However, the expulsion of the uterine endometrium is carried out by strong uterine contraction due to prostaglandin F2α hormone.
- Contrary to the cervical mucus changes seen during the proliferative phase and ovulation, progesterone decreases and thickens the cervical mucus making it non-elastic since the fertilization period is passed, and sperm entry is no longer a priority.
- At the end of the second half of the menstrual cycle, when the production of the progesterone is reduced, the FSH is triggered. Which in turn, stimulates the development and growth of ovarian follicle for the next cycle, concurrently proliferative phase in the uterus.
- If pregnancy occurs, a fertilized ovum is implanted within the endometrium, and the corpus luteum will persist and maintain the hormone levels. However, if no fertilized ovum is implanted, then the corpus luteum regresses, and the serum levels of 17-beta-estradiol and progesterone decrease rapidly.

Box 8.3 enlists some of the abnormalities related to menstruation. Few menstrual disorders have been described in Chapter 12: Gynecological Conditions: Clinical and Physiotherapy—Part I.

Box 8.3: Abnormalities related to menstruation.

- Amenorrhea: Absence of menstruation
- Hypomenorrhea: Decreased menstrual bleeding
- Menorrhagia: Excessive menstrual bleeding
- Oligomenorrhea: Decreased frequency of menstrual bleeding
- Polymenorrhea: Increased frequency of menstruation
- Dysmenorrhea: Menstruation with pain
- Metrorrhagia: Uterine bleeding in between menstruations

ROLE OF PHYSIOTHERAPY DURING ADOLESCENCE

Health Promotion

Health promotion comprises all the means utilized for strengthening and developing health reserve in order to keep the scales weighed on the side of good health. The World Health Organization (WHO) recommends for children and adolescents to accumulate at least 60 minutes of moderate to vigorous-intensity physical activity daily, which should include strengthening activities 3 times per week. All children and young people should minimize the amount of time spent being sedentary. Sleep is increasingly recognized as a component of good health. Children who do not get enough sleep are at increased risk for obesity, type 2 diabetes, attention and behavior problems, poor mental health, and injuries. Children aged 6 to 12 years need 9–12 hours of sleep a night. Teens aged 13 to 18 years need 8–10 hours of sleep a night.

Increasingly unhealthy diets, inactive lifestyles, mental ill-health, alcohol and tobacco use, and environmental risks such as air pollution are some of the most prominent issues facing adolescents today. Adolescent health should therefore become a lawful and clear concern of different contributing parties in this field, including parents, teachers, health professionals, counselors, the media and other community organizations.

Dysmenorrhea

Dysmenorrhea is a menstrual disorder defined by the presence of painful cramps of uterine origin that occur during menstruation. It is one of the most common causes of pelvic pain and short-term absenteeism from school or work, among young and adult women.

Based on its pathophysiology, dysmenorrhea is classified into two types:

1. **Primary dysmenorrhea (PD):** It is menstrual pain associated with normal ovulatory cycles, without pelvic pathology, and a clear physiological etiology. It is most common in adolescents and young adults.
2. **Secondary dysmenorrhea:** It is menstrual pain associated with an identifiable disease (endometriosis, fibroids, adenomyosis, pelvic adhesions, polyps in the endometrium, pelvic inflammatory disease) or use of an intrauterine contraceptive device.

Medical Management

Nonsteroidal anti-inflammatory drugs (NSAIDs) along with oral contraceptives help to relieve symptoms of primary dysmenorrhea by decreasing the excessive levels of prostaglandins present during menstruation.

Physiotherapy Management

- **Transcutaneous electrical nerve stimulation (TENS):** The application parameters for TENS can be: high frequency, in continuous mode, at 100 Hz and 200 μs, with a strong but comfortable intensity according to the sensations of each individual, for 30 min, in the lower abdomen.
- **Heating modalities:** Simple heating modalities like hot pack can be of help to reduce the pain. The proposed mechanism behind heat therapy is through the reduction of muscle tension and the promotion of abdominal muscle relaxation.

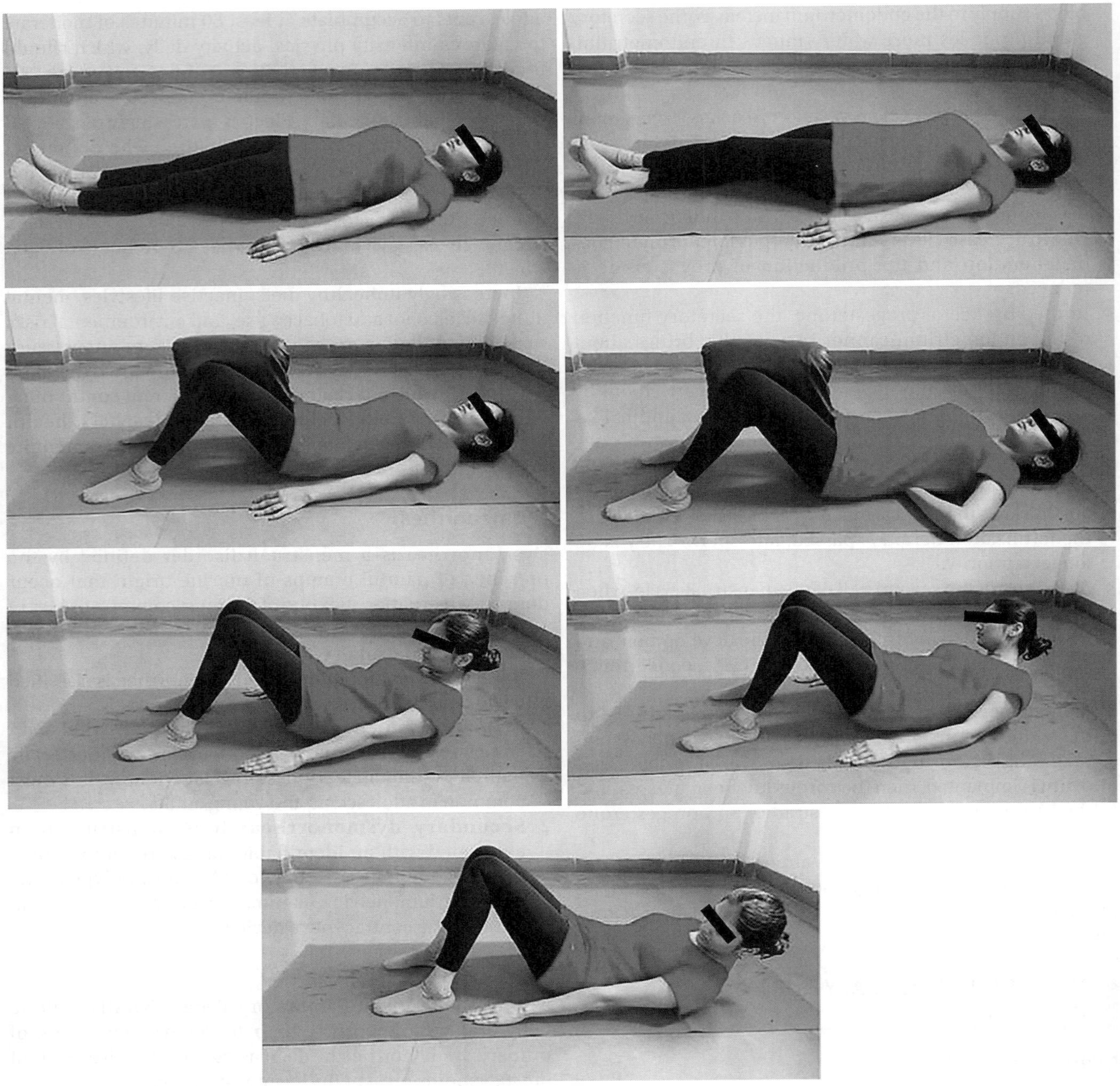

Fig. 8.9: General mobility and isometric exercises.

- **Exercises:** Regular practice of aerobic exercises, Suryanamaskar **(Fig. 34.1)**, Yogasanas **(Fig. 34.2)** and general stretching and mobility exercises as shown in **Figures 8.9 and 8.10**, have been found to be beneficial in reducing the symptoms of primary dysmenorrhea. Kegel exercises specifically may help to increase local blood supply to the uterus, allowing for the rapid elimination of prostaglandins and a decreased intensity of menstrual pain.

Obesity

This is covered in Chapter 30: Obesity in Women of the book.

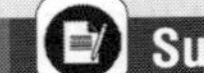

Summary

Every girl passes through the pubertal changes in her life, impacting her physical, mental and social health. The age at which puberty is achieved has lot of impact on overall health; early puberty or late puberty both can lead to associated health issues. Promoting healthy lifestyle at early age is one of the key factors to regularize pubertal age and should be kept at focus by all concerned stakeholders and policymakers. Adolescence is the right time to inculcate healthy habits.

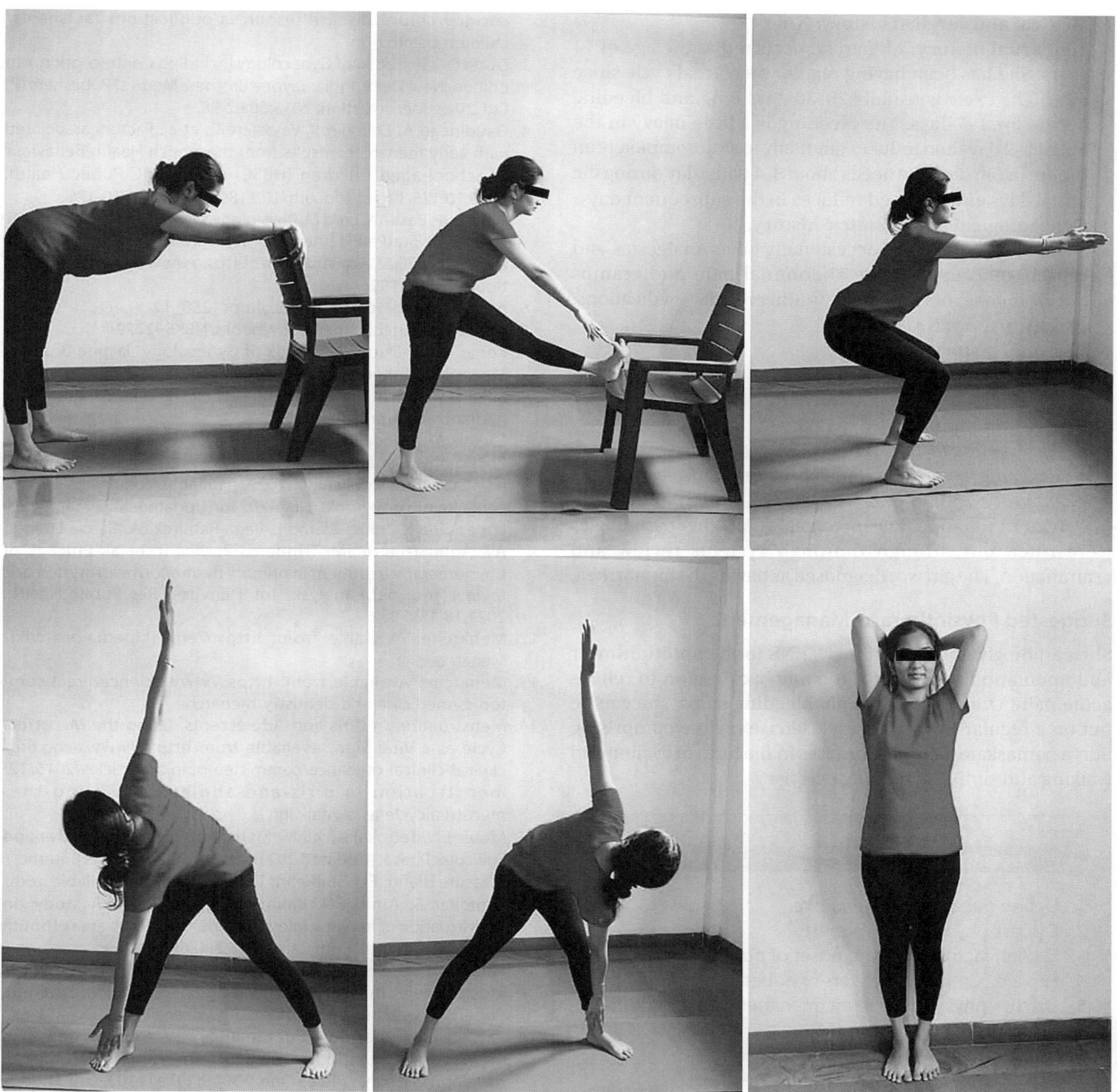

Fig. 8.10: Stretching exercises.

CLINICAL EXAMPLE

A 19-year-old girl comes to a physiotherapy clinic with complaints of severe abdominal pain and back pain during menstruation since 2 years with onset of symptoms at the age of 17, 4 years after menarche. Severe menstrual cramping and pain began a few months ago; the pain is so severe that she reported several instances of absence from college. Painful cramping starts 5–7 days before menses begin, with the worst pain experienced on the first day of flow; the pain disappears completely by the third day of flow.

She is gravida 0.

She had been treated conservatively by her primary care physician with nonsteroidal anti-inflammatory drugs (NSAIDs) for her dysmenorrhea with temporary relief.

Physiotherapy Assessment

- **History of presenting illness:** The girl complains of pain in the lower pelvic area during initial days of her menstrual cycle. The pain wears off gradually on its own. She has no such complaint between her menstrual bleeding.

- **Medical and surgical history:** NAD
- **Menstrual history:** Menarche occurred at the age of 14 years. She has been having regular menstrual cycle since then. The cycle is usually 28–30 days long and bleeding occurs for 4–5 days. The bleeding is a little heavy in the initial 2–3 days and reduces gradually to stop completely on the 4th or 5th day. She needs about 3–4 pads/day during the initial days and the need reduces in the subsequent days.
- **Gynecological and obstetric history:** NAD
- **Drug history:** The girl occasionally takes analgesics and muscle relaxants for the abdominal pain and cramps during menses but is not on any other regular medications.
- **Family history:** NAD
- **Personal history:** NAD
- **Pain examination:**
  - *Site:* Pelvic and low back areas
  - *Type:* Cramping type of pain
  - *Aggravating factors:* Activity
  - *Relieving factors:* Rest, analgesics and muscle relaxants
  - *Intensity:* 7/10

Pelvic examination was not required. All other pathologies were ruled out through thorough systems review and examination. The girl was diagnosed as having dysmenorrhea.

Suggested Physiotherapy Management

She can be given conventional TENS to the anterior lower abdomen and hot packs for the low back region to relieve acute pain. Once her menstrual bleeding stops, she can be put on a regular physiotherapy exercise regime comprising Surya namaskara, aerobic exercises in the form of cycling and walking and simple stretching exercises.

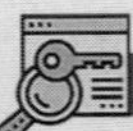

Review Questions

1. Define puberty and menarche.
2. Discuss physiology of puberty.
3. Explain factors affecting onset of puberty.
4. Explain common disorders of puberty.
5. Discuss physiotherapeutic management for common disorders of pubertal age.
6. What are the determinants of menarche?
7. Explain the physiology of menarche.
8. List out the causes for early menarche.
9. Define menstruation.
10. Explain the phases of menstruation.
11. Enumerate abnormal menstruation disorders.

Bibliography

1. Canelón SP, Boland MR. A systematic literature review of factors affecting the timing of menarche: The potential for climate change to impact women's health. Int J Environ Res Public Health. 2020;17(5):1703. https://doi.org/10.3390/ijerph17051703.
2. Centers for Disease Control and Prevention [Internet]. United States. [Cited on 2nd October 2022]. Available from https://www.cdc.gov/chronicdisease/resources/publications/factsheets/children-health.htm
3. Dutta DC. Textbook of Gynecology Including Contraception, 6th edition. New Delhi, India: Jaypee Brothers Medical Publishers (P) Ltd. 2013. Menstruation. 2013;80:82-98.
4. Gaudineau A, Ehlinger V, Vayssiere C, et al. Factors associated with early menarche: results from the French Health Behaviour in School-aged Children (HBSC) study. BMC Public Health. 2010;10:175. https://doi.org/10.1186/1471-2458-10-175
5. Holesh JE, Bass AN, Lord M. Physiology, Ovulation. [Updated 2022 May 8]. In: StatPearls [Internet]. Treasure Island (FL): StatPearls Publishing. 2022. Available from: https://www.ncbi.nlm.nih.gov/books/NBK441996/
6. https://doi.org/10.4103/jfmpc.jfmpc_258_17
7. https://www.ncbi.nlm.nih.gov/books/NBK542229/
8. Konar H. DC Dutta's Textbook of Gynecology. Jaypee Brothers Medical Publishers(P) Ltd: 2016.
9. Kukarni S. Age at menarche and secular trend in Maharashtrian (Indian) girls Amrita Bagga.
10. Lacroix AE, Gondal H, Karlie R. Shumway KR, Langaker MD, et al. Physiology, Menarche. In: StatPearls [Internet]. Treasure Island (FL): StatPearls Publishing. 2022. Available from: https://www.ncbi.nlm.nih.gov/books/NBK470216/[Updated 2022 Mar 17]
11. López-Liria R, Torres-Álamo L, Vega-Ramírez FA, García-Luengo AV, Aguilar-Parra JM, Trigueros-Ramos R, et al. Efficacy of physiotherapy treatment in primary dysmenorrhea: A systematic review and meta-analysis. Int J Environ Res Public Health. 2021;18(15):7832.
12. Menarche. Available from: https://en.wikipedia.org/wiki/Menarche
13. Menarche. Available from: https://www.sciencedirect.com/topics/medicine-and-dentistry/menarche
14. Menstruation in Girls and Adolescents: Using the Menstrual Cycle as a Vital Sign. Available from https://www.acog.org/clinical/clinical-guidance/committee-opinion/articles/2015/12/menstruation-in-girls-and-adolescents-using-the-menstrualcycle-as-a-vital-sign
15. Monis CN, Tetrokalashvili M. Menstrual Cycle Proliferative and Follicular Phase. [Updated 2021 Sep 14]. In: StatPearls [Internet]. Treasure Island (FL): StatPearls Publishing. 2022. Available from:
16. Omidvar S, Amiri FN, Bakhtiari A, Begum K. A study on menstruation of Indian adolescent girls in an urban area of South India. J Family Med Prim Care. 2018;7(4):698-702.
17. Padubidri VG, Shaw S. Textbook of Gynecology, 15th edition. India: Elsevier (A Divisionof Reed Elsevier India Pvt. Limited). Puberty, Paediatric and Adolescent Gynaecology. 2010;4:51-63.
18. Pathak PK, Tripathi N, Subramanian SV. Secular trends in menarcheal age in India—evidence from the Indian human development survey. PLoS One. 2014;9(11):e111027. https://doi.org/10.1371/journal.pone.0111027
19. Reed BG, Carr BR. The Normal Menstrual Cycle and the Control of Ovulation. [Updated 2018 Aug 5]. In: Feingold KR, Anawalt B, Boyce A, et al., (Eds). Endotext [Internet]. South Dartmouth (MA): MDText.com, Inc. 2000. Available from: https://www.ncbi.nlm.nih.gov/books/NBK279054/
20. Rosenbloom A. Physiology of Growth. Annales Nestle. 2007;65:97-108.
21. Ruble DN, Brooks-Gunn J. The experience of menarche. Child Dev. 1982;53(6):1557-66. PMID: 7172781.
22. Sapsford R, Bullock-Saxton J, Markwell S, (Eds). Women's Health: A Textbook for Physiotherapists. WB Saunders; 1998.
23. Sembulingam K. Essentials of Medical Physiology, 6th Edition, India: Jaypee Brothers Medical Publishers (P) Ltd. Menstruation Cycle. 2012;80:482-91.

24. Soliman A, De Sanctis V, Elalaily R. Nutrition and pubertal development. Indian J Endocr Metab. 2014;18:39-47.
25. Sultan C, Gaspari L, Maimoun L, Kalfa N, Paris F. Disorders of puberty. Best Pract Res Clin Obstet Gynaecol. 2018;48:62-89.
26. Thiyagarajan DK, Basit H, Jeanmonod R. Physiology, Menstrual Cycle. In: StatPearls [Internet]. Treasure Island (FL): StatPearls Publishing. 2022. PMID: 29763196.
27. World Health Organization [Internet] [Cited on 2nd October 2022]. Available from https://www.who.int/news-room/factsheets/detail/adolescents-health-risks-and-solutions
28. World Health Organization [Internet] Switzerland [PublisherUnknown] [Date Unknown] Available from: https://www.who.int/health-topics/adolescent-health#tab=tab_1

Multiple Choice Questions (MCQs)

To test your understanding and recall of key concepts.

1. **What is the physiological hallmark of puberty in females?**
   A. Ovulation
   B. Menarche
   C. Pubarche
   D. Thelarche

2. **Which hormone triggers the luteal phase of the menstrual cycle?**
   A. Estrogen
   B. Progesterone
   C. Luteinizing Hormone (LH)
   D. Follicle-Stimulating Hormone (FSH)

3. **What is the importance of the Tanner scale in clinical assessments during puberty?**
   A. It measures body fat percentage.
   B. It identifies chronological age
   C. It evaluates physical maturity stages based on secondary sexual characteristics.
   D. It calculates bone mineral density at menarche

4. **Which of the following is *not* a determinant of menarche?**
   A. Genetics
   B. Anthropometrics
   C. Nutrition
   D. BMI of parents

5. **The primary function of Kisspeptin in puberty is to:**
   A. Suppress the gonadotropin-releasing hormone (GnRH)
   B. Re-instate the gonadotropin-releasing hormone (GnRH)
   C. Inhibit the follicular development
   D. Promote the androgen production

6. **A 14-year-old girl presents with a history of intense athletic training and delayed menarche. What could be the likely cause?**
   A. Hormonal imbalances due to hypothyroidism
   B. Increased physical stress leading to delayed pubertal timing
   C. Precocious puberty from overactivation of hormones
   D. Genetic predisposition to early puberty

7. **Which of the following is *true* for dysmenorrhea?**
   A. Primary dysmenorrhea is associated with identifiable pelvic pathology
   B. Secondary dysmenorrhea is caused by systemic conditions like hypothyroidism
   C. Primary dysmenorrhea is associated with normal ovulatory cycles and no pelvic pathology
   D. Secondary dysmenorrhea is limited to adolescent girls

ANSWERS

1. B	2. C	3. C	4. D
5. B	6. B	7. C	

Chapter 9

Menopause

Priyasingh Rangey

LEARNING OBJECTIVES

At the end of the chapter, the reader will be able to:

- Understand menopause.
- Gain knowledge about the epidemiology and etiology behind menopause.
- Learn about the endocrinology of menopause.
- Know the symptoms of menopause.
- Discuss premature or early menopause.
- Learn the diagnosis and medical management for menopause.
- Conduct physiotherapy assessment and management for women with menopausal concerns.

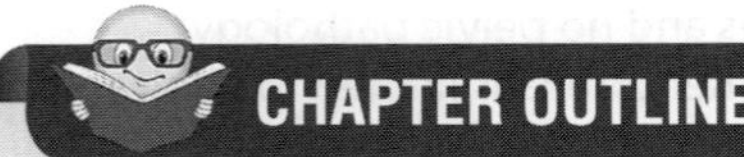

CHAPTER OUTLINE

- Introduction
- Epidemiology
- Etiology
- Endocrinology
  - Normal reproductive function
  - Ovarian aging in women
  - Changes in hypothalamus and pituitary with reproductive aging
  - Integration of hormonal changes with aging in women
  - Stability of hormones after menopause
- Menopausal symptoms
  - Vasomotor symptoms
  - Urogenital symptoms
  - Sleep
  - Psychological symptoms
  - Cognitive symptoms
  - Sexual dysfunction
- Premature or primary ovarian insufficiency
- Complications of menopause/disease risk associated with menopause
- Diagnosis
- Medical management
  - Hormone therapy
  - Selective estrogen receptor modulators (SERMs)
  - Nonhormonal treatment
- Nonpharmacological management
  - Patient education
  - Nonprescription remedies
  - Hypnosis
  - Yoga
  - Lifestyle modifications
- Physiotherapy assessment
- Physiotherapy management
  - American College of Sports Medicine (ACSM) recommendations
  - Physical activity
  - Blood flow restriction
  - Physiotherapy for vaginal health
  - Chinese vaginal geisha balls

INTRODUCTION

Menopause is associated with many changes: change in hormone secretion, reproductive status, appearance, bodily functions, expectations, social circumstances and relationships. It is a normal stage of a woman's life. Most women do not have any major problems and navigate through this phase without much difficulty. Many may welcome it and feel happy about the relief from monthly menses and risk of unwanted pregnancies; which is termed as 'postmenopausal zest'. On the other hand, there might be some who may face a lot of difficulties through this period. The social context on menopause also makes it difficult for such women to come forward and verbalize their problems.

The World Health Organization (WHO) defines menopause as "permanent cessation of menstruation resulting from loss of ovarian follicular activity". The American College of Obstetricians and Gynecologists (ACOG) defines menopause similarly as "time when a female stops having menstrual periods naturally as the ovaries stop making estrogen". "Menopause transition" denotes the period starting from the first irregular or skipped menstrual period to the final menstrual period (FMP). Other terms related to menopause **(Fig. 9.1)** are described in **Box 9.1**.

In 2001, the Stages of Reproductive Aging Workshop (STRAW) divided the adult female life into three phases—reproductive, menopausal transition and postmenopause. These three phases were subdivided into a total of seven stages, which were centered around the FMP **(Table 9.1)**. They were later changed in 2011 by STRAW+10.

Box 9.1: Terminologies related to menopause.

- **Premenopause:** Period of regular or irregular menses before menopause or perimenopause when the female is still capable of reproduction
- **Menopause:** Permanent cessation of menses for a year due to estrogen deficiency and not associated to any pathology
- **Perimenopause or climacteric:** Period from immediately prior to menopause (when endocrinological, biological and clinical features begin) to at least one year after menopause
- **Postmenopause:** Period after the menopause
- **Menopause transition:** Period starting from the first irregular or skipped menstrual period to the final menstrual period
- **Early menopause:** Time span between the onset of spontaneous or iatrogenic menopause before the age of 40 years and the typical accepted age of menopause for that given population
- **Delayed menopause:** Menopause beyond the age of 54 years or 2 standard deviations (SD) above the natural age of menopause for that given population
- **Postmenopausal bleeding:** Uterine bleeding occurring after 12 months of amenorrhea (should be investigated if lasts more than 6 months)

EPIDEMIOLOGY

The average age of menopause varies from one country to another and between different races or ethnic groups. There is also positive association between the age of menarche and the age of natural menopause. The median age of menopause is 51 years in high-income countries, with the range being quite wide 45–55 years.

The average age of menopause is much lower in India, around 46.6 years (JB Prasad, et al., 2021). Menopause is correlated with the following factors in India.

- **Marital status:** Unmarried women (45 ± 6.3 years) undergo menopause earlier compared to married (46.1 ± 4.9 years) or widowed (47.9 ± 4.8 years) women.
- **Education:** More educated women have higher menopausal age (46.1 ± 5.3 years in illiterate compared to 47.2 ± 4.4 years in graduates and higher educated women).
- **Socioeconomic status (SES):** Women belonging to higher SES (48.1 ± 4.2 years) have higher menopausal age compared to those belonging to lower SES (46.1 ± 5.2 years).
- **Body mass index (BMI):** Women with lower BMI have earlier menopause. This could be explained by the fact that BMI is a major determinant of endogenous estrogen levels. Women with higher BMI have higher levels of estradiol and esterone, leading to delayed menopause.
- **Parity:** Multiparous women usually have earlier menopause compared to women with lower parity.

Clinical Pointer

As there has been an increase in life expectancy due to advances in modern technology and healthcare, about one-third of a female's lifespan is spent in an estrogen-deficient stage causing long-term metabolic, cardiopulmonary and musculoskeletal complications.

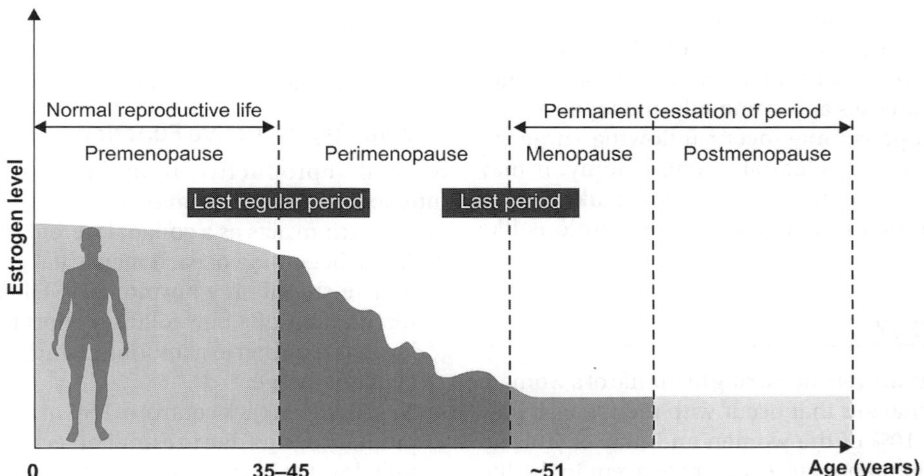

Fig. 9.1: Stages of menopause.

Table 9.1: Stages of adult female life.

Phase	***Stage***		***Characteristics***
Reproductive phase	Stage -5	Early reproductive stage	Variable or regular menstrual cycle
	Stage -4	Peak reproductive stage	Regular menstrual cycle
	Stage -3	Late reproductive stage	*Stage -3b* • Regular menstrual cycles • Normal FSH levels • Low AMH levels • Low antral follicle count
			Stage -3a • Subtle changes in flow or length of cycle • Variable levels of FSH • Low antral follicle count
Menopausal transition	Stage -2	Early menopausal transition	• Variable menstrual cycle length • Increased levels of FSH • Low antral follicle count
	Stage -1	Late menopausal transition	• Amenorrhea of at least 60 days • FSH levels >25 IU/L • Low antral follicle count
	Stage 0	Final menstrual period	
Postmenopause	Stage +1	Early postmenopause period	*Stage +1a* • Marks end of 12 month period of amenorrhea since FMP • Increased levels of FSH • Very low antral follicle count *Stage +1b* • Increased levels of FSH • Very low antral follicle count *Stage +1c* • Stable levels of FSH • Very low antral follicle count
	Stage +2	Late postmenopause period	Remaining lifespan

(FSH: follicle-stimulating hormone; AMH: anti-Müllerian hormone; FMP: final menstrual period; IU/L: international unit/liter)

ETIOLOGY

Menopause can be natural or iatrogenic (i.e., caused by a disease or treatment intervention):

- Natural menopause occurs due to a declining number of ovarian follicles with age. Granulosa cells in the ovary reduce causing a decline in the levels of estradiol and inhibin B. Subsequently levels of follicle-stimulating hormone and luteinizing hormone rise. All these changes lead to irregular menses and eventually, menopause.
- Iatrogenic menopause may occur following surgeries like hysterectomy and bilateral oophorectomy. It may be caused due to treatment of diseases like breast cancer, endometriosis or treatment interventions like chemotherapy.

ENDOCRINOLOGY

Menopause is a natural event occurring in the life of a woman. The physiological changes that occur with menopause may be subtle in about 10% of the women and may exhibit no symptoms. Although menopause is a single event in the life of a woman and is indicated retrospectively by the FMP, the process of reproductive aging is gradual and encompasses the following stages:

1. Initial period, where compensatory changes occur in the hypothalamus, pituitary glands and ovaries to help maintain reproductive competence and gonadal hormone secretion
2. Marked variability in follicle development, secretion from ovaries and subsequent symptoms leading to FMP
3. Low and stable ovarian secretion.

Normal Reproductive Function

Normal reproductive function is a tightly integrated interaction between hypothalamus, pituitary and ovary. The endometrium acts as a gonadal steroid end organ **(Fig. 9.2)**.

- At the beginning of each menstrual cycle, higher levels of follicle-stimulating hormone (FSH) are required for the recruitment of a new follicle cohort and restraint in FSH levels is required to allow only a single follicle to reach pre-ovulatory stage.
- Negative feedback control of FSH at the hypothalamus and pituitary occurs due to estradiol secretion from developing follicles. Ovarian secretion of inhibin B and inhibin A provides selective inhibition of FSH at pituitary.

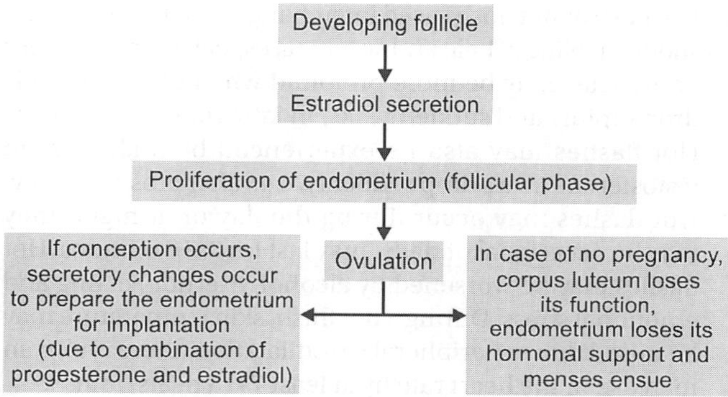

Fig. 9.2: Normal reproductive function.

- Estradiol levels rise in the late follicular phase, resulting in luteinizing hormone (LH) surge required for ovulation to occur. LH surge is dependent on ongoing pulsatile gonadotropin-releasing hormone (GnRH) secretion and increased gonadotropin response to GnRH occurring at the pituitary as a result of increased estradiol secretion from the dominant follicle.
- The progesterone released from corpus luteum inhibits the GnRH pulse frequency. In early and mid luteal phases, FSH synthesis increases in response to slow GnRH pulse frequency, although FSH secretion is inhibited by estradiol and inhibin A. In the late luteal phase, this negative feedback is lost due to the waning corpus luteum and FSH rises preferentially over LH. Negative feedback due to progesterone and estradiol is lost, resulting in increased hypothalamic GnRH secretion. This is essential to attain adequate levels of FSH for follicular recruitment of the next cycle.

Ovarian Aging in Women

- In women, the number of resting follicles is finite and it keeps reducing with age. There is no new production of follicles similar to men, who can produce sperms.
- The finite pool of resting ovarian follicles reaches maximum during intrauterine life. It decreases to one million at the time of birth and still reduces to 250,000 till puberty. The pool still decreases in number during and after puberty when the follicles leave the ovaries for further growth or degeneration.
- During early reproductive life, the number of growing follicles is correlated to the size of resting follicle pool. Between 30–35 years of age, there is an acceleration of follicle loss due to increasing percentage of growing follicles, till the number of follicles reduces to 100–1000, when cessation of reproductive cycles occurs.
- Age-related changes occur in the oocyte quality with the decrease in follicle number, leading to decrease in fertilization and conception and pregnancy loss. Chemotherapy, radiation and smoking damage the oocyte and/or dividing granulosa cells, thereby still accelerating follicle loss.

Changes in Hypothalamus and Pituitary with Reproductive Aging

- During normal reproductive function, ovarian hormones and peptides act at the hypothalamus and pituitary, regulating the secretion of gonadotropins (FSH and LH).
  - At the hypothalamus, progesterone inhibits LH secretion and GnRH pulse frequency. Estradiol influences the quantity of overall GnRH secreted and hence, the amount of GnRH secreted with each pulse.
  - At the pituitary, estradiol reduces the response of gonadotropes to GnRH such that the inhibition is greater for FSH than LH. Inhibin B causes selective inhibition of FSH over LH at the pituitary.
- With ovarian aging, there is a selective increase in FSH levels due to lower levels of inhibin B. With reduction in ovarian function and loss of ovulatory cycles, there is an increase in GnRH pulse frequency. Declining levels of estradiol result in increased levels of GnRH and increased gonadotropin response to GnRH. As a result of alterations in the isoform compositions of FSH and LH due to loss of estradiol, their half-life is prolonged. All these changes cause a 15-fold and 10-fold increase in FSH and LH levels respectively, in the early years after FMP.
- Between 50–75 years of age, FSH and LH levels decrease by 30–40% due to a 22% reduction in GnRH pulse frequency and subsequent reduction in the amount of GnRH. This is initially compensated by a 14% increase in the amount of GnRH secreted with each pulse. There is also a 30% reduction in the FSH and LH responses to GnRH at the pituitary.
- Estrogen negative feedback remains intact in older postmenopausal women and this can be demonstrated by the declining levels of FSH, LH and glycoprotein free alpha-subunit (FAS) and overall amount of GnRH with low-dose estrogen administration.

Integration of Hormonal Changes with Aging in Women

- There is an age-related decrease in the number of follicles as reflected by:
  - Decrease in number of antral follicles seen on ultrasound
  - Reducing levels of anti-Mullerian hormone (AMH)
  - Decreasing levels of inhibin B
- During stages of early ovarian aging, as inhibin B levels reduce, FSH levels rise and drive increased recruitment of follicles into the growing pool, creating increased follicular loss. AMH is responsible for restraining this activity of FSH and also restraining FSH dependent stimulation of aromatase (expressed in the ovaries and responsible for conversion of androgens to estrogens). AMH levels decline in menopause and hence, this restraint is reduced. Increased expression of aromatase is suggested by an increase in the ratio of estrogen to androstenedione in the follicular phase in regularly menstruating women ≥35 years of age and higher aromatase expression in granulosa cells

aspirated from the dominant follicle. Thus, falling AMH and rising FSH levels are responsible for the accelerated depletion of the pool of resting follicles after 35 years of age.

- As age and follicular loss advance, the compensatory changes prove insufficient and cycles become irregular, indicating the onset of menopause transition. In the year preceding FMP, most of the cycles are either anovulatory or have prolonged follicular phases. Asynchronous FSH and ovarian function hampers the preovulatory surge required for ovulation to occur. In addition to this, the pituitary response to GnRH is attenuated, further contributing to abnormal cycle dynamics. All these changes may cause irregular bleeding, hot flushes, breast tenderness, mood changes and sleeping problems.

Stability of Hormones after Menopause

- In the initial 1–2 years after FMP, occasional follicle development may occur.
- Estradiol levels reduce gradually up to estradiol nadir 2 years after FMP. After that, estradiol levels remain low and stable.
- FSH levels remain stable up to 8 years after FMP, then reduce by approximately 30% till the age of 75.
- LH levels also exhibit changes similar to FSH levels.
- All other menopausal symptoms may reduce, but hot flushes may persist. Hypoestrogenism may lead to genitourinary syndrome.

MENOPAUSAL SYMPTOMS

The menopausal transition defines a biopsychosocial phase where majority of the women face physiological changes influenced by a variety of social, cultural, ethnic and psychological factors. Reports of menopausal symptoms by females may be influenced by the following factors:

- Lifestyle—diet, smoking, reproductive history and exercise
- Body mass index
- Socioeconomic status
- Climate
- Mood
- Cognition (including beliefs and attitudes towards menopause, attribution of symptoms to menopause)

The four core symptoms of menopause include vasomotor and vaginal symptoms, insomnia and mood changes. Several other symptoms like sexual dysfunction, urinary incontinence, joint and muscle aches and changes in skin elasticity and body contour have also been reported by women.

Vasomotor Symptoms

- Vasomotor symptoms, vary in frequency, intensity and duration. These are the most bothersome symptoms in menopausal women.
- Almost 85% women report hot flashes during this period. Hot flashes may even be present before menstrual irregularities start and after the phase of menopausal transition.
- Hot flash or hot flush (used interchangeably) is defined as a sudden feeling of heat and sweating, especially in the upper body. They may be more profound when estrogen levels drop rapidly and suddenly, i.e., in iatrogenic menopause. Hot flashes may also be experienced by males, when testosterone levels drop suddenly, e.g., after prostatectomy.
- Hot flashes may occur during the day or at night, they may be occasional or daily, may last for 3–10 minutes. Hot flashes may be worsened by alcohol, exertion, eating and emotional stress. During a hot flush, skin temperature may be raised due to peripheral vasodilatation, there is also an increase in the heart rate by at least 7–15 beats/min.
- The exact pathophysiology behind vasomotor symptoms is not known, but they are hypothesized to occur due to estrogen withdrawal. They are linked with pulsatile pituitary LH secretion as well as decreased concentrations of endorphin in the hypothalamus. They are associated with increased release of norepinephrine, serotonin and other similar neuroregulators that cause upregulation of 5-hydroxytryptamine (serotonin) (5-HT_{2A}) receptor in the hypothalamus. This changes the set point temperature in the hypothalamus, triggering inappropriate heat loss. This results in peripheral vasodilation and excessive sweating.
- Along with hot flashes, women may complain of other vasomotor symptoms like chills, night sweats, anxiety, migraines and palpitations. Migraines without aura are commoner than migraines with aura (they may pose risk of stroke in females who smoke or are on oral contraceptives). Tension or cluster headaches may also occur.
- Vasomotor symptoms may improve with time even in absence of any treatment. Care should be taken to consider certain other conditions that masquerade as hot flushes **(Box 9.2)**.

Urogenital Symptoms

- Approximately 60% of the women experience some or the other form of urogenital symptoms. Urogenital tissues are extremely sensitive to estrogen. The fluctuations in estrogen levels that occur with menopausal transition and postmenopause render these tissues fragile and cause distressing symptoms. These symptoms may include vaginal and/or urethral atrophy and sexual dysfunction **(Box 9.3)**.

Box 9.2: Conditions that can masquerade as hot flushes.

- Epilepsy
- Anxiety disorders
- Infection
- Autoimmune disorders
- Thyroid disease
- Tuberculosis
- New-onset hypertension
- Carcinoid syndromes
- Diabetic autonomic dysfunction/hypoglycemia
- Insulinoma/pancreatic tumors
- Leukemia/lymphoma mast-cell disorders
- Use of selective-reuptake inhibitors or serotonin norepinephrine-reuptake inhibitors

Box 9.3: Genitourinary syndrome of menopause.

Vulvovaginal atrophy seen in menopause is also termed as 'Genitourinary syndrome of menopause' (GSM). It refers to the vulvar, vaginal and lower urinary tract changes that occur due to estrogen deficiency and may affect the health, sexuality and quality of life of the woman. The term 'vulvovaginal atrophy' does not encompass the changes occurring in the lower urinary tract and hence a consensus panel in 2013 with representation from the ACOG recommended the term—GSM.

- Vaginal atrophy can result in pruritus, dryness and dyspareunia. Almost 27–60% women complain of moderate or severe vaginal dryness or dyspareunia associated to menopause. Vaginal symptoms can also include narrowing and shortening of vagina and uterine prolapse in addition to vaginal atrophy.
- Urethral atrophy may result in stress incontinence, urgency, frequency and dysuria.
- Unlike vasomotor symptoms, urogenital symptoms do not improve with time, in absence of any treatment.

Sleep

- Insomnia occurs in 40–50% of the females during menopausal transition and this may or may not be related to mood disorders. However, there is a higher incidence of anxiety, stress, depression and tension in such females.
- It is still unclear whether these sleep problems are related to hormonal changes, age-related changes in sleep architecture or other menopausal symptoms. However, it has been observed that exogenous estrogen leads to improvement in subjective and objective sleep due to a decrease in hot flushes.

 **Clinical Pointer**

A study by Murphy and Campbell proposed that poor sleep quality can be attributed to higher core body temperatures due to elevated LH levels in late menopause.

- Increase in rates of sleep apnea have been observed. The pathophysiology behind this is thought to relate to:
  - Postmenopausal weight gain
  - Decreased levels of progesterone since it stimulates respiration
  - Decline in melatonin and growth hormone levels
- Polysomnography has become a useful tool in assessing sleep complaints. Sleep questionnaires can also be used.

Psychological Symptoms

- Several studies have shown that there is a rise in the likelihood of development of depressive episodes in the perimenopausal period. Also, there is an increased risk of depressed mood during menopausal transition. In some instances, anxiety precludes depression.
- Risk factors for the development of mood disorders in menopausal women include:
  - Poor sleep
  - Higher body mass index
  - Smoking
  - Age
  - Stressful or negative life events
  - Lack of employment
  - Associated vasomotor symptoms
  - Personal or family history of depression or premenstrual dysphoric disorder
- Estrogen has the following effects which may play role in causing depression:
  - Decreases monoamine oxidase (MAO) activity in the central nervous system (CNS), thereby hindering the breakdown of serotonin and norepinephrine
  - Increases synthesis of serotonin, causes upregulation of 5-hydroxytryptamine (5-HT1) receptors, and downregulation of 5-HT2 receptors
  - Increases activity of norepinephrine in the brain, possibly by decreasing reuptake and degradation due to inhibition of MAO and catechol-O-methyltransferase
- Depression is considered to occur due to dysregulation in the monoaminergic pathways in the CNS. Fluctuating estrogen levels seen during menopausal transition can alter these serotonergic and noradrenergic systems.
- Many theories have been proposed to explain depression during menopausal transition:
  - Empty nest syndrome (children become independent and no longer need their parents to help/support them)
  - Loss of fertility
  - Change in childbearing role
  - Societal value of youth (societies valuing age and experience tend to have women reporting less about depression)
- Screening tools can be used to identify women at risk of development of such disorders and they can then be referred to mental health specialists for further evaluation and management.

Cognitive Symptoms

- Perimenopausal and recently postmenopausal females may complain of memory problems. These problems are an outcome of menopausal transition and not normal aging. This can be explained by studies where improvement in memory was observed with administration of hormone replacement therapy. The risk of Alzheimer's also increases with menopause.
- Other cognitive challenges faced include trouble with organizing and planning or concentrating or executive function.
- Collectively, all these cognitive changes are termed as 'mild cognitive impairment' (MCI).
- It is hypothesized that these cognitive symptoms could be due to inadequate sleep resulting from hot flushes occurring at night or as a result of the changes in hormonal milieu that occurs with menopausal transition in parts of the brain related to cognition.

 **Clinical Pointer**

A SWAN study conducted in females aged 42–52 years concluded that repeated testing improved verbal memory and processing speed scores in pre-, peri-, early post- and late postmenopausal women. Hormone use before the final menses was associated with better scores in all groups.

- Evaluation for cognition should include a thorough history (medical, drug, family history), systems review and physical examination. Mini mental state examination (MMSE) can be used for complete objective evaluation of cognitive function.

 **Clinical Pointer**

Cognitive changes like loss of language skills or vocabulary, loss of older memories, impaired reading comprehension, disorientation and inability to perform independent activities of daily living (ADL) should be considered a warning sign and help from healthcare practitioner should be sought.

Sexual Dysfunction

- Sexual dysfunction is common among menopausal women, but it is rarely reported as the women are too reserved to complain about it.
- The etiology of sexual dysfunction in menopause can be multifactorial:
  - Psychological symptoms like anxiety and depression
  - Conflict with partner
  - Medication use
  - Physical problems like vaginitis, etc.
- Careful evaluation of physical, psychological, sociological and lifestyle variables should be done.

PREMATURE OR PRIMARY OVARIAN INSUFFICIENCY

Premature/primary ovarian insufficiency (POI) is the accelerated loss of ovarian function occurring well in advance of the destined timeline. It is characterized by reduction in number of residual ovarian follicles and resultant deficiency of female sex hormones, causing female subfertility and early menopause. Due to lack of awareness about this condition, the diagnosis and hence, the treatment are usually delayed, resulting in development of severe symptoms and long-term health consequences due to estrogen deficiency in females. POI can be spontaneous or iatrogenic due to procedures like bilateral oophorectomy, radiation therapy or chemotherapy. In cases of iatrogenic POI, the ovarian insufficiency is anticipated and hence, can be managed early. However, when POI is spontaneous, it is rarely diagnosed or managed early.

Etiology

Table 9.2 presents the causes of POI.

Clinical Presentation

Box 9.4 presents the clinical features of POI.

Diagnosis

POI should be considered in any healthy, nonpregnant female under the age of 40 presenting with more than 3 consecutive months of amenorrhea or infertility.

- A thorough medical and family history should be taken with particular focus on the chronology of events and personal exposures.
- Physical examination should focus on skin changes like hyperpigmentation or depigmentation which may reflect

Table 9.2: Causes of POI.

Spontaneous	Idiopathic	
	Genetic	Fragile X premutation
		Turner syndrome
		Aromatase deficiency
		Bloom syndrome
		Fanconi anemia
		FSH receptor mutations
		Autoimmune polyglandular syndrome
		Trisomy X
		Ataxia telangiectasia
		17α-hydroxylase deficiency
	Infections	Mumps oophoritis
		Malaria
		Tuberculosis
		Varicella
		Cytomegalovirus
		Shigella
	Autoimmune	
Induced	Bilateral oophorectomy	
	Chemotherapy	
	Radiation therapy	
	Environmental toxins	
	Pelvic vessel embolization	

(FSH: follicle-stimulating hormone)

Box 9.4: Clinical presentation of POI.

- Menstrual abnormalities—primary or secondary amenorrhea
- Subfertility/infertility
- Menopausal symptoms
- Goiter
- Changes in skin pigmentation
- Hair loss/alopecia
- Fatigue
- Anxiety/depression

any underlying autoimmune disorders. Examination of the genital organs may reveal signs of genital atrophy.

- Pathological investigations reveal:
  - Elevated levels of serum FSH> 25 IU/L on 2 separate occasions one month apart
  - Low levels of estradiol (E2) < 50 pg/mL
  - Low or absent levels of anti-Mullerian hormone (AMH)
- Radiological investigations reveal:
  - Imaging reveals small ovarian volumes, thin endometrial echo (<4 mm) and low antral follicle counts (<5)
  - Transvaginal pelvic ultrasonography may confirm signs of ovarian compromise

Complications or Sequelae of POI

Box 9.5 presents the complications of POI.

Management

- Hormone therapy using estrogen alone or a combination of estrogen and progesterone can be advised.
- Cessation of smoking should be advised to prevent bone loss and maintain cardiovascular health.
- Adequate dietary intake of calcium and vitamin D is advised.
- Females should be asked to maintain weight or lose weight if required, exercise regularly, maintain healthy diet and control their blood pressure, cholesterol and glucose levels.

COMPLICATIONS OF MENOPAUSE/DISEASE RISK ASSOCIATED WITH MENOPAUSE

Osteoporosis

Osteoporosis is a common complication of menopause that leads to several musculoskeletal disorders. It has been described in detail in Chapter 10: Osteoporosis.

Cardiovascular Diseases

- Declining levels of estrogen in menopause cause changes in a female's lipid profile as well as vasoconstriction, resulting in increased risk of cardiovascular diseases like coronary artery disease and stroke.
- A difference as high as 2- or 3- folds has been observed in women of the same age with and without menopause.
- Menopausal women, hence, should be advised to maintain their diet and exercise regularly.

Cancer

- Due to declining levels of estrogen, there is an increase in the risk of cancer in postmenopausal women.
- Risk of breast cancer, cervical cancer, endometrial cancer, vulvar cancer and ovarian cancer increase postmenopause.
- Screening tests and annual health check-ups help in early detection.

Box 9.5: Complications of POI.

- Menopausal symptoms
- Poor cardiovascular health
- Poor bone health
- Neurocognitive decline
- Anxiety
- Depression
- Infertility
- Decreased life expectancy

DIAGNOSIS

- Diagnosis of menopause is made clinically, if a healthy woman above 45 years of age presents with amenorrhea or irregular menses and has menopausal symptoms, after ruling out all other possibilities.
- No laboratory tests are routinely required to diagnose menopause; however, they may be required to rule out other pathologies. An elevated serum FSH (greater than 40 mIU/mL) is indicative of ovarian failure. An FSH test should not be used in females taking hormonal medications.
- A dual-energy X-ray absorptiometry (DEXA) scan can be done in postmenopausal females above 65 years of age to screen for osteoporosis.

MEDICAL MANAGEMENT

Management in menopause is focused on disruptive menopausal symptoms and prevention of long-term complications.

Hormone Therapy

- Hormone therapy has varied roles in menopause. It can:
  - Manage vasomotor symptoms
  - Prevent urogenital atrophy
  - Preserve a good lipoprotein profile
  - Prevent bone loss
- Hormone therapy can be given in various forms like creams, tablets or patches and can be continuous or cyclic. Hormone therapy can consist of systemic estrogen, estrogen-progestin, progestin alone, estrogen-bazedoxifene or combined oral contraceptives.
- Estrogen therapy is quite useful in relieving majority of the vasomotor symptoms, improving sleep and quality of life and reducing irritability. Common adverse effects of estrogen include breast tenderness, uterine bleeding and bloating. **Box 9.6** enlists the indications and contraindications of systemic estrogen therapy.
- A combination estrogen-progestin therapy in cyclic doses is recommended in women with an intact uterus, as there is a risk of developing uterine cancer or uterine hyperplasia if such women are administered unopposed estrogen. A combination treatment improves vasomotor, urogenital and sleep symptoms and prevents osteoporosis and associated fractures.
- Hormone therapy, whenever used, should be only for a short period of time and in low doses, as it has been associated with an increase in the risk of breast cancer, ovarian cancer, stroke, thromboembolism and coronary artery disease.

Box 9.6: Indications and contraindications of systemic estrogen therapy.

Indications:

Moderate to severe vasomotor symptoms

Absolute contraindications:

- History of deep vein thrombosis or pulmonary embolism
- Unexplained vaginal bleeding
- Known history of clotting disorder or thrombophilia
- History of breast, ovarian or endometrial cancer or other estrogen dependent neoplasia
- Untreated hypertension
- Known hypersensitivity to hormone therapy

Relative contraindications:

- High triglycerides (>400 mg/dL)
- Gallbladder disease
- Elevated risk of breast cancer

Clinical Pointer

A meta-analysis published in The Lancet in 2019 concluded that if hormone therapy is started at age of 50 years and continued for 5 years, it increases the incidence of development of breast cancer at age 50–69 years by approximately 1 in every 50 consumers of combination of estrogen and daily progestogen preparations; 1 in every 70 consumers of combination of estrogen and intermittent progestogen and 1 in every 200 consumers of estrogen-only preparations.

- Hormone therapy is contraindicated by people having history of:
  - Breast cancer
  - Endometrial cancer
  - Pulmonary embolism
  - Liver disease
  - Coronary heart disease
  - Deep vein thrombosis
  - Unexplained vaginal bleeding
- Local estrogen therapy using vaginal rings, creams or tablets can be used for atrophic vaginitis.
- Testosterone is prescribed concomitantly with estrogen therapy and hormone therapy occasionally to improve symptoms of sexual dysfunction. However, the doses required are quite high and may produce hyperandrogenic effects. It does not improve vasomotor symptoms.

Selective Estrogen Receptor Modulators (SERMs)

- SERMs like raloxifene, bazedoxifene, and ospemifene possess the ability to alter estrogen action without increasing the risk of cancer or stimulating endometrial growth.
- They have the same efficacy as estrogen therapy in preventing bone loss and promoting beneficial lipoprotein levels.
- Raloxifene prevents bone loss and reduces low density lipoprotein levels (proestrogen) and has antiestrogen effect on breast and uterus tissue.
- Bazedoxifene, when combined with estrogen[referred to as a tissue selective estrogen complex (TSEC)], can help in reducing vasomotor symptoms without influencing the endometrium.
- Ospemifene is effective in improving urogenital symptoms.
- Earlier, tamoxifen was used for prevention of breast cancer and osteoporosis in postmenopausal women but it increased the risk of endometrial cancer as it acted as an agonist for uterus endometrial hyperplasia and polyp production. Hence, its use was discontinued.

Nonhormonal Treatment

- Nonhormonal drugs like selective serotonin reuptake inhibitors (SSRIs), serotonin-norepinephrine reuptake inhibitors (SNRIs), clonidine and gabapentin can be used for short durations to manage menopausal symptoms.
- SSRI like paroxetine and SNRI like venlafaxine, are antidepressants that can be used to manage vasomotor symptoms like hot flashes. They are not much effective but can result in one lesser hot flash/day. The doses used are much lower compared to doses used for antipsychiatric purposes. Common side effects include nausea, dizziness and headache.
- Gabapentin and clonidine, too, have been proven to reduce the frequency of hot flashes in a day. Gabapentin reduces up to 2 hot flashes/day, whereas clonidine is used for mild symptoms. Pregabalin, too, has been proven to reduce vasomotor symptoms.
- A stellate ganglion block (SGB) has also been studied for its effects on vasomotor symptoms and several studies have concluded that it is effective in reducing vasomotor symptoms by 4–90%, with limited adverse effects. It involves blockade of the sympathetic ganglia located in the lower cervical and upper thoracic region using an anesthetic agent. The North American Menopause Society has recommended the use of SGB with caution in the treatment of moderate to severe vasomotor symptoms as it is invasive and there is lack of long-term studies.

NONPHARMACOLOGICAL MANAGEMENT

Patient Education

- Explain that menopause is a normal event in the life of a woman and help them maintain a positive attitude about it.
- Provide an explanation about the stages of menopause and related symptoms.
- Explain the long-term implications of menopause.
- Explain the lifestyle modifications that can be done (explained later in the chapter).
- Smoking cessation, especially if considering hormone therapy.
- The woman should involve in at least 150 minutes/week of cardiovascular exercise and at least 2–3 sessions of weight-bearing exercise.
- Maintenance of healthy weight using a healthy diet containing good amounts of calcium and vitamin D.

- The woman should believe that sexual activity is normal and if she has any pain or other symptoms during or related to intercourse, she should consult her health practitioner.
- If the woman is facing difficulties due to menopausal symptoms, she should consult her health practitioner.
- Avoid over-the-counter remedies for menopausal symptoms and seek guidance from the health practitioner.
- Yoga and meditation can be practised for stress management.

Nonprescription Remedies

- Complementary and alternative medicine options include vitamin E, phytoestrogens, and omega-3 fatty acids.
- Which help in managing vasomotor symptoms.
- Plant estrogens or phytoestrogens occur naturally in some foods. They are of two types—isoflavones and lignans. Sources of phytoestrogens are:
  - Isoflavones—lentils, soybeans, chickpeas and other legumes
  - Lignans—certain fruits and vegetables, flaxseed and whole grains
- Common sage or garden sage (an herb) is believed to contain compounds that have estrogen-like effects and has been proven to manage menopausal symptoms. It should be used with caution in females with hypertension or epilepsy.
- Red clover and soy have been proven to be effective in managing osteoporosis and high cholesterol.
- Studies have not concluded any significant effects of other phytoestrogens on menopausal symptoms.

Hypnosis

According to research from the National Center for Complementary and Integrative Health at the US National Institutes of Health, hypnotherapy helps in improving sleep and quality of life and reducing frequency of hot flashes.

Yoga

- Yoga has become a popular complementary way of achieving a healthy life **(Fig. 9.3)**.

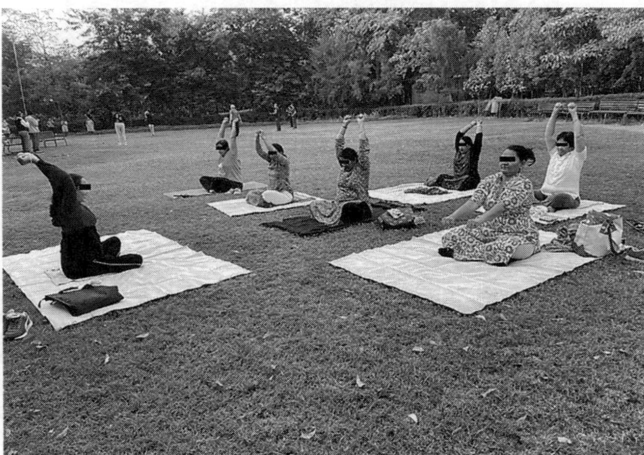

Fig. 9.3: Yoga.

- Several studies have proven the effects of Yoga in improving sleep quality and decreasing insomnia, vasomotor symptoms and osteoporosis.

Clinical Pointer

A systematic review in 2009 concluded that there was insufficient evidence to suggest that Yoga was an effective intervention for menopause. However, another systematic review in 2011 concluded that Yoga improved menopausal symptoms. There has been such conflicting evidence but since Yoga is a low cost intervention, has no adverse effects and is rather safe under the supervision of trained personnel, it can be used for menopausal women.

- Various Yogasanas that can be performed for menopause are described in Chapter 34: Yoga for Women's Health.

Lifestyle Modifications

- To cool hot flashes:
  - Wear layers, which can be removed
  - Drink cool water or go to a cooler area
  - Try to find out the trigger (spicy food, warm environment, warm beverages, etc.) for hot flashes and eliminate it
- To decrease vaginal discomfort:
  - Use over-the-counter water based vaginal lubricants or moisturizers
  - Staying sexually active helps keep the vagina moist and reduce discomfort
- To prevent menopause-related complications like heart disease, osteoporosis and urinary incontinence:
  - Eat a healthy and balanced diet containing adequate amounts of vitamin D and calcium
  - Eat foods that are rich in good cholesterol (high density lipoproteins) and help lower bad cholesterol low density lipoproteins and very low-density lipoproteins
  - Stop smoking
  - Exercise regularly, incorporating weight bearing exercises and pelvic floor strengthening exercises
- To improve sleep:
  - Practice relaxation using meditation or other techniques
  - Avoid caffeine and alcohol in large amounts

PHYSIOTHERAPY ASSESSMENT

Assessment follows the protocol described in Chapter 4: Assessment in Women's Health. **Box 9.7** describes physiotherapy assessment for menopause in brief. Certain outcome measures that can be used for menopause are presented in **Box 9.8**.

PHYSIOTHERAPY MANAGEMENT

Box 9.9 lists the benefits of exercise in menopausal women.

Box 9.7: Physiotherapy assessment for menopause.

- **Subjective examination:**
  - Age: Usually above 45 years of age
  - History of presenting illness: Ask regarding the presence of abnormal menses, period of abnormality, any associated symptoms like hot flushes, night sweats, sleeping disturbances, anxiety, depression, palpitations, headaches, Trophic changes
  - Medical and surgical history
  - Menstrual history: To determine the regularity of menses
  - Gynecological and obstetrical history: To determine whether the cause is natural or iatrogenic
  - Sexual activity: To determine the presence or absence of any sexual problems
  - Personal history: To determine the presence of any health concerning habits
  - Family history: May help in determining the likely time of menopause
  - Drug history
- **Objective examination:**
  - Body mass index: To determine body weight gain or loss
  - Range of motion of all major joints
  - Manual muscle testing or functional muscle tests to determine strength of major muscle groups
  - Pelvic floor assessment
  - Trophic changes
  - Posture
  - Gait
  - Assessment of cardiopulmonary endurance—six minute walk test or shuttle walk test can be used
  - Assessment of cognitive status—MMSE can be used
  - Assessment of psychological status—scales like beck depression inventory or Hamilton anxiety rating scale can be used
  - Assessment of quality of life—MENQOL or SF-36 can be used

Box 9.8: Outcome measures used for assessment of menopausal symptoms.

- **For vasomotor symptoms:**
  - Daily hot flash diary
  - Hot flush rating scale
  - Hot flush behavior scale or Hunter menopause scale
  - Hot flush related daily interference scale
- **For menopausal symptoms:**
  - Greene climacteric scale
  - Kupperman menopausal index
- **For health-related quality of life:**
  - Menopause rating scale (MRS)
  - Menopause specific quality of life (MENQOL)
  - Women's health questionnaire (WHQ)
  - Short form: 36 (SF-36)

Box 9.9: Benefits of exercise in menopausal women.

- Improves cardiorespiratory function
- Reduces metabolic risks associated with declining estrogen levels (increases HDL, reduces LDL, fibrinogen and triglycerides)
- Creates calorie deficit, thereby reducing the postmenopausal weight gain
- Increases bone mass, reducing the risk of osteoporosis
- Reduces stress and elevates mood
- Reduces hot flashes

American College of Sports Medicine (ACSM) Recommendations

American College of Sports Medicine (ACSM) recommendations for exercise program for menopausal years:

- **Cardiorespiratory exercises:**
  - Moderate intensity physical activity for 30–60 minutes for at least 5 days in a week

    OR

    Vigorous physical activity for 20–30 minutes for at least 3 days in a week
  - Combination of moderate and vigorous physical activity
  - Current physical activity levels, exercise history, health status, physical capabilities and feasibility should be taken into consideration while deciding the mode and intensity of aerobic exercise
  - Large muscle groups should be engaged for longer durations or by incorporating intervals of varying intensities or including simultaneous upper and lower extremity movements **(Fig. 9.4)**
  - At least 150 minutes of exercise per week to prevent weight gain and 250 minutes per week to promote long-term weight loss
- **Resistance exercises:**
  - Each muscle group should be exercised 2–3 days/week with 2–4 sets of 8–12 repetitions; 1 set of 8–12 or 12–15 repetitions for deconditioned women or those exercising for the first time
  - Freeweights, theraband or equipment can be used as resistance
  - Resistance exercises are especially helpful in improving and maintaining bone mineral density
- **Neuromotor exercises:**
  - Exercises focusing on agility, balance and coordination help in improving daily function and reduce falls **(Figs. 9.5A and B)**
  - These exercises should be adapted to the individual woman's needs
  - Yoga and Tai chi help too

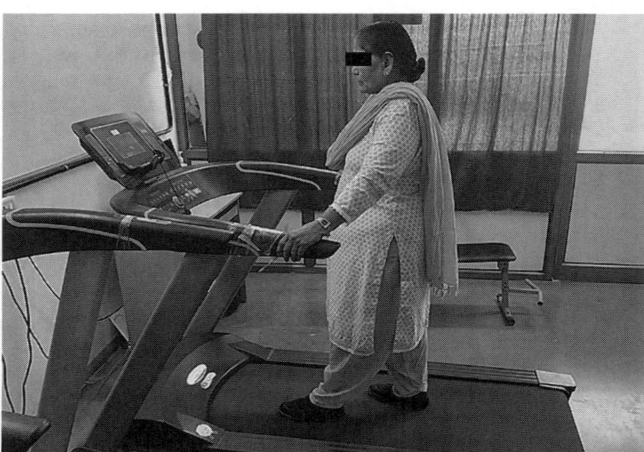

Fig. 9.4: Cardiorespiratory exercises.

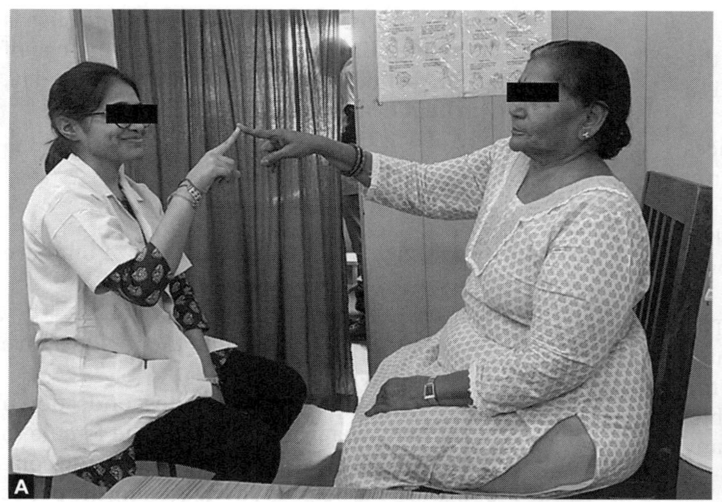

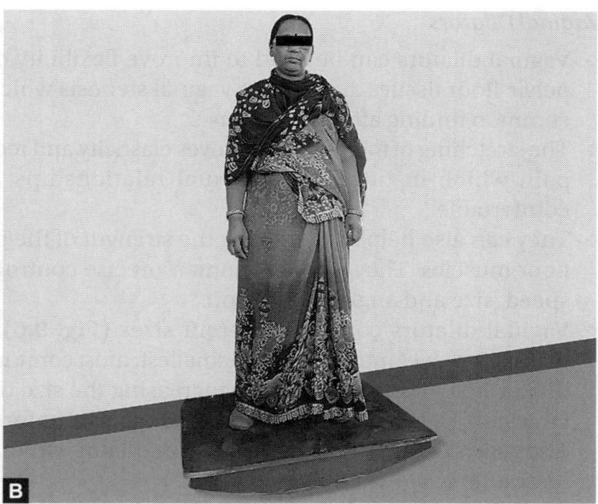

Figs. 9.5A and B: Neuromotor exercises.

- Duration and frequency of the exercises can be increased as tolerated
- **Flexibility exercises:**
  - Flexibility exercises should be performed at least 2–3 times/week
  - Each major muscle-tendon group should be stretched to improve and maintain range of motion

Physical Activity

Physical activity in menopause is aimed at:
- Achieving and maintaining a healthy weight
- Improving bone health
- Improving physical, mental and emotional health
- Improving menopausal symptoms
- Improving quality of life

Physical activity can include simple daily activities like walking or jogging, aerobic exercises like running, swimming, cycling, etc., resistance training using different forms of resistance, weight-bearing exercises, aquatic exercises, balance exercises, Yoga, Pilates and Tai chi.

Physical activity in any form has been proven to:
- Improve bone mineral density, enhance bone metabolism and reduce bone resorption
- Improve body fat and diastolic blood pressure
- Improve strength, endurance, balance and flexibility
- Improve blood brain derived neurotrophic factor (BDNF) levels, thereby improving memory and depression
- Improve sleep quality and anxiety
- Improve physical fitness, quality of life and functional capacity
- Improve overall health

Blood Flow Restriction

ACSM states that loads higher than 65% of 1 Repetition Maximum (1RM) are required to gain effective results with strength training. But sometimes, such high loads may not be tolerated by the subject, e.g., when the subject has chronic obstructive pulmonary disease or osteoporosis. A Japanese scientist, Yoshaki Sato, developed a method called blood flow restriction (BFR) consisting of low load exercises associated with a manual or pneumatically inflated cuff at the most proximal part of the limb. The device occludes venous flow but allows partial arterial flow. In elderly individuals, low intensity resistance training with blood flow restriction (LIBFR) improves bone markers, muscle strength and hormonal responses. Studies have shown improvement in muscle strength and balance in postmenopausal females too. However, it does not change body composition.

Physiotherapy for Vaginal Health

Physiotherapy for vaginal health incorporates pelvic floor physiotherapy which focuses on:
- Increasing knowledge and awareness regarding the pelvic floor
- Desensitization of painful areas
- Improving proprioception of the pelvic floor
- Improving muscle relaxation and tonification
- Increasing elasticity of tissues

Physiotherapy treatment also includes manual therapy, functional training using coordination, strengthening, flexibility and relaxation techniques and electrophysical agents. Physiotherapy management for vaginal and pelvic health is described in Chapter 15: Managing the Pelvic Floor.

Kegel Exercises

- Kegel exercises focus on augmenting the strength of the pelvic floor muscles.
- They can help in improving dyspareunia and prevent and improve symptoms of urinary incontinence.
- Kegel exercises alone or in combination with sex education can also improve sexual function (arousal, orgasm and satisfaction) in postmenopausal women.
- Kegel exercises can be done actively by the subject or can be done using devices like the Kegel master.

Vaginal Dilators

- Vaginal dilators can be used to improve flexibility of the pelvic floor tissues and reduce vaginal stenosis which is a common finding after menopause.
- The stretching of the vagina improves elasticity and reduces pain which in turn makes sexual relationships more comfortable.
- They can also help in improving the strength of the pelvic floor muscles. They give the woman precise control over speed, size and angle of insertion.
- Vaginal dilators come in different sizes **(Fig. 9.6)**. The therapy involves introducing the smallest, most comfortable dilator first and then gradually increasing the size till the largest size available, as the subject becomes comfortable. The goal is to introduce the largest size dilator without any discomfort.
- **Technique of use:**
  - The subject is in crook lying with the knees shoulder-width apart.
  - The subject may use a hand mirror to localize the vagina.
  - The vaginal opening and the dilator can be lubricated using a water-based jelly to ease the process of insertion. The subject inserts the smallest vaginal dilator into the vagina. Relaxation techniques can be used to increase comfort and relax the pelvic floor muscles.
  - The vaginal dilator should be inserted to the point of mild discomfort or muscle tension. No force should be used to go beyond this point.
  - No pain should be caused during insertion; the dilator should feel snug inside the vagina and not painful. If no pressure is felt, the next larger size dilator should be tried.
  - The dilator should be moved inside the vagina for 5–10 minutes. More lubricants can be added, if required. The dilator should be moved in and out and rotated in circles at the back, middle and opening of the vagina.
  - The dilator should be washed thoroughly with soap and hot water, dried using a clean towel or paper and stored safely in its kit.
  - A small amount of vaginal bleeding after dilator use is normal. If the bleeding is more (i.e., requiring use of a sanitary napkin) or continues for more than a day, contact with healthcare provider should be made.
  - A frequency of 3–4 times per week is recommended, with use not exceeding 2 days in a row.

Vaginal Cones

- Vaginal cones or weights come in the same size but have different weights.
- **Technique of use:**
  - Vaginal cones can be introduced into the vagina above the levator plate **(Fig. 9.7)**.
  - Once inside the vagina, the cone descends down slightly owing to its weight. This causes the female to contract the pelvic floor muscles to try to keep the cone inside the vagina. This helps in strengthening the pelvic floor muscles.
  - The weight of the vaginal cone can be gradually increased as the strength of the pelvic floor muscles develop.
  - The female has to maintain the cone inside the vagina for at least one minute during standing or walking. The time can be gradually increased.
- Improvements in muscle tone can be experienced after 2–3 weeks and the treatment should be continued for 2–3 months.

Chinese Vaginal Geisha Balls

- These are one, two or occasionally three balls **(Fig. 9.8)** attached with a string. Each ball contains a smaller ball inside it.
- **Technique of use:**
  - The Chinese vaginal balls are introduced into the vagina behind the pubococcygeus muscle.
  - The subject moves about, with the balls inside.
  - With movement, there is movement of the inner balls, creating vibrations that stimulate the vibrio-receptors present in the vagina. This provokes a contraction of pelvic floor muscles.

Fig. 9.6: Vaginal dilators.
(*Courtesy:* "File: Plastic and Silicone vaginal dilators.jpg" by Lloydjane is licensed under CC BY-SA 4.0.).

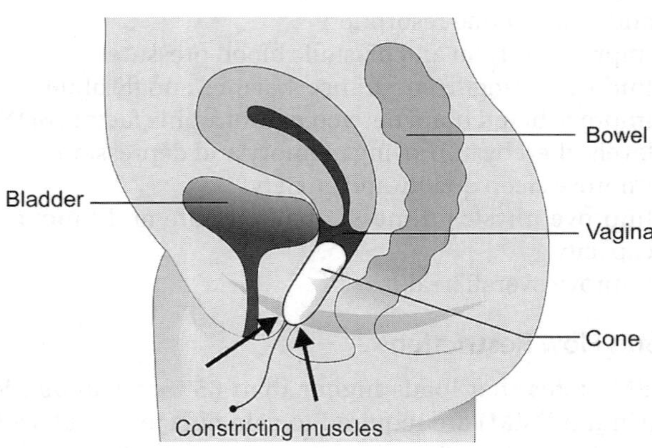

Fig. 9.7: Positioning vaginal cone inside the pelvic floor.

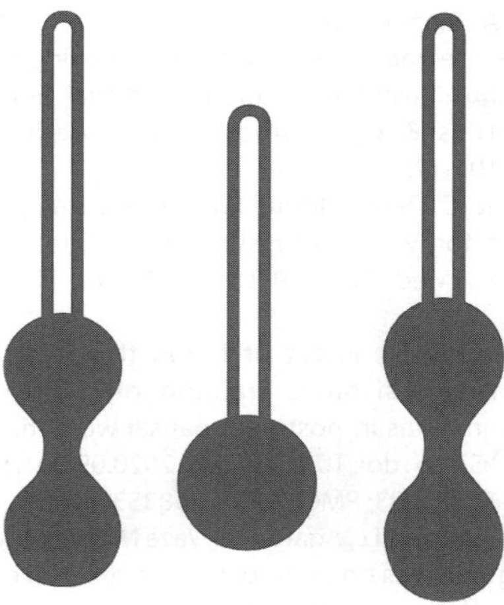

Fig. 9.8: Chinese vaginal geisha balls.

- The baroreceptors of the vagina are also stimulated due to the weight of the balls, this too, induces pelvic floor contraction.
- The balls are kept inside the vagina till the point of fatigue. Once the woman feels that she would not be able to retain the balls inside, they should be pulled out. The balls should not be kept inside for more than three consecutive hours.

❖ These balls help in improving the strength of the pelvic floor muscles and provide good proprioception.

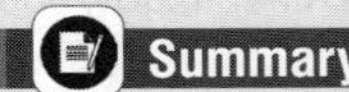

Summary

Menopause is a natural event occurring in the life of every woman. It may be an easy phase for some whereas difficult for some others. Many may present with certain symptoms which need to be managed. Diagnosis of menopause is based on history and exclusion of any other causes of amenorrhea. Usually, no laboratory tests are required. Medical management focuses on hormonal treatment; however, many nonhormonal alternatives are also available. Physiotherapy management focuses on exercises, physical activity, relaxation and improvement of vaginal health.

CLINICAL EXAMPLE

A 47-year-old female, 2.5 years postmenopausal, presents with complaint of dribbling of urine during coughing, sneezing and heavy weight lifting. She also complains of easy tiredness and sleep problems.

Physiotherapy Assessment

History reveals dribbling of urine since 6 months which has increased in severity gradually. She gets night sweats while sleeping since 2 years and gets easily tired since the same time. She had a gradual decline in her menses and they completely stopped 2.5 years ago. She has no history of any medical co-morbidities and is on no medication. She has no history of any surgery in the past. She has two children—one older son (25 years old) and a younger daughter (22 years old), both delivered vaginally without any complications. She has no history of abortions or miscarriages or still births.

Examination reveals weakness of pelvic floor muscles, reduced cardiopulmonary endurance and reduced muscle strength of major muscle groups of the body.

Suggested Physiotherapy Management

❖ Pelvic floor muscle exercises for pelvic floor muscle strengthening.
❖ Medical chair can be used for stimulation of the pelvic floor muscles.
❖ Aerobic exercises starting with moderate intensity 5 times a week and 30 minutes duration.
❖ Strengthening exercises for all major muscles of the body at 60–80% of 1RM.

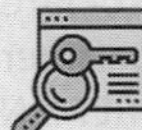

Review Questions

1. Discuss the physiotherapy assessment and management of a 43-year-old female presenting with amenorrhea for 13 months, hot flushes and lethargy.
2. Define menopause. Explain the endocrinology behind it.
3. Explain the symptoms of menopause in detail.
4. Write in detail about premature ovarian insufficiency.
5. Explain in detail the physiotherapy management of menopause.
6. Write short notes on:
   a. Genitourinary syndrome of menopause
   b. Stages of menopause
   c. Etiology of menopause
   d. Physiotherapy assessment of menopause
   e. Medical management of menopause
   f. Nonpharmacological management of menopause

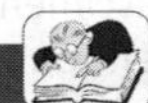

Bibliography

1. Ahuja M. Age of menopause and determinants of menopause age: A PAN India survey by IMS. J Midlife Health. 2016;7(3):126-31. doi: 10.4103/0976-7800.191012. PMID: 27721640; PMCID: PMC5051232.
2. Amarin Z. "Hysterectomy: Past, Present and Future". Hysterectomy- Past, Present and Future [Working Title], edited by Zouhair Amarin, IntechOpen, 2022. 10.5772/intechopen.103086.
3. An KC. Selective estrogen receptor modulators. Asian Spine J. 2016;10(4):787-91. doi: 10.4184/asj.2016.10.4.787. Epub 2016 Aug 16. PMID: 27559463; PMCID: PMC4995266.
4. Carugno J, Fatehi M. Abdominal Hysterectomy. [Updated 2021Dec 5]. In: StatPearls [Internet]. Treasure Island (FL): StatPearls Publishing. 2022. Available from: https://www.ncbi.nlm.nih.gov/books/NBK564366/.
5. Collaborative Group on Hormonal Factors in Breast Cancer. Type and timing of menopausal hormone therapy and breast cancer risk: individual participant meta-analysis of the worldwide epidemiological evidence. The Lancet. 2019;394(10204):1159-68.

6. Dalal PK, Agarwal M. Postmenopausal syndrome. Indian J Psychiatry. 2015;57(Suppl 2):S222-32. doi: 10.4103/0019-5545.161483. PMID: 26330639; PMCID: PMC4539866.
7. Darware M, Ghordadekar D, Dhole R, Noman O. Physiotherapy rehabilitation of post-hysterectomy geriatric patient: A case report. Bioscience Biotechnology Research Communications. 2021;SI 14(6): 71-6. http://dx.doi.org/10.21786/bbrc/14.6.17.
8. da Silva MDL, Pereira PMG, Geraldes AAR, de Farias RPGF, dos Santos JM, do Socorro Cirilo-Sousa M. Effects of resistance training with blood flow restriction on the body composition of postmenopausal women. International Physical Medicine & Rehabilitation Journal. 2018; 3(3): 195-98.
9. Fernandez-Rhodes L, Malinowski JR, Wang Y, Tao R, Pankratz N, Jeff JM, et al. The genetic underpinnings of variation in ages at menarche and natural menopause among women from the multi-ethnic population architecture using genomics and epidemiology (PAGE) study: A trans-ethnic meta-analysis. PLoS ONE. 2018;13(7):e0200486. https://doi.org/10.1371/journal.pone.0200486.
10. Goldstein KM, Coeytaux RR, Williams JW Jr, et al. Nonpharmacologic Treatments for Menopause-associated Vasomotor Symptoms [Internet]. Washington (DC): Department of Veterans Affairs (US); 2016. APPENDIX D, MEASUREMENT SCALES FOR MENOPAUSE. Available from: https://www.ncbi.nlm.nih.gov/books/NBK447620/.
11. Hall JE. Endocrinology of the menopause. Endocrinol Metab Clin North Am. 2015;44(3):485-96. doi: 10.1016/j.ecl.2015.05.010. PMID: 26316238; PMCID: PMC6983294.
12. Harlow SD, Gass M, Hall JE, Lobo R, Maki P, Rebar RW, et al. Executive summary of the Stages of Reproductive Aging Workshop +10: addressing the unfinished agenda of staging reproductive aging. Climacteric. 2012;15(2):105-14. doi: 10.3109/13697137.2011.650656. Epub 2012 Feb 16. PMID: 22338612; PMCID: PMC3580996.
13. https://www.acog.org/womens-health/faqs/the-menopauseyears#:~:text=Menopauseis%20the%20time%20in%20 your,through%20menopause%20is%2051%20years.
14. InformedHealth.org [Internet]. Cologne, Germany: Institute for Quality and Efficiency in Health Care (IQWiG); 2006. Hysterectomy (surgical removal of the womb) 2018. Available from: https://www.ncbi.nlm.nih.gov/books/NBK525761/
15. Jorge MP, Santaella DF, Pontes IMO, Shiramizu VKM, Nascimento EB, Cabral A. Hatha Yoga practice decreases menopause symptoms and improves quality of life: A randomized controlled trial. Complementary Therapies in Medicine. 2016;26: 128-35.
16. Joshi S, Khandwe R, Bapat D, Deshmukh U. Effect of yoga on menopausal symptoms. Menopause International. 2011;17(3):78-81. doi:10.1258/mi.2011.011020.
17. Kalra S, Yadav J, Ajmera P, Sindhu B, Pal S. Impact of physical activity on physical and mental health of postmenopausal women: A systematic review. J Clin of Diagn Res. 2022;16(2):YE01-YE08. https://www.doi.org/10.7860/JCDR/2022/52302/15974.
18. Kashanian M, Ali SS, Nazemi M, Bahasadri S. Evaluation of the effect of pelvic floor muscle training (PFMT or Kegel exercise) and assisted pelvic floor muscle training (APFMT) by a resistance device (Kegelmaster device) on urinary incontinence in women: a randomized trial. Eur J Obstet Gynecol Reprod Biol. 2011;159:218-23.
19. Kaunitz AM, Manson JE. Management of menopausal symptoms. Obstet Gynecol. 2015;126(4):859-76. doi: 10.1097/AOG.0000000000001058. PMID: 26348174; PMCID: PMC4594172.
20. Khosravi A, Riazi H, Simbar M, Montazeri A. Effectiveness of Kegel exercise and lubricant gel for improving sexual function in menopausal women: A randomized trial. European Journal of Obstetrics & Gynecology and Reproductive Biology. 2022;274:106-12.
21. Lee YS, Wie C, Pew S, Kling JM. Stellate ganglion block as a treatment for vasomotor symptoms: Clinical application. Cleve Clin J Med. 2022;89(3):147-53. doi: 10.3949/ccjm.89a.21032.
22. Linero C, Choi SJ. Effect of blood flow restriction during low-intensity resistance training on bone markers and physical functions in postmenopausal women. J Exerc Sci Fit. 2021;19(1):57-65. doi: 10.1016/j.jesf.2020.09.001. Epub 2020 Sep 25. PMID: 33293983; PMCID: PMC7683332.
23. Meeta M, Digumarti L, Agarwal N, Vaze N, Shah R, Malik S. Clinical practice guidelines on menopause: An executive summary and recommendations: Indian menopause society 2019–2020. J Midlife Health. 2020;11:55-95.
24. Menopause: diagnosis and management. London: National Institute for Health and Care Excellence (NICE); 2019 Dec. (NICE Guideline, No. 23.) Available from: https://www.ncbi.nlm.nih.gov/books/NBK552590/.
25. Nazarpour S, Simbar M, Tehrani FR, Majd HA. Effects of sex education and kegel exercises on the sexual function of postmenopausal women: A randomized clinical trial. J Sex Med. 2017;14 (7): 959-67.
26. O'Neill S, Eden J. The pathophysiology of menopausal symptoms. Obstetrics, Gynaecology & Reproductive Medicine. 2017; 27 (10):303-10.
27. Peacock K, Ketvertis KM. Menopause. [Updated 2022 Feb 2]. In: StatPearls [Internet]. Treasure Island (FL): StatPearls Publishing; 2022. Available from: https://www.ncbi.nlm.nih.gov/books/NBK507826/
28. Perez KS, Garber CE. Exercise prescription for the menopausal years: Promoting and Enhancing Well-Being. ACSM's Health & Fitness Journal. 2011;15(3):8-14. doi: 10.1249/FIT.0b013e3182160f2f.
29. Pillarisetty LS, Mahdy H. Vaginal Hysterectomy. [Updated 2022 May 8]. In: StatPearls [Internet]. Treasure Island (FL): StatPearls Publishing; 2022. Available from: https://www.ncbi.nlm.nih.gov/books/NBK554482/.
30. Prasad JB, Tyagi NK, Verma P. Age at menopause in India: A systematic review. Diabetes MetabSyndr. 2021;15(1):373-77. doi: 10.1016/j.dsx.2021.01.013. Epub 2021 Jan 20. PMID: 33524647.
31. Rochera M, Andreu C, Madrid Y, Bouallalene K, Pau E. Physiotherapy as a way to maintain vaginal health during menopause. Advances in sexual medicine. 2017; 7: 97-104. doi: 10.4236/asm.2017.72007.
32. Santoro N, Epperson CN, Mathews SB. Menopausal symptoms and their management. Endocrinol Metab Clin North Am. 2015;44(3):497-515. doi: 10.1016/j.ecl.2015.05.001. PMID: 26316239; PMCID: PMC4890704.
33. Simoni B, et al. The Benefits of Physical Activity on Climacteric Women. A Multidisciplinary Look at Menopause, edited by Juan Rodriguez-Landa, Jonathan Cueto-Escobedo, IntechOpen, 2017. 10.5772/intechopen.68829.
34. Soo LM, Jong-In K, Ha, Jeong Yong HJ, Kate B, Edzard E. Yoga for menopausal symptoms: a systematic review. Menopause. 2009;16(3):602-08. doi: 10.1097/gme.0b013e31818ffe39.
35. Torrealday S, Kodaman P, Pal L. Premature Ovarian Insufficiency—an update on recent advances in understanding and

management. F1000Res. 2017;29;6:2069. doi: 10.12688/f1000research.11948.1. PMID: 29225794; PMCID: PMC5710309.
36. Yilmaz S, Terzioğlu F. The effects of Kinesio taping and breathing exercises on pain management after gynaecological abdominal surgery: A randomized controlled study. International journal of nursing practice. 2022 https://doi.org/10.1111/ijn.13088.

Multiple Choice Questions (MCQs)

To test your understanding and recall of key concepts.

1. **Which hormone shows a 15-fold increase in levels during early years after menopause?**
   A. Progesterone
   B. Estrogen
   C. Follicle-stimulating hormone (FSH)
   D. Luteinizing hormone (LH)
2. **Why do women with higher BMI experience delayed menopause?**
   A. They have increased levels of endogenous estrogen
   B. They have fewer antral follicles
   C. They undergo earlier ovulation
   D. They experience faster follicle depletion
3. **How do vasomotor symptoms arise during menopause?**
   A. Due to elevated cortisol levels
   B. Due to estrogen withdrawal affecting the hypothalamus
   C. Due to the increase in GnRH pulse frequency
   D. Due to the decline in FSH levels
4. **A postmenopausal woman complains of frequent falls. Which physiotherapy intervention should be prioritized?**
   A. Resistance exercises for upper limbs
   B. Neuromotor exercises for balance and coordination
   C. Cardiovascular exercises to improve endurance
   D. Aquatic exercises to reduce joint stress
5. **Which of the following is *true* with respect to premature/primary ovarian insufficiency (POI)?**
   A. Delayed loss of ovarian function
   B. Abundant female sex hormones
   C. Estrogen deficiency
   D. Accelerated loss of ovarian function
6. **How does the decrease in anti-Müllerian hormone (AMH) influence ovarian aging?**
   A. It accelerates follicular loss by reducing restraint on FSH stimulation
   B. It increases ovulatory cycles, leading to higher conception rates
   C. It enhances estradiol secretion, stabilizing the menstrual cycle
   D. It decreases aromatase activity, reducing estrogen synthesis
7. **Which of the following is *not* a core symptom associated with menopause?**
   A. Vasomotor symptoms
   B. Vaginal symptoms
   C. Insomnia
   D. Changes in skin elasticity
8. **A physiotherapy intervention plan for a 55-year-old woman with menopausal urogenital symptoms should include____________________.**
   A. Pelvic floor muscle training
   B. Cardiovascular exercises for general health
   C. Neuromotor exercises for balance improvement
   D. All of the above

ANSWERS

1. C	2. A	3. B	4. B
5. D	6. A	7. D	8. D

Chapter 10

Osteoporosis

Anu Arora

LEARNING OBJECTIVES

At the end of the chapter, the reader will be able to:

- Understand and define osteoporosis.
- Gain knowledge about the epidemiology of osteoporosis and the reasons for gender and creed wise-bias in prevalence.
- Understand minutely the pathogenesis, types, diagnosis, risk assessment, prevention, and treatment of osteoporosis.
- Develop an understanding of various tools used in assessment of osteoporosis and learn their appropriate usage.
- Assess a subject with decreased BMD and provide physiotherapy management for the same.
- Learn about the role of exercise in the management of osteoporosis and understand the clinical rationale for the same.

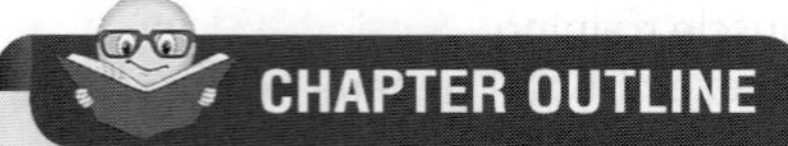

INTRODUCTION

Osteoporosis has been recognized as a progressive, systemic skeletal disorder, characterized by low bone mass and microarchitectural deterioration of bone tissue, leading to a consequent increase in bone fragility and susceptibility to fracture.

The fragility fractures, which are the focal consequences of the disease lead to detrimental repercussions on the mental and physical well-being of the affected subject in the form of pain, suffering, disability, and possibly even mortality in severe cases.

EPIDEMIOLOGY

Increase in the average life expectancy along with a greater proportion of the population over the age of 50 years are likely to result in an increased number of people affected by osteoporosis.

Indian Scenario

2013, estimates suggested that approximately 50 million people in India had T-scores of <–1 (below normal bone mineral density).

The situation is even more grave for the females with the evidence in various published literature suggestive of a prevalence of osteoporosis in about 40–50% of Indian postmenopausal women and about 20% of men above 50 years.

Qualitative studies have revealed that Indians have a low bone mineral density when compared to their Western Counterparts due to hereditary factors, nutritional deficiencies, and smaller skeletal size.

Global Scenario

With an estimate indicating an annual contribution of 8.9 million fractures worldwide, osteoporosis can eventually lead to reduced physical and psychological health, lower quality of life, and shorter life expectancy, thereby representing a major global health problem.

BONE PHYSIOLOGY

Bone is a complex, metabolically active and dynamic tissue that through its architecture and composition facilitates essential mechanical functions that it performs.

The skeletal system per se is responsible for many functions including:

- Providing framework for the muscular system
- Protection for the internal organs
- Site for major hematopoietic organ
- The mineral reservoir of calcium (storing 98% of the body's total calcium)

The human skeletal system comprises two types of bone (**Fig. 10.1**):

1. **Cortical bone**
2. **Cancellous bone**

The difference in the relative ratio of cancellous to the cortical bone at different skeletal sites makes some specific sites of some bones more likely to sustain **osteoporosis-induced fragility fractures** than others. These **vulnerable sites** include sites shown in **Figure 10.2**.

Trabecular bone has a higher surface-to-volume ratio than cortical bone and is thus potentially more sensitive to alterations in the rate of bone turnover, a process that occurs on the surface of the bone. This makes the **cancellous bone more susceptible to changes in metabolic or hormonal profile and thereby osteoporosis.**

Bone Homeostasis: Physiological Mechanisms

In spite of their apparently static appearance, bones are metabolically active and undergo a continuous process of formation and resorption through discrete bone-remodeling units.

Bone is a biphasic material that is made up of hydroxyapatite calcium phosphate embedded in a collagen matrix. While collagen makes the bone flexible, minerals provide stiffness. Throughout life, older bone is periodically resorbed by osteoclasts at discrete sites and replaced with new bone made by osteoblasts. This process is known as remodeling. Bone remodeling consists of two phases:

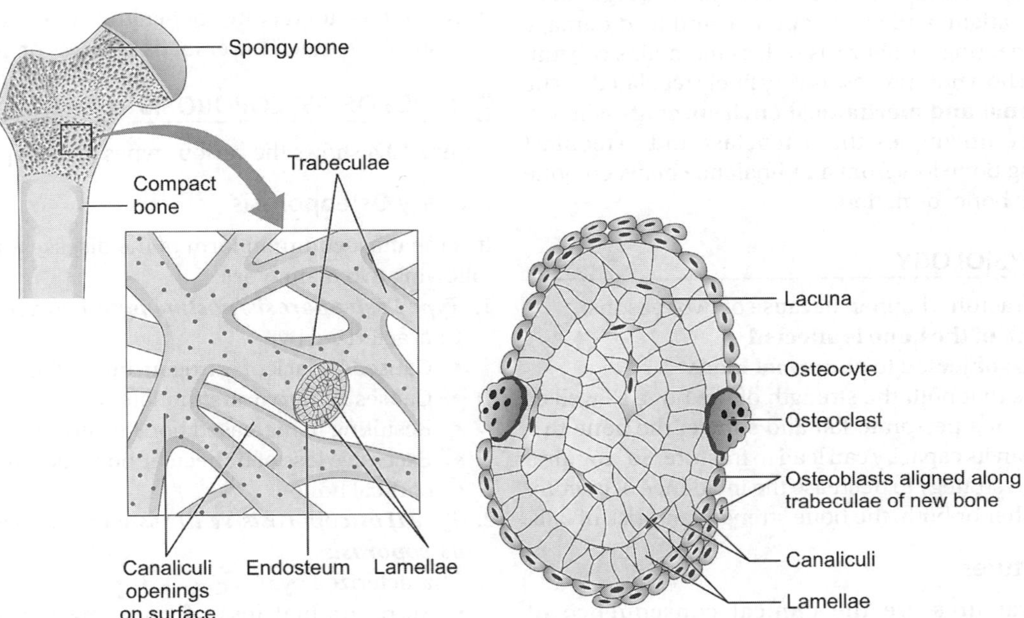

Fig. 10.1: Cortical bone and cancellous bone.

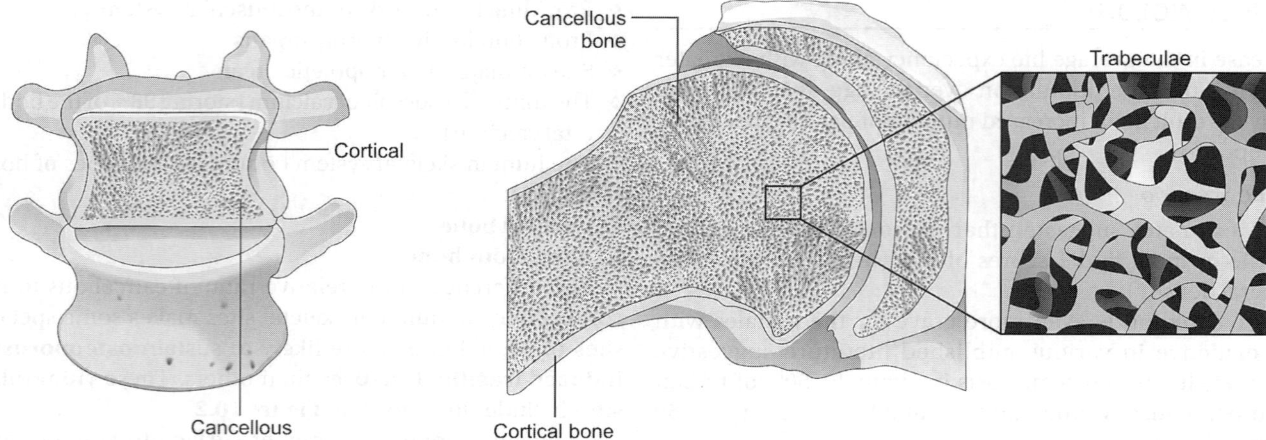

Fig. 10.2: Cortical and cancellous bone in the vertebral body and neck of femur *(For color version, see Plate 2).*

1. The **resorption phase** involves the removal of old, dead, or damaged bone
2. The **formation phase** occurs following resorption phase and produces new bone.

The cells involved in these processes are:
- Osteocytes
- Osteoblasts
- Osteoclasts

The osteocytes and osteoblasts are uninucleated cells of mesenchymal origin. Osteocytes have receptors for parathyroid hormone (PTH) and an abundance of ribosomes involved in the synthesis of collagen propeptides.

Osteoclasts are multinucleated cells found along the cortical endosteal surface and trabeculae in the Howship lacunae where the mineralized bone is being actively resorbed.

This continuous bone turnover or remodeling is vital for the mechanical integrity of the skeletal system **(Fig. 10.3)**, as it prevents fatigue and wears and tear-induced damage to the weight-bearing structure as well as maintains calcium homeostasis. The whole process is very finely regulated by the bone's **hormonal and mechanical environments** wherein any imbalance uncouples the osteoclast and osteoblast activity causing bone loss from an imbalance between bone resorption and bone formation.

PATHOPHYSIOLOGY

Osteoporotic fractures happen because of two reasons:
1. **The strength of the bone is affected**
2. **The bone is subjected to abnormal loads**

This implies that both the strength of the bone as well as the propensity of a person to fall and subject the bone to a load greater than its capacity can lead to fracture. So, any kind of management strategy to decrease the incidence of fracture must target either or both, the bone strength and risk of fall.

Fragility Fractures

- Fragility fractures are the clinical consequence of osteoporosis. Fragility fracture refers to those fractures that result from any low energy transfer trauma such as a fall from standing height or less.

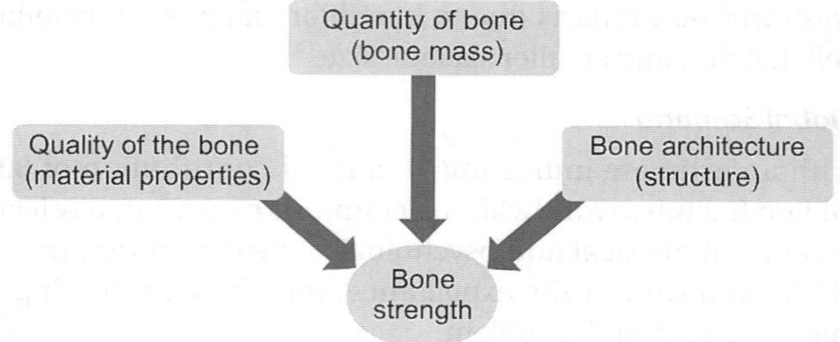

Fig. 10.3: Determinants of bone strength.

- They are often seen in the regions of the hip, wrist, and spine as fracture neck femur, wedge compression fractures of the vertebral bodies, and fractures of the distal end of the radius.
- In contrast to fractures of healthy bone, fragility fractures result from much lower loads or stress on the bone.

TYPES OF OSTEOPOROSIS

Figure 10.4 shows the various types of osteoporosis.

Primary Osteoporosis

It is the most common form of the disease and includes the following two main types:

1. ***Type I osteoporosis/postmenopausal osteoporosis***
   Characterized by:
   - Caused by lack of estrogen and androgen
   - Causes PTH to overstimulate osteoclasts
   - Resulting in increased bone turnover
   - Excessive loss of trabecular bone as compared with the cortical bone.
2. ***Type II osteoporosis/senile osteoporosis/age-associated osteoporosis***
   Characterized by:
   - More gradual loss of bone mass due to systemic senescence which is found equally in both genders.

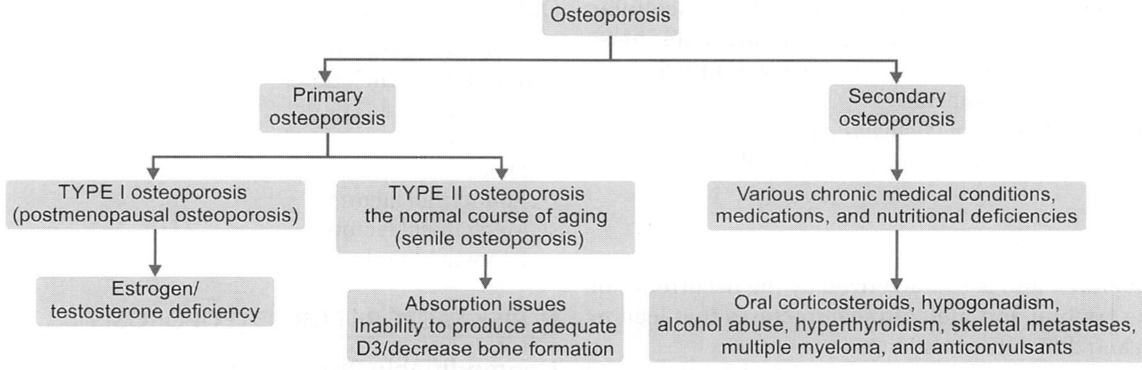

Fig. 10.4: Classification of osteoporosis.

Table 10.1: Causes of secondary osteoporosis.

Medical issues	***Medications***	***Endocrinal diseases***	***Lifestyle choices***
Eating disorder: Anorexia nervosa	Glucocorticoids	Hypogonadism	Low physical activity
Malnutrition	Antiepileptics	Hyperthyroidism	Excessive smoking, alcohol consumption
Chronic inflammatory diseases like RA	Anticoagulants (heparin)	Cushing's syndrome	Low body weight
Post-intestinal resection		Hyperparathyroidism	
Transplant patients			

(RA: rheumatoid arthritis)

- Age-induced loss of stem-cell precursors triggers this predominant loss of cortical bone.
- Bone loss due to increased bone turnover.

Secondary Osteoporosis

Secondary osteoporosis is characterized as having a clearly definable etiologic mechanism **(Table 10.1)**.

Osteoporosis of Pregnancy/Osteoporosis Postdelivery

- **Presentation:** Severe back pain and multiple vertebral fractures.
- **Etiology:** Osteoporosis of pregnancy is likely to be related to poor diet or calcium and vitamin D deficiency whereas post-delivery while breastfeeding could be related to excessive secretion of PTH-related peptide, which is accountable for calcium transport in the breast and for the deployment of calcium from bone to milk.
- The majority of cases resolve spontaneously with Bone mineral density (BMD) increasing with cessation of breastfeeding. Subjects with osteoporosis during pregnancy are at increased risk for postmenopausal osteoporosis.

Nutritional Deficiencies

- They may affect the skeleton by impairing the supply of calcium and vitamin D, leading to secondary hyperparathyroidism. Deficiencies are a common occurrence after gastric resection and in patients with short-bowel syndrome.
- In females with eating disorders (anorexia nervosa), nutritional deficiency is worsened by amenorrhea.

Immobilization

Temporary or permanent immobilization resulting from any condition musculoskeletal/neurological/systemic may cause bone loss from disuse.

Medication Use

Glucocorticoids-induced osteoporosis:

- Prolonged use of corticosteroids constitutes the most common cause of secondary osteoporosis irrespective of gender. Exogenous glucocorticoids (GC) are synthetic compounds (dexamethasone and methylprednisolone) used for the treatment of autoimmune diseases, rheumatism, gastrointestinal diseases, organ transplantation and to treat certain cancers.
- Two main mechanisms are responsible for GC mediated decrease in the calcium concentration:
  - Reduced intestinal calcium absorption by opposing the action of vitamin D and decreasing the expression of calcium channels in the duodenum
  - Increased renal calcium excretion by decreasing calcium reabsorption which leads to secondary hyperparathyroidism

Gonadotropin-releasing hormone agonists reduce circulating estrogen levels and thereby cause excessive bone loss.

Drugs like tamoxifen and raloxifene, interfere with the binding of estradiol (estrogen precursor) to nuclear receptors and thereby impair the cellular action of the hormone in premenopausal women.

Heparin reduces osteoblastic activity and decreases osteoblast adhesion to matrix proteins. Long-term treatment with heparin therefore causes osteoporosis.

Aluminum and lithium interfere with intracellular signaling. Additionally, aluminum impairs osteoblast function which may be responsible for osteoporosis with aluminum-containing antacids.

Antiepileptic drugs *like phenytoin*, interfere with vitamin D metabolism thereby increasing the risk of osteoporotic fractures.

Juvenile Osteoporosis

It affects children and is characterized by the occurrence of primarily vertebral and metaphyseal fractures that lead to back pain and difficulty in walking.

PEAK BONE MASS

- Peak bone mass (PBM) refers to the amount of bone present after skeletal maturation. It is alternately defined as the total quantity of bone gained by the time a steady skeletal state has been attained.
- PBM is broadly referred to as an umbrella term for *structural bone strength* and is determined by the bone mass density, microarchitecture, microscopic repair mechanisms and geometric properties of the bone. It is a crucial determinant of the risk of osteoporotic fracture.
- To reduce the risk of osteoporosis, one needs to **acquire as much bone mass as possible prior to menopause** and **reduce the rate at which bone is lost after menopause**.
- The greater the quantity of bone mineral at the time of peak bone mass achievement, the more bone an individual can afford to lose. In other words, greater the PBM, lesser is the risk of osteoporosis.
- The period of adolescence is an appropriate window of opportunity to maximize bone mass.

Time of Peak Bone Mass Attainment

Peak bone mass or calcium accretion in the bones is reached in the third decade of life. Reports of the age at peak bone mass vary from 20 to 30 years **(Fig. 10.5)**.

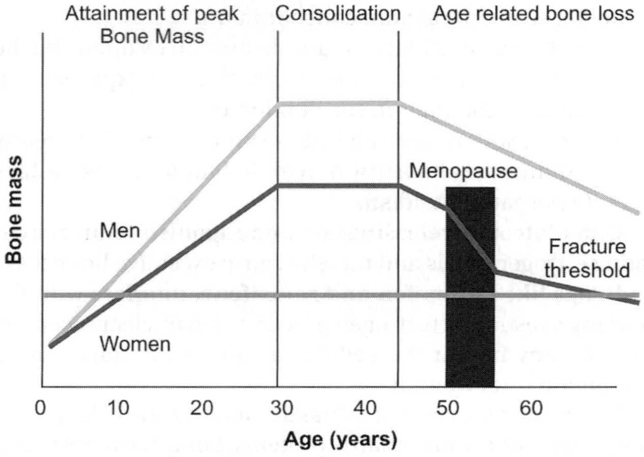

Fig. 10.5: Effect of age on accretion of bone mass.

Determinants of Peak Bone Mass

Bone mass accumulation during growth is influenced by various factors including:

- Genetics
- Gender
- Diet
- Endocrinal factors
- Mechanical factors
- Exposure to other risk factors

RISK FACTORS FOR OSTEOPOROSIS

Nonmodifiable Risk Factors

There are some nonmodifiable factors including **gender bias, advancing age, ethnicity, and genetic factors** which increase the risk of decline in BMD.

Gender Bias

In females: In comparison to their male counterparts, women have a relatively smaller body frame and therefore a narrower bone structure. In addition, females tend to consume smaller portions of food thereby ingesting less calcium-rich diets. Even their exposure to sunlight is lesser owing to sociocultural factors, making them probable candidates for vitamin D and consequentially calcium deficiency.

- Most importantly, estrogen levels in females are a major determinant of BMD. Therefore, making estrogen-deficient females (postmenopausal) more susceptible to osteoporosis.
- Indian females are relatively more vulnerable to this decrease in BMD, as even though the average age at menarche in Indian girls is 12.5 years, menopause in these females is seen earlier than in their Caucasian counterparts. While the average age of menopause in Indian women is 46.2 years, it is about 51 years in their Western counterparts.

In males: Hypogonadism in males caused by hypopituitarism, hyperprolactinemia, overtraining or inadequate energy intake can also lead to a decline in BMD.

Effect of Age and Gender on BMD

- Remodeling of bone is known as coupled activity of osteoclasts causing resorption of older bone and osteoblasts replacing it with new bone. However, till the achievement of PBM, cumulative bone formation is higher than bone resorption. But, in later life, the process of bone formation in each remodeling site can no longer match up to the bone that was resorbed, leading to a small amount of bone loss with each remodeling cycle. So, advancing age, after the achievement of PBM, implies a decreasing BMD. This effect is further amplified by the age-associated decline in levels of hormones.
- The skeleton, owing to its weight-bearing function is subjected to long periods of loading and fatigue-induced damage which is manifested in the form of microscopic cracks, that progressively increases with age.

Box 10.1: Rapid and slow-paced bone loss in females.

- After attaining PBM at the age of 30 years, there is a loss of bone at a rate of approximately 0.3% and 0.5% per year in males and females respectively.
- There is an accelerated loss of bone in females, at a rate of 2% per year during menopause, steered by estrogen deficiency.
- Age-related loss of bone mass is a universal phenomenon. However, the presence of any other insinuating factors may limit an individual's capacity to achieve PBM, thereby increasing the likelihood of developing osteoporosis later in life.

- Also, there is an age-wise and gender-wise discrepancy in the inherent cortical bone geometry. While males have greater increase in periosteal (outer) diameter, females have a narrow endocortical surface. This gender bias is seen as a greater overall bone mass in males as compared to females **(Box 10.1)**.

Effect of Ethnicity and Genetics on BMD

- Ethnicity and race may have an influence on the BMD.
- Indian women tend to have lower BMD than their Caucasian and Black counterparts.
- One of the factors responsible for this ethnic variation in BMD can be the polymorphisms in the gene for vitamin D receptors in different races.
- Apart from this, the factors mentioned above in the diet and nutrition section also explain the increased susceptibility of Indians to calcium deficiency and osteoporosis.
- Research has found that the prevalence of fractures is highest in white women while BMD is relatively higher in African Americans.
- National Osteoporosis Risk Assessment (NORA) Cohort is one of the largest multiethnic studies which revealed that in Asian women, the risk for osteoporosis was higher than in White women.
- Genetic variation in the various ethnic groups could be a potential explanation for the variability in different ethnic groups.

Effect of Puberty on BMD

- The gender bias in the bone mass becomes prominent during puberty. This difference can be attributed to the prolonged bone maturation period in males as compared to females leading to a relatively greater increase in bone size and cortical thickness.
- Puberty also witnesses an asynchrony between the gain in stature and bone mass. This phenomenon may be the probable reason for the occurrence of a brief period of relatively increased bone fragility during puberty that may account for the pattern of increased fracture incidence during adolescence.

Modifiable Risk Factors

Calcium Deficiency

- Calcium is deposited in the bone matrix in the form of hydroxyapatite crystals. This imparts the essential hardness of bone. The bioavailability of calcium in humans is from both dairy sources and non-dairy sources. Indian diets are traditionally known to fall short of the Indian Council of Medical Research's recommended dietary allowance of 600 mg/day of calcium for adult women.
- In addition, Indian diets are known to have a higher ratio of phytates to calcium, which may hinder calcium absorption from the already calcium-deficient diets. This may impede the bone remodeling process, resulting in lower BMD.

Vitamin D Deficiency/Hypovitaminosis D

- Vitamin D is obtained either from dietary sources or from cutaneous synthesis upon exposure to ultraviolet radiation from sunlight.
- Vitamin D stores can be assessed by measuring the serum concentration of 25-hydroxyvitamin D [25(OH)D], which is the most commonly used index of vitamin D status.
- Vitamin D is essential for the effective absorption of calcium from the gut. Therefore, a deficiency of vitamin D can lead to calcium deficiency and can thus adversely affect the mineralization of bones. When serum 25(OH) D decreases, parathyroid hormone (PTH) concentrations increase, which increases the risk of increased osteoclast activity and, ultimately, bone resorption.
- **Some significant factors which can lead to vitamin deficiency**, especially in Indians include:
  - Low sun exposure
  - Traditional Indian attire like saris, and salwar kameez
  - Inadequate calcium content in the diet
  - Poor vitamin D fortification of food
  - Use of sunscreens
  - Highly pigmented skin

Lifestyle

- Lifestyle has been defined as a distinctive pattern of personal and social behavior characteristic of an individual or a group. Lifestyle is referred to the characteristics of people including their day-to-day behaviors and functions of job, activities, fun, and diet.
- Urbanization has steadily made lifestyles more and more sedentary where decreased sun exposure coupled with low physical activity has progressively caused deterioration of bone health.

Nutritional Status

- Poor nutritional status wherein deficiency of calcium and vitamin D, the two main nutrients involved in bone health, play a major role in influencing the risk of osteoporosis.
- Recent systematic review and meta-analysis have provided evidence of an inverse association between a healthy dietary intake and risk of low BMD.
- There is a habitual low intake of calcium in women across the life span in India, from toddlers, adolescents, and pregnant and lactating mothers to postmenopausal women. The gender bias in calcium intake between sexes especially in the lower socioeconomic classes also makes a point of increased risk of calcium deficiency in females.

- The predominantly vegetarian Indian diet along with the phytates and oxalates in the fiber-rich diet which decrease the absorption of calcium make a case for calcium deficiency in Indians.
- Indians also have a higher level of the enzyme, 25(OH)-D-24-hydroxylase contributing to hypovitaminosis D. Several studies have demonstrated a positive correlation between body mass index and BMD. Research conducted in India has confirmed that a body weight of less than 60 kg and a height of less than 155 cm may significantly increase the risk of osteoporosis in women.

Previous History of Fractures

- Previous history of low impact fragility fractures increases the risk of having another fracture in near future and is therefore a significant predictor of subsequent osteoporotic fracture.
- Vertebral wedge compression fractures are strong predictors of more such pathological spinal fractures in times to come.
- The magnitude of association between prior fracture and subsequent fracture was more pronounced at specific sites such as hip, vertebrae, and wrist fracture in literature.

Tobacco Smoking

Tobacco smoke influences bone mass directly as well as indirectly as shown in **Figure 10.6**.

Alcohol Consumption

- Various researches have demonstrated that chronic, heavy alcohol consumption has detrimental effects on bone health and increases the risk of osteoporosis as it triggers a bone remodeling imbalance, with a predominant decrease in bone formation.
- Alcohol, is also believed to induce osteocyte apoptosis, oxidative stress, and wingless-related integration site (WNT) signaling pathway modulation which in turn causes remodeling imbalance.

Medications

- Drug-induced osteoporosis is seen as a side effect of various medications.
- Methotrexate (in very high doses), and loop diuretics (e.g., furosemide) may also decrease bone mass by increasing calcium excretion in the kidneys. Excess thyroid supplementation in cases of hypothyroidism, can also cause demineralization of the bone. Aluminum-containing antacids can bind calcium in the gastrointestinal tract and decrease calcium absorption.
- Lithium can also increase PTH secretion which in turn causes calcium release from the bone to raise serum calcium levels.

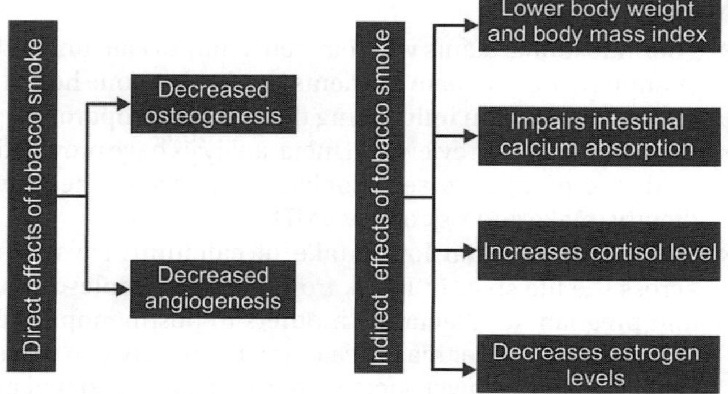

Fig. 10.6: Direct and indirect effects of tobacco smoke on bone.

 **Clinical Pointer**

Peak bone mass during childhood and adolescence and the rate of bone loss during aging are contributing factors for osteoporosis.

SIGNS AND SYMPTOMS

Osteoporosis has been often referred to in the literature as a **silent thief** because there are no specific visible symptoms associated with the decline in BMD until a fracture occurs. Some of the postural changes associated with osteoporosis include:

- **Kyphosis/Gibbus deformity or the Dowager's hump:** This is caused by vertebral compression fractures **(Fig. 10.7)**. With the hyperkyphosis and forward push of the head, the weight of the head will further augment the deforming forces of the spine and aggravate kyphosis **(Fig. 10.8)**. Kyphosis can also lead to a relative mismatch between the body's center of gravity and the base of support, which in turn makes the gait unsteady **(Box 10.2)**.

 **Clinical Pointer**

Clinically, a vertebra is considered fractured if the anterior height of the vertebral body is 80% or less of the posterior height. A new fracture requires loss of at least 20% of anterior height. In severe cases, the ribs contact the iliac crest and movement causes pain. This condition is called the **Iliocostal impingement syndrome** wherein the costal margin comes in contact with the iliac crest. The size of the gap between the costal margin and pelvic ridge (iliocostal distance) has been validated as a **clinical surrogate measure for the presence of osteoporosis and/or vertebral fragility fractures.**

- **Height loss:** Height loss is a frequent manifestation of vertebral osteoporosis. An irreversible height loss of 2 inches or more is a highly significant predictor of osteoporosis. However, some reversible height loss could also be seen due to poor posture.
- **Protruding abdomen:** The protruding abdomen which is a result of the kyphosis is a vastly under recognized consequence of osteoporosis.
- **Backache:** Back pain, caused by a fractured or collapsed vertebra.

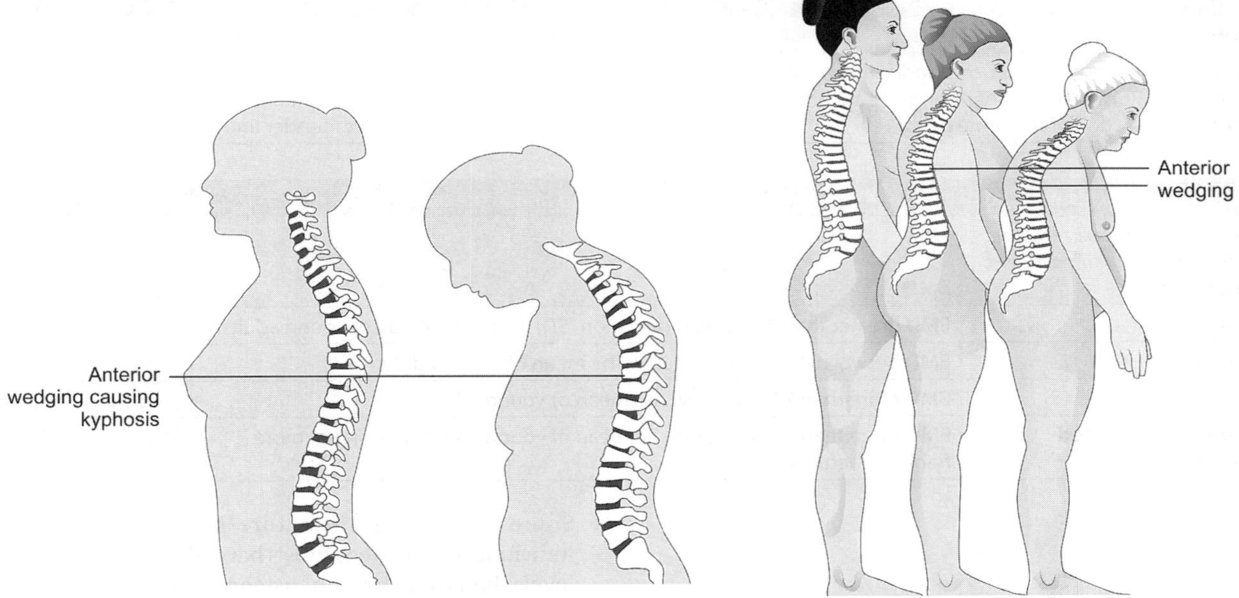

Fig. 10.7: Osteoporotic wedge compressions leading to Dowager's hump and reduced height.

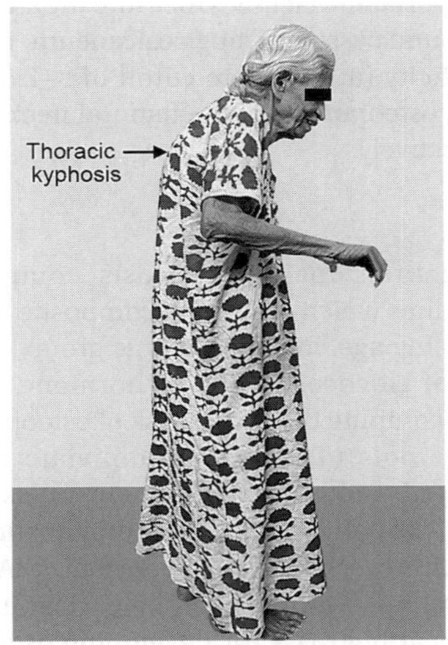

Fig. 10.8: Dorsal kyphosis in an elderly female causing Dowager's hump.

Box 10.2: Functional repercussions of kyphosis.

Difficulty in performing activities of daily living, a reduction in the balance, slower gait, respiratory concerns owing to impaired chest mobility, and higher postural sway which also augments the risk for falls.

- **Decreased pulmonary capacity:** Kyphosis seen in osteoporosis can lead to decreased lung volumes, which in severe cases can cause shortness of breath and pulmonary symptoms mimicking the restrictive lung disease.
- **Reflux esophagitis:** Seen in subjects with kyphosis due to the alterations in the abdominal space. Tight clothing can aggravate the problem.

DIAGNOSIS

Bone Mineral Density

Bone mineral density (BMD) is a measure for bone strength. It represents the amount of bone per unit area and is currently the most common surrogate of bone strength and gold standard for the diagnosis of osteoporosis and fracture risk assessment.

Table 10.2 shows difference between T-score and Z-score.

The World Health Organization (WHO) has defined osteopenia (low bone mass) as a site-specific bone density between 1.0 and 2.5 standard deviations less than the mean for young adults, and osteoporosis as a bone density that is 2.5 standard deviations less than the mean for young adult **(Table 10.3 and Fig. 10.9)**.

Clinical Pointer

Bone density test results are similar to interpreting an IQ score and the results are rated above, equal or below a statistically determined average. The **T-score** compares the subject's bone mass to that of an average young adult mean while the **Z-score** compares the subject's bone mass with that of individuals in a similar age group.

The bone mass of a given part of the skeleton is directly dependent upon both its volume or size and the density of the mineralized tissue contained within the periosteal envelope.

Table 10.2: Difference between T-score and the Z-score.

T-score	*Z-score*
The difference in the number of standard deviations between the mean BMD values of the patient and the mean of a young adult reference population of the same gender	The difference in the number of standard deviations between the mean BMD values of the patient and the mean of a reference population of the same race, gender and age

Table 10.3: WHO classification of low bone density and osteoporosis based on T-score.

Classification (Interpretation of T-Score for classification of Osteoporosis)	*BMD*	*T-score*
Normal	BMD greater than 1 standard deviation (SD) below the mean of young adults	(T-score: ≥ –1.0)
Osteopenia	BMD between 1 and 2.5 SD below the mean of young adults	(T-score: –1 to –2.5)
Osteoporosis	BMD more than 2.5 SD below the mean of young adults	(T-score: ≤ –2.5)
Severe or established osteoporosis	BMD more than 2.5 SD below the mean of young adults plus one or more fragility fractures	(T-score: ≤ –2.5)

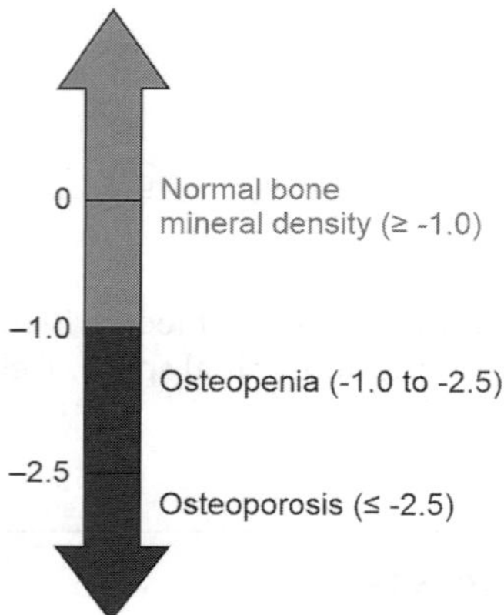

Fig. 10.9: WHO classification of low bone mineral density based on T-score *(For color version, see Plate 2).*

- Bone mineral density is measured through ***single and dual energy photon or X-ray absorptiometry*** **(SEXA and DEXA respectively).**
- **Dual-energy X-ray absorptiometry (DEXA)** imaging has a sentinel role in the evaluation of osteoporosis and is considered as the gold standard for diagnosing osteoporosis. *See* **Chapter 6:** Radiological Investigations in Women's Health.

Clinical Pointer

The International Society of Clinical Densitometry, the US Preventive Services Task Force (USPSTF), and the National Osteoporosis Foundation have all recommended an evaluation of BMD for all women over the age of 65 years.

Clinical Surrogate Measures that can Predict Osteoporosis

- **Dentition:** A decrease in bone density of the jaw may cause loosening of jawbone and loss of tooth may result due to poor anchoring of the teeth.
- Some evidence in literature has demonstrated that individuals with osteoporosis have **higher urinary calcium** levels than those without osteoporosis.
- **Quantitative ultrasound (QUS)** is used for measuring BMD in the peripheral skeleton. QUS for calcaneum is an inexpensive and safe screening tool for osteoporosis wherein small and portable machines measure the attenuation and speed of sound passing through calcaneum. The sensitivity and specificity (at a T-score cutoff of ≤–2.5) of QUS for predicting osteoporosis of the femoral neck are 82% and 50%, respectively.

Screening

- Screening tools for osteoporosis comprise simple questionnaires which evaluate a composite of risk factors viz. advancing age, high-risk ethnic group, weight, long-term use of glucocorticoids, or hormone replacement therapy to compute the overall risk of osteoporosis.
- Screening tools **(Table 10.4)** obliviate the need of sophisticated and costly equipment unless absolutely essential. Though they are not diagnostic tools, and therefore will never be a replacement for DEXA-based BMD assessment, however they can be crucial in identifying individuals at high-risk for developing osteoporosis. In addition, these tools are fast, easy to perform, cost effective, and possible to use in the rural Indian setting.

The Fracture Risk Assessment Tool (FRAX) predicts the risk of fractures with the aid of algorithms, excluding the measure of BMD, to identify those at risk for osteoporosis or fractures. The FRAX was implemented in 2008 by the World Health Organization and is used to calculate the chance of a fracture in a ten-year timeframe.

- The clinical risk factors included in FRAX are age, sex, race, height, weight, body mass index, a history of fracture, parent's history of hip fracture, use of oral glucocorticoids, rheumatoid arthritis, and other secondary causes of osteoporosis, smoking, alcohol use of three or more drinks daily, and the geographic area.

Table 10.4: Screening tools used for osteoporosis.

Name of the risk assessment tool	*Features*
Osteoporosis Self-Assessment Tool for Asians (OSTA)*	One-fifth of the difference between weight in kilogram and age in years (AUC** 0.806 in predicting femoral neck osteoporosis)
Osteoporosis Risk Assessment Instrument (ORAI)*	Age, weight, and estrogen therapy
Simple Calculated Osteoporosis Risk Estimation (SCORE)	Race, the presence of rheumatoid arthritis (RA), history of fractures, age, weight, and the use of estrogen therapy
Age, Bulk, One or Never Estrogen (ABONE)	Age, weight, and estrogen therapy
Male Osteoporosis Risk Estimation Score (MORES)*	To identify men at risk of osteoporosis

* Validated for use in the Indian population: The Indian Society for Bone and Mineral Research

**AUC: Area under the curve

- In the United States, the National Osteoporosis Foundation (NOF) recommends using FRAX to calculate fracture risk for patients who have T-scores between –1.0 and –2.5 in the spine, femoral neck, or total hip region.

Biochemical Investigations

The most common biochemical investigations used for the evaluation of osteoporosis (also *see* Chapter 5: Laboratory and Molecular Investigations in Women's Health) are the measurement of:

- Serum calcium
- Renal function
- Vitamin D3 levels
- Alkaline phosphatase levels
- Parathyroid hormone levels
- Thyroid function test

Osteoporosis-specific Quality of Life Questionnaires

- Quality of Life (QoL) is an assessment of an individual's self-perceptions in the context of their culture, value systems, personal goals, standards, and concerns which facilitate the aim of increasing life. Health-related QoL (HRQoL) is a subset of quality of life encompassing physical, mental, and social well-being.
- Physical, emotional, and psychological affliction along with the pain that results from fractures of the hip, spine or wrist, can alter the quality of life in the affected patients. Therefore, HRQoL is an important indicator of the clinical progression of patients with osteoporosis. **Table 10.5** enlists some common QoL assessment tools used in osteoporosis.

PREVENTION

Clinical Pointer

Prevention is the key: It's never too early and never too late.

In view of the fact that there are no safe and effective ways to rebuild the osteoporotic skeleton, prevention strategies emerge as a crucial pre-emptive method of limiting the incidence as well as the disability associated with osteoporosis.

Table 10.5: Commonly used QoL assessment tools in osteoporosis.

Name of QoL assessment tool	*Target population features*
Women's Health Questionnaire (WHQ)	Covers specific symptoms in menopausal and postmenopausal women
Osteoporosis Quality of Life Questionnaire (30 items)	Symptoms, physical function, activities of daily living, emotional function, and leisure
Mini-Osteoporosis Quality of Life Questionnaire (10 items)	Symptoms, physical function, activities of daily living, emotional function, and leisure
Osteoporosis Assessment Questionnaire	Overall well-being, Physical function, psychological status, symptoms, and social interaction
Osteoporosis Assessment Questionnaire Short Version	Physical function, emotional status, and symptoms
Osteoporosis Functional Disability Questionnaire	Pain, depression, functional status, social activities, and confidence
Quality of Life Questionnaire of the European Foundation for Osteoporosis	Pain, physical function, social function, general health perception, and mental function
Osteoporosis-targeted Quality of Life	Elderly women with or without clinical osteoporosis Domains of physical activity, adaptations for activities of daily living, and fears
16-item Assessment of Health-related Quality of Life in Osteoporosis	Physical function, disease-related fear, psychosocial status, and pain
Quality of Life Questionnaire in Osteoporosis	Fear of the future, self-image, well-being, mobility, localized pain, and specific mental repercussions

Primary Prevention

It involves identification of those at risk. It has following salient features:

- Begin early.
- Public awareness is crucial.
- Bone health can be optimized by creating an environment to achieve peak bone mass during adolescence, maintenance of healthy bone throughout the life cycle, and prevention of bone loss at menopause.
- **Minimize loss at menopause:** As bone is lost more rapidly in the years immediately after menopause, it is important to institute measures to reduce the loss of bone prior to or at the time of menopause.
- A variety of moderate-impact exercises and strength training have been shown to reduce the rate of loss of bone mass in the postmenopausal period even in those with low BMD.
- Ensure adequate calcium intake.
- Ensure adequate vitamin D intake. Minimum of 5–15 minutes of exposure to sunshine on hands, arms, and face is essential.
- **Physical activity:** Avoid a sedentary lifestyle. Get plenty of weight-bearing exercise, such as walking, aerobics, etc. Exercise three days a week, 30 minutes each time, or in three 10-minute segments over the course of the day.
- Gain weight if underweight.
- No smoking and limiting alcohol and caffeine-rich foods and drinks.
- Reduce bone loss by:
  - Hormone replacement therapy (HRT)
  - Regular exercise
  - Lifestyle modification
  - Adequate calcium intake

Secondary Prevention

It involves treatment of those who have already had an osteoporotic fracture.

ICF AND OSTEOPOROSIS

The tiered structure of the ICF provides an explicit list of health and health-related categories affected in patients with osteoporosis. ICF in osteoporosis **(Table 10.6)** represents the typical spectrum of problems in functioning and contextual factors that may influence the functioning of patients with osteoporosis. The domains include physical health, social health, mental health, and handicap/participation. Along with this are the subdomains with different levels of importance, such as pain, mobility, self-care, activities/roles, and need for support, as well as anxiety/depression and loss of self-esteem.

MANAGEMENT

Osteoporosis can be managed through the following measures:

- Pharmacological (antiresorptive and anabolic drugs)
- Relief of symptoms—e.g., pain relief
- Lifestyle modifications (dietary intake, weight-bearing exercise, hip protectors, and fall prevention measures).

Pharmacological Management

The primary aim of pharmacotherapy in osteoporosis is to increase bone density and reduce the incidence of future fracture risk. The drugs used for these purposes can be broadly classified into two types:

1. **Drugs that retard bone resorption** (estrogens, calcitonin, and bisphosphonates)
2. **Drugs that stimulate bone formation** (teriparatide and strontium ranelate).

PHYSIOTHERAPY ASSESSMENT

- *Risk factors*
- *Current pain levels*
- *Musculoskeletal:* Strength, ROM, posture, mobility and gait
- *Balance and coordination*
- *Cardiovascular assessment*
- *Current activity levels*
- *Quality of life*
- *Psychosocial assessment:* Decreased functional status and independence, social relationships, emotional well-being, depression, sleep problems, reduced appetite.

Exercise Testing in Osteoporosis

Exercise testing (ET) in osteoporosis as per standard ET guidelines for exercise prescription.

Box 10.3 enlists some precautions that need to be followed during exercise testing in subjects suspected of having osteoporosis.

PHYSIOTHERAPY MANAGEMENT

Managing a patient with a confirmed diagnosis of osteoporosis/osteopenia encompasses:

- Fracture risk assessment
- Assessment of any secondary causes of skeletal fragility

Table 10.6: International classification of functioning, disability, and health (ICF): Some domains from the comprehensive ICF core set for osteoporosis.

Body functions	*Body structure*	*Activities and participation*	*Environmental factors*
• Sensation of pain • Muscle power functions • Mobility of joint functions • Emotional functions	• Structure of trunk • Structure of lower extremity	• Walking • Lifting and carrying objects • Recreation and leisure	• Health services, systems and policies • Products or substances for personal consumption • Health professionals

Box 10.3: Some precautions to be followed during the testing procedure

- In patients with severe vertebral osteoporosis, for whom walking is painful, cycle ergometer is preferred as an alternative to treadmill exercise testing to assess cardiovascular function.
- In cases with a risk of osteoporosis, when using Treadmill for exercise tolerance, use a walking protocol instead of running to reduce the impact forces.
- In all protocols, as a precaution—keep the spine upright as flexion might increase the strain on the anterior wall of weakened vertebral bodies, thus increasing the likelihood of fracture.
- Vertebral compression fractures leading to a loss of height and spinal deformation can compromise ventilatory capacity.
- Forward shift in the center of gravity owing to hyperkyphosis, may affect balance during treadmill walking.
- Pre-exercise evaluation
- Screening programs such as the Physical Activity Readiness Questionnaire (PAR-Q) can be used to identify any abnormalities in the cardiovascular, pulmonary, musculoskeletal, metabolic or endocrine systems that should prevent physical activity.
- A companion tool to the PAR-Q, the Physical Activity Readiness Medical Examination (PARmed-X) is intended for use by physicians whose patients have been referred because of a positive response to one or more questions on the PAR-Q.
- Previous and current physical activity levels, use of medications, alcohol and cigarettes are reviewed.
- To facilitate better compliance, the exercise program must be tailored as per the patient's interests in form of sporting and activity preferences. A questionnaire on lifestyle would help in developing an individually appropriate and interesting program.

- Clinical decision-making on most efficient treatment
- Identification and management of all relevant clinical factors that may influence patient management.

General Aims of Physiotherapy Management

- To decrease pain
- To improve mobility
- To increase bone density
- To improve muscle strength, fitness, agility, endurance, balance
- To improve chest mobility and ventilation
- To decrease risk of fractures by falls prevention
- To improve activity and participation with or without assistive devices
- To improve mental health profile

Managing Pain in Osteoporosis

- While osteoporosis-related fractures may lead to acute pain, chronic pain, especially back pain, is a characteristic feature of severe osteoporosis.
- Bodily changes in patients with osteoporosis, joint imbalance, and muscular tension, may also lead to pain thus emphasizing the need for a multidimensional approach to decrease pain, and preserve and improve quality of life.
- Fragility fractures can cause a progressive loss of height and prolonged contraction of the paravertebral muscles in maintaining posture. These static postures can also cause muscle fatigue and pain.
- Chronic pain in subjects with osteoporosis can have origin from myriad sensory inputs including postural alterations, fractures, and muscle atrophy along with features of nociceptive and neuropathic pain.
- The evaluation of pain in patients with osteoporosis entails a holistic approach that includes the specific characteristics of the target population, and assesses their comorbidities, mental status and functional status (ability to carry activities as well as participation).
- Pain management may include pharmacological approaches, physiotherapy interventions, and some alternative therapies including Yoga, Tai Chi, etc.
- Postural taping can be used to increase proprioceptive feedback on correct postural alignment, improve thoracic extension, reduce pain, facilitate muscle activity and improve postural balance.
- In addition, soft manual tissue manipulation techniques and central posterior-anterior mobilization techniques have been found to be effective in managing pain.
- Low-frequency pulsed electromagnetic fields have found support in literature to relieve the pain of primary osteoporosis.
- Whole-body vibrations have been found effective in enhancing physical fitness by improving muscle strength and axial stability, neuromuscular coordination, and balance and reducing the risk of falls.
- Cognitive-behavioral therapy and mindfulness-based interventions are used to aid the subject to understand and accept the pain and promote self-control and coping strategies.

Braces for Osteoporotic Spine

- Orthoses play a vital role in stabilizing the compromised spine and providing adequate support for correct vertical alignment of the spine.
- They combine a **tension belt system** and anatomically shaped **adjustable rods**. This system helps alleviate pain and discomfort by relieving the excessive anterior compression of the vertebrae. The added stability has a positive effect on the psychological state of patients.

Anterior Spinal Hyperextension Brace (ASH Brace) (Fig. 10.10)

Functions:

- To immobilize the vertebral column
- To stabilize and maintain the spine in neutral/slight hyperextension
- To facilitate cervical and lumbar lordosis, relieving pressure on the anterior vertebral bodies

Dynamic hyperextension brace (DHB), is a novel dynamic orthosis introduced by Dr Sinaki. This brace focuses on strengthening the spinal extensors using a weighted kypho-orthosis and postural and proprioceptive training.

The unremitting pressure of the weight of DHB on the spine induces osteogenesis and subsequently decrease the rate of osteoporosis and kyphosis by improving the bone mineral density.

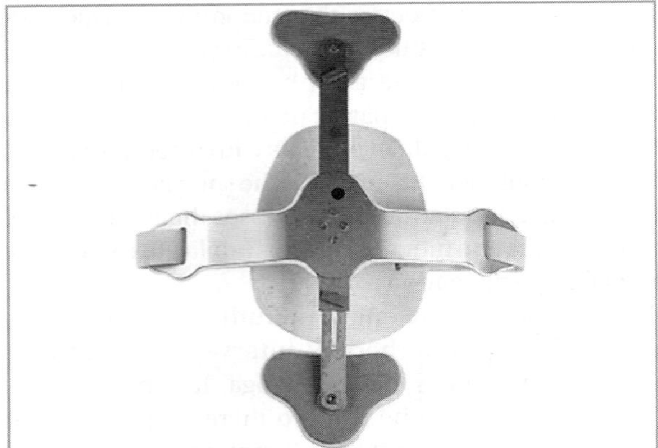

Fig. 10.10: Anterior spinal hyperextension (ASH) brace.

Role of Exercise in the Management of Osteoporosis

The rationale for the type of exercise in osteoporosis: In the late eighteenth century, Julius Wolff found that the bones adapt their microstructure according to the external mechanical environment. This hypothesis formed the basis of the mechanostat (mechanotransduction) theory of bone adaptation which states that bone deforms as a result of mechanical loading (compressive or tensile strains) which in turn, triggers an osteogenic bone response. Revolutionary research by Hert et al. documented that bone tissue responds best to dynamic rather than static loading. This implies that static loads (even those that produce fairly large stresses or strains) do not initiate osteogenesis. Therefore, stress or strain in the tissue cannot by itself be the primary stimulus for a cellular response. On the other hand, dynamic loading creates fluid movement generating shear stresses on the plasma membranes of resident osteocytes, bone lining cells, and osteoblasts. In response to this shear stress, the bone cells respond by initiating a cascade of cellular events.

High-impact exercises that produce large rates of deformation of the bone matrix best drive fluid through the lacunar-canalicular network system. Therefore, increasing the loading rate is an effective application of mechanical forces to promote osteogenesis.

Moreover, to stimulate the osteogenic effects for bone mass accretion, **the bone tissues must be exposed to unusual mechanical load exceeding those experienced during daily living activities.** Walking as an exercise is generally not effective in preventing bone loss in healthy ambulant individuals. This is because walking does not impart high loading forces onto the bone, nor does it represent a unique loading stimulus, both of which are important pre-requisites for osteogenic exercises **(Box 10.4)**. However, this does not exclude the possibility that long-term habitual walking for many years helps to preserve bone mass.

Strengthening through Resistance and Weight-bearing Exercises

- Exercise training in the form of resistance exercise (RE) has been recommended as an effective therapeutic strategy to encounter the loss of bone and muscle mass due to osteosarcopenia.

Box 10.4: Osteogenic exercises.

A rehabilitative exercise method carried out with the goal of stimulating osteogenesis that improves bone mineral density and helps prevent fragility fracture.

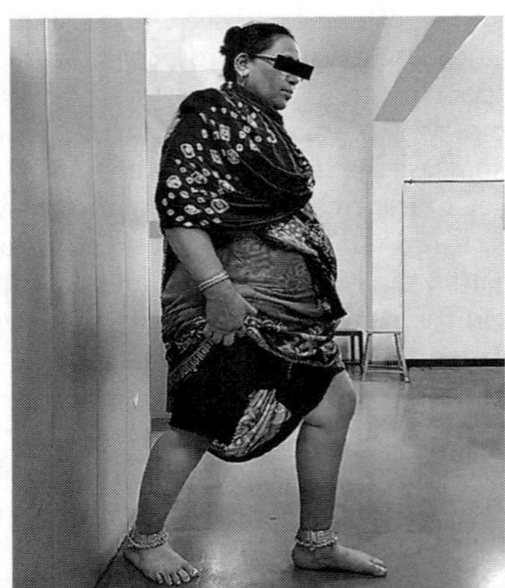

Fig. 10.11: Weight-bearing exercise.

- The benefits from RE in terms of BMD gain/preservation are achieved when the resistance is progressively increased over time and the magnitude of load is high (around 80–85% 1 RM). **Figure 10.11** shows a weight bearing (WB) exercise.

Tai Chi

Tai chi (TC) is a traditional systematic physical activity of Chinese origin, that employs specific regimens of physical movement, breathing techniques, and cognitive exercises (both visualization and focused internal awareness) with the aim of strengthening, relaxation, and optimum physical functioning and mental health. Evidence in literature is supportive of the role of TC as one of the nonpharmacological therapy treatments of osteoporosis.

Reducing Falls Risk

- Falling is an important risk factor for fracture. Though skeletal fragility causes increased susceptibility to fracture, however, it would be of little concern if potentially damaging loads, like those generated in a fall, were prevented.
- The incidence of falls **(Fig. 10.12)** increases with age because several sensory systems that control posture (vestibular, visual, and somatosensory) become compromised with advancing age and risk of falling increases rapidly with age.
- Muscle mass and muscle strength are known to increase stability, and can therefore be worked upon through appropriate exercises to counter instability and loss of balance which may lead to falls.

Clinical Pointer

Aquatic exercise may be utilized as a viable exercise option along with Land exercises to improve function and balance, thus ultimately decreasing risk of fall and any subsequent hip fractures in osteopenic and osteoporotic subjects.

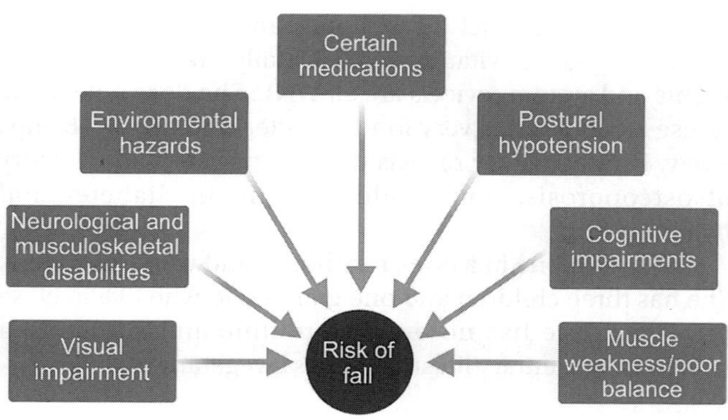

Fig. 10.12: Risk factors for fall.

Dietary Modifications

Calcium Intake

- An adequate calcium intake is considered essential for the positive effects of exercise to occur. Postmenopausal women, require greater calcium intake to retain calcium balance because of increased urinary calcium losses associated with low estrogen levels.
- The recommended daily intake (RDA) of calcium in postmenopausal women is 1,200 mg per day.

Vitamin D

Oral vitamin D supplementation of 700–800 IU/day appears to reduce the risk of hip and any nonvertebral fractures.

Table 10.7 provides the physiotherapy management of osteoporosis as per the BMD status of the subject.

Community Approach for Management of Osteoporosis

- One of the prominent regimes which have proven to be effective in this domain is the Osteofit exercise-based program, designed by the staff of the British Columbia Women's Hospital Centre Osteoporosis Program in Vancouver, Canada.
- Osteofit targets the following realms: Posture, balance, gait, coordination, and hip and trunk stabilization.
- Benefits of osteofit:
  - Improved performance in ADLs
  - Reduced backache
  - Improved general well-being
  - Lessened risk as well as fear of fall in subjects with decreased BMD

Box 10.5 provides a sample program for a female at risk of osteoporosis.

Box 10.5: Sample program for a female with risk of osteoporosis.

- **Warm up:** 20-minute (10 minutes of gentle stretching and Mobility+ 10 minutes of aerobic exercises)
- **Cardiovascular exercises:** Target heart rate 60% of HR_{Max} (220 – age) for a deconditioned woman and 70–75% for intermediate health
- **Resistance training:** Light free weights and rubber tubing, calisthenics targeting the major muscle groups. Examples:
  - Upper arm exercises—pushing/pulling/twisting against a wall
  - Quadriceps strengthening: Wall slide (squat) exercise or standing from a seated position.
  - Trunk stabilization: (i.e., core stability) exercises progressed from crook lying position to sitting and standing.
- **Posture correction:** Back posture correction exercises in standing, in a chair or prone.
- **Balance exercises:**
  - Hold a tandem stance for 10 seconds with their eyes open while holding onto the support.
  - Single leg stance with eyes open (then eyes closed), tandem forward walking, walking backward, and tandem backwards walking.
- **Functional activities:** Stair climbing, chair sit to stand to improve ADLs
- **Cool-down period:** 15-minute stretches sitting on the floor.

Table 10.7: Physiotherapy management of osteoporosis as per BMD status.

Category	*Subjects with positive risk of osteoporosis*	*Subjects with osteoporosis*	*Subjects with severe osteoporosis*
Aim	• General aims • Increase/maintain bone mass	• General aims • Maintain bone mass • Prevent fractures • Prevent falls	• General aims • Control pain • Maintain bone mass • Prevent further fractures • Reduce risk of falls • Improve balance
Exercises	• Brisk walk • Jogging • Aerobics • Cycling **(Fig. 10.13)** • Any other high impact physical activity	• Postural correction • Aerobic training • Strength training • Brisk walk • Balance exercises • Aquatherapy	• Slow walking • Swimming • Balance training • Pain management • Aquatherapy
	Special considerations/precautions		
	Pelvic floor muscle weakness	• No high impact exercise/physical activity • Avoid trunk flexion, lifting weights	
	Inability to perform with correct technique		

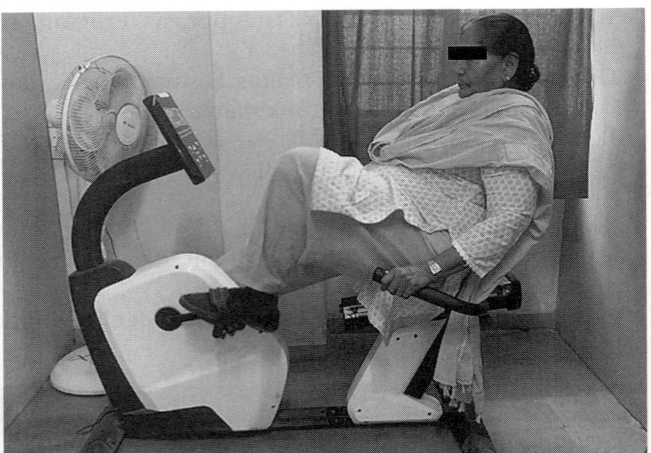

Fig. 10.13: Cycling.

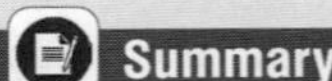

Summary

Osteoporosis is a syndrome of dysadaptation which leads to low bone mass, bone microarchitecture disruption of bone tissue, decreased skeletal strength, and increased redisposition to fractures at different sites such as the spine, hip, or wrist.

Evidence in the literature is suggestive of a great lack of knowledge about the awareness of osteoporosis. Healthcare professionals need to be more interested in initiating primary prevention, screening and prevention of osteoporosis among people who are at high risk. The key to long-term decline in incidence of osteoporosis is through prevention and screening. The aim of management in osteoporosis is geared towards improving/maintaining BMD and preventing any potential fall which might fracture the susceptible bone.

CLINICAL EXAMPLE

Mrs XYZ is a 52-year-old female experiencing diffuse bone pain over the past several years after menopause (5 years back). She has a history of fractures to her left hip and wrist. She complains that her back pain is becoming worse and is now hindering her daily activities such as lifting grocery bags and her grandchild without pain. She is not on any medication except vitamin E 400 IU daily. Her gynecological exams and system reviews are all WNL. She does not smoke or use alcohol but is very fond of coffee and takes 7–8 cups a day. Family history reveals that her mother had a history of osteoporosis, non-insulin dependent diabetes and hypertension.

She lives alone in a one-story house and works as a clerk. She has three children and one grandchild who live in close proximity. She has no exercise routine and admits to a somewhat sedentary lifestyle. She is a vegetarian.

Physical Examination

- Afebrile with unremarkable findings with exception to the musculoskeletal system.
- She weighs 50 kg and is 5 feet 3 inches. At her last exam 18 months ago, she was 5 feet 4 inches.
- On observation and palpation: Mild Dowager's hump, no edema, redness or heat present in joint areas.
- Mobility: Muscle guarding and tenderness are present in the thoracic and lumbar spine with limited range of motion.

Investigation

DEXA scan showed a T score of -2.2.

Positive Risk Factors

Postmenopausal; therefore, estrogen deficient, heredity, small body size, thin stature and lifestyle choices (sedentary, deficient diet, no exercise or sun exposure, excessive coffee intake).

Provisional Diagnosis

Postmenopausal osteoporosis

Suggested Management

- Diet and supplements: Avoid excessive coffee intake.
- Exercises **(Table 10.8)**: Brisk walking, weight-bearing exercises, resistance exercises (osteogenic exercises) to improve BMD.
- Tai Chi initiated to increase bone mass and balance.

Table 10.8: Exercise considerations for osteoporosis.

Training method	*Mode*	*Frequency, intensity, and time*	*Progression*	*Goals*	*Special considerations/ comments*
Aerobic	Walking or stationary cycling	4–5 times per week at a moderate intensity; start at 20 min/session if the patient has a minimal history of exercise	Increase speed and distance gradually after initial 2 weeks	30–45 min at ≥ 3.0 mph for walking; ≥70 rpm for cycling	Avoid jogging and activities that increase fall risk like step aerobics

Contd...

Contd...

Training method	***Mode***	***Frequency, intensity, and time***	***Progression***	***Goals***	***Special considerations/ comments***
Strength	Resistance training	Start at 1–2 days/week depending on the client; 15 repetitions of 8–10 exercise (may require less strenuous program initially)	Add a set after initial 2 weeks	3–4 days/week at 10–12 repetition/set	Avoid spinal flexion during all exercises; use slow and controlled movements; target legs and back
Range of motion	Stretching	5–7 days/week for 10–12 minutes; hold each stretch for approximately 15–20 seconds		Increase or maintain range of motion	Stretching exercises involving spinal flexion should be avoided

Review Questions

1. What are the factors that make Indian females more vulnerable to a decline in BMD?
2. Enlist the differences between cortical and cancellous bones.
3. Why are the cancellous bones at a greater risk of osteoporosis?
4. List three common sites of osteoporotic fractures.
5. Describe the physiology of bone remodeling process.
6. List any three determinants of bone strength.
7. What are the two major types of osteoporosis?
8. What is secondary osteoporosis? Describe four major reasons that can cause secondary osteoporosis.
9. What is PBM? Give its significance for future risk of fragility fractures.
10. Describe modifiable and nonmodifiable risk factors for osteoporosis.
11. Discuss the direct and indirect effect of tobacco smoke on bone
12. Write a short note on drug-induced osteoporosis.
13. Discuss the various signs and symptoms of osteoporosis.
14. Why is osteoporosis referred to as a "silent killer"?
15. What is the gold standard for assessment of osteoporosis.
16. Differentiate between T-score and Z-score.
17. Write briefly about the WHO classification of low bone density and osteoporosis based on BMD.
18. What are various valid tools for assessment of risk factors for osteoporosis in Indian subjects?
19. Write a short note on primary prevention of osteoporosis.
20. Discuss in detail the physiotherapy management of osteopenic and osteoporotic females.
21. Discuss the role of weight-bearing/resistance exercise for the management of BMD deficits.
22. Enlist the precautions to be followed during the testing procedure in females suspected with osteoporosis.
23. Write a short note on: "osteogenic exercises" for the management of osteoporosis.

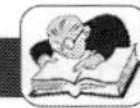

Bibliography

1. Ahuja M. Age of menopause and determinants of menopause age: A PAN India survey by IMS. J Midlife Health. 2016;7(3):126-31. doi: 10.4103/0976-7800.191012. PMID: 27721640; PMCID: PMC5051232
2. Al-Bashaireh AM, Haddad LG, Weaver M, Chengguo X, Kelly DL, et al. The effect of tobacco smoking on bone mass: An overview of pathophysiologic mechanisms. J Osteoporos. 2018;2018:17. Article ID 1206235, *https*://doi.org/10.1155/2018/1206235
3. Mahan LK, Escott-Stump S, Raymond JL. Krause's Food and the Nutrition Care Process,13th edition. St Louis: Elsevier; 2012.
4. Malhotra A, Mithal A. Osteoporosis in Indians. Indian J Med Res. 2008;127:263-68.
5. Meeta M, Harinarayan CV, Marwah R, Sahay R, Kalra S, Babhulkar S. Clinical practice guidelines on postmenopausal osteoporosis: *An executive summary and recommendations – Update 20192020. J Midlife Health. 2020;11:96-112.
6. Mithal A, Kaur P. Osteoporosis in Asia: a call to action. Current Osteoporosis Reports. 2012;10(4):245-47.
7. Panday K, Gona A, Humphrey MB. Medication-induced osteoporosis: screening and treatment strategies. Ther Adv Musculoskelet Dis. 2014;6(5):185-202. https://doi.org/10.1177/1759720X14546350
8. Population based reference standards of Peak Bone Mineral Density of Indian males and females–an ICMR multi-centre task force study. New Delhi; 2010. www.icmr.nic.in
9. Salari N, Ghasemi H, Mohammadi L, et al. The global prevalence of osteoporosis in the world: a comprehensive systematic review and meta-analysis. J Orthop Surg Res. 2021;16(1):609. DOI: 10.1186/s13018-021-02772-0. PMID: 34657598; PMCID: PMC8522202.
10. Weaver CM, Gordon CM, Janz KF, et al. The National Osteoporosis Foundation's position statement on peak bone mass development and lifestyle factors: a systematic review and implementation recommendations. Osteoporos Int. 2016;27:1281-1386. https://doi.org/10.1007/s00198-015-3440-3.

Multiple Choice Questions (MCQs)

To test your understanding and recall of key concepts.

1. **Which of the following statements is correct with respect to osteoporosis?**
   A. Increased bone density
   B. Microarchitectural deterioration of bones
   C. Inflammatory condition of the joints
   D. Excessive calcium deposition in the bones

2. **Which type of bone is most susceptible to osteoporosis-related changes?**
   A. Cortical bone
   B. Cancellous bone
   C. Compact bone
   D. Osteoid bone
3. **Which of the following is the gold standard test for evaluation of osteoporosis?**
   A. Bone scintigraphy
   B. Dual-energy X-ray absorptiometry (DEXA)
   C. Quantitative ultrasound (QUS)
   D. Computed tomography (CT)
4. **Why are postmenopausal women at higher risk for osteoporosis?**
   A. Increased calcium absorption from the gut
   B. Estrogen deficiency leads to increased osteoclastic activity
   C. Testosterone suppresses bone formation in women
   D. Estrogen enhances renal calcium excretion
5. **What role does vitamin D play in bone health?**
   A. Inhibits bone resorption by osteoclasts
   B. Enhances calcium absorption in the gut
   C. Increases urinary calcium excretion
   D. Stimulates osteoclastogenesis
6. **A 60-year-old woman presents with back pain and a history of low-impact fractures. Her DEXA T-score is -2.8. Which of the following would be the best initial management?**
   A. High-impact aerobic exercise
   B. Calcium, vitamin D, and bisphosphonates
   C. Complete bed rest to prevent further fractures
   D. Anabolic steroids and complete bed rest
7. **A patient with low bone mineral density and back pain seeks physiotherapy management. Which of the following exercises should be avoided?**
   A. Resistance training
   B. Weight-bearing exercises
   C. Trunk flexion exercises
   D. Aerobic exercises
8. **A healthcare program proposes an osteoporosis prevention strategy focusing on public awareness, dietary supplementation, and lifestyle modification. Which element is *most* critical for primary prevention?**
   A. Screening postmenopausal women for osteoporosis
   B. Educating adolescents about peak bone mass attainment
   C. Promoting surgical interventions for high-risk individuals
   D. Encouraging bed rest in elderly individuals
9. **A patient with osteoporosis experiences frequent falls due to poor balance and muscle weakness. Which combination of interventions is *most* effective?**
   A. Tai Chi, balance training, and resistance exercises
   B. Bed rest, analgesics, and high-impact exercises
   C. Cycling, aerobic training, and vitamin C supplements
   D. Postural taping, aquatic exercises, and meditation

ANSWERS

1. B	2. B	3. B	4. B	5. B
6. B	7. C	8. B	9. A	

Chapter 11

The Elderly Female

Apurv Shimpi, Anu Arora

"Aging is Gendered"

LEARNING OBJECTIVES

At the end of the chapter, the reader will be able to:

- Understand the need to address the female geriatric population as a unique entity.
- Understand the concept of evidence-based practice in the domain of geriatric physiotherapy.
- Evaluate an older adult using appropriate functional measures with an understanding of contraindications and concerns.
- Understand and assess the impact on bone health, pelvic floor muscle, and cognition in elderly women and devise appropriate screening and intervention measures.
- Understand the concept of neuromotor exercise training for older adults.
- Gain an insight into strategies to improve compliance to exercise regime in older adults.

CHAPTER OUTLINE

INTRODUCTION

Aging is defined as a decline in functional capacity and resistance to various stressors with the passage of time, leading to an increased risk of morbidity and mortality in subjects of advancing age.

Demographic transitions over the years have favored a unidirectional rise in the life expectancy of the population across the barriers of geography, caste, culture, and even the socio-economic strata. These transitions are a direct consequence of improved healthcare delivery services and the adoption of healthy lifestyles.

However, the demographic changes are impacting the genders in very distinctive manners and have forced gerontologists to focus attention on the gender bias in population aging. Epidemiological studies have found females to be the leading gender among the aged in terms of sheer numbers. Even though there exists some mutual fundamental needs and concerns for both elderly males as well as females, however, the fact remains that women and men age differently—not just physically and physiologically, but emotionally and socially as well.

Society world over, witnesses a level of discrimination against the older people for both women and men, however when the gender-based discrimination further adds to aging bias, it creates a "double whammy", especially for the females. Globally, the gender gap in life expectancy is 4.2 years wherein the male has an average life expectancy of 68, while the women's life expectancy is 72.2 years.

While it is widely accepted that decline in health parameters positively correlates with age in both men and women, there is limited awareness of the distinctiveness of the health-related changes in elderly females as compared to elderly males.

REPERCUSSIONS OF ADVANCING AGE ON PHYSICAL AND MENTAL HEALTH

The musculoskeletal system is often the first to be affected by age. The eyes, followed by the ears, begin to decline in function early in midlife. Most of the internal physiological functions also tend to decline with age gradually but continuously after the age of 30.

Aging can also affect sex hormones. This effect is much more pronounced in females than males because of the dramatic decline in estrogen with menopause. In comparison, the level of testosterone in males also decreases with age, but the transition is much more gradual.

Mental health is essential to overall health and well-being. A large proportion (almost 20%) of older adults experience some type of mental health concern. These could include anxiety, severe cognitive impairment, and even mood disorders (like depression or bipolar disorder).

These mental health concerns not only are associated with distress and suffering but can also lead to impairments in physical, mental, and social functioning.

Despite the decline in functions and capacities with age, most organs possess much more functional capacity than the body's current **needs (functional reserve)**. Therefore comorbidities, rather than changes brought by normal aging, are usually accountable for age-associated functional decline.

This functional decline makes older adults more susceptible to various stressors, like physical stresses in form of strenuous physical activity or environmental stresses like extreme temperature variations.

Vulnerability of females to the above further increases in view of:

- Financial dependence on others
- Dependence on the dynamic hormonal milieu
- Sociocultural factors promoting malnutrition
- Higher psychological distress

Furthermore, in comparison to males, elderly females fare poorly on most indicators of subjective well-being and mental health.

GENDER BIAS IN DIFFERENTIAL EPIDEMIOLOGY OF CHRONIC DISEASES

There exists a difference in the prevalence of chronic diseases and other health conditions suffered by each gender.

- While men suffer more than women from cancer and heart disease, which are key factors of mortality, women, in turn, have higher rates of chronic conditions, such as arthritis, depression, osteoporosis, and related fractures.
- Evidence in literature has also shown that women suffer from higher morbidity than men due to acute and chronic physical and psychiatric diseases.
- In addition, at age 60 and over, men have greater incidence of hearing loss, injuries resulting from falls, and neck and back pain, while women suffer more than men from problems of vision loss, depressive disorders, osteoarthritis, urinary incontinence, and frailty.
- The incidence and prevalence of dementia is higher among women, partially due to women's greater longevity, and the increased chance of dementia onset with aging.

Disability is evaluated by measures of difficulties in performing personal care-related activities of daily living (ADL) including basic personal activities, such as eating, getting dressed, washing, and using the toilet, and instrumental activities of daily living (IADL), such as home maintenance activities, managing money, walking and climbing stairs. "Life expectancy with disability" is the measure used to assess functioning throughout the life course. According to evaluations based on this measure, women on average live more years with disability than men, and the years lived with disabilities accumulate in old age.

National and international comparisons indicate that women have an advantage over men in life expectancy, but they are disadvantaged in almost all dimensions of quality of life-related to health, functioning, and subjective well-being. Yet, there are indications that personal, family, and national orientations regarding gender roles influence gender equality in health.

This susceptibility of the women of advancing age and the special types of problems they are likely to come across over their lifespan, which could possibly even marginalize them, make it imperative to treat this subgroup of women, with greater sensitivity and knowledge and focus on differences in the aging experience of females compared to males.

HEALTH AFFECTION IN ELDERLY FEMALES

World Health Organization has defined Health as a state of complete physical, mental and social well-being and not merely the absence of disease or infirmity. This definition makes health a multifaceted phenomenon, which alludes to a lack of physical and mental disease along with dimensions of quality of life as perceived and facilitated by society.

Physical Health in Aging Females

Physical functioning is an important marker of healthy aging. Physical health is a reflection of the health parameters of life expectancy, lack of disease, and infirmity. Physical functions, such as muscle function, ability to walk, soft tissue flexibility, balance, respiratory function, and bone mineral density decline with age.

- Comparative evaluation of age-related strength loss in human females and males revealed that though the age-related loss in isometric strength does not show any gender bias, the peak torque decline is gender-related, which could be the reason behind differential rate of age-related functional decline. On one hand, while it is established that women generally live longer than men, it also leads to more years of their lives with functional limitations.
- Older women score significantly lower on most indicators of subjective well-being.
- There is a higher rate of decline in flexibility in men compared to women requiring an early intervention for flexibility enhancement strategy.

The gender-specific decline in physical functions calls for appropriate timing and gender-based interventions for older people **(Fig. 11.1)**.

Sarcopenia and Sarcopenic Obesity in Elderly Females

Sarcopenia is age-related loss of lean body mass which is associated with many adverse health outcomes, such as:

- Increased risk of falls and fractures
- Impaired aerobic performance
- Disability
- Mortality

Sarcopenic obesity (SO) on the other hand is a combination of sarcopenia and obesity which is characterized by excess body fat and reduced muscle mass and strength. In SO, there is a synergistic negative influence of obesity with reduced muscle mass in older adults, leading to sarcopenic obesity. Therefore, sarcopenic obesity is aptly considered as the confluence of two current epidemics—rise in obesity and aging population.

It has been found that sarcopenic obesity has been associated with an amplified risk of disability in daily living, mortality, metabolic syndrome, and cardiovascular disease along with some other co-existing concerns like osteoarthritis, osteoporosis, and depression in elderly populations.

In a recently conducted systematic review and meta-analysis, it was indicated that, SO affects more than one in ten older adults globally.

Biological Causes for SO

The primary biological factors that lead to sarcopenic obesity are age-associated changes in metabolism and body composition. These are augmented by coexisting obesogenic environmental factors and concomitant physical concerns that develop with normal aging.

Gender-specific Hormonal Variation: Role of Estrogen

Estrogen deficiency post menopause causes an increase in body weight and fat mass, specifically in the visceral region along with age-associated decline in muscle. Estrogen can attenuate this through modulation of inflammation in skeletal muscle through satellite cell activation.

Assessment and Management

Figure 11.2 describes assessment of sarcopenia.

Exercise can attenuate some hormonal imbalance, lessen oxidative stress, and encourage mitochondrial synthesis along with altering the immunological and motor function and improving muscle oxidative capacity. In a prefrail and frail population, a strategy combining exercises (Resistance + Aerobics) along with appropriate and adequate nutritional interventions are effective in combating SO **(Fig. 11.3)**.

Cardiovascular Health in Aging Females

Coronary artery disease is much more prevalent in males under the age of 40 years as compared to females. Though the gender bias in the prevalence disappears in those aged 40–60 years, however, it shoots up in elderly women (>60 years) wherein the prevalence of CAD is even greater than in males. Evidence suggests that the clinical indicators of CHD appear

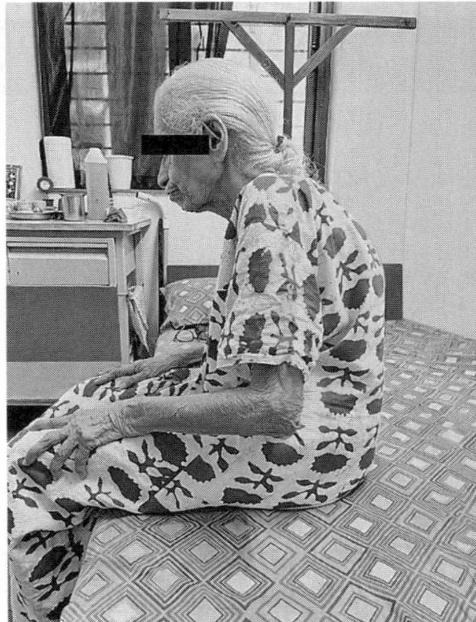
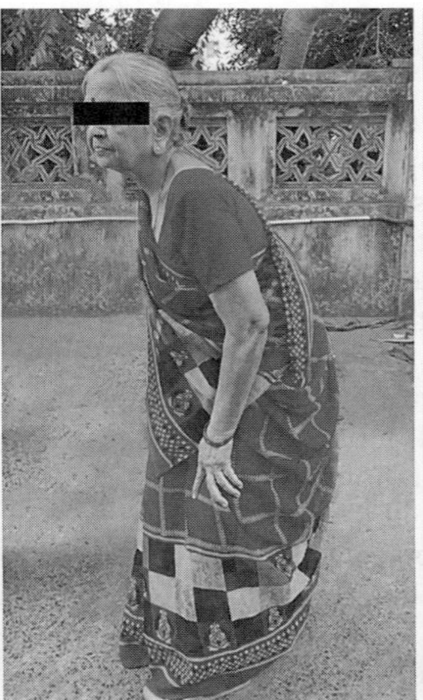
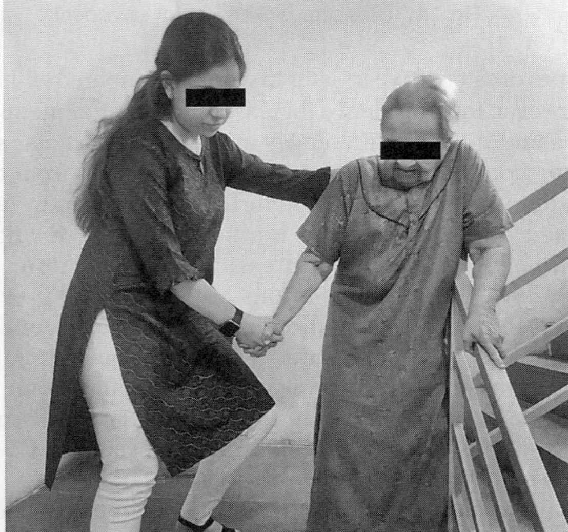

Fig. 11.1: Physical health.

Screening

- **Increased body mass index (BMI) or waist circumference**
- **Surrogate indicators of sarcopenia** (e.g., clinical symptoms, risk factors or validated questionnaires like SARC-F*)

Diagnosis

- **Skeletal muscle function (SMF):** Hand grip strength, knee extensor strength or chair-stand test
- **Body composition (BC):** Increased fat mass and reduced muscle mass

Staging

- **Stage I:** No complications
- **Stage II:** Presence of at least one complication because of altered BC or SMF parameters (e.g., metabolic cardiovascular, respiratory diseases and disabilities)

*SARC-F questionnaire: Strength, assistance with walking, rising from a chair, climbing stairs, and falls to screen probable sarcopenia

Fig. 11.2: The European Society for Clinical Nutrition and Metabolism (ESPEN) and the European Association for the Study of Obesity (EASO) Consensus Statement for Screening, Diagnosis and Staging of Sarcopenic Obesity.

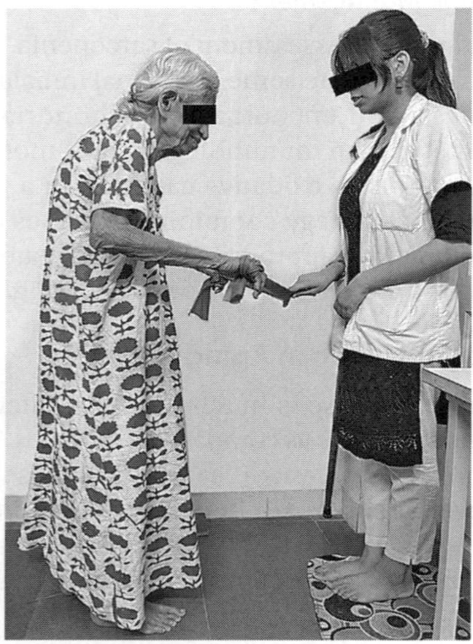

Fig. 11.3: Resistance exercises for sarcopenia.

approximately 10 years later in women compared with males. However, the prevalence increases rapidly after menopause.

Gender-based differences in the cardiovascular system stem from the differences in gene expression from the sex chromosomes. This may be further augmented by gender-based differences in the hormonal milieu, resulting in gender-unique gene expression and function. These differences result in variations not only in the prevalence but also in the presentation of cardiovascular conditions, including those associated with autonomic regulation, hypertension, DM, and vascular remodeling. Some of the notable sex-based differences in the risk factors associated with atherosclerotic cardiovascular disease (ASCVD) are shown in **Box 11.1**.

In terms of primary prevention of the disease, it is important to delineate the significant risk factors for coronary artery disease in women. The National Cholesterol Education Program (NCEP) and scientific statements from the AHA and the American College of Cardiology (ACC) have identified risk factors as shown in **Box 11.2** as part of a women's risk assessment. **Box 11.3** provides the global cardiovascular risk prediction for women.

Box 11.1: Gender-based differences in the risk factors associated with atherosclerotic cardiovascular disease.

- **Myocardial infarction:** Earlier occurrence and higher mortality in diabetic women compared with diabetic men.
- **Heart failure (HF):** Diabetic women have a higher risk of developing HF compared with diabetic men.
- **Stroke:** DM is a stronger risk factor for stroke in women compared with men.
- **Peripheral artery disease:** DM is a stronger risk factor for the development of claudication in women compared with men.
- **Hypertension:** Higher prevalence of HTN in women over age 60 than in men.
- **Obesity:** The impact of obesity on the development of CAD appears to be greater in women than in men. According to the Framingham heart study, obesity elevated the risk of CAD by 64% in women compared with 46% in men.
- **Sedentary behavior:** Prevalence of inactivity and sedentary behaviors is higher among women than men.

Box 11.2: Significant risk factors for coronary artery disease in women.

- Age >55 years
- Dyslipidemia
- Family history of premature CHD
- Smoking
- Hypertension
- Risk equivalents of peripheral arterial disease
- History of diabetes mellitus
- Elevated triglycerides
- Obesity
- Glucose intolerance
- Sedentary lifestyle

Box 11.3: Global cardiovascular risk prediction.

The Reynolds risk score for women: Estimates risk of adverse cardiovascular event (ischemic stroke, myocardial infarction, need for coronary revascularization, or cardiovascular death) in women over age 45.

Pelvic Floor and Aging

Pelvic floor musculature (PFM) is a challenging area with distinct functions in health and disease. The incidence of pelvic floor dysfunction increases steadily during the aging process in women. The estimated prevalence of pelvic floor dysfunction may vary widely because of various reasons. Though the absence of standardized and well-validated definitions and measures is definitely to be blamed for the inconsistency, so is the reluctance of the females to come out in open and report the problem and seek appropriate management for the same.

The functional and structural deviations of the pelvic floor in elderly women are summative effects of factors shown in **Box 11.4**.

Pelvic floor dysfunction may be associated with dysfunctions of micturition, defecation, prolapse, and sexual intercourse. Condition-specific standardized assessment tools can be used to assess symptoms, distress associated with the condition and quality of life as shown in **Box 11.5**.

Management: Has been dealt in Chapter 15: Managing the Pelvic Floor.

Empathetic approach to the patient is the touchstone of effective management of PF dysfunction which begins with patient education on the function of the pelvic floor muscle and the role of exercise to strengthen and alleviate the unwanted symptoms.

Some strategies that can be adopted for easier and clear understanding:

- Make the patient visualize the pelvic floor as a hammock/trampoline which when contracted would lift up. The use of images and videos can aid this understanding.
- Discuss the mechanism of insult to the pelvic floor with your patient as to how the strain that is put on the hammock/trampoline with repeated pregnancies/certain positions and occupations could cause stretch weakness. This context-specific teaching will enhance understanding, motivation, and eventual compliance with the exercise regime.
- Take the patient in confidence about the frequency, intensity, and type of exercise required for desired benefits. This will help set realistic goals for effective results from the management without burnout or dropouts.
- Incorporate functional goals for all the exercise protocols which would make the benefits of the therapy appealing to the patients.
- Advice use of knack/counter bracing technique (CBT) as a strong and well-timed, premeditated, preventative contraction of the pelvic floor muscles to control leaking during any activity which increases the intra-abdominal pressure like coughing, sneezing and lifting heavy objects.
- Last but not least, the verbal and nonverbal communication of the therapist which ensures care, empathy, and concern will boost patient confidence to pursue treatment.

Box 11.4: Factors leading to changes in the PF in elderly women.

- Parity
- Mode of delivery
- Postmenopausal estrogen deficiency
- Higher BMI
- History of pelvic surgery
- Medical history (comorbidities: DM, HTN, etc.)
- Age-related systemic changes in neurological and cardiovascular systems—urethral sphincteric muscle dysfunction
- Overactive bladder
- Incomplete bladder emptying—elevates post-void residual
- Detrusor instability
- Under perfusion of the frontal lobes of the cerebral cortex (regional impairment of function) causing urge incontinence and reduced bladder sensation
- Peripheral nervous system: ↓ acetylcholinesterase-positive nerves, ↓ number of nerve axons in detrusor muscle with increasing age
- ↓maximal urethral closure pressure

Box 11.5: Tools to assess PF and its associated problems.

- The Brink scale
- PERFECT score-modified Oxford grading
- Incontinence impact questionnaire (IIQ)
- The pelvic floor distress inventory (PFDI)
- The pelvic floor impact questionnaire (PFIQ)

Clinical Pointer

Avoid stopping the flow of urine in the midflow while urinating as this may lead to difficulty in fully emptying the bladder, leaving residual urine and detrusor instability in the long run.

Mental Health and Elderly Female

Mental health in general refers to a lack of mental illness and dementia, as well as any psychological characteristics and coping resources, such as self-esteem, self-efficacy, hardiness, and sense-of-coherence. Optimal mental health is central to full social participation.

- Evidence suggests that in comparison to men, elderly women score significantly lower on most indicators of subjective well-being and mental health. This is because men and women are different, not just in their physical characteristics, but also in their psychological makeup. Alpha bias in psychological theories presents a gender-sensitive viewpoint and acknowledges the difference between men and women. Therefore, gender is a critical determinant of mental health and mental illness.

- Depressive disorders account for close to 41.9% of the disability from neuropsychiatric disorders among women compared to 29.3% among men. Depression can present in conjunction with dementia but may also occur as a separate entity. This can lead to significant cognitive changes. The depressed elderly may be more irritable, have a decrease or loss of interest in day-to-day activities, and may even show weight gain or loss and sleep disorders.

Cognitive Health in Females

Aging brings about structural and functional changes in the brain including alterations in neuronal structure without neuronal death, loss of synapses, and dysfunction of neuronal networks all lead to cognitive decline which is further augmented by age-related diseases. Epidemiological studies have found that women are more likely than men to be diagnosed with any dementia and Alzheimer's disease. Through a systematic review in 2013, the author showed that the prevalence of dementia was higher in women than in men, with a ratio of 1.65:1. This could be a direct outcome of the fact that, globally, life expectancy in females is greater than in males.

Normal Aging and Cognitive Functioning

Though the rate of aging may differ amongst individuals, dementia is a common finding in very elderly individuals. However, dementia is not an essential part of the normal aging process. The normal aging process involves both preserved and declining cognitive functions. Dementia is a major cause of morbidity and mortality among elderly people. Unfortunately, dementia is incurable, and the existing pharmacological and nonpharmacological interventions can only delay its progression.

Social Health in Elderly Subjects

Traditionally, our culture is more of a male-dominated society. How much ever we talk of gender equity, females still remain or prefer to remain on a back seat in many situations. As the age advances, these elderly females are somehow pushed more behind, being dormant and unattended to by the family. This is more seen in situations when her husband, the once upon man of the house, is not alive. From a physiotherapist's perspective, it is of utmost importance to not just understand the state of physical deconditioning of this population but also understand the mental and social deconditioning as well.

Old age comes with its own set of issues and concerns. There is a rapid deterioration in the physical and cognitive functioning of the elderly leading to the affection of their health and quality of life as well. Males also show deterioration in their physical functioning and vitality by a condition termed andropause. This andropause is gradual and very commonly slow in transition over a period of 10–15 years, starting from around 40 to 59 years of age. Concurrently there is also a gradual decline in physical functioning, especially with dual-tasking or multitasking activities. This automatically predisposes a person to decline in activities and a silent predisposition to postural deficits and risk of falls over time. These changes are seen much faster in females by virtue of menopause and hence bring about rapid changes in their physical function and health, including bone mineral density, muscle cross-sectional area and strength, metabolic functioning as well as cognitive functions, complex tasks, and decision-making abilities, and self-confidence and control.

THE ELDERLY FEMALE AND FINANCIAL STABILITY

CLINICAL EXAMPLE 1

> Mrs ECG is a 75-year-old lady who was a novel writer. She earns royalty income from the novels she writes but her son does not give her any money from that. Her husband passed away with a huge bank balance and property in her name but neither is she aware of the same nor does she get any money in her hands. She is dependent on her accountant son for her daily needs and expenses and is ill-treated by her daughter-in-law as well.

Most of the times as per the cultural norms' females are given a secondary position in the family. The husband is usually the one who looks at financial implications and hence in case of demise of the husband the females find it extremely difficult to manage the financial provisions. Although this may not be true in totality, this is the commonest situation observed. In case of an elderly female there is a loss of not just financial stability, but also loss of confidence in handling any financial concerns as well as loss of the primary earning position in the family which predisposes them to a dependent position. Hence when such a patient or client is seen by a physiotherapist, the expenses on healthcare are routinely looked at as a major concern rather than the health of the concerned individual.

THE ELDERLY FEMALE AND TECHNOLOGY

CLINICAL EXAMPLE 2

> Mrs PVD is a 68-year-old lady. She is literate till the 3rd standard of schooling. Her son works as a medical representative in a company. She has a 17-year-old grandson and she feels she is unable to understand any of the aspects of communication with him making her feel helpless and hopeless. She just lands up sitting in a corner of her house cursing life.

The upgradation of technology and progress in the field of medicine has brought the whole world closer. The newer generations are becoming more and more techno-savvy and updated. But throughout these rapid advancements and changes, something which does not change is the perspectives of the elderly, especially the elderly females. There is an extreme challenge for them to catch up even with updates, like even using a basic feature of a smartphone.

The general understanding of the current elderly female population is that they are not very well versed with latest technological aspects that are being used. Video chatting, text messages, net banking, phone banking, etc., are being used quite a lot. But most elderly females are either not well-versed with this or are apprehensive to use this particular technological domain. Today's world is a world of a digital era wherein being connected by virtue of social media is equally important. But many of the elderly population especially females depict social isolation and lack of functioning.

Many elderly females are not aware of what technology is available. The level of ignorance can be as low as not knowing what cell phone they are using or what features the phone has. Although this is not a very important aspect, this certainly denotes an ignorance towards technological advances which are important to stay in communication, do online transactions, or simply express emotions.

Education of the girl child is now given importance. But if we look at the elderly population, many of them are not necessarily educated or literate to have their own financial independence. In fact, in the rural set up, still a girl child is not given a priority to be educated as against a male child. Considering elderly females, not just at the rural, but even at the urban setup it is quite frequently observed that many of them have a low literacy rate thereby causing an inhibition in socialization. In today's era where social media is becoming a strong platform for connection lack of education and technical knowledge makes this elderly female feel more restrained and restricted and hence give the feeling of dependency isolation and depression.

THE ELDERLY FEMALE AND HEALTHCARE SYSTEMS

Today most of the healthcare system is based on digital components, for example, the Government of India has launched the Ayushman Bharat digital health program which uses technology in understanding health domains across the country. Insurance coverage has become a necessity for most of the health care aspects. The government has launched numerous schemes for the elderly population like the following among others:

- Pradhan Mantri Vaya Vandana scheme
- Rashtriya Vayashri Yojana
- National Old age pension scheme
- National program for the healthcare of the elderly

But it is observed that many of the senior citizens, especially females, do not have their own insurance or are unaware of the possible schemes and benefits that are offered by the government for the Healthcare system for their well-being.

THE ELDERLY FEMALE AND SOCIAL ASPECTS

Clinical Example 3

Mrs MRI is a 76-year-old lady. She is a retired primary school teacher teaching students in a local language school. She had a fracture intercondylar right femur 3 months ago and is not very compliant with her physiotherapy for rehabilitation. She is staying with her son in another city and feels depressed as she has limited communication with people. She does not like to use smartphones for communication and feels left out.

Social isolation is one of the important causes of acceleration of aging. Non-involvement in social activities or being away from peers causes a rapid deterioration in the health of the elderly population. It is quite frequently observed that elderly males have some or the other friend circle as against elderly females who tend to be more alone and focus only on family and their well-being. This social isolation is a significant cause of deterioration in health and its functioning in elderly females. It is quite usually seen that elderly males may be involved in social activities like laughter club, social gatherings. Elderly females are also preparing to do this but there is a lot of variability in the urban versus the rural setup **(Fig. 11.4)**.

The Social Outlook towards the health and functioning of the elderly population plays a very important role in their personal health care, for example, an elderly female is expected to be at home and be involved in social aspects and social domains like family care, taking care of the grandchildren and being involved in social and religious aspects.

THE ELDERLY FEMALE LIVING ALONE

Clinical Example 4

Mrs ABG is a 63-year-old was widow 20 years ago when she lost her husband in a train accident. She has a married daughter who stays close by. Mrs ABG had a compound ankle fracture in the same train accident and is surviving with a deformity. She does not want to stay with the daughter as she does not want to be a burden on her and does not want her deformity to be an issue at her daughter's place.

It is quite frequently found that senior citizens tend to stay alone. Even in the case of the male child, the preference is to keep the elderly parents away, either due to challenges in managing senior citizens or lack of family commitment. In case of female child, cultural barriers make it quite evident for the elderly parents to stay alone. The prevalent sociocultural factors may contribute to perceptions of the mother-in-law as intrusive and thus lead to isolation.

Presence of any associated health concerns lead to further social isolation. Hence in such situation the support of the

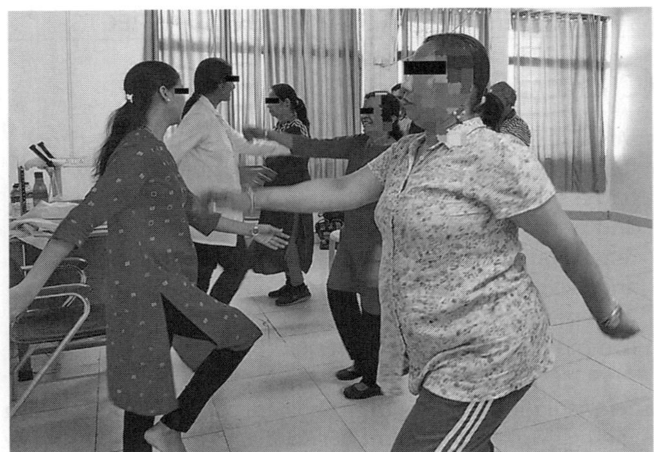

Fig. 11.4: Group exercises to counter social isolation in elderly females.

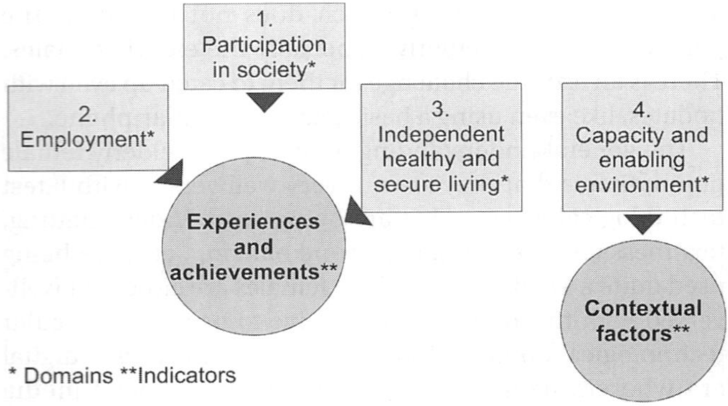

Fig. 11.5: Active aging index—indicators and domains for active aging.

family is extremely crucial and this will lead to betterment in functioning as well as social acceptance.

MENOPAUSE AND OSTEOPOROSIS

Menopause and osteoporosis are described in detail in Chapter 9: Menopause and Chapter 10: Osteoporosis respectively.

MEASUREMENT TOOLS

Assessment of Elderly Women is described in Chapter 4: Assessment in Women's Health. Active Aging Index (AAI) devised by the United Nations is an important tool to measure the untapped potential of older people for active and healthy aging. This in turn proves to be a marker for the level of preparedness for aging **(Fig. 11.5)**.

SOME NOVEL APPROACHES TO AGE-RELATED IMPAIRMENTS

In addition to the standard of care for managing elderly subjects, some novel techniques are gaining popularity because of their effectiveness and acceptability amongst older adults. These include:

Neuromotor Exercise Training for Older Adults

Neuromotor exercise training involving motor skills such as balance, coordination **(Fig. 11.6)**, gait and agility, and proprioceptive training is also called **functional fitness training**. Cardinal features of these exercises are:

- Progressively difficult postures that gradually reduce the base of support (e.g., two-legged stand, semi tandem stand, tandem stand, one-legged stand)
- Dynamic movements that perturb the center of gravity (e.g., tandem walk, circle turns)
- Stressing postural muscle groups (e.g., heel, toe stands)

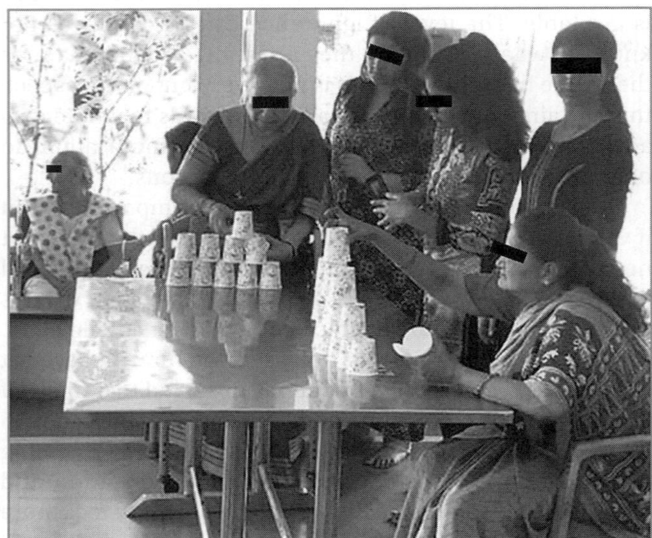

Fig. 11.6: Neuromotor coordination exercises.

- Reducing sensory input (e.g., standing with eyes closed)
- Tai chi

Art-based Therapy

Art-based therapy (ABT) has been defined by the British Association of Art Therapists as a form of psychotherapy that uses the medium of art as its primary mode of communication.

Process of ABT

- It involves a wide range of individually appealing creative activities and art-creating methods which target the elderly subjects' functioning at cognitive, motor, emotional and sometimes even at interpersonal levels.
- Based on the activity undertaken, ABT may also serve as a non-verbal expressive medium which enlightens the therapist about the patient's 'inner world' through the interaction between the patient, the therapist, and art materials (object or image).

- ABT has been found to be very effective in managing the manifestations of the disease. ABT may help to slow cognitive deterioration and improve quality of life.
- Choosing an activity or medium that commensurate with the competency of the subject, invokes her interest and actively engages her through sensory and intellectual stimulation are some fundamental prerequisites for the success of the therapy.

Lifestyle Modifications for Healthy Aging

Advancing age results in a reduced adaptability of the body to adapt to physiological stresses and maintain homeostasis. This in turn would make the elderly subject more susceptible to illness and injury. However, the good news is that as one ages, the capability to tolerate stresses is still partially modifiable with positive lifestyle adaptations.

The physical stress theory (PST) proposed by Mueller and Maluf demonstrates the effect of physical stress on tissue adaptation. The older adults with very low tolerance to physiological stresses are more amenable to disease and have reduced capability to counter the effects of even most benign diseases like diarrhea. On the contrary, in a person in homeostasis, the outcome of exercise is a definitive positive change followed by systemic adaptation.

Many age-related issues are amenable to change with regular adequate and appropriate exercise: sleep, sexual function, depression, gastroesophageal reflux disease (GERD), gastric motility, and constipation.

Improving Compliance in Older Adults

Provided the older adults are under a therapist with appropriate attitude, knowledge and skills in treatment techniques, the success of any rehabilitation protocol with older subjects will depend on:

- Client's physical condition
- Level of motivation
- Caregivers and support systems
- Skill of the therapist as a patient educator/counselor

Following can help improve adherence to exercise schedules in elderly subjects:

- Regular feedback
- Positive reinforcement
- Behavioral strategies: Social support, self-efficacy, the ability to make healthy choices, and perceived safety to enhance adherence
- Expose older adult to role models
- Decrease unpleasant sensations associated with the activity
- Group therapy

If the efforts to promote women's overall health focus solely on physical and mental health then they maybe at a risk of neglecting the very factors that bring these individualistic factors into being. Hence there is an imminent need to recognize the broader, social, economic, and legal factors that may affect women's lives and thereby health. So there is need to look into the sociocultural, economic, legal, infrastructural, and environmental factors that may have a bearing on women's health in the community setting.

Summary

Differences on the basis of gender, are part of human existence, that is expressed in terms of both biological structure and functions. In view of the anticipated gravity of the population of elderly women across the world, it is imperative to take stock of this occurrence, highlight the scale and significance of the issues, acknowledge and appreciate, the differences between the aging elderly, and take specific and pre-emptive actions to ensure their physical, mental and social well-being as well continued functional independence and enriched quality of life.

With more than 50% contribution to the total population, women truly represent the greater half. So, the empowerment of women and promotion of gender equality in the domain of health and well-being will not only benefit womenfolk but communities at large.

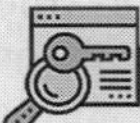

Review Questions

1. How does epidemiology of chronic diseases differ between genders?
2. Explain health affection in elderly females.
3. What is sarcopenia and sarcopenic obesity?
4. How is the pelvic floor affected with aging?
5. How does aging affect mental and cognitive health?
6. Describe approaches used to manage age-related impairments.
7. Write short notes on:
   a. The elderly female and technology
   b. The elderly female and healthcare systems
   c. Measurement tools used for aging female
   d. Social health in elderly females

Bibliography

1. Arber S, Ginn J. Gender and inequalities in health in later life. Soc Sci Med. 1993;36(1):33-46. doi:10.1016/0277-9536(93)90303-L.
2. Beam CR, Kaneshiro C, Jang JY, Reynolds CA, Pedersen NL, Gatz M. Differences between women and men in incidence rates of dementia and Alzheimer's disease. J Alzheimers Dis. 2018;64(4):1077-83. doi:10.3233/JAD-180141.
3. Centers for Disease Control and Prevention. Loneliness and social isolation linked to serious health conditions [Internet]. 2020 [cited 2025 Jan 10]. Available from: https://www.cdc.gov/aging/publications/features/lonely-olderadults.html
4. Cerrato J, Cifre E. Gender inequality in household chores and work–family conflict. Front Psychol. 2018;9:1330. doi:10.3389/fpsyg.2018.01330.
5. Chadda RK, Deb KS. Indian family systems, collectivistic society and psychotherapy. Indian J Psychiatry. 2013;55(Suppl 2):S299-309. doi:10.4103/0019-5545.105555.

6. Choi NG, Dinitto DM. The digital divide among low-income homebound older adults: Internet use patterns, eHealth literacy, and attitudes toward computer/Internet use. J Med Internet Res. 2013;15(5):e93. doi:10.2196/jmir.2645.
7. Donovan NJ, Blazer D. Social isolation and loneliness in older adults: Review and commentary of a National Academies report. Am J Geriatr Psychiatry. 2020;28(12):1233-44. doi:10.1016/j.jagp.2020.08.005.
8. Fiske A, Wetherell JL, Gatz M. Depression in older adults. Annu Rev Clin Psychol. 2009;5:363–89. doi:10.1146/annurev.clinpsy.032408.153621.
9. Flett GL, Heisel MJ. Aging and feeling valued versus expendable during the COVID-19 pandemic and beyond: A review and commentary of why mattering is fundamental to the health and well-being of older adults. Int J Ment Health Addict. 2021;19(6):2443–69. doi:10.1007/s11469-020-00339-4.
10. Gao Q, Mei F, Shang Y, Hu K, Chen F, et al. Global prevalence of sarcopenic obesity in older adults: A systematic review and meta-analysis. Clin Nutr. 2021;40(7):4633–41. doi:10.1016/j.clnu.2021.06.009.
11. Goswami S, Deshmukh PR. How "elderly staying alone" cope up with their age and deteriorating health: A qualitative exploration from rural Wardha, Central India. Indian J Palliat Care. 2018;24(4):465–71. doi:10.4103/IJPC.IJPC_87_18.
12. Government of India. Ayushman Bharat Digital Mission [Internet]. 2021 [cited 2025 Jan 10]. Available from: https://www.india.gov.in/spotlight/ayushman-bharat-digitalmission-abdm
13. Haase KR, Cosco T, Kervin L, Riadi I, O'Connell ME. Older adults' experiences with using technology for socialization during the COVID-19 pandemic: Cross-sectional survey study. JMIR Aging. 2021;4(2):e28010. doi:10.2196/28010.
14. Halaweh H, Dahlin-Ivanoff S, Svantesson U, Willén C. Perspectives of older adults on aging well: A focus group study. J Aging Res. 2018;2018:9858252. doi:10.1155/2018/9858252.
15. Hastings JS, Madrian BC, Skimmyhorn WL. Financial literacy, financial education and economic outcomes. Annu Rev Econ. 2013;5:347-73. doi:10.1146/annurev-economics-082312-125807.
16. Hatcher D, Chang E, Schmied V, Garrido S. Exploring the perspectives of older people on the concept of home. J Aging Res. 2019;2019:2679680. doi:10.1155/2019/2679680.
17. Kasthuri A. Challenges to healthcare in India – The five A's. Indian J Community Med. 2018;43(3):141-3. doi:10.4103/ijcm.IJCM_194_18.
18. Marston HR, Genoe R, Freeman S, Kulczycki C, Musselwhite C. Older adults' perceptions of ICT: Main findings from the Technology in Later Life (TILL) study. Healthcare (Basel). 2019;7(3):86. doi:10.3390/healthcare7030086.
19. Mitzner TL, Boron JB, Fausset CB, Adams AE, Charness N, Czaja SJ, et al. Older adults talk technology: Technology usage and attitudes. Comput Human Behav. 2010;26(6):1710-21. doi:10.1016/j.chb.2010.06.020.
20. Molina-Mula J, Gallo-Estrada J, González-Trujillo A. Self-perceptions and behavior of older people living alone. Int J Environ Res Public Health. 2020;17(23):8739. doi:10.3390/ijerph17238739.
21. National Academies of Sciences, Engineering, and Medicine. Families caring for an aging America. Schulz R, Eden J, editors. Washington (DC): National Academies Press; 2016. doi:10.17226/23606.
22. Peek ST, Luijkx KG, Rijnaard MD, Nieboer ME, van der Voort CS, Aarts S. Older adults' reasons for using technology while aging in place. Gerontology. 2016;62(2):226-37. doi:10.1159/000430949.
23. Ram Prakash R, Lingam L. Why is women's utilization of a publicly funded health insurance low? A qualitative study in Tamil Nadu, India. BMC Public Health. 2021;21(1):350. doi:10.1186/s12889-021-10311-6.
24. Saurabh S, Sarkar S, Pandey DK. Female literacy rate is a better predictor of birth rate and infant mortality rate in India. J Family Med Prim Care. 2013;2(4):349-53. doi:10.4103/2249-4863.123911.
25. Seyfzadeh A, Haghighatian M, Mohajerani A. Social isolation in the elderly: The neglected issue. Iran J Public Health. 2019;48(2):365–6.
26. Sharma N, Chakrabarti S, Grover S. Gender differences in caregiving among family caregivers of people with mental illnesses. World J Psychiatry. 2016;6(1):7–17. doi:10.5498/wjp.v6.i1.7.
27. Sipilä S, Törmäkangas T, Sillanpää E, Aukee P, Kujala UM, Kovanen V, et al. Muscle and bone mass in middle-aged women: Role of menopausal status and physical activity. J Cachexia Sarcopenia Muscle. 2020;11(3):698–709. doi:10.1002/jcsm.12546.
28. Tiwari SC, Pandey NM. The Indian concepts of lifestyle and mental health in old age. Indian J Psychiatry. 2013;55(Suppl 2):S288-92. doi:10.4103/0019-5545.105538.
29. Vaportzis E, Clausen MG, Gow AJ. Older adults' perceptions of technology and barriers to interacting with tablet computers: A focus group study. Front Psychol. 2017;8:1687. doi:10.3389/fpsyg.2017.01687.
30. VikasPedia. Senior citizens welfare schemes [Internet]. 2021 [cited 2025 Jan 10]. Available from: https://vikaspedia.in/social-welfare/senior-citizens-welfare
31. Wang MT, Degol JL. Gender gap in science, technology, engineering, and mathematics (STEM): Current knowledge, implications for practice, policy, and future directions. Educ Psychol Rev. 2017;29(1):119-40. doi:10.1007/s10648-015-9355-x.
32. Zhang Y, Harper S. Son or daughter care in relation to self-reported health outcomes for older adults in China. Front Public Health. 2022;9:793873. doi:10.3389/fpubh.2021.793873.
33. Zunzunegui MV, Alvarado BE, Guerra R, Gómez JF, Ylli A, Guralnik JM, et al. The mobility gap between older men and women: The embodiment of gender. Arch Gerontol Geriatr. 2015;61(2):140-8. doi:10.1016/j.archger.2015.06.018.

Multiple Choice Questions (MCQs)

To test your understanding and recall of key concepts.

1. Which factor significantly contributes to sarcopenic obesity in elderly females?

A. Lack of exercise
B. Estrogen deficiency
C. Increased testosterone
D. High bone mineral density

2. The concept of 'functional reserve' in aging refers to_______________.

A. The body's resilience to recover from chronic illnesses
B. The remaining capacity of organs to meet increased demand under stress
C. The energy reserve stored for strenuous physical activity
D. The immune system's backup capacity

3. **Which strategy would best help an elderly female with pelvic floor dysfunction regain functional independence?**
   A. Regularly practicing Kegel exercises with visual aids
   B. Adopting a sedentary lifestyle to reduce strain
   C. Using intermittent urinary catheters as needed
   D. Implementing hormonal therapy without exercise

4. **A 70-year-old female with sarcopenic obesity has difficulty climbing stairs and walking long distances. Which combination is the most effective initial intervention?**
   A. High-protein diet and resistance exercises
   B. Aerobic exercises with flexibility training
   C. Cognitive-behavioral therapy and balance exercises
   D. Prolonged rest and low-intensity walking

5. **Which of the following is *true* with respect to the difference in the aging process between males and females, specifically in terms of andropause and menopause?**
   A. Both processes occur gradually with similar physical changes
   B. Menopause leads to rapid bone density loss, while andropause causes a slower decline in vitality
   C. Andropause predominantly affects cognition, while menopause only impacts physical health
   D. Both processes equally contribute to the onset of sarcopenic obesity

6. **Which intervention plan is most suitable for managing sarcopenic obesity in elderly females while addressing compliance issues?**
   A. Emphasize regular aerobic exercise alongwith individual diet plans
   B. Introduce group-based resistance training alongwith tailored nutritional support
   C. Focus solely on dietary modifications to reduce obesity
   D. Prescribe pharmacological solutions for weight management

7. **A community health initiative is planning to improve exercise adherence among elderly females in a rural area with low literacy levels. Which of the following plans would be most effective?**
   A. Establish peer-led group exercise sessions with simple visual instructions
   B. Provide smartphones preloaded with exercise applications in the local language
   C. Organize weekly seminars on the importance of exercise with PowerPoint presentations
   D. Build a central fitness facility with advanced exercise equipment

ANSWERS

1. B	2. B	3. A	4. A	5. B
6. B	7. A			

Chapter 12

Gynecologic Conditions: Clinical and Physiotherapy—Part I

Ami Vishal Mehta, Shivani Sheth, Priyasingh Rangey

LEARNING OBJECTIVES

At the end of the chapter, the reader will be able to:
- Understand and enlist menstrual disorders.
- Describe the etiology, clinical features and management of amenorrhea in detail.
- Describe pelvic infections—clinical features, diagnosis, management.
- Explain abnormal uterine bleeding—its types.
- Learn about pelvic and low back pain.

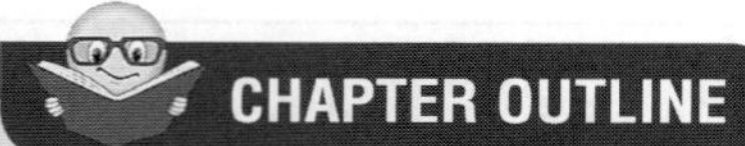

CHAPTER OUTLINE

- Introduction
- Menstrual disorders
  - Dysmenorrhea
  - Premenstrual syndrome (PMS)
  - Mittelschmerz's syndrome
- Amenorrhea
- Abnormal uterine bleeding
  - Hypermenorrhea (Menorrhagia)
  - Polymenorrhea
  - Metrorrhagia
  - Oligomenorrhea
  - Hypomenorrhea
  - Dysfunctional uterine bleeding (DUB)
- Pelvic Infections
  - Genital tuberculosis
  - Pelvic inflammatory disease
  - Sexually transmitted infections
- Pelvic pain and low back pain
  - Acute pelvic pain
  - Chronic pelvic pain
  - Low back pain

INTRODUCTION

Gynecological conditions are quite common among the female population. They consist of a variety of conditions ranging from menstrual disorders, abnormal uterine bleeding, pelvic infections, pelvic inflammatory disease to infertility and prolapse of pelvic organs. The role of physiotherapy has grown from being just a part of the obstetric team to helping manage gynecological disorders as well. There are many gynecological conditions where physiotherapy plays a crucial role in managing pain, healing of tissues, developing pelvic floor muscle strength and improving the quality of life of patients.

With recent developments in science, it has come to knowledge that even with proper medical care and treatment; patients suffer from chronic pains after certain gynecologic conditions and interventions. Physiotherapy helps in managing these chronic disorders as well and improves the daily function of such individuals.

MENSTRUAL DISORDERS

Dysmenorrhea

Dysmenorrhea is a Greek term for "painful monthly bleeding." Dysmenorrhea is a common complaint among women during their reproductive age. There are two types:
1. Primary dysmenorrhea
2. Secondary dysmenorrhea

Primary Dysmenorrhea

It is common in adolescents and the incidence reduces as age increases. It is common within 2 years of menarche, and it becomes negligible postdelivery. Common causes include:

- Psychosomatic factors: Lower pain threshold among adolescents
- Abnormal anatomical and functional aspects of myometrium
- Imbalance in the autonomic nervous control of the uterine muscle
- Increased production of prostaglandins or increased sensitivity of myometrium to the normal production of prostaglandins which causes increased contraction of myometrium.
- Increased vasopressin is found during menstruation in women having dysmenorrhea. Vasopressin increases prostaglandin synthesis which increases myometrial activity and dysrhythmic contraction which leads to ischemia and hypoxia and ultimately causes pain.

Clinical features

- Pain begins a few hours before or with onset of menstruation
- Severity of pain lasts for 24 hours but seldom lasts beyond 48 hours
- **Type of pain:** Spasmodic
- **Site:** Confined to lower abdomen, may radiate to the posterior and medial aspects of thigh
- **Associated factors:** Nausea, vomiting, fatigue, diarrhea, headache and tachycardia
- **Vasomotor changes:** Pallor, cold sweats, occasional fainting, in severe cases syncope and collapse may occur.

Diagnosis

- Abdominal and pelvic examination would not reveal any abnormal finding.
- For detection of pelvic abnormalities ultrasonography (USG) is gold standard.

Medical and surgical management

- Analgesics and antispasmodics can be prescribed.
- Prostaglandin inhibitors, oral contraceptives and NSAIDs can be used.
- Nerve ablation can be used as a last resort.

Secondary Dysmenorrhea

In this, the menstrual pain is due to an underlying disease, disorder, or structural abnormality either within or outside the uterus.

Causes

- Cervical stenosis
- Chronic pelvic infection
- Pelvic endometriosis
- Pelvic adhesions
- Adenomyosis
- Uterine fibroid
- Endometrial polyp
- Intrauterine contraceptive device (IUCD) causing uterine and pelvic congestion.

Clinical features

- **Pain site:** Anterior and posterior aspect of back usually without any radiation
- **Type of pain:** Dull
- **Time:** It usually appears 3–5 days prior to periods and relieves as menstruation starts
- **Associated factors:** There are no systemic discomforts.

Diagnosis

- Abdominal and pelvic examinations would reveal the causative factor.
- USG, laparoscopy, hysteroscopy, or laparotomy would also help to reveal the offending lesions.

Medical and surgical management

The treatment of secondary dysmenorrhea is aimed at cause and not the symptoms. The treatment of dysmenorrhea depends on age, severity, and parity of the female.

Physiotherapy Management of Dysmenorrhea

Physiotherapy management of dysmenorrhea includes:

- Conventional transcutaneous electrical nerve stimulation (TENS) to reduce menstrual pain
- Thermotherapy to reduce menstrual pain, cramps, and provide muscle relaxation
- Stretching **(Figs. 12.1 and 12.2)**, aerobic exercises and Yoga help in improving the general well-being of the female and reduce muscle cramps occurring during menstruation.
- Kegel exercises help in improving pelvic floor muscle strength and endurance, improve blood circulation to the uterus and reduce muscle cramps.
- Recent studies have used Kinesio-taping (over T11–12 dermatome, suprapubic region or lower abdomen, sacral region and low back) for dysmenorrhea from the probable day of ovulation to the end of menstruation and found it to be effective.

Premenstrual Syndrome (PMS)

This is an endocrine disorder with psychological implications and has no known etiology. It occurs prior to the menstruation cycle. As per American College of Obstetricians and Gynecologists (ACOG) it is:

- Unrelated to organic lesion
- Occurs regularly during the luteal phase of each ovulatory menstrual cycle
- Symptoms disturb the lifestyle of the female
- Symptom free period during rest of the cycle

Clinical Features

PMS symptoms **(Table 12.1)** are cyclic in nature and occur during the last 7–10 days of the cycle.

Premenstrual dysphoric disorder (PMDD), earlier known as late luteal dysphoric disorder (LLDD), is the most severe form of PMS, which greatly affects the daily functioning and perceived quality of life of a woman.

Diagnosis

Diagnosis of PMDD can be stipulated by the presence of all of the following criteria:

- Presence of a minimum of five luteal-phase symptoms (from **Table 12.1**), at least one of which must be a mood

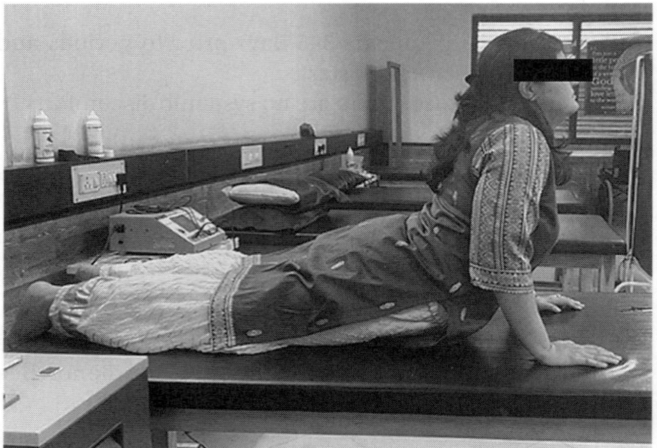

Fig. 12.1: Stretching of abdominal muscles.

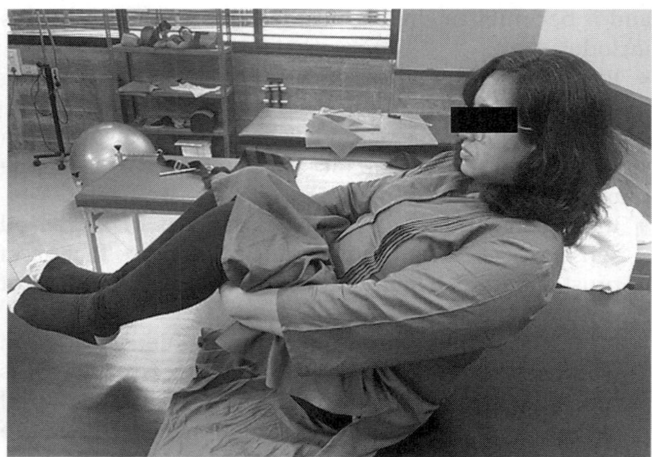

Fig. 12.2: Stretching of back muscles with rhythmic rocking.

Table 12.1: Clinical features of premenstrual syndrome.

Related to water retention	Abdominal bloating
	Breast tenderness
	Weight gain
	Swelling of extremities
Neuropsychiatric symptoms	Mood swings
	Irritability
	Depression
	Anxiety
	Confusion
	Increased appetite
	Anger
	Headache
	Restlessness
	Forgetfulness
General symptoms	Dyspareunia
	Fatigue
	Tiredness
	Insomnia

symptom (i.e., anxiety or tension, depressed mood, affect lability, or persistent anger and irritability)

- Two cycles of daily charting to confirm the timing of symptoms
- Evidence of impairment of function

Symptoms must not be an exacerbation of another psychiatric condition.

Management

General management

Nonpharmacological management: Lifestyle and dietary modifications like yoga, stress management, psychological counseling, avoidance of use of excessive salt, caffeine and alcohol can be tried.

Pharmacological management:

- Antidepressants such as selective serotonin reuptake inhibitors (SSRI) and noradrenaline reuptake inhibitors (SNRI) can be used. Fluoxetine which is a SSRI given orally 20 mg is found to significantly improve psychiatric and behavioral symptoms.
- Anxiolytic agents such as Alprazolam.
- Diuretics—to manage water retention can be given especially in second half of cycle. Frusemide 20 mg daily for 5 days a week is found to be effective.

Clinical Pointer

Drugs must be prescribed at least two days prior to onset of symptoms and should be continued till menstruation starts.

Hormonal medications like oral contraceptive pills (OCPs), progesterone, spironolactone and bromocriptine can be prescribed.

Physiotherapy Management

- Regular aerobic exercises help increase red blood cells (RBCs), decrease the levels of progesterone and increase beta-endorphin level and increase pain tolerance, resulting in improvement of concentration, fatigue, and the majority of PMS symptoms.
- Yoga reduces stress, by reducing inflammatory mediators, and regulates levels of immunoglobulin A (IgA). Beneficial effects have been found when yoga was performed for 10 weeks, 3 sessions per week for 60 minutes.

Alternative Therapy

- **Cognitive behavioral therapy (CBT):** Royal College of Obstetricians and Gynecologists (RCOG) guidelines state that "When treating women with severe PMS, CBT should be considered routinely as a treatment option".
- **Aromatherapy:** Aromatherapy is found to be effective in improving physical and emotional symptoms associated with PMS. It can be used one week before the menstruation.

❖ **Acupuncture and acupressure:** Acupuncture provides greater reduction in mood-related PMS symptoms whereas acupressure improves both physical and mental health and in general improves the quality of life in females with PMS.

Mittelschmerz's Syndrome

Mittelschmerz—or ovulation pain, as it is commonly known today—is a benign preovulatory lower abdominal pain that occurs midcycle (between days 7 and 24) in women. Mittelschmerz may affect over 40% of women of reproductive age, and it occurs almost every month in these patients.

Causes

The exact causes are unknown, but some probable factors are:

❖ Increased tension of the graafian follicle, prior to rupture
❖ The follicular fluid following ovulation causes peritoneal irritation
❖ Contraction of fallopian tubes and uterus

Clinical Features

Mittelschmerz can present as pain in hypogastrium or in either iliac fossa, and it will generally be on the same side as the developing follicle. The pain usually ceases within three to twelve hours, although patients who have undergone ovarian surgery may experience Mittelschmerz that persists until the onset of menstruation. It may be associated with vaginal bleeding or excessive mucoid vaginal discharge. The patient may also report mild backache.

Management

Analgesics and giving assurance to the patients is found to be effective. In obstinate cases, cure is absolute by making cycle anovular with contraceptive pills.

AMENORRHEA

The absence of menstruation in a female of reproductive age is termed as 'Amenorrhea'. It is not a disease, but a symptom.

Amenorrhea can be—primary or secondary. Primary amenorrhea is absence of initiation of menses, whereas secondary amenorrhea is the absence of menses in a previously menstruating female.

 **Clinical Pointer**

The most common cause of amenorrhea is pregnancy and it should be the first cause to be ruled out before moving to other etiologies.

Types of Amenorrhea

Clinically, there are two types of amenorrhea **(Fig. 12.3)**:

1. Physiological
2. Pathological

Physiological Amenorrhea

The following are situations where amenorrhea is present and physiological in nature and considered normal or non-pathological:

❖ **Primary:** Before puberty
❖ **Secondary:**
  - During pregnancy
  - During lactation
  - After menopause

Pathological Amenorrhea

Cryptomenorrhea

Periodic shedding of the endometrium and bleeding occurs, but the blood fails to come out through the genital tract because of obstruction in the passage.

Causes:

❖ Congenital
  - Transverse vaginal septum
  - Imperforate hymen
  - Atresia of upper third vagina and cervix
❖ Acquired
  - Secondary vaginal atresia
  - Cervical stenosis

Clinical features:

❖ History of amenorrhea
❖ Periodic lower abdominal pain
❖ Symmetric enlargement of the uterus

Management:

❖ Cervical dilatation to drain collected blood
❖ Reconstructive surgery for secondary atresia of vagina

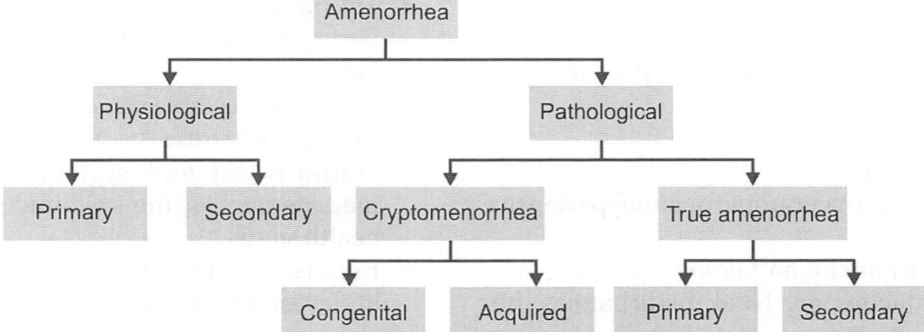

Fig. 12.3: Types of amenorrhea.

True Amenorrhea

- True primary amenorrhea is primary amenorrhea with absent or poor secondary sex characteristics.
- True secondary amenorrhea is amenorrhea secondary to some pathology not related to anatomical obstruction.

Primary Amenorrhea

Primary amenorrhea is absence of menstruation by 16 years of age.

Etiology

Abnormal chromosomal pattern, hypergonadotropic hypogonadism, hypogonadotropic hypogonadism, developmental defect of genital tract, thyroid and adrenal cortex disorders, unresponsive endometrium, metabolic disorders like juvenile diabetes and systemic illnesses like malnutrition, anemia, tuberculosis, etc., may contribute as etiological factors.

Investigations

- Pelvic ultrasonography (USG), karyotyping, CT scan can be performed for differential diagnosis.
- Follicle-stimulating hormone (FSH), luteinizing hormone (LH), thyroid stimulating hormone (TSH) and prolactin levels
  - Low or normal FSH and LH levels—physiological delay
  - Elevated LH:FSH ratio—polycystic ovarian syndrome
  - Elevated LH and FSH levels—premature ovarian failure, gonadal dysgenesis, resistant ovary
  - Abnormal TSH levels—hypo- or hyperthyroidism
  - Increased prolactin levels—hyperprolactinemia

Management

Management is usually medical or surgical depending on the etiology.

Secondary Amenorrhea

It is defined as absence of menstruation in a previously menstruating female for >6 months.

Etiology

Table 12.2 presents the probable causes of true secondary amenorrhea.

Other causes of secondary amenorrhea can include stress, body weight, psychotropic and antihypertensive drugs, contraceptive pills, malnutrition and diabetes.

Table 12.2: Etiology of true secondary amenorrhea.

Anatomical structure	*Pathology*
Uterus	• Postradiation therapy • Hysterectomy • Tubercular endometritis • Synechiae
Ovaries	• Premature ovarian failure • Polycystic ovarian syndrome • Chemotherapy • Resistant ovarian syndrome • Ovarian tumors • Hyperandrogenism • Oophorectomy • Pelvic radiation
Pituitary gland	• Adenoma • Acromegaly • Cushing's disease • Simmond's disease
Adrenal gland	• Adrenal tumor • Cushing's syndrome

History

- Mode of onset—sudden or gradual; hypo- or oligomenorrhea
- Sudden change in body weight
- Presence of eating disorders
- Intake of contraceptives, psychotropic or antihypertensive drugs
- History of radiotherapy or chemotherapy
- Symptoms like headaches or visual disturbances, hot flashes, vaginal dryness, inappropriate lactation, acne or hirsutism
- History of curettage, cesarean section, severe postpartum hemorrhage or prolonged lactation
- Positive family history

Examination

Examination may reveal following findings:
- Nutritional status
- Reduced skin temperature
- Presence of acne or hirsutism
- Discharge of milk from breasts
- Mass in lower abdomen
- Presence of striae (may point towards Cushing disease)
- Clitoral enlargement
- Adnexal mass

Management

- If no abnormality is detected and:
  - The patient is not anxious about the amenorrhea, then no treatment is required.
  - The patient is not anxious for fertility but about amenorrhea, oral combined steroidal contraceptives should be prescribed for at least 3 cycles with normal endogenous estrogen and ethinyl estradiol should be prescribed for those with low endogenous estrogen.
  - The patient is anxious about fertility, the couple should undergo evaluation for primary infertility and tubal factor.
- If there is a detectable cause:
  - Anxiety and stress—assurance and psychotherapy
  - Malnutrition and systemic illness—appropriate management of the systemic illness and improving health status
  - Exercise induced amenorrhea—appropriate diet and limitation of activity
- Medical and surgical management is decided depending on the underlying pathology.

ABNORMAL UTERINE BLEEDING

Uterine bleeding which is more or less than the normal volume, regularity, duration, or frequency **(Table 12.3)** is known as abnormal uterine bleeding (AUB). One-third of women experience AUB at least once in their life.

Etiology

International Federation of Obstetrics and Gynecology (FIGO) gave the acronym PALM-COEIN which describes the cause of AUB. The first portion, PALM, describes structural issues. The second portion, COEI, describes nonstructural issues. The N stands for "not otherwise classified."

- P: Polyp
- A: Adenomyosis
- L: Leiomyoma
- M: Malignancy and hyperplasia
- C: Coagulopathy
- O: Ovulatory dysfunction
- E: Endometrial disorders
- I: Iatrogenic
- N: Not otherwise classified

Examination

Bimanual examination should be done, including speculum examinations to exclude any palpable pathology of pelvis.

Investigations

- Laboratory tests: A urine pregnancy test, complete blood count, serum ferritin test (not done in routine), coagulation panel, thyroid function tests, gonadotropins, prolactin.
- Ultrasound and color Doppler
- Saline infusion sonography
- Hysteroscopy
- Endometrial sampling
- Laparoscopy
- Diagnostic dilatation and curettage

Management

For acute abnormal uterine bleeding, hormonal methods are the first line medical management. Intravenous (IV) conjugated equine estrogen, combined oral contraceptive pills (OCPs), and oral progestins are all options for treating acute AUB.

Based on the PALM-COEIN acronym for etiologies of chronic AUB, specific treatment options for each category exist which may be decided by the concerned medical professional.

Table 12.3: Characteristics of normal menstruation.

Interval between two cycles	28 days (21–35 days)
Menstrual flow	4–5 days
Menstrual blood	35 mL (20–80 mL)

Complications

Complications of chronic abnormal uterine bleeding can include anemia, infertility, and endometrial cancer. With acute abnormal uterine bleeding, severe anemia, hypotension, shock, and even death may result if prompt treatment and supportive care are not initiated.

Hypermenorrhea (Menorrhagia)

This is defined as excessive (>80 mL) and/or extensive (>7 days) bleeding.

Causes

Table 12.4 enlists the causes of hypermenorrhea.

Diagnosis

- Increased duration of flow
- Passage of clots in blood flow
- Increased number of sanitary pads used
- Pallor
- Low hemoglobin

Management

- Nonsteroidal anti-inflammatory drugs (NSAIDs), such as ibuprofen or naproxen sodium help in reducing menstrual blood loss. NSAIDs have the added benefit of relieving painful menstruation.
- Tranexamic acid (Lysteda)
- Oral contraceptives

Polymenorrhea

It is defined as cyclic bleeding in which cycle in reduced to less than 21 days and remains constant at that frequency. If the frequency of cycle is associated with prolonged bleeding it is known as epimenorrhea. It is commonly seen in adolescence, prior to menopause and following delivery and abortion, in PID or ovarian endometriosis.

Table 12.4: Causes of hypermenorrhea.

Organic causes		***Functional causes***
Pelvis	Fibroid uterus, adenomyosis, pelvic endometriosis, IUCD in utero, retroverted uterus, granulosa cell tumor of ovary	Adenomyosis
Systemic	Liver dysfunction, congestive cardiac failure, severe hypertension	Fibroid uterus
Endocrinal	Hyperthyroidism or hypothyroidism	Dysfunctional uterine bleeding
Hematological	Platelet deficiency, leukemia, thrombocytopenia, von Willebrand's disease	Chronic tubo-ovarian mass
Emotional and psychological issues		

(IUCD: intrauterine contraceptive device)

Metrorrhagia

Menometrorrhagia is the term used when bleeding becomes irregular and excessive, making it difficult to identify the periods. It is defined as irregular, acyclic bleeding from the uterus.

Causes

- Pregnancy
- Use of contraceptives
- Intrauterine devices
- Sexually transmitted infections (STIs)
- Coagulation disorders
- Genital trauma
- Neoplasms
- Infections such as genital tuberculosis
- Submucous fibroid
- Uterine polyp

Treatment

It depends on the underlying causative pathology.

Oligomenorrhea

This condition is defined as menstrual bleeding occurring at regular frequency of more than 35 days apart. Causes include age (adolescence and preceding menopause), obesity, endocrine disorders, androgen producing tumor, tubercular endometritis, drug induced. Oral contraceptives and hormonal therapy form the mainstay of medical management. Surgery may be necessary in case of adnexal and adrenal tumors.

Hypomenorrhea

In this condition menstrual bleeding becomes unduly scanty and lasting less than 2 days.

Causes

Table 12.5 enlists causes of hypomenorrhea.

Management

Medical management is needed only if a significant abnormality is found. Medical management will depend on cause. Iron tablets and hormonal therapy have been found to be efficient.

Dysfunctional Uterine Bleeding (DUB)

- This is defined as abnormal uterine bleeding, in absence of any detectable organic, systemic and iatrogenic cause.
- Heavy menstrual bleeding is a condition where the bleeding interferes with a female's physical, emotional, social, and mental quality of life.

Table 12.5: Causes of hypomenorrhea.

Local	Uterine synechiae, endometrial tuberculosis
Endocrinal	Thyroid dysfunctions, premenopausal period, use of oral contraceptives
Systemic	Malnutrition

- **There are two types of DUB:**
  1. Ovulatory DUB accounts for about 80% of cases. In ovulatory DUB the menstruation is regular, preceded by ovulation and heavy but of normal duration. It is most common in women in their 30s.
  2. Anovulatory DUB is more likely to occur at the beginning and end of the reproductive years. The menstrual cycle is irregular, and the bleeding is heavy and may be prolonged. Polycystic ovary syndrome may be associated with chronic anovulation.

Diagnosis

- Dysfunctional uterine bleeding is a diagnosis of exclusion. Uterine and systemic causes must be excluded before the diagnosis is made.
- A careful history and examination should be performed to exclude organic disease and to determine the extent of lifestyle impairment, what previous treatments have been used, and the woman's expectations from treatment.
- The assessment of heavy menstrual bleeding is quite subjective, and women may over or underestimate their menstrual loss. The symptoms and signs that may signify heavy menstrual bleeding include:
  - An unusual increase in blood loss
  - More than 7 days of bleeding
  - Bleeding or flooding not contained within pads or tampons (particularly if wearing the largest size)
  - Clots greater than 3 cm
  - The presence of signs of anemia or iron deficiency on blood testing
- Apart from laboratory examinations, transvaginal ultrasound (except in the adolescent woman) will aid in excluding pelvic causes of heavy bleeding. Hysteroscopy with dilation and curettage or endometrial biopsy, or laparoscopy if there is associated pain, will be diagnostic but not curative for DUB.

Management

- Medical treatment consists of antifibrinolytic tranexamic acid, nonsteroidal anti-inflammatory drugs, the combined contraception pill, progestogen, danazol, or analogues of gonadotrophin releasing hormone. The levonorgestrel releasing intrauterine device is developed for contraception but is also effective in the treatment of dysfunctional uterine bleeding.
- Surgical treatment includes endometrial ablation of the first and second-generation, and hysterectomy.

PELVIC INFECTIONS

Infections can affect the following structures of the female reproductive system:

- Vulva
- Vagina
- Cervix
- Uterus
- Fallopian tubes

The commonly seen infections are as follows:

Genital Tuberculosis

Tuberculosis (TB) is a worldwide health problem, though it has a declining mortality rate. The presence of genital tuberculosis (TB) varies with the patient's environment and social status. With the increase in prevalence of human immunodeficiency virus the prevalence of TB is rising.

Etiology and Pathogenesis

- *Mycobacterium bacillus* is the common causative agent for genital tuberculosis.
- **Mode of transmission:** Genital tuberculosis usually develops secondary to pulmonary tuberculosis via hematogenous route. It can also occur secondary to infections in the kidney, skeletal system, or gastrointestinal tract via lymphatic route. Rarely, it can also occur due to infection of genitalia through sexual transmission.
- The most common organs affected due to genital TB **(Table 12.6)** are fallopian tubes, followed by endometrium, ovaries, cervix, and vagina/vulva.
- Genital TB is common in females, especially of reproductive age (15–45 years). Genital TB can mimic or coexist with other gynecological and abdominal pathologies such as genital carcinomas, acute appendicitis, ovarian cysts, or ectopic pregnancy.

Clinical Presentation

Genital tuberculosis usually is asymptomatic or presents with very few symptoms. The most common clinical symptom is infertility, other signs and symptoms are listed in **Table 12.7**.

Diagnosis

Genital TB is paucibacillary in nature. So, a positive test of M bacillus is not necessary, a detailed examination, history is needed for the correct diagnosis of this condition.

- **A detailed history:** Medical history of tuberculosis (lung, kidney, skeletal tissues), HIV positive, family history of tuberculosis, or history of antituberculosis therapy (ATT)

Table 12.6: Genital tuberculosis (TB).

Type of TB	*Characteristics*
Fallopian tube TB	Often leads to infertility
Uterine TB	• Endometrium is affected in 50–80% patients through hematogenous, lymphatic or contagious route • May lead to amenorrhea and infertility
Ovarian TB	• Comprises 20–30% of total genital TB • Can cause defects in ovarian function and sometimes complete destruction of ovaries **(Fig. 12.4)**
Cervical TB	• Rarely involved (less than 5%) in genital TB • Usually secondary to TB of fallopian tube or uterus
Vulval and vaginal TB	• Can occur secondary to TB of uterus or cervix • Clinically manifests as hypertrophic ulcer or growth on the vulva or vagina • Rarely can occur via sexually transmitted infected semen of partner

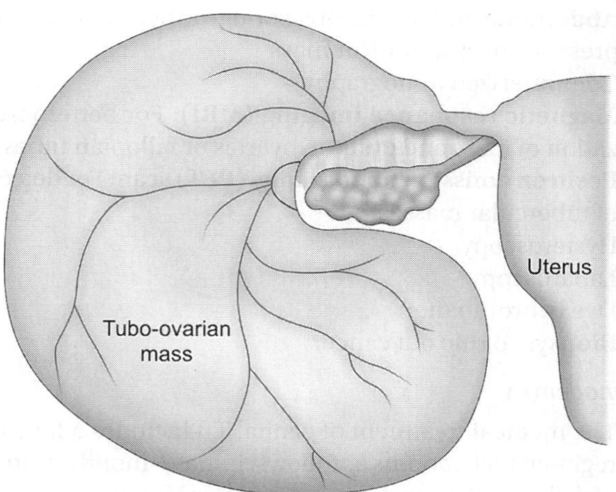

Fig. 12.4: Tubo-ovarian mass.

Table 12.7: Signs and symptoms of genital TB.

General symptoms	*Systemic signs*
Fever	Increased body temperature
Loss of appetite	Lymphadenopathy
Unintentional weight loss	Crackles on chest auscultation
Fatigue, malaise, weakness	
Menstrual symptoms	***Abdominal/pelvic examination***
Menorrhagia (heavy menstrual flow)	Vague or definite abdominal or pelvic lump
Postmenopausal bleeding	Ascites
• Oligomenorrhea (infrequent and irregular menstrual flow) • Hypomenorrhea (scanty menstruation flow)	Doughy feel of abdomen
Amenorrhea	
Dysmenorrhea	Soft, tender enlarged uterus
Infertility	Lump in adnexa
Abdominal or pelvic pain	Fullness in pouch of Douglas
Abdominal or pelvic mass	Tenderness in pouch of Douglas
Ulcers on genitals or pelvic organs	Solid lesions on external genitals
Urinary or fecal incontinence	Ulcers or fistula on genitals

- **Physical examination:** Both pelvic and abdominal examination **(Table 12.7)**.
- **Investigations:**
  - Blood tests—anemia, leukocytosis with lymphocytosis and raised erythrocyte sedimentation rate (ESR)
  - Serological tests like ELISA
  - Mantoux (tuberculin) test and interferon gamma release assays; poor sensitivity and specificity
  - Mycobacterial smear and culture
  - Polymerase chain reaction test
- **Chest radiographs:** For diagnosis of pulmonary TB

- **Abdominal and pelvic ultrasonography:** For detection of presence of cysts and/or mass
- Computerized tomography
- **Magnetic resonance imaging (MRI):** For better visualization of mass and cysts on ovaries or fallopian tubes
- **Positron emission tomography (PET) scan:** For detection of tubercular masses
- Hysteroscopy
- Laparoscopy
- Dye hydrotubation
- **Biopsy:** To rule out cancer

Management

- The medical treatment of genital TB includes a four-drug regimen for 6 months as follows: initial 2-month treatment of daily rifampin, isoniazid, pyrazinamide, and ethambutol, followed by 4-month treatment of daily isoniazid, rifampin, and ethambutol.
- Recent report of WHO suggested bedaquiline and delamanid as an injection-free regimen for all types of TB, including multidrug-resistant TB.
- Along with the comprehensive ATT management, females who are facing infertility due to tubal tuberculosis can opt for assisted reproductive technology (ART), such as *in vitro* fertilization and embryo transfer.
- Recent development of biotechniques have led to successful treatment options of stem cell transplantation and nanomaterials, regenerative ovaries, the fallopian tubes, or the endometrium to treat permanent injuries.

Physiotherapy Management

- Aerobic exercise plans with adequate warm-up can be given to maintain and improve endurance and quality of life.
- Symptomatic relief from dysmenorrhea can be obtained with stretching and relaxation exercises.

Clinical Pointer

Caution should be taken while inculcating electrotherapy in physiotherapy plan as it may worsen the infection. For active genital TB, electrophoresis can be given with 3% sodium thiosulphate along with ATT. For chronic TB ultrasound hydrocortisone therapy can be given.

Pelvic Inflammatory Disease

Pelvic inflammatory disease (PID) is a disorder of upper genital tract. It is infection and inflammation of the uterus, fallopian tubes and other adjacent pelvic organs. Various terms which describe the pelvic organ infections are:

- Salpingitis
- Salpingo-oophoritis
- Endometritis
- Adnexitis
- Parametritis
- Pyosalpinx
- Tubo-ovarian abscess
- Tubo-ovarian complex
- Pelvic peritonitis
- Perihepatitis
- Periappendicitis

Etiology and Pathogenesis

- The most common causative organisms in India are *Neisseria gonorrhoeae, Chlamydia trachomatis. Mycoplasma genitalium, Mycoplasma hominis*, and *Ureaplasma urealyticum* are also found in people having PID.
- The risk factors associated with PIDs are menstruating teenagers, multiple sex partners, absence of contraceptive pill, previous history of acute PID, intrauterine device (IUD) users, and is common in regions with high prevalence of sexually transmitted disease.
- In PID infective organisms often ascend from lower genital tract (cervical or cervicovaginal infections) to the upper genital tract. Endometritis can lead to salpingitis, pyosalpinx and sometimes tubo-ovarian abscess formation. Perihepatitis (Fitz-Hugh-Curtis syndrome) also often occurs with infection that is associated with PID.

Clinical Presentation

Symptoms

Majority of people having PID remain asymptomatic or are subclinical (60%). As per ACOG, the symptoms of PID are:

- Abnormal vaginal discharge
- Pain in the lower abdomen (often a mild ache)
- Pain in the upper right abdomen
- Abnormal menstrual bleeding
- Fever and chills
- Dysuria
- Nausea and vomiting
- Dyspareunia

Diagnosis and Investigations

The diagnosis of PID is usually through clinical suspicion. History of unprotected sex with varied or new partner(s), puberty, lack of hygiene and having unexplained lower abdominal or pelvic pain often suggests the need to start empiric treatment for PID. It is essential to diagnose and treat PID early because untreated PID can lead to infertility, ectopic pregnancy and/or chronic pelvic pain. This fact has led to the recommendation of "**Syndromic diagnosis**".

In syndromic diagnosis women with lower abdominal tenderness, adnexal tenderness or cervical motion tenderness should be treated for PID if there is no other diagnosis.

Signs

- Low abdominal tenderness
- Adnexal tenderness on bimanual vaginal examination
- Cervical motion tenderness on bimanual vaginal examination
- Oral temperature >38.3°C (>101°F)
- Abnormal cervical mucopurulent discharge or cervical friability

Investigations

- Blood investigations in PID would reveal increased number of white blood cells on saline microscopy of vaginal fluid
- Elevated erythrocyte sedimentation rate
- Elevated C-reactive protein
- Laboratory documentation of cervical infection with *N. gonorrhoeae* or *C. trachomatis*
- CT scan will help to diagnose perihepatic inflammation.
- Laparoscopy is useful for diagnosis of salpingitis, tubo-ovarian abscess, peritonitis, and possibly perihepatitis.
- Endovaginal power-Doppler ultrasonography
- MRI seems to be as accurate as endovaginal ultrasonography in the diagnosis of in-patient PID. It helps to diagnose any type of tubo-ovarian abscess or inflammation.
- Endometrial biopsy with histopathologic evidence of endometritis.

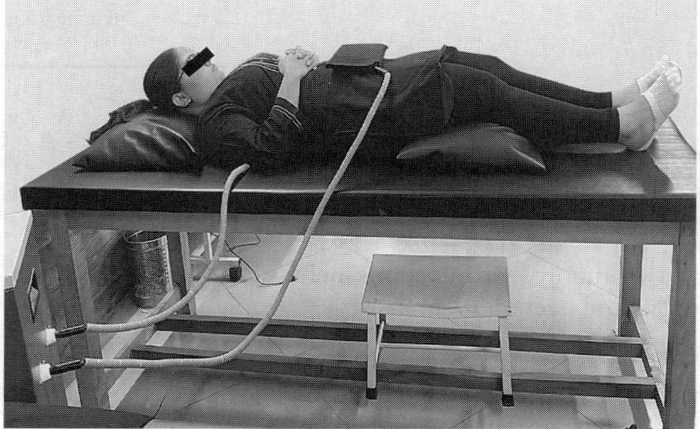

Fig. 12.5: SWD application in supine lying (first half of the treatment).

Treatment

Prevention

- Community based approach to increase awareness among people about safe sex. This will also help to prevent sexually transmitted infections.
- Routine screening of high-risk population
- Methods to inculcate awareness about improving health.

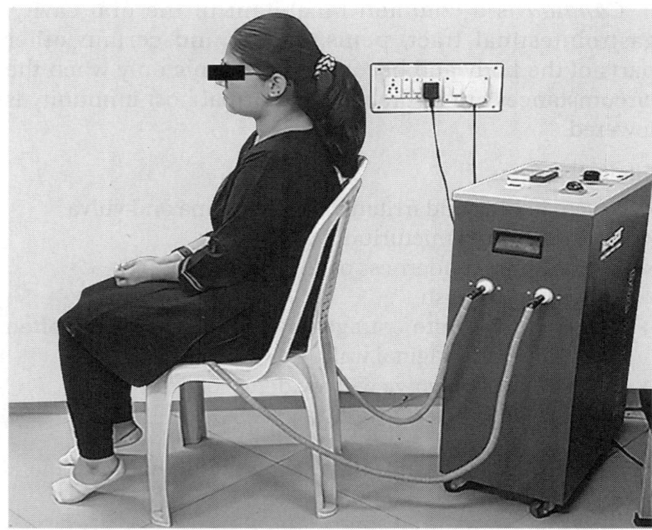

Fig. 12.6: SWD application in sitting (second half of the treatment).

Medical Management

Current treatment guidelines suggest use of broad-spectrum antibiotic agents to treat PID. Effective combination treatment strategy includes doxycycline plus metronidazole. Along with starting any antimicrobial treatment for PID, any intrauterine contraceptive device should be removed, and other methods of contraception should be initiated.

Physiotherapy Management

Management of symptoms of pelvic pain and tenderness can be obtained by proper pelvic rehabilitation. The rehabilitation techniques which can be used are:

- Pelvic floor muscle exercises: Kegel exercises
- Myofascial release of painful trigger points
- Core stabilization exercises in form of Pilates or Swiss ball exercise
- Electromyography (EMG) biofeedback of pelvic muscles
- Relaxation techniques can also be included
- Stretching of pelvic floor muscle, hip adductors and iliopsoas can also be added
- Short wave diathermy has been found to be helpful in symptomatic treatment of PID **(Figs. 12.5 to 12.7)**. SWD using crossfire technique for 15 sessions in a month on alternate days for 20 minutes is found effective in control of pain and inflammation.

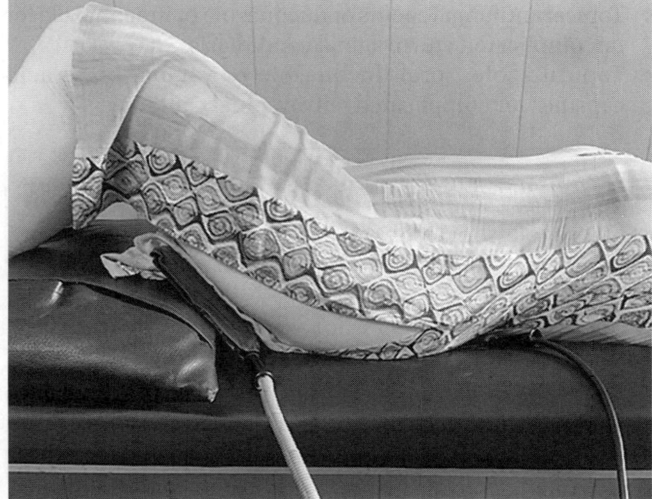

Fig. 12.7: SWD application in crook lying (second half of the treatment) (alternate position)

Sexually Transmitted Infections

Sexually transmitted infections (STIs) **(Fig. 12.8)** include the infections which are predominantly transmitted via sexual contact with an infected person. It is common in younger age group.

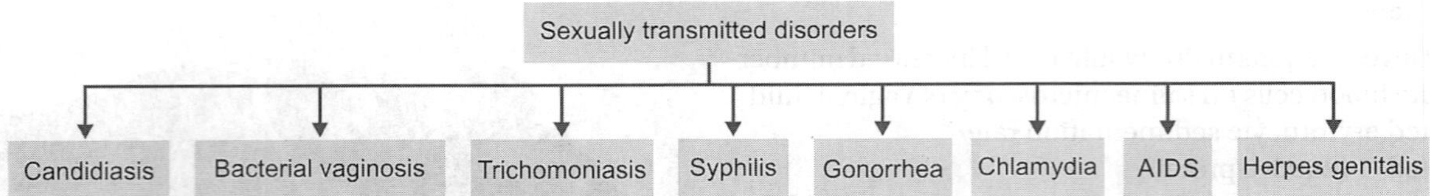

Fig. 12.8: Classification of STI.

Commonly seen infections include candidiasis, trichomoniasis and bacterial vaginosis.

Candidiasis

Candidiasis is an opportunistic infection caused by a fungal organism named *Candida*. It is an yeast infection, also called moniliasis, candidosis or thrush. It usually occurs as a secondary infection in immunocompromised individuals. **Box 12.1** gives risk factors for *Candida vaginitis*.

Candida is a common inhabitant of the oral cavity, gastrointestinal tract, penis, vagina and certain other parts of the body and becomes pathogenic only when the circumstances are favorable, i.e., normal host immunity is lowered.

Box 12.1: Risk factors for *Candida vaginitis*.

- Diabetes
- Pregnancy
- Broad spectrum antibiotics
- Thyroid or parathyroid disorders
- Obesity
- Drugs like steroids or combined oral contraceptive pills
- Immunosuppressed state

Clinical features

- Severe itching and irritation in the vagina and vulva
- Burning during micturition
- Vaginal pain, tenderness or soreness
- Erythematous rash
- Thick, curdy white cottage cheese like discharge often adherent to the vaginal wall
- Red and swollen vulva with evidence of pruritus.

Diagnosis

Microscopy of vaginal discharge shows budding yeast.

Management

- Intravaginal fungal preparations
- Vaginal cream or pessary composed of nystatin, clotrimazole, terconazole and miconazole
- Topical antifungal agents or fluconazole or itraconazole for uncomplicated vulvovaginal candidiasis
- Topical azoles, oral fluconazole or vaginal boric acid capsules for complicated vulvovaginal candidiasis

Clinical Pointer

Fluconazole should be avoided in the first trimester of pregnancy.

Bacterial Vaginosis

Bacterial vaginosis is caused by *Gardnerella vaginalis (G. vaginalis)*, the *Bacteroides* species, *Mobiluncus, Peptococcus species, Mycoplasma hominis* and *Prevotella*. A significant decrease in Lactobacilli is seen among such females.

Risk factors

- New or multiple sexual partners
- Cigarette smoking
- Immunosuppression
- Intrauterine copper device
- Sexual intercourse at an early age

Diagnosis

- Creamy vaginal discharge with fishy odor
- Homogenous grayish white discharge that is adherent to the vaginal wall
- Vaginal pH >4.5
- No inflammation of the vagina as observed by biopsy

Management

Metronidazole and tinidazole or oral and intravaginal Clindamycin.

Trichomoniasis

Trichomoniasis is a protozoan infection caused by *Trichomonas vaginalis* that commonly occurs in the child bearing period. *T. vaginalis* is a motile organism that lives in the prostate and urethra of males and the lower genitourinary tract of females. It increases the risk of human immunodeficiency virus (HIV) infection in both males and females and is associated with adverse outcomes during pregnancy.

Clinical features

- Thin, greenish yellow or gray, frothy, offensive vaginal discharge
- Itching and irritation around the introitus
- Dysuria with increased frequency of micturition
- Inflammation of vulva with evidence of pruritus
- Vaginal examination shows red discoloration with inflammation and multiple punctate hemorrhagic spots giving appearance of a strawberry (classic but rare sign)
- Mild tenderness of the pelvis

Diagnosis

- Trichomonads can be visualized on wet prep microscopy
- Nucleic acid amplification tests (NAATs) with vaginal discharge
- Vaginal pH > 4.5

Management

The CDC recommends three strategies—a single 2-gram dose of tinidazole, a single 2-gram dose of metronidazole or a seven-day course of 500 mg metronidazole twice daily.

Gonorrhea

Neisseria gonorrhoeae is the causative gram-negative bacteria having incubation period of 3–7 days.

Clinical features

Approximately 50% of people with gonorrhea are asymptomatic and if symptoms are present they are usually very non-specific **(Table 12.8)**.

Diagnosis

Laboratory confirmation of *N. gonorrhoeae* infection's diagnosis is made by direct detection of the gonococcal pathogen in urogenital, anorectal, pharyngeal, or conjunctival swab specimens. NAATs are now used for detection of gonococci.

Medical management

Single dose of any of the following can be done:
- Ceftriaxone
- Ciprofloxacin
- Ofloxacin
- Cefixime
- Levofloxacin

Clinical Pointer

Regular follow-up with blood culture should be done a week after therapy and then again should be repeated at monthly intervals, if the reports are negative, it can be said the patient is cured.

Syphilis

It is a systemic bacterial infection caused by *Treponema pallidum*. It is a common infection in people with multiple partners.

Clinical features

Primary stage: A single chancre marks the onset of the primary (first) stage of syphilis, but there may be multiple sores. The chancre is usually firm, and painless. These painless chancres can occur in locations that make them difficult to notice (e.g., the vagina or anus). The chancre lasts 3–6 weeks and heals regardless of whether a person receives treatment. However, the infection will progress to the secondary stage if the person with syphilis does not receive treatment.

Table 12.8: Clinical features of gonorrhea.

Local	*Distant*
• Dysuria • Excessive vaginal discharge • Involvement of Bartholin's gland can cause pain and swelling over labia • Rectal discomfort maybe present	• Infection may spread to liver capsule causing perihepatitis • Adhesions of abdominal walls • Septicemia which can be characterized by low grade fever, skin rash, endocarditis, tenosynovitis, perihepatitis, septic arthritis, polyarthralgia • Pelvic inflammatory disease

Secondary stage: Skin rashes and/or mucous membrane lesions (sores in the mouth, vagina, or anus) mark the second stage of symptoms. This stage typically starts with the development of a rash on one or more areas of the body. Rashes during the secondary stage:
- Can appear when the primary chancre is healing or several weeks after the chancre heals.
- Usually do not cause itching.
- May appear as rough, red, or reddish-brown spots on the palm of the hands and bottoms of the feet. However, rashes with a different appearance may occur on other parts of the body. Sometimes they resemble rashes caused by other diseases.
- May be so faint they are hard to notice.

Condyloma lata are large, raised, gray or white lesions. They may develop in warm, moist areas like the mouth, underarm or groin region.

In addition to rashes, signs and symptoms of secondary syphilis may include:
- Fever
- Swollen lymph nodes
- Sore throat
- Patchy hair loss
- Headaches
- Weight loss
- Muscle aches
- Fatigue

The symptoms of secondary syphilis will go away with or without treatment. However, without treatment, the infection will progress to the latent and possibly tertiary stage of disease.

Latent stage: The latent (hidden) stage of syphilis is a period when there are no visible signs or symptoms of syphilis. Without treatment, syphilis will remain in the body even though there are no signs or symptoms. *Early latent syphilis* is latent syphilis where infection occurs within the past 12 months. *Late latent syphilis* is latent syphilis where infection occurs more than 12 months ago. *Latent syphilis of unknown duration* is when there is not enough evidence to confirm initial infection was within the previous 12 months. Latent syphilis can last for years.

Tertiary syphilis

Tertiary syphilis is rare and develops in cases of untreated syphilis. It can appear 10–30 years after a person gets the infection, and it can be fatal. Tertiary syphilis can affect multiple organ systems, including:
- Brain
- Nerves
- Eyes
- Heart
- Blood vessels

- Liver
- Bones
- Joints

Symptoms of tertiary syphilis vary depending on the organ system affected.

Diagnosis

- Testing strategies for syphilis consist of dark-field microscopy and serological tests.
- As per CDC people with neurologic symptoms should undergo cerebrospinal fluid (CSF) examination.

Treatment

Single dose of intramuscular (IM) penicillin G benzathine 2.4 million units.

Clinical Pointer

Patients need to be followed post-treatment at 3, 6, 9, 12, and 24 months with serial nontreponemal tests. A 4-fold decline in these tests indicates successful treatment.

Chlamydial Infections

Chlamydia is a common STD caused by infection with Chlamydia trachomatis. It can cause cervicitis, urethritis, and proctitis.

In women, these infections can lead to:

- Pelvic inflammatory disease (PID)
- Tubal factor infertility
- Ectopic pregnancy
- Chronic pelvic pain

Herpes Genitalis

It is caused by Herpes simplex virus (HSV) type I and II.

Clinical features

Symptoms usually appear less than 7 days after contact with infected person. There is inflammation of clitoris, vagina, vestibule, labia, perineum and cervix. The vesicles progress into shallow ulcers which spontaneously heal by crusting. This entire process takes about 3 weeks.

Constitutional symptoms such as fever, malaise, headache with vulvar burning, pruritus, dysuria or retention of urine maybe present.

Diagnosis

- Virus tissue culture is done
- Detection of antigen by **enzyme-linked immunoassay (ELISA)** or immunofluorescent method can be done
- Polymerase chain reaction (PCR) test to identify the HSV DNA is the rapid, specific and most accurate test.

Treatment

- Acyclovir which inhibits synthesis of DNA by virus is effective in acute attack.
- Prophylactic use of acyclovir reduces recurrence.
- Valacyclovir or famciclovir given orally thrice daily can also be used.
- Saline bath would help to reduce the local pain.

Acquired Immunodeficiency Syndrome (AIDS)

Human immunodeficiency virus (HIV) has infected >60 million people since its discovery and 30 million people have died since the pandemic began. HIV can be transmitted via the exchange of a variety of body fluids from infected people, such as blood, breast milk, semen and vaginal secretions.

Clinical features

The first signs of HIV infection may be flu-like symptoms:

- Fever
- Chills
- Rash
- Night sweats
- Muscle aches
- Sore throat
- Fatigue
- Swollen lymph nodes
- Mouth ulcers

These symptoms may come and go within two to four weeks. This stage is called acute HIV infection. If the infection is not treated, it becomes chronic HIV infection.

Medical management

HIV disease can be managed by treatment regimens composed of a combination of antiretroviral (ARV) drugs.

- Current antiretroviral therapy (ART) does not cure HIV infection but suppresses viral replication and allows an individual's immune system recovery to strengthen and regain the capacity to fight off opportunistic infections and some cancers.
- WHO has recommended *Treat All*: that all people living with HIV be provided with lifelong ART, including children, adolescents, adults and pregnant and breastfeeding women, regardless of clinical status or CD4 cell count.

Physiotherapy management

The primary goals (depending on the stage of the disease) for prescribing exercise in HIV-infected patients are:

- To improve quality of life (QoL)
- To improve physical tolerance
- To improve neuromuscular function
- To promote long-term exercise compliance

Therefore, we should include both short- and long-term individualized goals based on the subjective and objective findings in the patient's assessment.

Most HIV studies have used a three times weekly intervention with success or three/four times per week. Type or mode of aerobic exercises to improve the cardiovascular system includes running, walking, swimming, aerobics classes, circuit training, and cycling, whereas exercises to stress the neuromuscular system include progressive resisted exercises (PRE) involving weights, cables/pulleys/resistance bands, body weight, and plyometrics.

Prevention and control of STIs are based on the following five major strategies (CDC guidelines of 2021):

1. Accurate risk assessment and education and counseling of persons at risk regarding ways to avoid STIs through changes in sexual behaviors and use of recommended prevention services

2. Pre-exposure vaccination for vaccine preventable STIs
3. Identification of persons with an asymptomatic infection and persons with symptoms associated with an STI
4. Effective diagnosis, treatment, counseling, and follow up of persons who are infected with an STI
5. Evaluation, treatment, and counseling of sex partners of persons who are infected with an STI.

PELVIC PAIN AND LOW BACK PAIN

Pelvic pain is the most common symptom that the patient presents with in gynecology. It may be acute or chronic. Pelvic pain can be—splanchnic or referred **(Table 12.9)**. It can be acute or chronic. Acute pelvic pain is easy to diagnose, however, chronic pelvic pain often goes undiagnosed.

Clinical Pointer

A trigger point tenderness suggests ilioinguinal nerve entrapment whereas, ovarian point tenderness is suggestive of pelvic congestion syndrome.

Acute Pelvic Pain

- Acute pelvic pain is defined as lower abdominal or pelvic pain lasting less than 6 months.
- It is of short duration and the intensity of symptoms is proportionate to the extent of tissue damage.
- The basic mechanism underlying most causes of acute pelvic pain is irritation of the peritoneum by infection or blood.

Table 12.10 presents some of the causes of acute pelvic pain.

Diagnosis

Table 12.11 shows history taking and physical examination findings and their probable diagnoses.

Investigations

- Blood investigations—Hb estimation, differential and total WBC count and packed cell volume are important. Infection is suggested by an increased WBC count.
- Microscopic examination of midstream urine—pus cells, RBCs and bacteria suggest UTI.
- Urine pregnancy test for pregnancy
- Nucleic acid amplification tests (NAATs) to detect chlamydia and gonorrhea infections
- Erythrocyte sedimentation rate (ESR) may be raised with inflammatory conditions.

Table 12.9: Referred pelvic pain.

Structure	***Site of pain***
Cervix	Upper sacral region
Body of uterus	Hypogastrium, medial and anterior aspects of thighs
Fallopian tubes and ovaries	Above the midinguinal point
Uterosacral ligament	Lower sacral region

Table 12.10: Causes of acute pelvic pain in women.

Reproductive age	Gynecologic	• Endometriosis • Ectopic pregnancy • Pelvic inflammatory disease (PID) • Adenomyosis • Ruptured ovarian cyst • Ovarian torsion • Tubo-ovarian abscess • Uterine fibroid • Abortion
	Gastrointestinal	• Gastritis • Appendicitis • Diverticulitis • Bowel obstruction • Irritable bowel syndrome • Perirectal abscess • Mesenteric venous thrombosis
	Urinary	• Cystitis • Ureterolithiasis • Pyelonephritis
	Other causes	• Lead poisoning • Porphyria • Narcotic seeking • Sickle cell crisis • Dissecting aortic aneurysm • Malingering • Somatization disorder
Adolescence	Most causes same as females of reproductive age	• Imperforate hymen • Transverse vaginal septum
Pregnancy		• Endometriosis • Ectopic pregnancy • Ovarian torsion • Corpus luteum hematoma • Placental abruption • Ovarian vein thrombosis • Uterine impaction
Post-menopause	Most causes same as females of reproductive age except ectopic pregnancy and ovarian torsion	

Imaging

- X-ray abdomen to diagnose intestinal perforation or obstruction; free fluid suggests ruptured cyst
- Ultrasonography to diagnose pelvic mass or pregnancy
- Laparoscopy to visualize any pelvic pathology
- When ultrasonography is indeterminate, computed tomography (CT) or magnetic resonance imaging should be considered.

Management

- Medical management would suffice for urinary tract infection, PID, gastroenteritis and hyperstimulation syndrome.
- Laparotomy may be required for hemoperitoneum, twisted ovarian cyst, ruptured tubo-ovarian abscess and in case of acute surgical condition.

Table 12.11: History taking and physical examination findings and their probable diagnoses.

History	Dysmenorrhea	Endometriosis, uterine fibroid
	Dysuria	Urinary tract infection (UTI), PID
	Dyspareunia	Endometriosis, ovarian cyst
	Bilateral pelvic pain	PID
	Left-sided pelvic pain	Ruptured ovarian cyst, kidney stone, diverticulitis
	Right-sided pelvic pain	Ruptured ovarian cyst, kidney stone, ovarian torsion, appendicitis
	Radiation of pain to groin	Kidney stone, ovarian torsion
	Mid-cycle pain	Mittelschmerz
	Gross hematuria	UTI, kidney stone
	Nausea and vomiting	Ovarian torsion, appendicitis
	Vaginal discharge	PID
	Vaginal bleeding	Uterine fibroid, ectopic pregnancy
	Urinary frequency	UTI
Physical examination	Fever	PID, appendicitis, pyelonephritis
	Bilateral abdominal tenderness	PID
	Left lower quadrant abdominal tenderness	Diverticulitis
	Right lower quadrant abdominal tenderness	Appendicitis
	Hypotension	Ruptured hemorrhagic ovarian cyst, ectopic pregnancy
	Adnexal mass	PID, ectopic pregnancy, uterine fibroid, corpus luteum cyst, follicular cyst, diverticula of colon
	Cervical motion, adnexal or uterine tenderness	PID
	Vaginal discharge of mucopurulent quality	PID

Chronic Pelvic Pain

Chronic pelvic pain (CPP) is pelvic pain that lasts for six months or more. It is a chronic, disabling and persistent problem that is relatively common in women. It may be associated with PID, irritable bowel syndrome or a major depressive disorder. It is a form of centralized pain where the pain threshold of the body is lowered. Central pain is characterized be hyperalgesia or allodynia. Management of CPP is complex and requires multidisciplinary approach where some patients may benefit from cognitive behavioral therapy (CBT) or hormone replacement, whereas some others may require invasive procedures like spinal cord stimulation or total hysterectomy.

Diagnosis

- History may present signs of hyperalgesia and allodynia which may suggest central sensitization. Cotton tip applicator test (application of cotton swab to abdominal region) can be done to assess allodynia.
- Pain is located in the pelvic region and has lasted for at least six months.
- Pain is usually unrelated to pregnancy and may be constant or episodic.
- History taking should include questions regarding association between menses and the pelvic pain, sexual activity, bowel movements and urination.
- Quality of life should be assessed, as it is usually affected.
- Motor or autonomic dysfunction may be present.
- Initial diagnostic work up includes urine analysis, urine pregnancy test, complete blood count, erythrocyte sedimentation rate, testing for gonorrhea or chlamydia and pelvic ultrasonography.
- Transvaginal ultrasonography may be required for masses, cysts and adenomyosis.

Box 12.2 presents some red flags for CPP.

Management

- Conservative or radical surgery to remove the causative pathology. Hysterectomy for pelvic endometriosis or adenomyosis once the female has completed child-bearing or does not wish to bear child.
- Pain management can be done using nonsteroidal anti-inflammatory agents (NSAIDs) like ibuprofen, naproxen and COX-2 inhibitors; neurolytic agents like tricyclic anti-depressants, serotonin uptake inhibitors and ion channel blockers; narcotics or oral contraceptive pills.

Box 12.2: Red flags for chronic pelvic pain.

- Postmenopausal bleeding or onset of pain
- Postcoital bleeding
- Pelvic mass
- Unexplained weight loss
- Hematuria

Box 12.3: Factors associated with gynecologic LBP.

- LBP related to child birth or some gynecological procedure
- Symptoms aggravated during menses
- Pain does not go beyond L4 vertebra
- Diffuse and dull pain

- Pelvic floor physiotherapy (included in Chapter 15: Managing the Pelvic Floor) is beneficial in relieving CPP.
- CBT relieves pain and stress and improves function in CPP.
- Other management options include peripheral nerve blocks, radiofrequency ablation and neuromodulation using spinal cord stimulator.

Low Back Pain

Low back pain (LBP) is a common complaint among parous women. It is crucial to differentiate LBP due to gynecologic reasons from musculoskeletal reasons **(Box 12.3)**.

Common causes of LBP include:

- Uterine displacement (prolapse or retroversion)
- Chronic pelvic infection
- Neoplasm
- Endometriosis

Management of LBP involves managing the underlying causative pathology.

Summary

Several gynecological conditions exist that can affect the female body. Most common of these are—menstrual disorders, low back pain and pelvic pain, pelvic infections including sexually transmitted infections, inflammatory disorders and uterine bleeding disorders. Among menstrual disorders, dysmenorrhea is the most common complaint. It can be primary or secondary in character. Management of primary dysmenorrhea is aimed at managing the symptoms and comprises of analgesics, antispasmodics, oral contraceptives and NSAIDs; whereas management of secondary dysmenorrhea is aimed at managing the cause rather than the symptoms. Premenstrual syndrome affects the female a lot psychologically and can be managed by lifestyle and diet modifications, antidepressants, anxiolytics and diuretics. Physiotherapy management comprises aerobic exercises and Yoga. CBT, aromatherapy and acupuncture and acupressure. Mittelschmerz's syndrome or ovulation pain can be managed using analgesics and contraceptive pills. Amenorrhea is absence of menstruation, which can be physiological or pathological. Physiological amenorrhea occurs before puberty, during pregnancy and lactation and after menopause, and does not need to be managed. Pathological amenorrhea can be primary or secondary and needs to be managed. Uterine bleeding which is more or less than the normal volume, regularity, duration, or frequency is known as abnormal uterine bleeding (AUB). Medical management includes hormonal methods, whereas surgical options include removal of polyps, hysterectomy or adenomyomectomy. Such disorders also include hypermenorrhea, polymenorrhea, metrorrhagia, hypomenorrhea and dysfunctional uterine bleeding. Pelvic infections are also quite commonly seen in the female population. They can affect any of the female reproductive structures such as vulva, vagina, fallopian tubes, uterus and cervix. Pelvic inflammatory disorder, genital tuberculosis and sexually transmitted infections like candidiasis, gonorrhea, chlamydial infections, syphilis, trichomoniasis, HIV/AIDS and bacterial vaginosis are included in pelvic infections. Most of the gynecological patients present with pelvic or low back pain which can be managed by treating the underlying cause.

CLINICAL EXAMPLE FOR PRIMARY DYSMENORRHEA

A 20-year-old female having primary dysmenorrhea since past two years reported to the clinic. Her chief complaint is severe disabling pain with menstruation in lower abdomen lasting 24 hours. The severity of pain is such she needs leave from work. She described the nature of pain as spasmodic. She also complained of nausea, vomiting and fatigue. Last month she went to the gynecologist who did pelvic and abdominal examination and found no pathology. She was diagnosed with primary dysmenorrhea and was prescribed antispasmodic. Physiotherapist found the girl has a sedentary lifestyle and is obese.

Suggested Physiotherapy Management

- Regular aerobic exercises with 15-minutes warm, 45 minutes moderate intensity exercise and 10 minutes of cool down which will include stretching. This must be done on alternate days every week for 12 weeks.
- Yoga poses such as cobra pose should be done regularly for 10 weeks.

Review Questions

1. What is genital tuberculosis?
2. Discuss various menstrual disorders in detail.
3. Describe in detail: Amenorrhea.
4. Describe in detail: Dysmenorrhea.
5. Write short notes on:
   a. Sexually transmitted infections
   b. Dysfunctional uterine bleeding
   c. Low backache
   d. Trichomoniasis of vagina
   e. Vaginal candidiasis
   f. AIDS

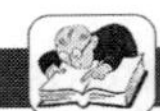

Bibliography

1. ACOG Practice Bulletin No. 198. (2018). Obstetrics & Gynecology. 2018;132(3), e87–e102. doi:10.1097/aog.0000000000002841
2. American College of Obstetricians and Gynecologists. (Updated 2018). Practice Bulletin No. 114: Management of endometriosis. Obst Gynecol. 2010;116(1), 223–36.
3. American Society for Reproductive Medicine. (n.d.). Quick facts about infertility. http://connect.asrm.org/srs/about/newitem9?ssopc=1
4. Armour M, Ee CC, Hao J, Wilson TM, Yao SS, Smith CA. Acupuncture and acupressure for premenstrual syndrome. Cochrane Database Syst Rev. 2018(8):CD005290.pub2.
5. Bongers MY, Mol BW, Brolmann HA. Current treatment of dysfunctional uterine bleeding. Maturitas 2004;47(3):159-74.
6. Brinson Z, Tang VL, Finlayson E. Postoperative functional outcomes in older adults. Curr Surg Rep. 2016;4(6):21. doi: 10.1007/s40137-016-0140-7. Epub 2016 May 4. PMID: 28344894; PMCID: PMC5362160.
7. Buck Louis GM. Persistent environmental pollutants and couple fecundity: An overview. Reproduction. 2014;147(4):R97-R104.
8. Buck Louis GM, Barr DB, Kannan K, Chen Z, Kim S, Sundaram R. Paternal exposures to environmental chemicals and time-to-pregnancy: Overview of results from the LIFE Study. Andrology. 2016;4(4):639-47.
9. Dydyk AM, Gupta N. Chronic Pelvic Pain. [Updated 2022 May 29]. In: StatPearls [Internet]. Treasure Island (FL): StatPearls Publishing. 2022. Available from: https://www.ncbi.nlm.nih.gov/books/NBK554585/.
10. Es-Haghee S, Shabani F, Hawkins J, Zareian MA, Nejatbakhsh F, Qaraaty M. The effects of aromatherapy on premenstrual syndrome symptoms: A systematic review and meta-analysis of randomized clinical trials. Evidence-based complementary and alternative medicine. 2020;2020.
11. Grace GA, Devaleenal DB, Natrajan M. Genital tuberculosis in females. Indian J Med Res. 2017;145(4):425-36. doi: 10.4103/ijmr.IJMR_1550_15. PMID: 28862174; PMCID: PMC5663156.
12. Guidelines for the management of heavy menstrual bleeding. National Health Committee New Zealand, 1998.
13. Hess CL, Howard MA, Attinger CE. A review of mechanical adjuncts in wound healing: Hydrotherapy, ultrasound, negative pressure therapy, hyperbaric oxygen, and electrostimulation. Ann Plast Surg. 2003;51(2):210-18. doi: 10.1097/01.SAP.0000058513.10033.6B.
14. Heydari N, Abootalebi M, Tayebi N, Hassanzadeh F, Kasraeian M, Emamghoreishi M, et al. The effect of aromatherapy on mental, physical symptoms, and social functions of females with premenstrual syndrome: A randomized clinical trial. J Family Med Prim Care. 2019;8(9):2990.
15. Howkins and Bourne Shaw's Textbook of Gynecology. 17th edition. Elsevier Publications; 2018.
16. Konar H. DC Dutta's Textbook of Gynecology, 8th edition. New Delhi: Jaypee Brothers Medical Publishers Ltd; 2020.
17. Li C, Gong Y, Wang B. The efficacy of pelvic floor muscle training for pelvic organ prolapse: a systematic review and meta-analysis. Int Urogynecol J. 2016;27(7):981-92. [PubMed]
18. Linda McIntosh RN. Abnormal vs. dysfunctional uterine bleeding: What's the difference?. Nursing. 2004;34:11-14.
19. Montenegro ML, Vasconcelos EC, Candido Dos Reis FJ, Nogueira AA, Poli-Neto OB. Physical therapy in the management of women with chronic pelvic pain. Int J Clin Pract. 2008;62(2):263-9.
20. Mrugacz G, Grygoruk C, Sieczyński P, Grusza M, Bołkun I, Pietrewicz P. [Etiopathogenesis of dysmenorrhea]. Med Wieku Rozwoj. 2013;17(1):85-9.
21. Nawaz G, Rogol AD. Amenorrhea. [Updated 2022 Jun 21]. In: StatPearls [Internet]. Treasure Island (FL): StatPearls Publishing. 2022. Available from: https://www.ncbi.nlm.nih.gov/books/NBK482168/.
22. NICHD. Physical labor, hypertension and multiple meds may reduce male fertility. 2015. Retrieved December 19, 2016, from https://www.nichd.nih.gov/news/releases/Pages/030915-male-fertility.aspx
23. Nichite S, Tripathi P, Mehta A. Passing DNB Obstetrics and Gynecology, 2nd edition. New Delhi: Jaypee Brothers Medical Publishers Ltd; 2017.
24. Paavonen J. Pelvic inflammatory disease. Medicine. 2005;33(10):43-46. doi:10.1383/medc.2005.33.10.43
25. Patel DR. Management of pelvic inflammatory disease in adolescents. Indian J Pediatr. 2004;71(9):845-47. doi:10.1007/bf02730726
26. R AN, Rafiq NB. Candidiasis. In: StatPearls [Internet]. Treasure Island (FL): StatPearls Publishing. 2022. [Updated 2022 Aug 7]. Available from: https://www.ncbi.nlm.nih.gov/books/NBK560624/.
27. Schumann JA, Plasner S. Trichomoniasis. In: StatPearls [Internet]. Treasure Island (FL): StatPearls Publishing. 2022. [Updated 2022 Jun 21]. Available from: https://www.ncbi.nlm.nih.gov/books/NBK534826/.
28. Sharma JB, Sharma E, Sharma S, Dharmendra S. Female genital tuberculosis: Revisited. Indian J Med Res. 2018;148(Suppl):S71-S83. doi: 10.4103/ijmr.IJMR_648_18. PMID: 30964083; PMCID: PMC6469382.
29. Sharma R, Biedenharn KR, Fedor JM, Agarwal A. Lifestyle factors and reproductive health: Taking control of your fertility. Reprod Biol Endocrin. 2013;11:66.
30. Smarr MM, Sundaram R, Honda M, Kannan K, Buck Louis G. Urinary concentrations of parabens and other antimicrobial chemicals and their association with couples' fecundity. Environmental Health Perspectives. 2016. Advance online publication. doi:10.1289/EHP189
31. The initial management of menorrhagia: evidence based clinical guidelines. No 1. Royal College of Obstetricians and Gynaecologists, 1998.
32. Uzuncakmak T, Alkaya SA. Effect of aromatherapy on coping with premenstrual syndrome: A randomized controlled trial. Complement Ther Med. 2018;36:63-7.
33. Wang Y, Shao R, He C, Chen L. Emerging progress on diagnosis and treatment of female genital tuberculosis. J Int Med Res. 2021. doi:10.1177/03000605211014999
34. Wiegersma M, Panman CMCR, Hesselink LC, et al. Predictors of success for pelvic floor muscle training in pelvic organ prolapse. Phys Ther. 99.1. 2019;99(1):109-17. Web.
35. Wurn BF, Wurn LJ, King CR, Heuer MA, Roscow AS, Scharf ES, et al. Treating female infertility and improving IVF pregnancy rates with a manual physical therapy technique. Med GenMed. 2004;18;6(2):51. PMID: 15266276; PMCID: PMC1395760.
36. Yilmaz S, Terzioğlu F. The effects of Kinesio taping and breathing exercises on pain management after gynaecological abdominal surgery: A randomized controlled study. Int J Nurs Practice. 2022. https://doi.org/10.1111/ijn.13088.

Multiple Choice Questions (MCQs)

To test your understanding and recall of key concepts.

1. **An endocrine disorder with psychological implications, unrelated to organic lesion and occurring regularly during the luteal phase of each ovulatory menstrual cycle is__________.**
   A. Secondary dysmenorrhea
   B. Primary dysmenorrhea
   C. Premenstrual syndrome (PMS)
   D. Mittelschmerz's syndrome
2. **How does prostaglandin imbalance contribute to primary dysmenorrhea?**
   A. It increases pain tolerance by lowering prostaglandin levels
   B. It causes vasodilation, reducing oxygen supply to the myometrium
   C. It enhances uterine contractions leading to ischemia and hypoxia
   D. It inhibits myometrial activity, leading to muscle relaxation
3. **Which of the following statement is accurate in the context of dysmenorrhea?**
   A. Primary dysmenorrhea is associated with systemic symptoms like nausea, while secondary dysmenorrhea lacks systemic symptoms
   B. Secondary dysmenorrhea is caused by psychological factors, while primary dysmenorrhea is structural
   C. Primary dysmenorrhea pain occurs before menstruation, while secondary dysmenorrhea starts after menstruation
   D. Secondary dysmenorrhea is caused by underlying pathologies, unlike primary dysmenorrhea
4. **Which prescription would be most effective for a patient with premenstrual syndrome (PMS) experiencing significant mood swings that affect her daily life?**
   A. NSAIDs and yoga sessions
   B. Selective serotonin reuptake inhibitors (SSRIs)
   C. Diuretics during the luteal phase
   D. Cognitive-behavioral therapy (CBT) combined with dietary modifications
5. **Why is ultrasound considered the gold standard in the diagnosis of pelvic abnormalities?**
   A. It identifies hormonal imbalances
   B. It provides clear imaging of pelvic structures and abnormalities
   C. It confirms systemic infections
   D. It assesses the functionality of the hypothalamic-pituitary-ovarian axis

ANSWERS

1. C	2. C	3. D	4. B	5. B

Chapter 13

Gynecologic Conditions: Clinical and Physiotherapy–Part II

Ami Vishal Mehta, Priyasingh Rangey, Shivani Sheth

LEARNING OBJECTIVES

At the end of the chapter, the reader will be able to:

- Gain knowledge about infertility and endometriosis.
- Discuss uterine prolapse, its types, diagnosis and management.
- Describe genital tract injuries in detail.
- Understand gynecological surgeries.
- Know about the various investigative procedures used in women's health.
- Learn about the physiotherapy assessment and management in the commonly used investigative procedures and gynecological surgeries.
- Gain knowledge about the importance of each surgery and procedure in women's health.

CHAPTER OUTLINE

INTRODUCTION

The field of gynecology deals with female healthcare concerns particularly related to the female reproductive system. This may require several investigations and interventions to be performed for the diagnosis and management of such conditions. Gynecological investigations and interventions can help in early diagnosis and management which can significantly improve the quality of life of the female and reduce morbidity and mortality to a huge extent.

Physiotherapy helps in improving outcomes in almost all of the gynecological surgeries as well as conditions. It helps in improving fertility by improving the lifestyle and hormonal levels, helps with healing in case of tissue injuries, reduces pain, improves mobility and enhances physical activity levels, thereby improving quality of life.

The previous chapter dealt with menstrual disorders, infections and bleeding abnormalities. This chapter will deal with infertility, endometriosis, uterine prolapse, genital tract injuries and gynecological investigations and interventions.

ENDOMETRIOSIS

This is a non-neoplastic condition where endometrium is present in regions of body other than uterine mucosa. When the ectopic endometrial tissues are found in myometrium, it is called endometriosis interna or adenomyosis. Other common and rare sites for endometriosis are as shown in **Table 13.1** and **Figure 13.1**.

Prevalence of endometriosis is 6–10% worldwide, however, it is more common in infertile women.

Pathogenesis

According to the retrograde menstruation theory by Sampson, ectopic endometrium is sloughed via patent fallopian tubes into the peritoneal cavity during menstruation.

Though retrograde menstruation explains the physical displacement of endometrial fragments into the peritoneal cavity, additional steps are necessary for the development of endometriotic implants. Escape from immune clearance, attachment to peritoneal epithelium, invasion of the epithelium, establishment of local neurovascularity and continued growth and survival are necessary if endometriosis is to develop from retrograde passage of endometrium. Collectively, investigations involving the pathophysiology of endometriosis have revealed several well supported molecular hallmarks of this disease:

- ❖ Genetic predisposition
- ❖ Estrogen dependence
- ❖ Progesterone resistance
- ❖ Inflammation

Table 13.1: Sites of endometriosis.

Common sites	*Rare sites*
Ovaries	Nasal mucosa
Fallopian tubes	Arms
Pelvic lymph nodes	Legs
Pouch of Douglas	Lungs
Uterosacral ligaments	Umbilicus
Sigmoid colon	Abdominal scar
Appendix	Episiotomy scar

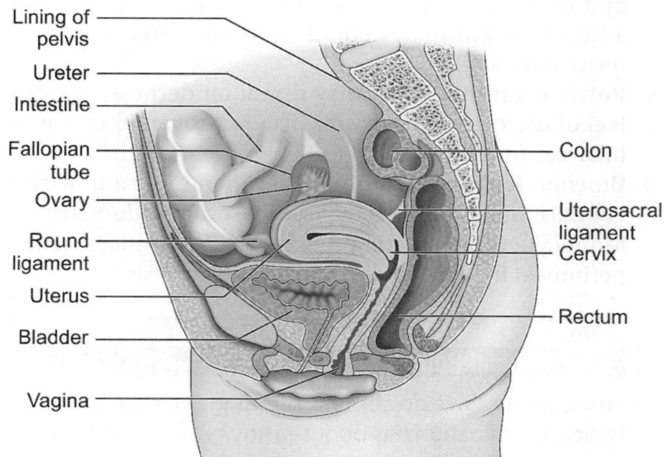

Fig. 13.1: Possible sites of endometriosis *(For color version, see Plate 2)*.

Table 13.2: Symptoms related to various sites of lesion of endometriosis.

Site	*Symptoms*
Urinary system	Dysuria, back pain or even hematuria
Sigmoid colon and rectum	Dyschezia, diarrhea, constipation, rectal bleeding or melena
Surgical scar	Cyclical pain, bleeding

Clinical Features

About one-fourth of patients with endometriosis are asymptomatic. It is common in ages 3–45 years and in nulliparous females.

Symptoms are related to the site of lesion and the ability of the area to respond to hormones (as shown in **Table 13.2**). Midline lesions are common, and the degree of severity is not related to the severity of endometriosis.

- ❖ Dysmenorrhea
- ❖ Abnormal menstruation
- ❖ Infertility
- ❖ Dyspareunia
- ❖ Chronic pelvic pain
- ❖ Abdominal pain
- ❖ Chronic fatigue
- ❖ Perimenstrual symptoms
- ❖ Catamenial chest pain
- ❖ Rarely hemoptysis

Clinical Pointer

Diagnosis is made from the classical symptoms of secondary dysmenorrhea, infertility and dyspareunia.

Examination and Investigations

- ❖ **Abdominal examination:** A mass may be felt in lower abdomen which arises from the pelvis—it may be chocolate cyst or tubo-ovarian mass arising from endometriotic adhesions. The mass could be tender and may have restricted mobility.

- **Pelvic examination:** It may reveal tenderness, nodular feel of uterosacral ligaments, fixed retroverted uterus or bilateral adnexal mass.
- **Biochemical investigations:** Elevation of serum marker CA 125 is often seen in females with severe endometriosis. Monocyte Chemotactic Protein (MCP-1) is increased in peritoneal fluid of females with endometriosis.

 **Clinical Pointer**

Many patients have no abnormal findings on examination. Physical examination has poor sensitivity and specificity.

Imaging

- **Ultrasonography:** Transvaginal and endorectal ultrasound are helpful for diagnosis of rectosigmoid endometriosis.
- **CT scan:** It is better than ultrasound for diagnosis.
- **MRI:** It shows characteristic hyperintensity on T1 weighted image and hypointensity on T2 weighted image. It is helpful for diagnosis of deep infiltrating endometriosis.
- Laparoscopy is the gold standard and confirmation is often done by laparoscopy or laparotomy.
- Biopsy of excised lesion is ideal but negative histology does not rule out the diagnosis.

Medical Management

This is a progressive disease; hence it is imperative to understand the possible treatment options.

- Hormone therapy is used to treat endometriosis-associated pain. Hormones come in the form of a pill, a shot or injection, or a nasal spray. This may help slow the growth and local activity of both the endometrium and the endometrial lesions. Treatment also prevents new areas and scars (adhesions) from growing, but it will not make existing adhesions go away.

The possible options of hormone treatments to treat pain from endometriosis:

- **Gonadotropin-releasing hormone (GnRH) medicines:** They stop the production of hormones to prevent menstruation, and the growth of endometriosis.
  - *Mode of delivery:* Some GnRH medicines come in a nasal spray taken daily, as an injection given once a month, or as an injection given every 3 months.
  - Most healthcare providers recommend staying on GnRH medicine for only about 6 months at a time, with several months between treatments if they are repeated. The risk for heart complications and bone loss can increase in case of prolonged use.
  - *Side effects:* These medications also have side effects, including hot flashes, tiredness, problems sleeping, headache, depression, joint and muscle stiffness, bone loss, and vaginal dryness.

 **Clinical Pointer**

After stopping the GnRH medicine, the body comes out of the menopausal state, menstruation begins, and pregnancy is possible.

- **Oral contraceptives:** These help make a woman's period lighter, shorter, and more regular. Women prescribed contraceptives also report relief from pain.
  - *Side effects:* These hormones can have some mild side effects such as weight gain, bloating, and bleeding between periods, especially when women first start to take the pills continuously.
- Progesterone and progestin, taken as a pill, by injection, or through an intrauterine device (IUD), improve symptoms by reducing a woman's period or stopping it completely.
  - As a pill taken daily, these hormones reduce menstrual flow without causing the uterine lining to grow. As soon as a woman stops taking the progestin pill, symptoms may return, and pregnancy is possible.
  - An IUD containing progestin is useful in reducing endometriosis-associated pain. It reduces the size of lesions and reduces menstrual flow.
  - *Side effects:* Women taking these hormones may gain weight, feel depressed, or have irregular vaginal bleeding.
- **Danazol:** This medication is usually started from the 5th day of menstrual cycle. While taking this drug, women will have a period only occasionally or not at all.
  - *Side effects:* Common side effects include oily skin, pimples or acne, weight gain, muscle cramps, tiredness, smaller breasts, and sore breasts. Headaches, dizziness, weakness, hot flashes, or a deepening of the voice may also occur while on this treatment.

 **Clinical Pointer**

Danazol's side effects are more severe than those from other hormone treatment options.

 **Clinical Pointer**

Danazol can harm a developing fetus. Therefore, it is important to prevent pregnancy while on this medication. Hormonal birth control methods are not recommended for women taking danazol. Instead, healthcare providers recommend using barrier methods of birth control, such as condoms or a diaphragm.

- **Pain medications:** Pain medications may work well if pain or other symptoms are mild. These medications range from over-the-counter pain relievers to strong prescription pain relievers. The most common types of pain relievers are NSAIDs.

Surgical Management

Research shows that some surgical treatments can provide significant relief from endometriosis-related pain.

- **Laparoscopy:** To remove the endometriosis, the surgeon makes at least two or more small cuts in the abdomen and does excision of the lesion or destruction of the lesion called cauterizing or vaporizing. Scar tissue may also be removed at this time because it may contribute to endometriosis-associated pain.
- **Laparotomy:** In this, the surgeon may remove the endometriosis patches. Hysterectomy or total hysterectomy with bilateral salpingo-oophorectomy may also be considered by the surgeon if ovaries and uterus are found to be affected.
- **Surgery to sever pelvic nerves:** If the pain is in the centre of the abdomen, healthcare providers may recommend cutting nerves in the pelvis to lessen the pain during either laparoscopy or laparotomy. The American College of Obstetricians and Gynecologists (ACOG) reports several clinical trials that showed these procedures to be ineffective at relieving pain from endometriosis. These procedures are not currently included in the ACOG recommendations for management of endometriosis.
    - Two procedures are used to sever different nerves in the pelvis:
        1. Presacral neurectomy severs the nerves connected to the uterus.
        2. Laparoscopic uterine nerve ablation (LUNA) severs nerves in the ligaments that secure the uterus.

In some cases, hormone therapy is used before or after surgery to reduce pain and/or continue treatment. Current evidence supports the use of an IUD containing progestin after surgery to reduce pain.

Physiotherapy Management

Physiotherapists play a crucial role in management of secondary musculoskeletal impairments associated with endometriosis and in management of pelvic pain associated with this disorder.

Impairments

- Lumbar, sacroiliac, and pelvic floor pain
- Muscle spasms
- Trigger points (common in the pelvic floor and lumbar spine)
- Connective tissue dysfunction
- Urinary urgency
- Scar tissue adhesion

Management

- Pelvic floor strengthening
- Internal and external trigger point management
- Myofascial manual therapy
- Stretching and flexibility exercises **(Figs. 13.2 to 13.4)**
- Spinal mobilizations
- Nerve glides
- Relaxation exercises

INFERTILITY

This is defined as the inability to have clinical pregnancy within a year or more of well-timed unprotected coitus.

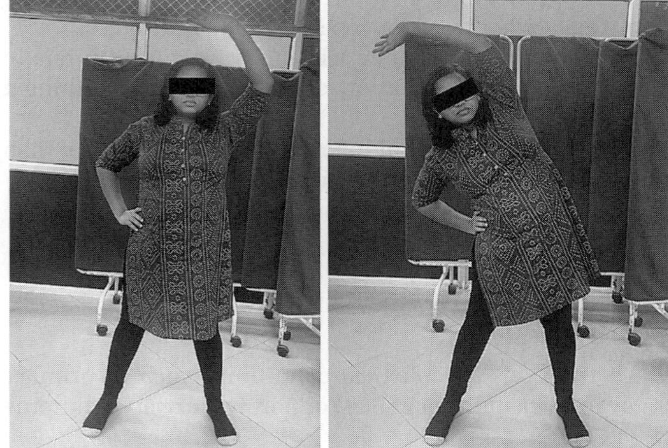

Fig. 13.2: Stretching of quadratus lumborum.

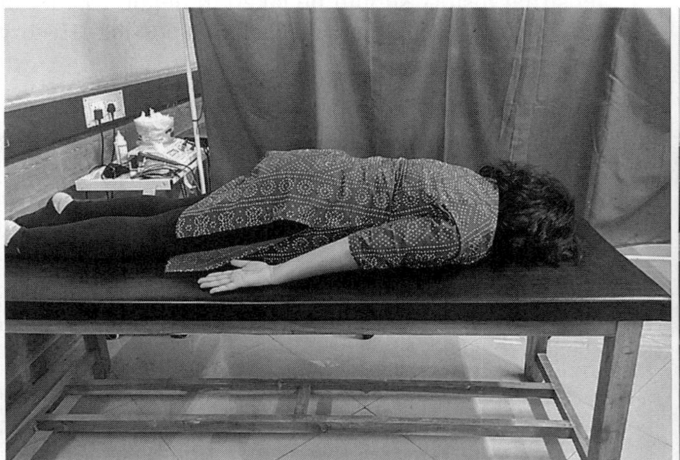
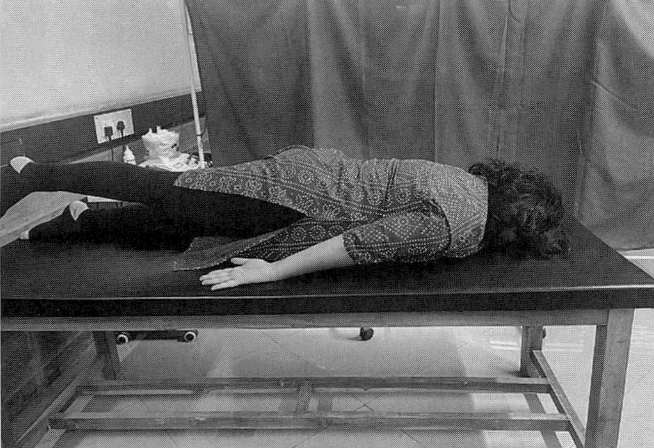

Fig. 13.3: Alternate leg raise.

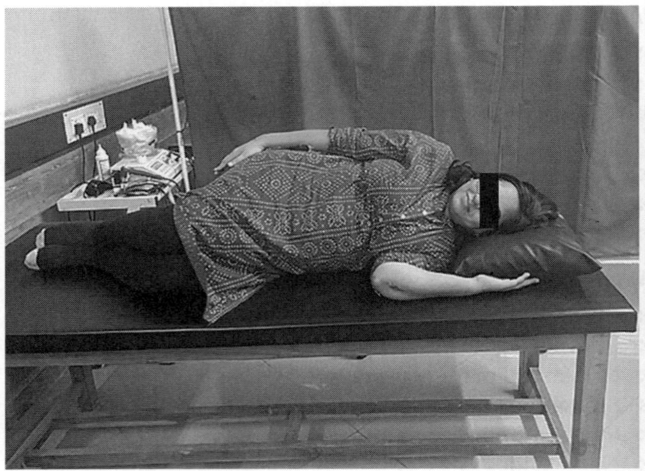
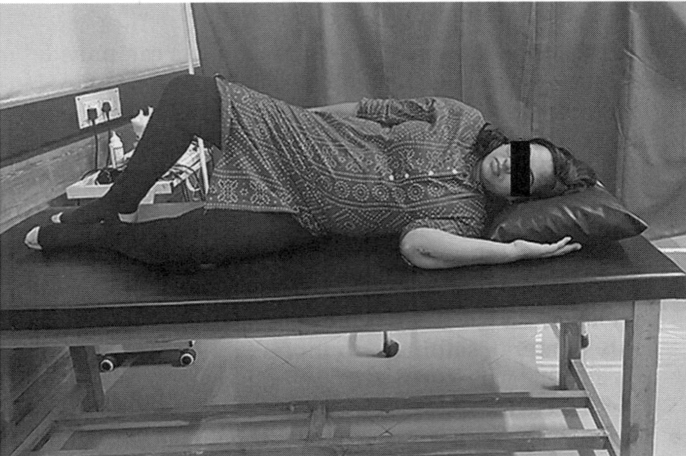

Fig. 13.4: Hip clam exercise.

According to the American Society of Reproductive Medicine:
- Infertility affects females and males equally.
- Male partner is the sole cause or contributory to the cause in 40% of the infertile couples.
- Twelve percent of all infertility cases are a result of the woman either weighing too little or too much.
- It is possible for women with body weight disorders to reverse their infertility by attaining and maintaining a healthy weight.
- Twenty-five percent of infertile couples have more than one factor that contributes to their infertility.

According to the WHO, estimate of the overall prevalence of primary infertility in India is between 3.9 to 16.8%.

Causes of Female Infertility

Failure to Ovulate

- Ovarian or gynecological conditions, such as primary ovarian insufficiency (POI) or polycystic ovary syndrome (PCOS)
- "Diminished ovarian reserve," which could be due to aging
- Endocrine disorders, such as thyroid disease or problems with the hypothalamus.

Structural

- Endometriosis
- Blocked tubes
- Uterine fibroids
- Polyps
- Scarring in the uterus from previous injuries, infections, or surgery
- An unusually shaped uterus, which can affect implantation and the ability to carry a pregnancy to term

Implantation Failure

- Genetic defects in the embryo
- Thin endometrium
- Embryonic defects
- Endometriosis
- Progesterone resistance
- Scar tissue in the endometrial cavity

> **Clinical Pointer**
>
> Lifestyle factors which impact fertility in both men and women are smoking, drug use such as cocaine, heroin, marijuana, obesity, being underweight, and environmental factors such as exposure to chemotherapy, radiation, and organic pesticides.

Infections can also cause infertility in men and women **(Box 13.1)**.

Investigations and Diagnosis of Female Infertility

History

Age, duration of marriage should be noted. Surgical history should be noted especially if there is any pelvic and/or abdominal surgery as it can lead to peritubal adhesions.

Menstrual history should be taken in detail. History of contraceptive practice should be elicited if possible. History of dyspareunia can be taken.

Box 13.1: Infections causing infertility.

- Untreated gonorrhea and chlamydia in women can lead to pelvic inflammatory disease, which leads to scarring and blockage of the fallopian tubes.
- Untreated syphilis increases the risk for a pregnant woman to have a stillbirth.
- Chronic infections in the cervix and surgical treatment of cervical lesions associated with human papillomavirus (HPV) infection can also reduce the chances of conception.
- The CDC recommends that all boys and girls aged 11 or 12 be vaccinated against HPV. Men and women who were not vaccinated as preteens can also get the vaccine into their early to mid-20s.

Examination

- **General examination:** BMI, check for acne, hirsutism as it can indicate PCOS.
- **Systemic examination:** To rule out presence of hypertension, thyroid disorder, or any infection.
- **Gynecological examination:** Inspect the presence of any vaginal infections, cervical tears, uterine size, position and mobility, presence of any adnexal masses.

Investigations

- Examples of lab tests include thyroid testing, prolactin levels, tests of ovarian reserve and progesterone
- X-ray hysterosalpingogram (HSG)
- Laparoscopy
- Transvaginal ultrasound
- Saline sonohysterogram (SIS)
- Hysteroscopy
- Endometrial biopsy
- Rubin's test (insufflation test)
- Sims-Huhner test is done to assess the quality of cervical mucus and capacity of sperm to survive in it
- Falloposcopy

Treatment of Infertility

- Education and assurance
- Maintaining body weight
- Advice to avoid smoking, alcohol, excessive caffeine
- Intrauterine insemination (IUI) involves the placement of washed sperm into the uterine cavity around the time of ovulation.
- **Fallopian tube sperm perfusion:** Large volume of washed and processed sperm is injected in the uterine cavity around the time of ovulation.
- **Assisted reproductive technology (ART):** The most expensive, but also most successful treatment of unexplained infertility consists of the spectrum of assisted reproductive technology including IVF (in-vitro fertilization), with or without ICSI (intracytoplasmic sperm injection)
- Controlled ovarian hyperstimulation
- Gamete intrafallopian transfer (GIFT)
- Gestational surrogacy

Physiotherapy Management

- In Czech Republic, the Mojzisovà method was used for management of infertility. The belief was that the state of lumbar muscles is associated with the functioning of the reproductive organs. This method included a combination of soft tissue and osseous mobilization techniques, post-isometric relaxation, and a home exercise program over a 6-month treatment period.
- It is found that giving site-specific manual soft-tissue therapy improves soft-tissue mobility, elasticity, and distensibility of the soft tissues. Theoretically, mobilization of the soft tissue may break collagenous cross-links and adhesions in the uterine wall that cause pain and dysfunction and improve chances of conception.
- This method is found to have low risks and side effects and appears to be an effective treatment for facilitating natural fertility and improving pregnancy rates/embryo transfer in women undergoing subsequent IVF.
- Physiotherapy for weight loss can be added in the plan if the female/male is obese/overweight. Further details can be found in Chapter 30: Obesity in Women.

UTERINE PROLAPSE

Uterine prolapse as the word suggests is the herniation of uterus into the vagina or beyond. This prolapse is often due to failure of ligamentous support of uterus and fascial support. According to the report of World Health Organization (WHO), the global prevalence of uterine prolapse is 2–20% among females of 45 years of age or below.

Degrees of Prolapse (Fig. 13.5)

- **First degree:** Uterus herniates inferiorly from its normal position but the external os will be inside the vagina.
- **Second degree:** The uterus goes inside the vagina, and the external os protrudes outside the vaginal introitus.
- **Third degree:** The uterus and cervix prolapse to lie outside the introitus.

Morbid changes seen in uterine prolapse:

- The vaginal mucosa becomes stretched and there may be some pigmentation.
- Initially on the prolapsed mass there will be keratinization, followed by cracks, infection, sloughing and ulceration. A trophic ulcer may develop on dependent part of the mass that is prolapsed, lying outside the introitus.
- The chronic congestion may lead to hyperplasia and hypertrophy of vaginal glandular components. This makes the vagina bulky and congested.
- Supravaginal part tends to become stretched or elongated due to strain by pull of ligaments to maintain cervix in position.

Symptoms

- While moving, patient may feel something is coming down from the vagina

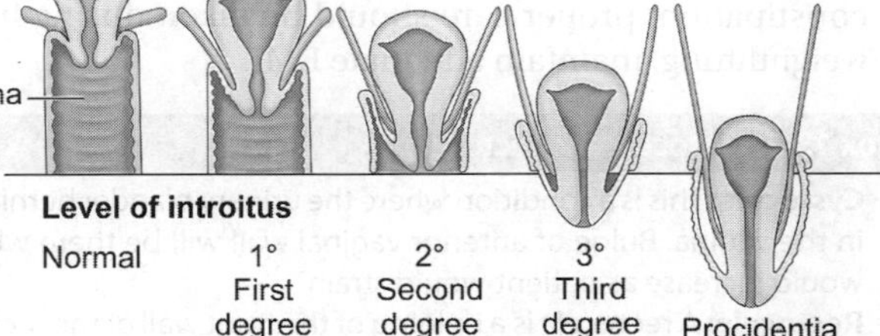

Fig. 13.5: Degrees of uterine prolapse *(For color version, see Plate 2).*

- Pelvic pain and/or back pain
- Dyspareunia
- White or blood-stained discharge may be present

Examination

General Examination

- Age—chances of prolapse increase with age
- Parity
- Occupation—history of heavy weightlifting
- History or presence of asthma, chronic obstructive pulmonary disease (COPD), cardiac disease
- History of abdominal, vaginal surgery
- Body mass index (BMI)—overweight/obese
- Examination of abdominal scar, mass in pelvis/abdomen

Palpation

- Inspection and palpation of abdomen, pelvis, rectal, vaginal and rectovaginal region
- Pelvic examination should be done in both dorsal and standing position
- If inspection in dorsal position yields negative results, patient can be asked to strain as if performing Valsalva maneuver in squatting position
- Examination of tone of levator ani muscle

Clinical Pointer

In first degree of uterine prolapse, diagnosis is made through speculum examination, the cervical descent can be found below the ischial spines on straining. In second or third degree prolapse, palpation can reveal a mass protruding through the introitus.

Clinical Pointer

Prolapse of uterus is often associated with prolapse of adjacent organs such as bladder and rectum.

Box 13.2 describes rectocele and cystocele.

Management

Preventive

- **Antenatal care:** To prevent any strain or injury to the supporting soft tissues during vaginal delivery.
- **Postnatal care:** To maintain and improve tone of pelvic floor muscles.
- **General measures:** Manage chronic cough, avoid constipation, proper care should be taken during heavy weightlifting, maintain adequate BMI.

Box 13.2: Cystocele and rectocele.

- **Cystocele:** This is a condition where the urinary bladder herniates in the vagina. Bulge of anterior vaginal wall will be there which would increase as patient would strain.
- **Rectocele:** A rectocele is a bulging of the front wall of the rectum into the back wall of the vagina.

Conservative

Indications of conservative management:

- Asymptomatic women
- Mild to moderate prolapse
- Medically not fit for surgery
- Desires to conceive in future

Types of conservative management:

- Pelvic floor muscle exercises
  - Physiotherapists play a crucial role to train the patient for pelvic floor muscle strengthening and conditioning. Kegel's exercises should be initiated after referral from gynecologist for management of prolapse. These exercises are helpful in first to third degree of prolapse.
  - The females have to be instructed on how to contract and relax the pelvic muscles through feedback given during digital palpation or through application of myofeedback or electrical stimulation (if necessary). Kegel's exercise must be performed 3 to 5 times per week, 2 or 3 times per day; and females should be taught to contract their pelvic floor muscles before and during any increases in abdominal pressure.
- Pessaries
  - These are mechanical devices which do not provide curative relief for prolapse but are used for symptomatic relief. These devices are available in various shapes and sizes. **Figure 13.6** shows donut-shaped pessary and **Figure 13.7** shows ring pessary.
  - A pessary can be used in early pregnancy (up to 18 weeks), then the uterus becomes enlarged enough to fit in properly in the brim of the pelvis. It is also suggested as a management technique for females who are unwilling to undergo operation or are unfit for operation. The patient should be trained in placing and removing the pessary. Follow-up should be done initially in 1–2 weeks and then 3–4 weeks.
  - Complications:
    - Vaginal discharge and odor
    - Vaginal and/or cervical mucosal erosions and abrasions

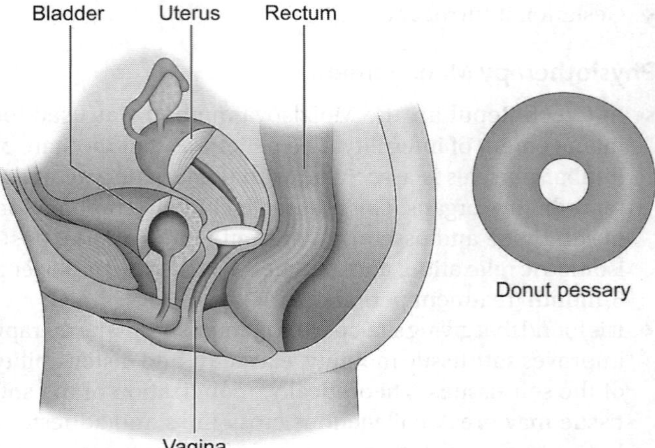

Fig. 13.6: Donut pessary.

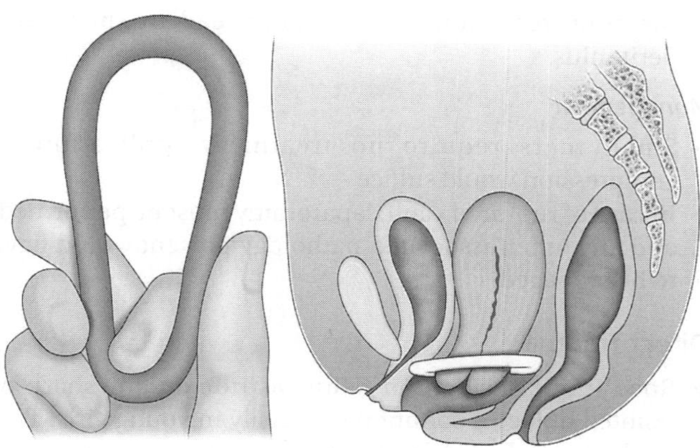

Fig. 13.7: Ring pessary.

  - Pessary incarceration within vagina with formation of adhesions
  - Neglected pessary for many years can lead to infection, sepsis, cancer, fistulae, etc.
- Hormonal replacement therapy (HRT) helps to improve minor prolapse in postmenopausal females.

Surgical Management

- Fothergill's operation
- Vaginal hysterectomy with pelvic floor repair
- Shirodkar's modification of Fothergill's
- Cervicopexy or sling operations (Purandare's operation)
- Colpocleisis
- Total vaginal mesh.

GENITAL TRACT INJURIES

- Genital tract injuries refer to injuries to the labia, vulva or vagina, urethra and anus and internal injuries to the bony pelvis, bladder, bowels and reproductive organs.
- Most common causes of genital tract injury are vaginal delivery, sexual violence and genital mutilation.
- **Complete perineal tear (CPT):** Tear of perineal body involving the sphincter ani externus with or without anorectal mucosa is called complete perineal tear.

According to ACOG (2014) criteria the classification of perineal tears **(Fig. 13.8)** is as shown in **Box 13.3**.

Etiology

- **Obstetrical:** It may result from sudden stretching and/or over stretching of perineum during childbirth. It can occur during forceps delivery, vacuum assisted delivery, or in case of increased birth weight (>3 kg). Midline episiotomy combined with forceps delivery substantially increases the risk of third-degree and fourth degree laceration. The risk of anal sphincter trauma with operative delivery and episiotomy is increased in primigravid women.
- **Gynecological:** Direct trauma to the perineum could be due to fall.

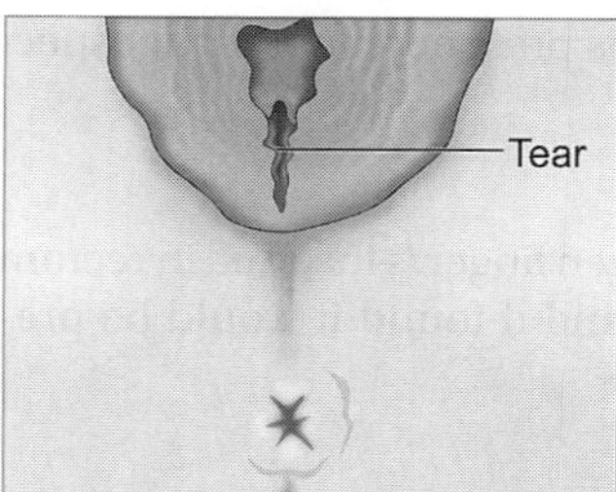

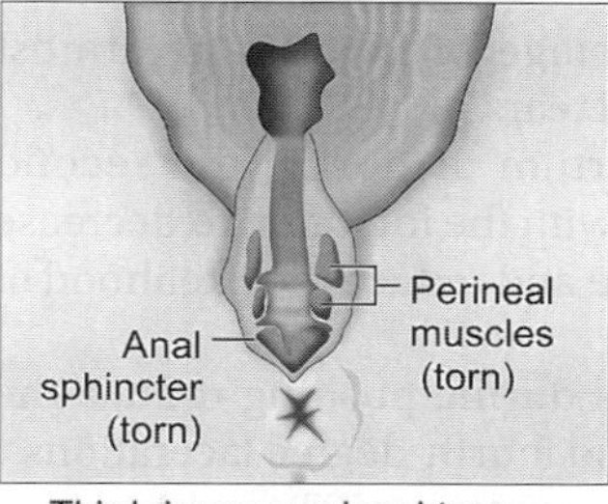

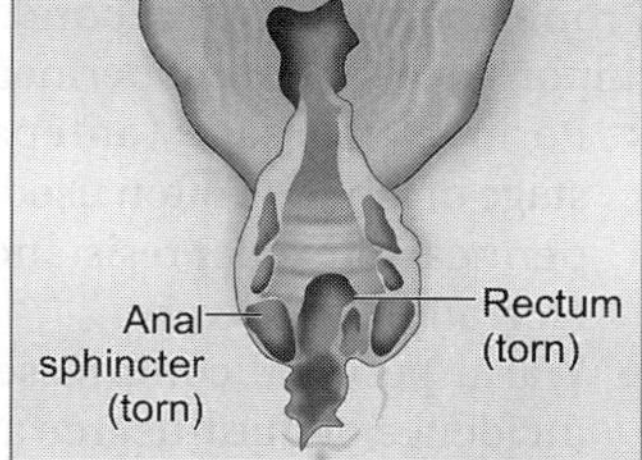

Fig. 13.8: Classification of perineal tears *(For color version, see Plate 2)*.

Box 13.3: Classification of perineal tears.

- **First degree:** Injury to perineal skin only.
- **Second degree:** Injury to perineum involving perineal muscles but not involving anal sphincter.
- **Third degree:** Injury to perineum involving anal sphincter complex.
  - *3a:* Less than 50% of external anal sphincter thickness torn **(Fig. 13.8)**.
  - *3b:* More than 50% external anal sphincter thickness torn.
  - *3c:* Both external anal sphincter and internal sphincter torn.
- **Fourth degree:** Injury to perineum involving anal sphincter complex (external anal sphincter and internal anal sphincter) and anal epithelium.

Clinical Features

The common symptoms of complete perineal tear are:

- The perianal region would be sore and painful
- If damage is mild, there would be incontinence of loose stool and if damage is severe there would be incontinence of hard stool as well.
- Urinary incontinence
- Vaginal bleeding
- Infection.

Clinical Pointer

The condition may remain asymptomatic for many years and may get discovered accidentally during a pelvic examination.

Signs

- Absence of perineum
- Dimples on the skin of either side of fused mucosa

- Radial wrinkling of the skin is present on posterior aspect of anal opening.

Palpation

- Absence of sphincter grip when finger is inserted in rectum
- There will be no prolapse, and if found it would be pre-existing

Management

Prevention

Proper care during second stage of labor is of utmost importance to prevent perineal tears.

- Perineal massage (antepartum or during the second stage of labor) is often used with the intention to decrease perineal muscular resistance and reduce the likelihood of laceration at delivery
- Warm perineal compresses during pushing reduce the incidence of third-degree and fourth-degree lacerations
- Timely episiotomy would also prevent CPT

Clinical Pointer

More care should be taken for controlled delivery of head than on the perineum.

- Delivery by extension should be avoided and flexion of the head should be maintained till sub-occiput comes under symphysis pubis so that lesser diameter of sub-occipital frontal region comes out (10 cm).
- Spontaneous forcible delivery of the head should be avoided by helping patient not to bear down during contractions. Delivery of the head should be in between the contractions.

Surgical Management

- A definitive surgery for repair of anal sphincter complex is sphincteroplasty with perineorrhaphy (restoration of perineal body). The best time for this is within 24 hours of injury but can be done within 3–6 months.
- By 3 months the local infection would subside, and general condition of the patient would improve.

Clinical Pointer

If surgery is delayed by more than 6 months, there is fibrosis on the margins and inconvenience of the patient is prolonged.

Coital Injuries

- Tearing of hymen may lead to mild hemorrhage or bruising of the vagina or urethra.
- If there is tearing of the vestibule or clitoris, it may cause severe hemorrhage.
- In case of rape, young girls or in case of postmenopausal atrophy there may be rupture of the vault of vagina. This may lead to prolapse of bowels and omentum through the ruptured vault, and it could lead to shock and peritonitis.

Management

- Small tears require no treatment-application of compression would suffice.
- In case of ruptured vault, laparotomy must be performed, and any other associated pathology present would have to be managed.

Direct Trauma

- Road traffic accident or falling astride on any sharp or pointed object is common especially in young girls. This could cause bruising of the vulva, and at times vulval hematoma.
- A major accident could also cause fracture of pelvis and associated injuries to pelvic organs such as bladder or rectum or vagina. It could also cause supralevator hematoma.
- Perforation of the vaginal wall with injury to the surrounding viscera could occur in case of fall on sharp objects.

Management

- Small vulval hematoma can heal itself but patient should be kept under observation for 24 hours. If not progressing it should be drained under anesthesia. But in case of large hematoma, which is spreading, it should be drained under general anesthesia. An incision is made, and the blood clots are scooped, hemostasis is secured, and obliteration of dead space is done by sutures.
- In case of suspected gut injuries or supralevator hematoma, laparotomy is indicated.

Instrument-induced Injury

Uterine injury can happen with all sorts of instruments used in gynecological operations such as cervical dilatation and uterine curettage. Cervical injuries by a dilator or vulsellum are common in nulliparous cervix. This may lead to hemorrhage and cervical incompetency.

Along with the inadvertent injuries the likely susceptible conditions are:

- Postmenopausal uterus
- Small and soft uterus such as during lactation
- Pyometra
- Malignancy

Management

Once the injury is detected during operation, the operation has to be stopped immediately. Further management will depend on the:

- Type of instrument which caused the injury
- Pathology in the uterus
- Impact on patient

Monitor pulse and blood pressure of the patient periodically and administer antibiotics when infection is suspected.

In infective uterus if antibiotics do not produce a change, laparotomy is to be done.

In case of malignancy or pyometra, laparotomy and definitive surgery have to be considered seriously.

Foreign Bodies

- Foreign bodies placed in uterus or vagina and retained for a long period of time could cause tissue damage.
- Any foreign body retained inside the human body can cause infection. This is common with rubber goods, swabs and gauze pieces. Very often this is associated with foul smelling discharge.
- A pessary retained and forgotten for a long time would cause vaginitis, ulceration and sloughing. It may also lead to vesicovaginal fistula which could lead to carcinoma. Prolonged retention of IUD could cause menorrhagia, irregular bleeding and if retained in postmenopausal females, it can produce pyometra or postmenopausal bleeding.

Management

Usually in young females, under general anesthesia the vagina is exposed, and the foreign body is removed through aural or nasal speculum.

INVESTIGATIVE PROCEDURES

Cervical Biopsy

This is defined as removal of small tissue from the cervix for further examination. This test is done to check abnormalities of precancerous conditions or cervical cancer.

Indications

- Positive PAP smear test.
- This is an outpatient procedure that can be used for removal of cervical polyps and genital warts.
- Positive test for presence of human papillomavirus (HPV).
- In case of suspicion of cervical cancer based on CT, MRI or USG investigations.
- It can be done when symptoms such as vaginal bleeding, heavy menstruation, pelvic pain and/or dyspareunia are suggestive of cervical cancer.

Types of Cervical Biopsies

- **Colposcopy (punch) biopsy:** In this procedure a circular blade (similar to a paper hole puncher) is used to remove a sample of tissue. A dye is often used for easy visualization of abnormal cervical tissue.
- **Cone biopsy:** In this procedure a scalpel or electric loop is used for removal of large cone-shaped pieces of cervical tissues.
- **Endocervical curettage (ECC):** In this procedure a curette is used to scrape and remove cells from the lining of the endocervical canal.

Complications

The most common complication following a cervical biopsy is light bleeding. Other possible complications (though rare) are:

- Heavy bleeding
- Infection
- Cervical stenosis due to scarring which can impair the menstrual flow
- Perforation of uterus
- Vaginal tear
- Incompetent cervix

Contraindications

- Acute pelvic inflammation
- Late pregnancy
- Labor
- Active/acute cervical or vaginal infection
- Patient is already in palliative care

Prior to Biopsy

These pre-requisites should be fulfilled before all investigative procedures.

- Ensure proper drug history is taken before biopsy.
- A patient on aspirin or warfarin may be required to take a lower dosage or miss the dose 24 hours before the biopsy.
- The healthcare provider may suggest to refrain from use of vaginal cream/tampons 24 hours prior to biopsy.
- A proper signed informed consent is taken before the procedure.

PAP Test

The Papanicolaou test is commonly abbreviated as PAP test. It is an exfoliative cytopathology test, done using a specimen of spontaneously exfoliated or mechanically dislodged cells and used for detection and diagnosis of precancerous or cancerous lesion, infection or abnormal hormonal activity.

Technique (Fig. 13.9)

- The sample should be adequate and well preserved.
- Specimen should be obtained without using a lubricant, as a lubricant can stain dark purple and hide several cells. Saline solution can be used for moistening the area and the speculum can be introduced after that.
- A wooden or plastic spatula, dipped in saline to prevent rapid dehydration of scraped cells should be used for scraping.
- After smearing, the slide should be immediately dipped in or sprayed with 95% ethyl alcohol solution before it dries.
- It is transported with a liquid medium to the laboratory where slide preparation is done for liquid-based cytology.
- Cervical cytology is reported using The Bethesda System (TBS), which is described in *Chapter 5: Laboratory and Molecular Investigations in Women's Health.*

Indications

Box 13.4 presents a cervical cytology screening program based on ACOG recommendations, Federation of Obstetric and Gynecological Societies of India, American Cancer Society and United States Preventive Services Task Force.

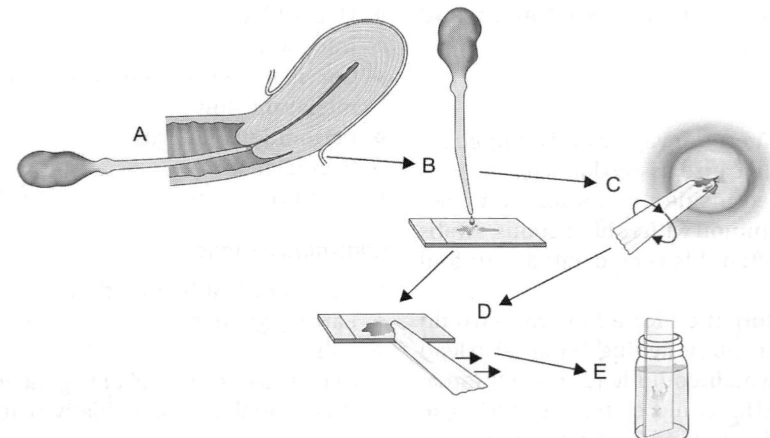

Fig. 13.9: PAP Test technique: (A) Aspiration of endocervical secretions; (B) Drops of endocervical secretion placed (not smeared) on labelled slide; (C) Scraping of cervix and endocervical os; (D) Mixing of scraped cells with endocervical secretion and smearing by a lateral motion; (E) Slide immediately placed in 95% ethyl alcohol solution.

Box 13.4: Cervical cytology screening program.

- Initial screening—to begin at 30 years according to the Government of India (25 years according to United States) and to be continued till 65 years of age regardless of sexual activity
- Screening interval
  - Women aged 25–29 years: Every 3 years
  - Women aged 30–66 years:
    - Pap testing alone every 3 years
    - Co-testing (Pap testing with high-risk HPV) every 5 years
  - Women aged >65 years:
    - If the female tests normal over past 10 years or no high-grade dysplasia (CIN 2/3) for past 20 years—no screening to be provided
    - Annual screening for females who are HIV seropositive, immunosuppressed, exposed to diethylstilbestrol (DES) in utero
- Women undergone total hysterectomy: No screening when hysterectomy done for benign conditions
- Women undergone subtotal hysterectomy: Usual screening as per above criteria

Contraindications

This test is not indicated for women without a cervix, or who have undergone total hysterectomy and/or those without a history of a high-grade precancerous lesion or any sign of cervical cancer in the last 20 years.

Complications

Complications are very rare with PAP smear. But patients should be educated about possible vaginal spotting immediately after the test. Minor bleeding or infection may also occur.

Hysteroscopy

Hysteroscopy is an investigative procedure for visualization of the endometrial cavity with an endoscopic device known as a "hysteroscope". This procedure is used for diagnosis and treatment of various endometrial abnormalities. This is a gold standard technique for diagnosis and treatment of intrauterine pathology.

Indications

- ❖ Abnormal uterine bleeding
- ❖ Infertility
- ❖ Postmenopausa bleeding
- ❖ Mullerian duct anomaly
- ❖ Endometrial thickening
- ❖ Suspicion of intracavitary lesion
- ❖ Presence of foreign bodies.

Contraindications

- ❖ Acute/active pelvic infection/inflammation
- ❖ Diagnosed endometrial or cervical cancer
- ❖ Pregnancy.

Clinical Pointer

In case of moderate vaginal bleeding, copious irrigation should be done for proper visualization.

Complications

The chances of complications are rare with hysteroscopy, but if they occur, it may prove fatal for the patient.

- ❖ Uterine perforations
- ❖ Hemorrhage
- ❖ Gas embolism: When hysteroscopy is performed with carbon dioxide as a distending medium
- ❖ Hyponatremia
- ❖ Increased intrauterine pressure can occur which would lead to fluid overload

Hysterosalpingography (HSG)

This is a radiologic procedure for visualization of uterus and fallopian tubes. In this radiographic study a radiopaque dye or contrast media is injected in the uterus and then X-ray is used to carry out investigative procedures. This is the second step after pelvic ultrasound which is used for investigation in females reporting with infertility.

Indications

- To find the cause of infertility
- Examination of tubal patency
- Examination of uterine malformations
- To detect any IUD
- In case of suspected secondary abdominal pregnancy
- Diagnosis of uterine synechiae
- To detect any structural endometrial abnormalities

Contraindications

- Acute pelvic infection
- True pregnancy
- **Contraindications to media:** In people with known or diagnosed Graves' disease, iodine allergies or history of thyroid disease—iodine media should not be used.

Complications

- Abdominal cramping
- Vaginal bleeding
- Vasovagal attack
- Physiological reactions such as nausea, vomiting, chills, flushing may occur in response to the media used

GYNECOLOGICAL SURGERIES

Hysterectomy

Hysterectomy is the surgical removal of the whole or part of the uterus. The rates of hysterectomy have comparatively reduced in recent years due to development of alternative modern techniques like uterine artery embolization for uterine leiomyomas and endometrial ablation for symptomatic uterine bleeding.

Clinical Pointer

Length of hospital stay is around 2–3 days in absence of any complications and complete recovery takes around 6–12 weeks. Patients should be asked not to drive till 2 weeks postprocedure and not to lift heavy weights till 6 weeks posthysterectomy. In case of abdominal hysterectomy, driving and swimming should be avoided for 4 weeks. Strenuous exercises should be avoided for 2 weeks after vaginal hysterectomy and 4 weeks after abdominal hysterectomy.

Hysterectomy can be performed through various routes and using various procedures:

- **Vaginal:** Uterus is removed through the vagina; no incisions are made in the abdomen wall; least invasive.
- **Abdominal:** Transverse incision (usually a Pfannenstiel incision) is made across the abdomen and uterus is removed through it; rates have declined as it is more invasive, requires longer hospitalization, has poorer outcomes and more risk of complications.
- **Laparoscopic:** Small incisions are made in the abdomen; surgical instruments and laparoscope are inserted through these small incisions; uterus is cut into small pieces inside the abdominal cavity and then removed using the surgical devices; vaginal hysterectomy can also be done laparoscopically.
- **Robot-assisted:** Robotic devices are used in the surgical procedure to gain better precision and accuracy.

Types

There are different types of hysterectomy **(Fig. 13.10)** depending on the extent of removal of the uterus and its adjacent tissues.

- **Sub-total hysterectomy:** Only the upper part of the uterus is removed. The cervix remains intact.
- **Total hysterectomy:** The whole uterus along with the cervix is removed.
- **Radical hysterectomy:** In this procedure the whole uterus, along with the adjacent tissues (such as fallopian tubes, ovaries) and the upper one third of the vagina are removed.

Indications

- Uterine fibroids/leiomyoma
- Pelvic organ prolapse
- Adenomyosis
- Abnormal uterine bleeding
- Endometriosis
- Chronic pelvic pain
- Malignancy and premalignant disease of uterus or ovaries

The vaginal route is the most preferred route for hysterectomy. Abdominal hysterectomy is usually performed in case of an enlarged, bulky uterus (uterine size larger than 12 weeks of gestation is used as a measure for qualification) or if the subject has a past history of abdominal surgery or in case of extrauterine disease, gynecological malignancies and severe adhesions or endometriosis.

Contraindications

Contraindications for abdominal hysterectomy are any conditions where a simpler approach can be favored and conditions where a more invasive approach may not be beneficial to the patient.

There are no absolute contraindications for vaginal hysterectomy but relative contraindications include:

- Morbid obesity
- Large, bulky uterus
- Lack of uterine descent
- Nulliparity
- Pelvic radiation
- Suspected severe pelvic adhesion and anatomical distortion from pelvic inflammatory disease (PID) or endometriosis
- Prior pelvic surgeries

Risks and Complications

Intraoperative complications

- Intraoperative bleeding
- Injury to surrounding structures—commonly genitourinary and gastrointestinal tract injuries

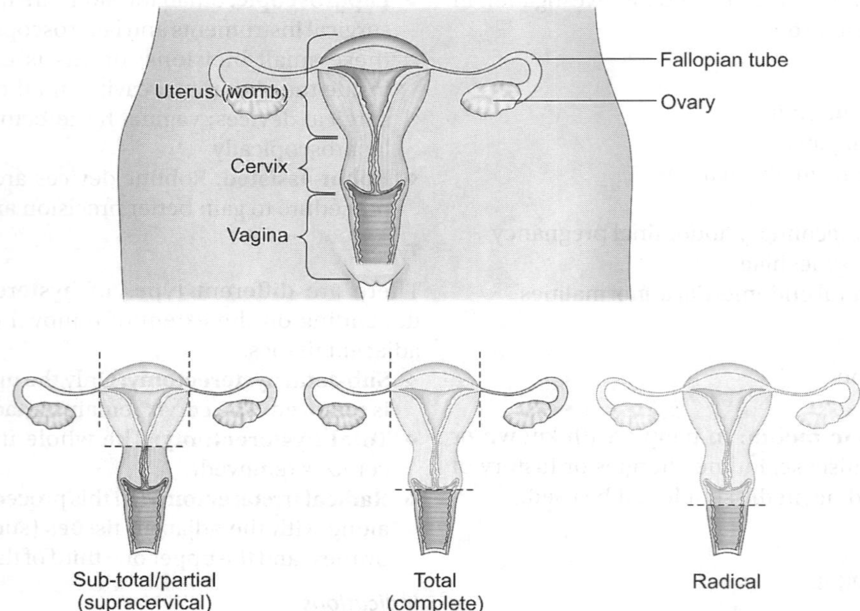

Fig. 13.10: Types of hysterectomy *(For color version, see Plate 3).*

- Nerve injury—femoral nerve, obturator nerve, iliohypogastric and ilioinguinal nerves, and occasionally peroneal nerve due to the positioning during the surgery
- Adverse reaction to anesthesia

Postoperative complications

- Pain
- Infection—vaginal cuff cellulitis, wound infection, pelvic abscess or infected hematoma, and urinary tract infection
- Venous thromboembolism—deep vein thrombosis (DVT) and pulmonary embolism (PE)
- Delayed wound healing
- Pelvic organ prolapse
- Ileus
- Bowel obstruction and urinary retention
- Scar tissue and adhesion formation in the abdominal cavity
- Fistulas—vesicovaginal, ureterovaginal, and rectovaginal fistulas
- Menopause
- Vaginal cuff dehiscence

Preoperative Physiotherapy Care

Preoperative physiotherapy will focus on initial assessment, instructions, warnings and sometimes, treatment.

Preoperative physiotherapy assessment

History should be taken and medical records should be referred to gain the following information:

- Risk of postoperative complications
- Pre-existing medical conditions
- History of previous surgery or physiotherapy for the same condition
- Status of continence

Preoperative physiotherapy management

- Patient education
  - Educate the patient regarding the basics of the procedure, need of the procedure, prognosis, possible complications and need of physiotherapy in the postoperative period (to avoid complications, improve pain and wound healing, improve pelvic floor muscle strength and endurance, improve function and quality of life)
  - Importance of early ambulation to reduce risks of deep vein thrombosis and pulmonary embolism
  - Leaflets, videos or audio tapes may be provided along with verbal instructions
  - Patient education helps in developing rapport with the patient, reducing their anxiety and ease their concerns
- Active cycle of breathing techniques (ACBT), Forced expiratory technique (FET) and supported coughing to prevent respiratory complications
- Active movements of the extremities and trunk
- Weight transfer and pressure relief techniques
- Pelvic floor muscle exercises
- Abdominal muscle exercises—pelvic tilting, transversus abdominis contractions, etc. **(Figs. 13.11 and 13.12)**

Postoperative Physiotherapy Care

Postoperative physiotherapy assessment

- History including the chief complaint, the reason for hysterectomy and details from the medical chart
- Drugs administered to the patient
- Assessment of vitals, mental status, breathing pattern and trophic changes
- Scar examination including the status of healing, adherence and pain (pain can be measured using an objective measure like visual analog scale or numerical pain rating scale)

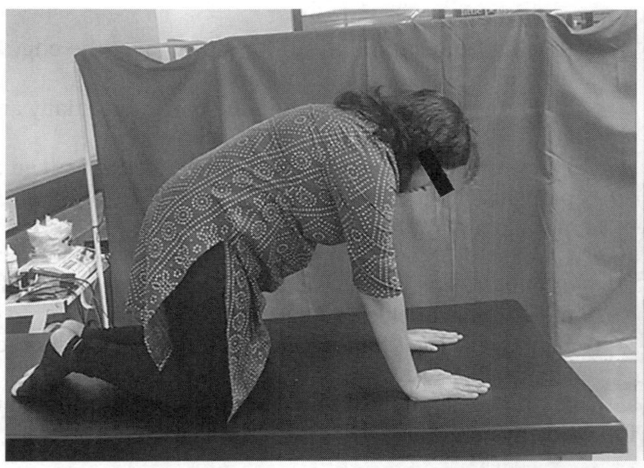
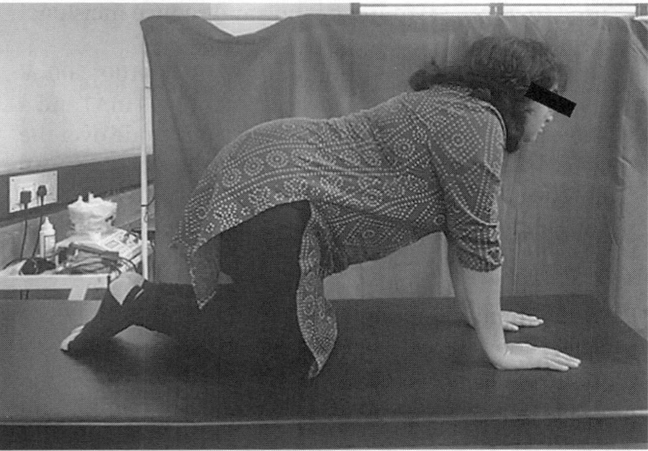

Fig. 13.11: Pelvic tilt in quadruped position.

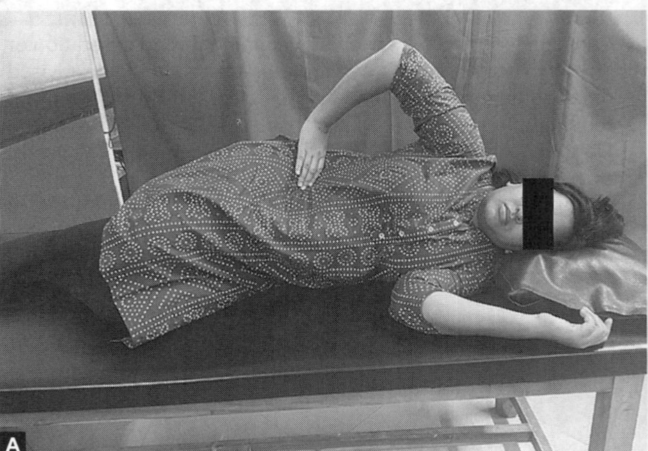
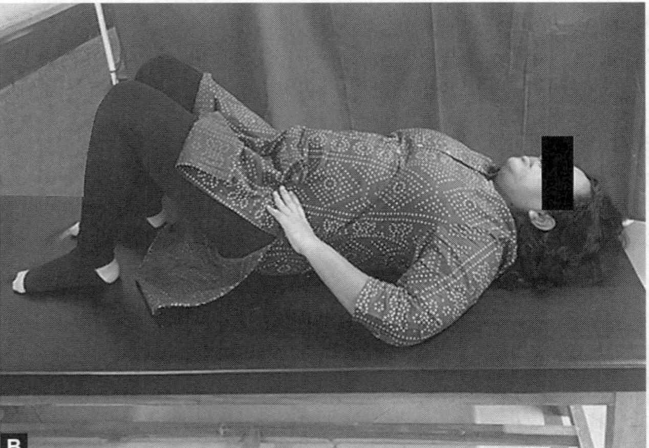

Figs. 13.12A and B: Transversus abdominis activation (A) in side lying and (B) in crook lying.

- Cardiorespiratory assessment including auscultation of breath sounds
- Examination of the musculoskeletal system including signs of muscle wasting, posture, muscle strength and endurance and tightness of any structures
- Functional assessment using scales like Functional Independence Measure (FIM), Activities Assessment Scale (AAS) or Katz Index of Activities of Daily Living

Postoperative physiotherapy management

- Patient education
  - Education regarding possible postoperative complications.
  - Implications of hysterectomy (mainly menopause) in the future.
  - Importance of physiotherapy and regular mobility.
- Prevention of complications
  - Breathing exercises and other breathing techniques like ACBT and FET will help in preventing any respiratory complications.
  - Care should be taken to support the incision (splinting) during any respiratory technique or whenever there is any increase in intra-abdominal pressure.
  - Ankle pump exercises, early ambulation and mobility will help in preventing DVT and PE.
  - Regular position changes to prevent accumulation of secretions and improve mobility.
- Abdominal incision care
  - Abdominal incisions should be washed with warm water and soap.
  - They should be patted dry and not rubbed vigorously.
  - Hydrogen peroxide or alcohol should be avoided as it may slow incision healing.
  - The incision should be covered with gauze bandage which should be changed regularly.
- Incision healing (in case of abdominal hysterectomy) and pain relief
  - Transcutaneous electrical nerve stimulation (TENS) can be applied surrounding the incision to relieve the pain.
  - Low level LASER therapy (LLLT) (doses ranging from 3–6 J/cm^2) has also shown promising results in improving wound healing.
  - Ultrasound therapy (low intensity, high frequency and pulsed mode) using the waterbag method can be

used to improve wound healing and reduce incisional pain.
- High voltage pulsed current (HVPC) [100–500 V (typically <200 V) with a low current (15–40 mA) and a short pulse duration] using negative electrode over the incision and positive electrode near the skin edge can also be used to improve incision healing.
- Kinesiotaping immediately after the surgery can help in relieving incisional pain and reducing time to passage of gas and defecation post-surgery.

❖ Pelvic floor muscle strengthening
- Pelvic floor muscle exercises should be started as early as the pain allows.
- A combination of fast and slow (maximal and submaximal) contractions should be performed.
- More details can be found in Chapter 15: Managing the Pelvic Floor.

❖ Abdominal exercises
- Pelvic tilting, knee rolling exercises **(Figs. 13.13A to C)** and transversus abdominis activation should be done in crook lying.

❖ Posture and back care
- Patients should be encouraged to sit, stand and walk tall.
- Posture correction using a biofeedback mirror and verbal cueing can be done.

❖ General mobility
- Moving from supine to sitting, sitting over the edge of bed, standing and marching on spot.
- Walking around the bed or in the corridor initially and gradually progressing to short distances.
- Patients can gradually increase the distance walked as pain and fatigue allow.

❖ Femoral nerve injury
- Care needs to be taken while making the woman stand as Quadriceps will be weak and there is a risk that the patient may buckle and fall.
- Management of femoral nerve injury should include Quadriceps exercises and electrical stimulation.

Box 13.5 presents advice to be provided to the patient following hysterectomy.

Box 13.5: Advices to be provided to the patient following hysterectomy.

- Constipation should be avoided. Straining during defecation or any other activity should be avoided. Patients should be advised to consume more fluids and fiber or use a short-term laxative if required.
- Light household activities can be commenced after 1–2 weeks but prolonged standing should be avoided.
- Lifting more than 1 kg should be avoided till 4 weeks. Heavy weight lifting should be resumed gradually at least 3 months after hysterectomy.

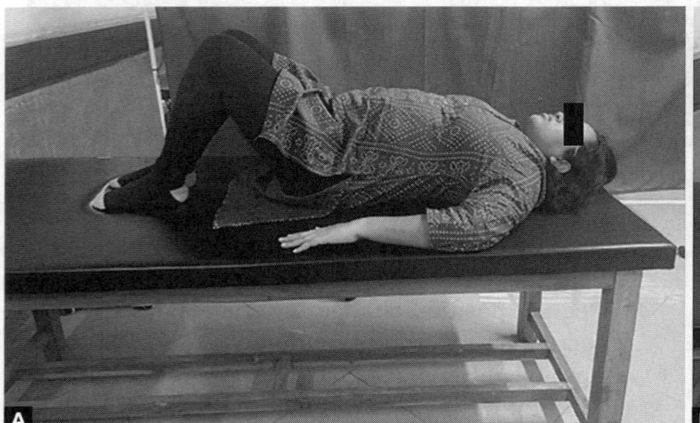

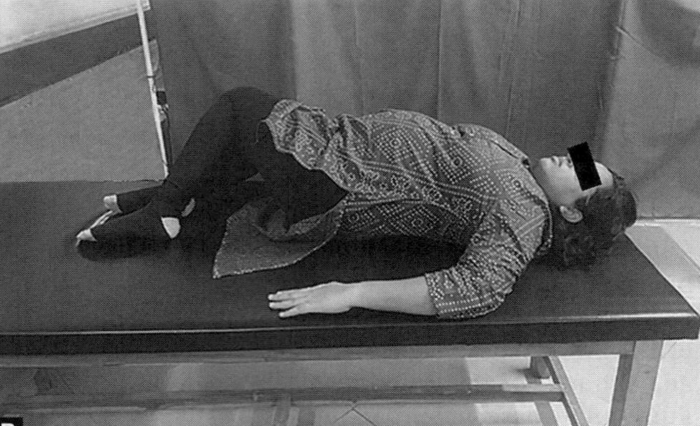

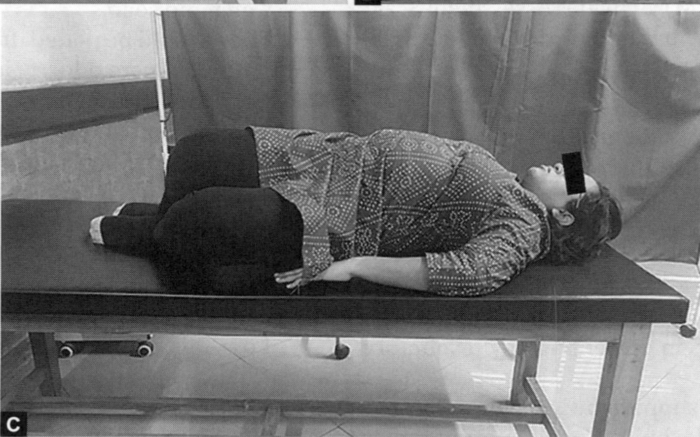

Figs. 13.13A to C: Spine twisting exercises: (A) Starting position; (B) Twist to right; (C) Twist to left.

Ovarian Cystectomy

This is a surgical removal of an ovarian cyst, while leaving the healthy ovarian tissue behind.

Routes

There are two routes of ovarian cystectomies.

1. *Laparoscopic ovarian cystectomy*
2. *Laparotomy*

Ovarian cystectomy can also be done in association with some other surgery.

Clinical Pointer

Patients can resume their normal activity 24 hours after a laparoscopic ovarian cystectomy. But strenuous activities are usually to be avoided for at least a week after surgery.

Clinical Pointer

After a laparotomy, normal activities can be resumed after 2–4 weeks.

Advantages

Laparoscopic ovarian cystectomy is preferred to laparotomy because of decreased postoperative morbidity, less pain, lower analgesia requirements, and earlier recovery to normal bowel function. In turn, this leads to a shorter hospital stay and earlier return to normal activity and mobility.

Indications

- Diagnosed definitive ovarian cyst
- Removal of symptomatic cysts
- Cyst of larger than 5 cm
- Investigation findings that deviate from functional cyst

Contraindications

Laparoscopic ovarian cystectomy is contraindicated:

- If the lesion is suspected to be malignant
- In presence of extensive anterior abdominal wall scarring
- High risk of anesthesia-related complications
- In case of bleeding diathesis

In such cases, laparotomy should be the preferred choice (except bleeding diathesis).

Postoperative Physiotherapy Management

- Instructions about method of getting out of bed should be given.
- Scheduled time of getting out of bed should increase from 3 hours on the first postoperative day to 8 hours on the fourth postoperative day.
- Walking distance should be increased from 125 m on day 1 to 1,000 m on fourth postoperative day.
- Respiratory and circulatory exercises should be done to avoid any complications of anesthesia.
- Splinting of incision while moving around, using washroom, coughing should be taught to the patient.
- Progressive muscle strengthening and endurance training should be included in the programme while giving a home exercise plan.

Salpingo-oophorectomy

This is the surgical removal of fallopian tubes (salpingectomy) and ovaries (oophorectomy). This can be bilateral or unilateral. A bilateral salpingo-oophorectomy is of three types:

1. Elective at time of hysterectomy for benign conditions
2. Prophylactic in women with increased risk of ovarian cancer
3. Therapeutic for treatment of malignancy

Types of Approach for Surgery

- Abdominal approach
- Laparoscopic approach
- Robotic approach

Indications

- Ruptured ectopic pregnancy
- Adnexal torsion with necrosis of ovary and fallopian tubes
- Tubo-ovarian abscess (non-responding to antibiotic treatment)
- Endometriosis
- Ovarian cancer or uterine cancer [ovarian cancer could be secondary to metastasis from distant malignancy (e.g., GI tract cancer)]
- Benign adnexal mass
- Ectopic pregnancy

Clinical Pointer

Salpingo-oophorectomy has been shown to increase survival for women who carry BRCA gene mutations.

Contraindications

There are no absolute contraindications for this surgery. The relative contraindication is pelvic adhesive disease.

Complications

This is a relatively safe procedure but some common complications include infection, bleeding and/or a bad reaction to anesthesia.

Other potential risks are:

- Blood clots
- Injury to urinary tract or surrounding organs
- Incisional hernia
- Formation of scar tissue—adhesion formation
- Bowel obstruction
- Nerve injuries—iliohypogastric and ilioinguinal, genitofemoral, femoral nerves

- Deep venous thrombosis
- Ovarian remnant syndrome

Clinical Pointer

Women who undergo bilateral salpingo-oopherectomy will have surgical menopause.

So, such women have to be monitored for risks associated with lack of oestrogen such as:
- Hot flushes
- Vaginal dryness
- Anxiety and/or depression
- Insomnia osteoporosis and cardiac disorders

Physiotherapy Management

Physiotherapy management would remain similar to the management post-hysterectomy as discussed in Chapter 12: *Gynecological Conditions: Clinical and Physiotherapy—Part I.*

Postoperative physiotherapy management

- For prevention of respiratory and circulatory complications—early mobilization in the form of training of getting out of bed. Walking 100–125 m on the first postoperative day. Splinting of incision should be done while walking, deep breathing and coughing to prevent hernia.
- Back hollowing exercises should be done to prevent postoperative back pain.
- Relaxation exercises should be inculcated in the plan to reduce postoperative anxiety, insomnia.
- Pelvic floor muscle exercise should be initiated after the pain subsides.

Pelvic Repair

This is a major surgical procedure done for repair or treatment of prolapse of pelvic organs. A pelvic repair can be:
- Anterior—for the anterior vaginal wall
- Posterior—for the posterior vaginal wall.

Types of Pelvic Repair

According to ACOG there are two types of pelvic repair surgery:
1. **Reconstructive:** This surgery is done for repair and/or restoration. This is done to restore the organs to the original position. Most reconstructive repair surgeries are done via a vaginal incision, at times abdominal or laparoscopic incision may also be used.
2. **Obliterative:** This type of surgery is done by removal and/or closure of all or a part of the vaginal canal (colpocleisis), this is done to restore the viscera back into the pelvis.

The types of reconstructive surgery include the following:
- **Fixation or suspension** using pelvic soft tissues, e.g., uterosacral ligament suspension and sacrospinous fixation. This is also known as "native tissue repair". It is done through an incision in the vagina. The prolapsed part is attached with stitches to a ligament or to a muscle in the pelvis. A procedure to prevent urinary incontinence may be done at the same time.
- **Colporrhaphy:** This procedure is used to treat prolapse of the anterior (front) wall of the vagina and prolapse of the posterior (back) wall of the vagina using vaginal incisions.
- **Sacrocolpopexy:** This surgery is used to treat vaginal vault prolapse and enterocele. It can be done with an abdominal incision or with laparoscopy. Surgical mesh is attached to the front and back walls of the vagina and then to the sacrum (tail bone). This lifts the vagina back into place.
- **Sacrohysteropexy:** This surgical procedure is used to treat uterine prolapse. Surgical mesh is attached to the cervix and then to the sacrum, lifting the uterus back into place.
- **Surgery using vaginally placed mesh:** Vaginally placed mesh has a significant risk of severe complications, including mesh erosion, pain, infection, and bladder or bowel injury. This type of surgery should be reserved for when the benefits may justify the risks. This may include women with anterior prolapse that has come back after a previous surgery. It may also include women who have a medical condition that prevents them from having a longer operation done through an incision in the abdomen.

Complications

- Abdominal incisions may cause damage to intestines or adhesions.
- After surgery with mesh placed in the abdomen, there is a small risk that the mesh will erode (wear through the tissues) into the vagina. Mesh erosion can cause scarring and pain that can be long-lasting. Additional surgery may be needed to remove the mesh.

Clinical Pointer

Postoperatively patients should be advised to avoid activities that can increase abdominal and pelvic pressure such as constipation and lifting heavy objects.

Physiotherapy Management

Preoperative management

- **Patient education:** The patient should be explained the surgical procedure and information should be provided about recovery and return to normal activities of daily living (ADL).
- Women should be taught (by digital palpation) how to correctly contract their PFMs and how to pre-contract against increases in intra-abdominal pressure (the knack). Women can be advised to do three sets of ten maximum contractions (up to 10-s hold) per day with 4-s rest between sets, followed by a 1-min rest followed by ten fast contractions.

Postoperative physiotherapy management

- Advice should be given to avoid constipation, heavy lifting.
- Patients should be taught correct technique of defaecation and bracing before coughing and lifting.

- Progressive pelvic floor muscle training:
  - Most women commence pelvic floor training approximately 4–6 weeks after prolapse surgery however this varies according to the surgical procedure, postoperative complications and the surgeon's protocol. Some women are advised to wait longer before recommencing pelvic floor exercises.
  - Pelvic floor training starts with brief gentle pelvic floor exercises lying down. Exercises are then progressed and training in upright positions (sitting and standing) are encouraged. Pelvic floor exercises after prolapse surgery should always feel comfortable and pain free.
  - Training progresses to maximize your pelvic floor strength and support before prescription of a long-term maintenance program.
  - Adjuncts such as biofeedback, electrical stimulation and exercise balls can be used.

Dilation and Curettage

It is a common diagnostic and treatment procedure. It is commonly known as D&C. In this, the cervix is dilated and then a uterine layer is scraped with a curette (curettage) . This can be performed on non-pregnant females.

Indications

For diagnostic purposes

- An Endometrial biopsy (EMB) is now preferred over D&C. But D&C is done for diagnosis if a patient has intolerance to EMB.
- Patients having endometrial hyperplasia, persistent abnormal bleeding or postmenopausal bleeding after a benign office biopsy warrant a D&C.
- Diagnostic D&C is also indicated in patients with cervical stenosis.
- It is also indicated for exclusion of endometrial cancer.
- For detection of cause in case of abnormal bleeding in postmenopausal women.

For therapeutic purposes

- As a temporary management of excessive and prolonged vaginal bleeding
- For removal of embedded IUD
- Dysmenorrhea

Contraindications

- Females who take anticoagulants
- Women who have bleeding diathesis

Clinical Pointer

D&C should be delayed in patients with active pelvic infection. However, in the circumstance of a septic abortion or endometritis with possible retained products of conception, the surgeon should proceed with uterine evacuation.

Complications

- Intrauterine perforation—most common site is the fundus
- Bleeding
- Cervical lacerations
- Infections

Summary

Infertility is on the rise in recent times due to poor eating and lifestyle habits. Males and females both are affected due to infertility. However, if diagnosed early, it can be managed easily and conception rates among couples can be improved drastically. Endometriosis is a common cause of infertility among females which can be managed medically or surgically. Due to increased violence, cases of genital tract injuries are also increasing nowadays which require psychological treatment as well along with medical, surgical and physiotherapy interventions. Many investigative procedures are used for women's health. The physiotherapist should understand the role of each procedure in the diagnostic process and clinical decision making. PAP test, hysteroscopy, HSG are some of the common diagnostic and surgical procedures. Hysterectomy is the most common and major gynaecological surgery. It is imperative to understand the role of physiotherapist in pre and postoperative management of hysterectomy and other gynecological surgeries.

CLINICAL EXAMPLE FOR HYSTERECTOMY

A 50-year-old female had undergone total abdominal hysterectomy with bilateral salphingo-oophorectomy. She was referred to physiotherapy department after her surgery. Her chief complaints are pain in lower abdomen and pelvis, difficulty in bed mobility. Physiotherapy management was given for 5 days a week for 2 weeks in the physiotherapy OPD. It helped to restore daily activities rapidly and improve the quality of life of the female.

Physiotherapy Management

Pre-treatment, complete physical examination of patient was done. The perineometer pre-treatment was 15 mm Hg deflection. After two physiotherapy sessions the perineometer showed 30 mm Hg which suggests improvement in the strength of pelvic floor muscles.

- Education about the prognosis of the condition was given. Respiratory exercises, coughing with splinting and ankle toe movements were taught on day 1.
- Along with this walking in the ward was done on first day.
- Transcutaneous electrical nerve stimulation (TENS) around the incision was given to relieve the pain.
- Pelvic floor exercises were started in first week with 10 repetitions and 2 sets. Repetitions and speed of contraction and relaxation were increased in the 2nd week (30 repetitions and 3 sets).
- She was encouraged to sit, stand, and walk 'tall.'

- In the first week, in crook lying-pelvic tilting, knee rolling and pelvic rotations on both sides were done. Gentle rolling and getting up from supine to side-lying were trained.
- Pelvic bridging, marching on the spot, stair climbing, tightening stomach while doing ADL was taught from the 2nd week.
- Home exercise plan with list of dos and don'ts were given after completion of two weeks of physiotherapy.

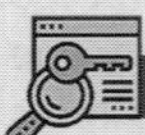

Review Questions

1. Discuss causes, investigations and management of infertility.
2. Enlist the types of cervical biopsy and its indications.
3. Describe the physiotherapy management posthysterectomy.
4. Define endometriosis. Discuss its etiology, clinical features, diagnosis and management.
5. Write about etiology, clinical features, diagnosis and management of pelvic inflammatory disorders.
6. What are the causes of uterine prolapse? Describe prophylaxis of uterine prolapse.
7. Write short notes on:
   a. Hysterectomy
   b. Complete perineal tear
   c. Pap smear
   d. D&C

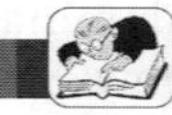

Bibliography

1. ACR Committee on Drugs and Contrast Media. ACR Manual on Contrast Media. American College of Radiology. 2021.
2. Amarin Z. Hysterectomy: Past, Present and Future. Hysterectomy—Past, Present and Future [Working Title], Zouhair Amarin (ed). IntechOpen. 2022. 10.5772/intechopen.103086.
3. American College of Obstetricians and Gynecologists. Cervical cancer screening and prevention. Practice Bulletin No. 157. Obstet Gynecol. 2016;127:e1-20.
4. Andrade Fdo S, Clark RM, Ferreira ML. Effects of low-level laser therapy on wound healing. Rev Col Bras Cir. 2014;41(2):129-33. English, Portuguese. doi: 10.1590/s0100-69912014000200010. PMID: 24918727.
5. Bachmann GA. Hysterectomy: A critical review. J Reprod Med. 1990;35(9):839-62. PMID: 2231559.
6. Broeze KA, Opmeer BC, Van Geloven N, Coppus SF, Collins JA, Den Hartog JE, et al. Are patient characteristics associated with the accuracy of hysterosalpingography in diagnosing tubal pathology? An individual patient data meta-analysis. Hum Reprod Update. 2011;17(3):293-300.
7. Carugno J, Fatehi M. Abdominal Hysterectomy. In: StatPearls [Internet]. Treasure Island (FL): StatPearls Publishing; 2022. [Updated 2021Dec 5]. Available from: https://www.ncbi.nlm.nih.gov/books/NBK564366/.
8. Clayton RD. Hysterectomy. Best Pract Res Clin Obstet Gynaecol. 2006;20(1):73-87. doi:10.1016/j.bpobgyn.2005.09.007. Epub 2005 Nov 7. PMID: 16275095.
9. Cooper DB, Menefee GW. Dilation and Curettage. In: StatPearls [Internet]. Treasure Island (FL): StatPearls Publishing. 2022. [Updated 2022Mar 9]. Available from: https://www.ncbi.nlm.nih.gov/books/NBK568791/
10. Darware M, Ghordadekar D, Dhole R, Noman O. Physiotherapy rehabilitation of post-hysterectomy geriatric patient: A case report. Bioscience Biotechnology Research Communications. 2021;SI14(6):71-6. http://dx.doi.org/10.21786/bbrc/14.6.17.
11. Djurasić L, Crnomarković D, Pejcić T, Jovanović M, Palibrk I, Grajić M, et al. The importance of physical therapy in the postoperative period after total cystectomy of bladder carcinoma. Acta Chirlugosl. 2011;58(1):103-5. doi: 10.2298/aci1101103d. PMID: 21630555.
12. Edelman A, Kapp N. Dilatation & Evacuation (D&E) Reference Guide: Induced abortion and postabortion care at or after 13 weeks gestation ('second trimester'). 2018. Chapel Hill, NC: Ipas.
13. Fahey MR, Irwig L, Macaskill P. Meta-analysis of Pap test accuracy. Am J Epidemiol. 1995;141:680-9.
14. Fahey MT, Irwig L, Petra Macaskill P. Meta-analysis of Pap Test Accuracy. Am J Epidemiol. 1995;141(7):680-80.
15. https://onlinelibrary.wiley.com/doi/abs/10.1002/pri.473
16. https://www.cdc.gov/cancer/cervical/basic_info/screening.htm
17. https://www.dovepress.com/cr_data/article_fulltext/s62000/62172/img/Table1.jpg
18. https://www.healthline.com/health/cervical-biopsy#purpose
19. https://www.sciencedirect.com/topics/medicine-and-dentistry/dilation-and-evacuation
20. https://www.urmc.rochester.edu/encyclopedia/content.aspx?ContentTypeID=92&ContentID=p07767
21. https://www. ver ywellhealth.com/cer vical-biopsy-513848#:~:text=A%20cervical%20biopsy%20is%20important,strains%20of%20human%20papillomavirus%20(HPV)
22. InformedHealth.org [Internet]. Cologne, Germany: Institute for Quality and Efficiency in Health Care (IQWiG). 2006. Hysterectomy (surgical removal of the womb). Updated 2018 Aug 23. Available from: https://www.ncbi.nlm.nih.gov/books/NBK525761/
23. Ingale G, Patil S, Thorat, R. Physiotherapy intervention in post-hysterectomy patient with urinary incontinence: A case report. J Pharm Res Int. 2021;33(60B):1652-8. doi: 10.9734/jpri/2021/v33i60B34790.
24. Kaunitz AM, Kapoor E, Faubion S. Treatment of women after bilateral salpingo-oophorectomy performed prior to natural menopause. JAMA. 2021;12;326(14):1429-30. doi: 10.1001/jama.2021.3305. PMID: 34636868; PMCID: PMC8792973.
25. Kruszka PS, Kruszka SJ. Evaluation of acute pelvic pain in women. Am Fam Physician. 2010;15;82(2):141-7. PMID: 20642266.
26. Moore JF, Carugno J. Hysteroscopy. In: StatPearls [Internet]. Treasure Island (FL): StatPearls Publishing. 2022. [Updated 2022 May 10].
27. Naib ZM. Pap Test. In: Walker HK, Hall WD, Hurst JW (eds). Clinical Methods: The History, Physical, and Laboratory Examinations. 3rd edition. Boston: Butterworths; 1990. Chapter 178. Available from: https://www.ncbi.nlm.nih.gov/books/NBK287/.
28. Nanda K, McCrory DC, Myers ER, Bastian LA, Hasselblad V, Hickey JD, et al. Accuracy of the Papanicolaou test in screening for and follow-up of cervical cytologic abnormalities: a systematic review. Ann Intern Med. 2000;132(10):810-9.
29. Paschopoulos M, Polyzos NP, Iavasidis LG, Vrekoussis T, Dalkalitsis N, Paraskevaidis E. Safety Issues of hysteroscopic surgery. Annals of the New York Academy of Sciences. 2006;1092(1):229-34.

30. Pillarisetty LS, Mahdy H. Vaginal Hysterectomy. In: StatPearls [Internet]. Treasure Island (FL): StatPearls Publishing. 2022. [Updated 2022 May 8]. Available from: https://www.ncbi.nlm.nih.gov/books/NBK554482/.
31. Robson J, van der Merwe C, Walters L, Noack L, Giles SM. The occasional cervical biopsy. Can J Rural Med. 2022;27:72-6.
32. Zhang FW, Wei F, Wang HL, Pan YQ, Zhen JY, Zhang JX, et al. Does pelvic floor muscle training augment the effect of surgery in women with pelvic organ prolapse? A systematic review of randomized controlled trials. Neurourol Urodyn. 2016;35(6):666-74. [PubMed]

Multiple Choice Questions (MCQs)

To test your understanding and recall of key concepts.

1. **What is the most common site for endometriosis?**
   A. Ovaries
   B. Pelvic lymph nodes
   C. Uterosacral ligaments
   D. Sigmoid colon

2. **Which serum marker is often elevated in severe endometriosis?**
   A. CA 125
   B. Beta-hCG
   C. LDH
   D. FSH

3. **Why is laparoscopy considered the gold standard for diagnosing endometriosis?**
   A. It directly visualizes endometriotic lesions and allows for biopsy
   B. It evaluates hormonal levels associated with the condition
   C. It identifies genetic predisposition
   D. It measures CA 125 levels accurately

4. **The primary goal of hormone therapy in managing endometriosis is______________.**
   A. To increase the menstrual flow and reduce symptoms
   B. To stop the production of hormones and growth of endometriosis
   C. To enhance the immune clearance of lesions
   D. To Promote retrograde menstruation for hormonal balance

5. **A 45-year-old female patient, known case of endometriosis, complains of pelvic floor pain. Which of the following physiotherapy intervention is most appropriate for her symptoms?**
   A. Electrical stimulation with high-intensity current
   B. Internal trigger point release combined with relaxation techniques
   C. High-impact aerobic exercises
   D. Short-wave diathermy applied to the abdomen

6. **Which of the following does *not* cause implantation failure thus leading to female infertility?**
   A. Genetic defects in the embryo
   B. Thin endometrium
   C. Embryonic defects
   D. Primary ovarian insufficiency (POI)

7. **Which of the following is *not* a type of cervical biopsy?**
   A. Colposcopy
   B. Cone biopsy
   C. Endocervical curettage (ECC)
   D. Hysteroscopy

ANSWERS

1. A	2. A	3. A	4. B	5. B
6. D	7. D			

Chapter 14

Simplifying the Enigma: Pelvic Floor

✍ *Suroshree Mitra, Anu Arora*

The mystery of the female pelvis is deeply rooted in the bowels of the two hip bones filled by the constituent urogenital system made up of the bladder and urethra, uterus, ovaries and vagina, and colon and rectum.

LEARNING OBJECTIVES

At the end of the chapter, the reader will be able to:

- Acquire detailed knowledge about pelvic floor anatomy, physiology.
- Learn about pelvic floor dysfunction and its types.
- Understand the urologic, gynecologic, colorectal, or generic clinical correlates of the PFD.
- Understand the application of ICF in PFD.

CHAPTER OUTLINE

INTRODUCTION

The human pelvis is a unique albeit complex anatomical structure that is central to many critical biological functions including bipedal ambulation, thermoregulation, continence and parturition (childbirth).

The female pelvic floor embraces a bladder with a urethra that functions towards storage and evacuation of urine; a uterus with cervix, a vaginal orifice, for reproductive and sexual function, and a rectum with an anus that serves for storage and removal of the stool. The pelvic floor is embedded with an intricate and interdependent muscular web along with its essential neuronal innervation and flexible connective tissue. The pelvic floor (PF) is structurally dependent on the surrounding pelvic bones which also serve to protect it. The multitasking and interdependence of the structures constituting the pelvic floor make it natural for the various pelvic floor disease conditions to be often interrelated.

Anatomically, the PF constitutes a complex assembly of connective tissues and striated muscles that must concurrently respond to multiple forces exerted by gravity, inertia, and varying intra-abdominal pressure as they uphold the appropriate position of the pelvic organs.

At a macroscopic level, the female PF multitasks to carry out various biomechanical functions like micturition, defecation, intercourse, pregnancy, and childbirth. In these functions, the contractile structures, i.e., the muscles act as the drivers needed to release or apply pressure for specific task completion. On the other hand, the non-contractile structures, i.e., the connective tissues maintain the constituent pelvic organs in their proper spatial orientation which in turn facilitates the optimum force of contraction by the pelvic floor muscle (PFM).

The pelvis can thus be visualized as being the home to the organs of bladder, uterus (or prostate in men), and the rectum while the pelvic floor muscles form the foundation of this home. Pelvic floor, acts as a supporting and suspensory structure that comprises ligaments and muscles that provide dynamic support to the urethra, bladder, vagina and rectum **(Table 14.1)**.

The structure and function of the pelvic floor go hand in hand for smooth and accurate functioning. The female pelvic floor is an entity that holds special importance during all stages from childhood to childbearing age, from menopause to PF in older adults. Therefore, to understand its dynamics thoroughly, is a mandate for all physiotherapists, to better educate and guide their patients. Also *see* Chapter 3: Anatomy and Biomechanics of the Female Body.

Table 14.1: Supportive and suspensory role of pelvic floor.

Function	*Supportive (contractile structures)*	*Suspensory (non-contractile structures)*
Structures Involved	Muscles: Coccygeus and Levator ani	Fibrous (endopelvic fascia): pubocervical fascia, rectovaginal fascia, cardinal and sacrouterine ligaments

ANATOMY OF BONY PELVIC FLOOR

The pelvic floor is a muscular sheath which also provides passage to urethral, vaginal and anal openings. The female pelvic floor consists of organs as shown in **Figures 14.1A to F and Figures 3.4, 3.6, 15.2**.

The female pelvic floor has a distinctive structure and function, which has to support vital organs and at the same time counter work against gravity as well as increased intra-abdominal pressure.

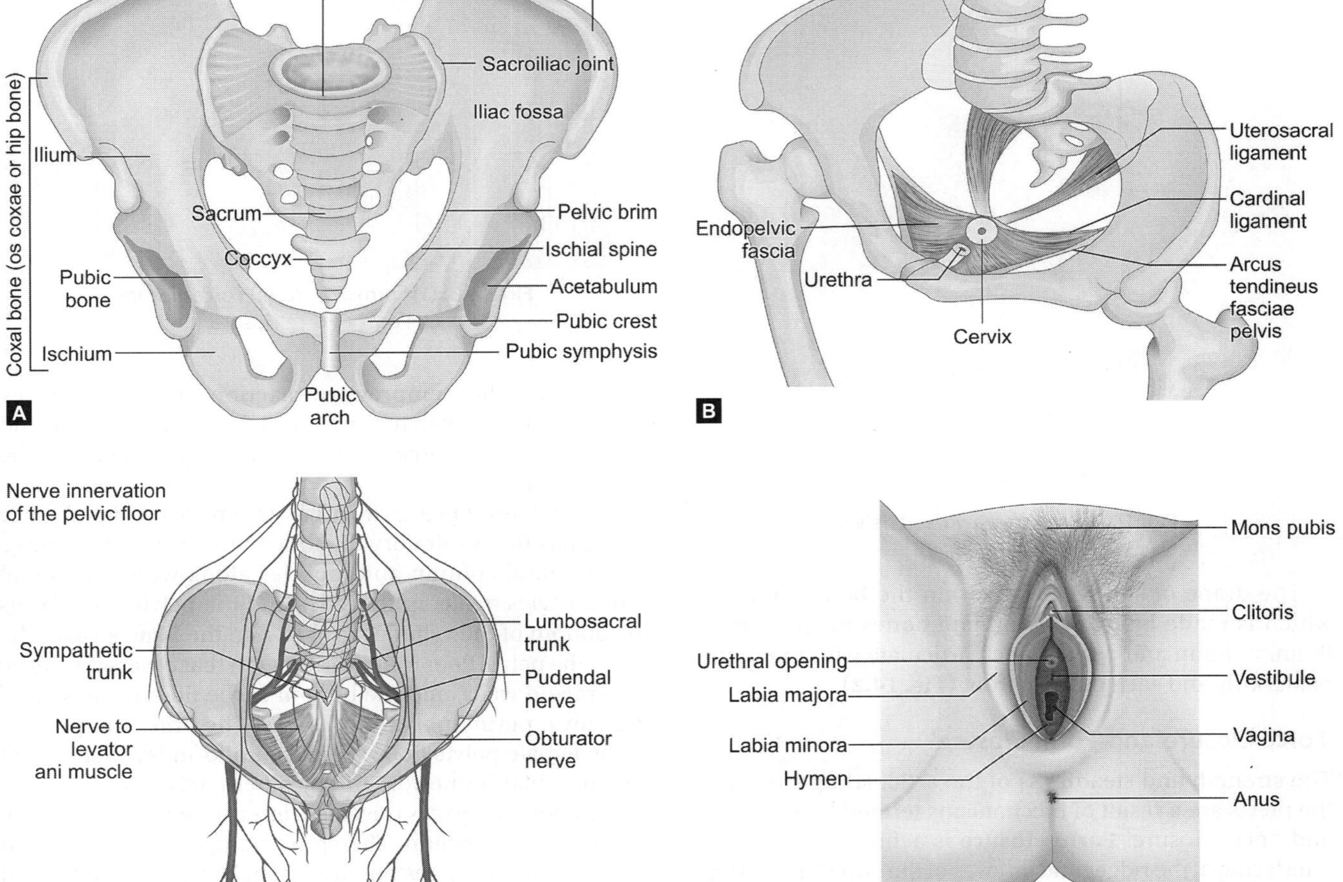

Figs. 14.1A to D

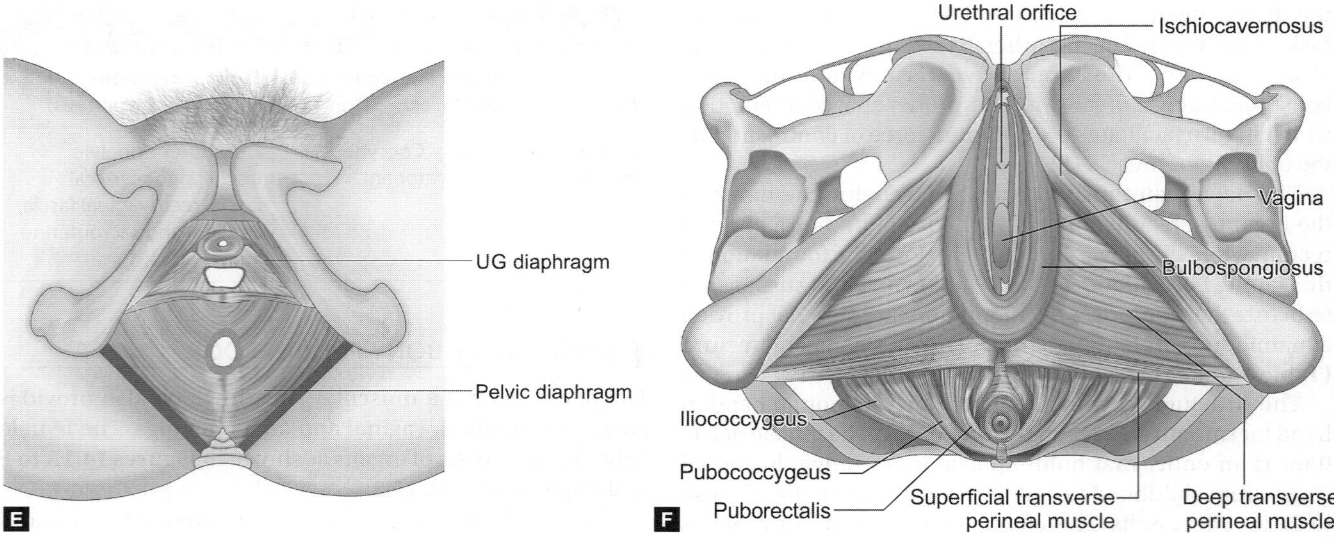

Figs. 14.1E and F

Figs. 14.1A to F. Organs in the pelvis: (A) The pelvis itself including pelvic ring and pelvic joints; (B) Endopelvic fascia and connective tissues (pelvic viscera), along with their attachments to the pelvic walls through the endopelvic fascia, forms first layer; (C) The nerves, blood vessels and lymphatic tissue; (D) External genitalia; (E) The urogenital (UG) diaphragm (perineal membrane) that spans the anterior portion of the pelvic outlet and connects the perineal body to the ischiopubic rami; (F) The bulbocavernosus, ischiocavernosus, and superficial transverse perineal muscles lie in superficial area of anterior outlet (urogenital hiatus) and posterior outlet (anal hiatus) *(For color version, see Plate 3 and 4).*

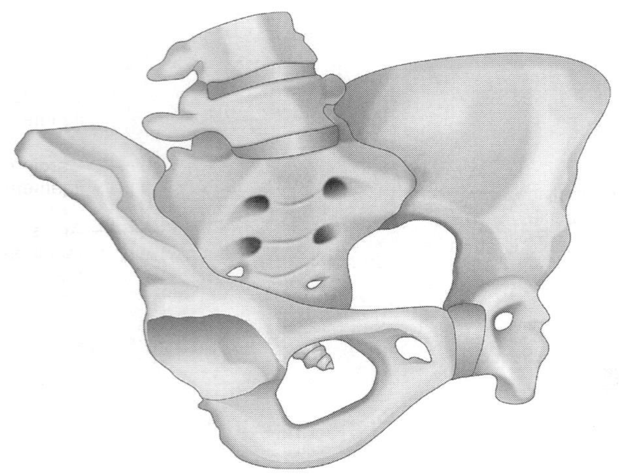

Fig. 14.2: Bony framework of pelvis.

The drape of soft tissue is within the bony framework which is made by two innominate bones made from the ilium, ischium and pubis, which articulate with the sacrum posteriorly and each other in front **(Fig. 14.2)**.

'Force Closure' and 'Form Closure'

The strength and steadiness of the articulating surfaces of the pelvis are a result of mechanisms termed 'force closure' and 'form closure'. **Form closure** is achieved through the interlacing of the ridges and grooves of the bony joint surfaces in the pelvis, **whereas force closure** is achieved through the compressive forces of the muscles, ligaments, and fascia, providing passive stability **(Fig. 14.3)**. Force closure creates a perpendicular compressive reaction force followed by sacral nutation that in turn prepares the pelvis to absorb and increase in load. Force closure, therefore supplements the form closure.

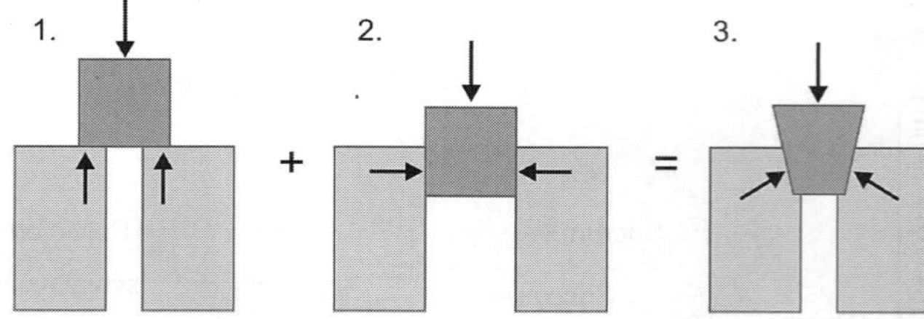

Fig. 14.3: (1) Form closure; (2) Force closure; (3) Form + Force closure.

The abdominopelvic cavity has a cylindrical shaped space which has the respiratory diaphragm muscle as the ceiling, the vertebral column and muscles along with abdominal wall muscles make up the sides and the pelvic floor forms the bottom of the cylinder as shown in the **Figure 14.4**. The top of the pelvic floor is the peritoneum that covers the pelvic viscera and walls, and the bottom of the floor is the skin of the vulva, perineum, and buttocks. The other uniqueness of the female pelvic floor is, unlike uniform layer/sheath of any muscular framework in any other part of the body, the pelvic floor has spaces traversed/interrupted by the urethra, vagina and the rectum. Therefore, along with the support it gives to the organs rested on it especially during increased intra-abdominal pressure, it must also allow for opening of the pelvic floor to accommodate various excretory and reproductive functions.

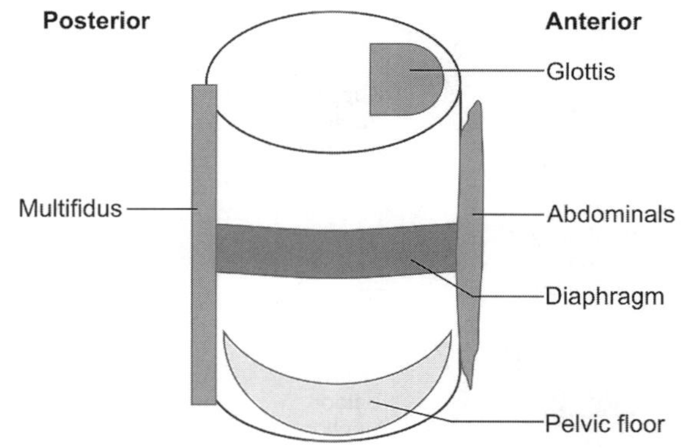

Fig. 14.4: Visualizing the abdominopelvic cavity.

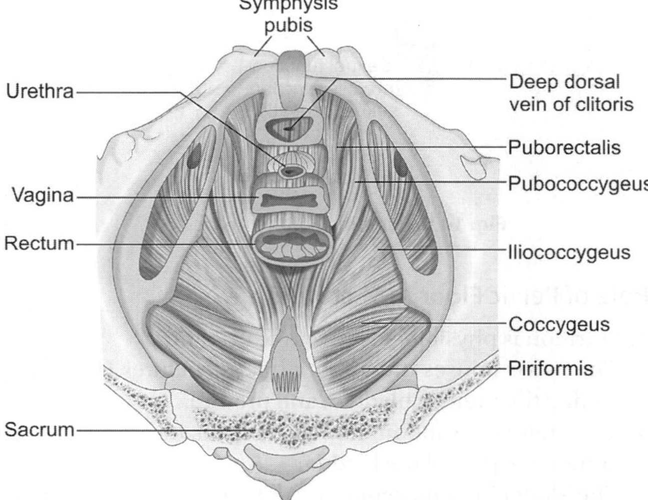

Fig. 14.5: Muscles of the pelvic floor *(For color version, see Plate 4).*

LAYERS OF PELVIC FLOOR AND KINESIOLOGY OF THE GENITAL SUPPORT

The three layers of the pelvic floor are made up of:

1. Striated muscle (under voluntary control)
2. Fibromuscular tissue (smooth muscles)
3. Fibrous tissue

The striated muscle can withstand and contract against loads along with the external anal sphincter which has resting activity too (provides constant support even at rest).

The endopelvic fascia and the visceral ligaments are the fibromuscular tissue origin as they have smooth muscles.

There are certain areas of the pelvic connective tissue, where pure dense regular collagen is found which are truly fibrous and include the tendinous arch of the pelvic fascia and the fasciae over the obturator internus muscle.

There are superficial and deep muscle layers of pelvic floor as shown in **Figure 14.5**.

- The superficial layer of muscles includes bulbocavernosus and ischiocavernosus, superficial transverse perineal muscles, external anal sphincter. The superficial layer has muscles relevant to the anal canal function namely, the external anal sphincter, perineal body and puboperineal muscles. The superficial transverse perinei have a supportive function, the bulbospongiosus and the ischiocavernosus play a role in sexual function.
- The deep pelvic floor muscles that line the inner walls of the pelvis are the levator ani and coccygeus that along with the endopelvic fascia comprise the pelvic diaphragm.
- The superficial layer has more fast twitch fibers than the deep layer. The striated muscles of levator ani and associated muscles of the urogenital diaphragm make the major active contraction bulk of the pelvic floor. The sphincteric muscles of the anus also have smooth muscle component.
- The deep pelvic floor muscles formed by Levator ani consist of:
  - Pubococcygeus (also known as the pubovisceral muscle)—originates from internal surface of pubic ramus and inserts into the lower sacral and coccygeal vertebra
  - Iliococcygeus—originates at the arcus tendinous levator ani and fuses with the pubococcygeus
  - Puborectalis—originates at inner surface of the right and left sides of the pubic bone.
- ***Pubococcygeus*** is located most anteriorly, arising from the pubic bone on either side, attaching to the walls of the pelvic organs and perineal body. Its fibers are directed posteriorly inserting into the anococcygeal raphe and coccygeus.
- ***Iliococcygeus*** is the posterior part of the levator ani. It forms a relatively flat, horizontal shelf spanning the potential gap from one pelvic sidewall to the other. Elevation and support of the pelvic organs are associated with the pubococcygeus and the iliococcygeus.
- ***Puborectalis*** muscle (can be viewed as middle muscle layer) is in between superficial and deep layer. Puborectalis is located below the pubococcygeus and forms a U-shaped sling around the rectum just cephalad to the external anal sphincter. Its sphincter-like action pulls the anorectal junction forward, accentuating the anorectal angle during contraction and is a primary contributor to fecal continence.
- The ***coccygeus*** muscle is also known as the ischiococcygeus (from ischial spine to lateral aspect of coccygeal vertebra).
- The ***pelvic diaphragm*** is wide and thin muscular layer (fascia and muscle) of tissue that forms the inferior border of the abdominopelvic cavity, extending from symphysis pubis to coccyx and from one lateral sidewall to the other.
- The ***urogenital diaphragm*** (triangular ligament), external and inferior to the pelvic diaphragm, is also a strong muscular membrane that occupies the area between the symphysis pubis and ischial tuberosities and stretches across the triangular anterior portion of the pelvic outlet. The constant muscle tone of the levator ani and coccygeus muscle by type I striated muscle fibers prevents the ligaments from becoming over stretched and damaged by constant tension.

Pelvic Ligaments

The pelvic ligaments are not classical ligaments but thickenings of retroperitoneal fascia (endopelvic fascia) and consist primarily of blood and lymphatic vessels, nerves and fatty connective tissue.

- The broad ligaments are thin, mesenteric like double reflection of peritoneum stretching from the lateral pelvic sidewalls to the uterus.
- The cardinal or Mackenrodt's ligaments extend from the lateral aspects of the upper part of the cervix and the vagina to the pelvic wall. The uterosacral ligaments extend from the upper portion of the cervix posteriorly to the third sacral vertebra.

Functions of the Muscles of the Pelvic Floor

The pelvic floor serves various functions as depicted in the **Figure 14.6**. These are performed basically by acting as a support or sling for the abdominal viscera including the rectum, constrictor, or continence mechanism to the urethra, vagina, and anal openings.

Role of Fast Versus Slow Fibers

The pelvic floor has both types of muscle fibers (fast as well as slow twitch). The slow twitch are more (approximately 70%) than the fast twitch fibers, to maintain urine and faecal continence. On the other hand, the fast twitch fibers contract as per need (whenever there is any rise in intra-abdominal pressure).

Clinical Pointer

Kegel has defined the pelvic floor functions as supportive, sphincteric and sexual.

Supportive Function

The pelvic floor supports the vital organs.

- *In males:* Bladder, urethra and prostate.
- *In females:* Vagina and uterus (females), anus, and rectum, along with the general support of the intra-abdominal contents.

The ligaments play a major role in this function along with the PFM. There is a normal resting tone in PFM at rest. The muscle activity of PFM rises with increase in intra-abdominal pressure (laugh, cough, sneeze, vomit, lift). Therefore, PFM needs to be strong enough to counteract the increase in the pressure time to time during daily routine activity. This supportive function is the primary function of the tonic, slow twitch fibers.

Sphincteric Function

The PFM ensures the continence of both urethrae as well as rectum. The phasic, fast-twitch fibers (30%) ensure quick closure of orifices during the function and at rest, the slow-twitch fibers (70%) ensure resting tone. When the pressure in the urethra is more than the pressure in the bladder there is continence. Loss of sphincter function may lead to incontinence.

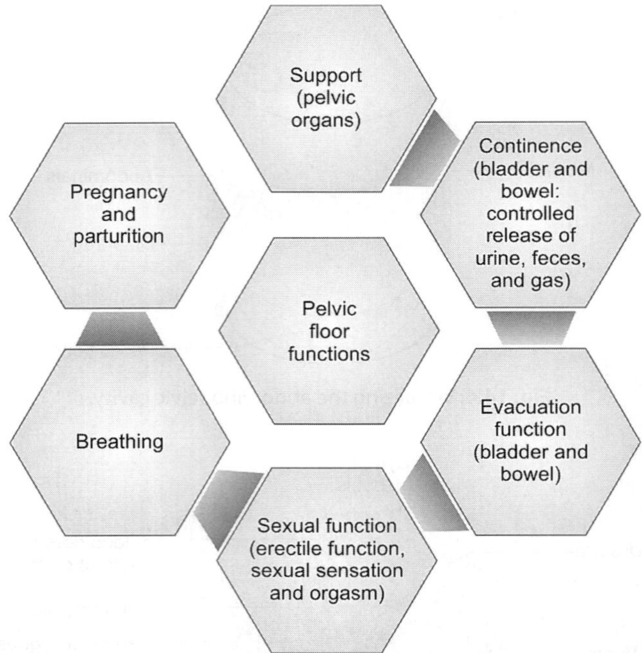

Fig. 14.6: Functions of the pelvic floor.

Role of Pelvic Floor in Micturition

Micturition is physiologic process of urination.

The pelvis houses the urinary tract structures **(Fig. 14.7)** including the ureters, bladder, and urethra.

- The ureters are abdominopelvic organs inserting into the superior aspect of the bladder.
- The bladder is a muscular organ that serves as a reservoir for urine. The bladder is fairly distensible, having a flat shape when empty to globular when full. The base of the bladder has the bladder neck, which acts to prevent the flow of urine, and pubovesical muscle works to open it during voiding.
- The urethra extends from the bladder neck and is central to urinary continence.

Urinary continence is an output of the functioning of the muscles and supportive structures which carry out the functions of urinary storage and evacuation. Normal pelvic floor function is a prerequisite for urine storage that demands that continence be maintained with normal urethral closure and urethral support. The endopelvic fascia (anterior vaginal wall) along with its connections to the arcus tendinous fascia pelvis (ATFP), and levator ani muscles (medial part) must be intact to provide normal urethral support.

Normal evacuation of urine requires a series of coordinated events, the first of which involves complete relaxation of the external urethral sphincter and levator ani muscles.

The muscles contribute to the sphincter mechanism comprised of the internal urethral sphincter mechanism (urethral smooth muscle and detrusor muscle), which work to shorten and widen the urethra, while contraction

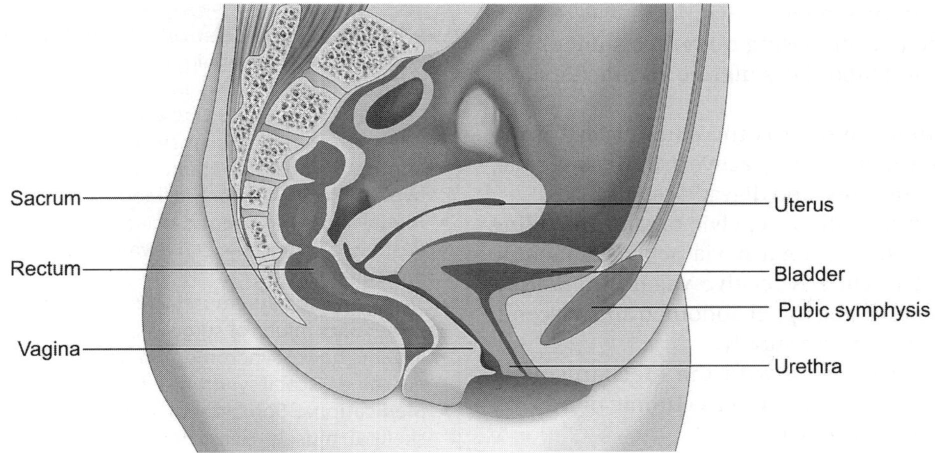

Fig. 14.7: Urinary tract.

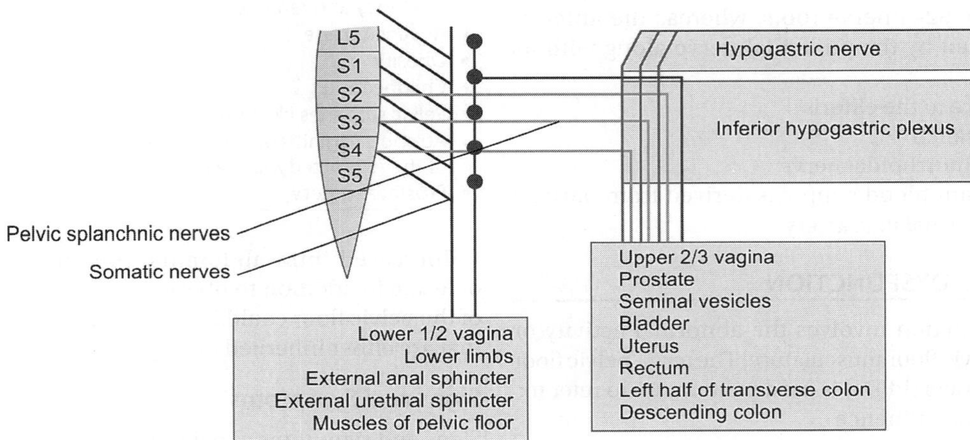

Fig. 14.8: Schematic diagram of somatic and autonomic pelvic nerves.

of circular smooth muscle provides resistance to flow. At the distal end, the external sphincter mechanism formed by the sphincter urethrae, compressor urethrae, and urethrovaginal sphincter muscles function to maintain closure of the urethra and permit voluntary interruption of urine flow. The sling-like vaginal base forms the base on which the urethra sits and compresses the bladder neck and urethra. If this vaginal support is disrupted, urinary incontinence may ensue. In normal state, the lower one-third of the vagina is approximately 45° from the horizontal. During voiding of urine, the PFM relaxes and detrusor muscle contracts.

The PFM contribute to resting continence till bladder fills to its capacity (commonly ~300–600 mL). Coordinated detrusor and sphincter function along with structural support, result in continence.

Sexual Function

The PFM also provides a proprioceptive sensation that contributes to sexual arousal. PFM are vital to pregnancy, childbirth and breathing process.

NEUROANATOMY OF THE PELVIC FLOOR

Detailed knowledge of the neuroanatomy of the pelvis (**Fig. 14.8**), and understanding the potential somatic and visceral sources of pelvic pain, is the foundation for the clinical decision-making for the management of PFD of neurological origin.

Neural control of pelvic organs is affected by a unique coordination of somatic and autonomic motor nervous systems; sensory information and feedback are supplied by both visceral and somatic sensory fiber systems.

- The motor neurons that contribute to the external rhabdosphincters and parts of the pelvic floor are located in Onuf's nucleus (ventral horn at S2–S4) and project via the pudendal nerve and sacral motor branches.
- The autonomic (parasympathetic) fibers constitute the pelvic plexus, while the somatic fibers from the ventral rami (sacral plexus) form the pudendal nerve.
- External anal sphincter muscle is innervated by the pudendal nerves.
- The sympathetic part of the autonomic nervous system is activated during stress and controls "fight or flight"

responses of the pelvic functions. Sympathetic activation promotes storage (by increasing outlet resistance) and inhibits voiding, and modulates uterine contractility and blood flow.

- The parasympathetic system is the counterpart of the sympathetic system that is usually active in the resting state, it is also known as the "rest and digest" system.
- Parasympathetic innervation to pelvic organs, including the uterus and cervix, is primarily via pelvic splanchnic nerves (S2–S4). The gonads receive vagal innervation because they develop in the upper abdomen and descend, retaining their original nerve supply.
- Pelvic nerves are associated with the mechanisms of defecation and micturition, as well as chronic pelvic and visceral pain and sexual activity.

Neurovascular Supply of the Pelvic Floor

The pelvic floor muscles are posteriorly innervated by direct efferents from the S2–4 nerve roots, whereas the anterior pelvis is innervated by the pudendal nerve along with its three branches:

1. The dorsal nerve to the clitoris
2. The perineal branch
3. The inferior hemorrhoidal nerve

The predominant blood supply is derived from parietal branches of the internal iliac artery.

PELVIC FLOOR DYSFUNCTION

Pelvic floor dysfunction involves the abnormal activity or function of the pelvic floor musculature. The term 'pelvic floor dysfunction/disorders (PFDs) is used in literature to refer to:

- Stress urinary incontinence
- Overactive bladder syndrome
- Pelvic organ prolapse (POP)
- Fecal incontinence

Epidemiology

There is a considerable variation of the prevalence of PFD. A meta-analysis of the prevalence of symptomatic pelvic floor disorders in community-dwelling women in low and middle-income countries found that the overall pooled prevalence of PFDs was 25%.

Etiology

Box 14.1 shows the factors that may contribute to PFD.

Box 14.1: Etiological factors of PFD.

- Poor evacuation techniques causing hypertonicity symptoms associated with voiding and defecation difficulties
- Lifestyle: Habitual efforts to avoid urination or bowel movements
- Dyssynergic defecation may begin in childhood
- Surgical or obstetric trauma may lead to muscular pain with hypertonicity of the pelvic floor
- Sexual abuse has been associated with chronic pelvic pain
- Posture, gait, and skeletal asymmetry may contribute to pelvic muscular pain
- Degenerative neuromuscular disease, spinal nerve injury
- Lower back injury, or surgery
- Irritable bowel syndrome, endometriosis, and interstitial cystitis are some visceral syndromes that might contribute to PFD pain
- Medications: Some medications can increase smooth and skeletal muscle relaxation, for example, muscle relaxants, narcotics, alpha-blocking agents, calcium-channel blockers, and methyldopa, thus contributing to incontinence
- Antihistamines and anticholinergics may also lead to urinary hesitancy and retention
- Advancing age
- Obesity
- Childbearing
- Pelvic surgeries like hysterectomy or pelvic trauma
- Atrophic vaginitis or vulvodynia may cause dyspareunia because of the reinforced muscle contraction causing pelvic pain
- Prostate surgery

Pathophysiology

The mechanical correlates of pelvic organ prolapse are related to the widening of the levator hiatus and laxity of the pelvic floor with a descent that is relative to the pubococcygeal line. These changes might be triggered by a myriad of risk factors in singular or multiple existence. They include:

- Obesity
- Menopause
- Pregnancy
- Childbearing

Increased intra-abdominal pressure with straining to defecate in addition to obesity might trigger POP. The laxity of the pelvic floor could be related to collagen abnormalities that are either inherited or acquired during pregnancy.

Signs and Symptoms

Signs and symptoms of pelvic floor dysfunction may include one or more of following:

- Frequent need to use the restroom
- Constipation or a straining pain during bowel movements
- Straining/difficulty to defecate
- Leaking stool or urine (incontinence)
- Painful urination
- Pain in the lower back with no other discernible cause
- Constant pain in the pelvic region, genitals, or rectum—with or without a bowel movement
- Dyspareunia

Clinical Pointer

Chronic pelvic pain:

- Chronic pelvic pain lasting for three to six months can be a disabling, persistent pain concern that presents with characteristic hyperalgesia and allodynia.
- Chronic pelvic pain can be attributed to deviant motor control strategies which are maladaptive in nature and lead to ongoing pain and disability.
- These faulty patterns may have negative repercussions on pelvic loading and stability, breathing, continence, pain, and even disability.

- Most common etiologies of chronic pelvic pain: Irritable bowel syndrome, musculoskeletal pelvic floor pain, painful bladder syndrome, peripheral neuropathy, and chronic uterine pain disorder.
- It responds positively to cognitive-behavioral therapy, mindfulness, and PF physiotherapy, along with pharmacological management.

Types of Pelvic Floor Dysfunction

On the basis of the tone of the pelvic floor muscles, two types of PFD can be identified as shown in **Table 14.2**.

Clinical Correlates of PFD

The clinical correlates of PFD can be urologic, gynecologic, colorectal, or generic and are quite often interrelated. Cross-talk in the course of normal regulation of the bowel, bladder, and sexual function may explain the involvement of these structures in pelvic pain syndromes. Therefore, concerns about all these systems can be associated with the PFD owing to hypertonicity, hypotonicity, loss of pelvic support, or mixed concerns **(Fig. 14.9)**.

Here are some urologic, gynecologic, colorectal, or generic correlates of PFD.

- **Urological concerns:**
  - Difficulty in urination which could be seen as hesitancy, delay in the urinary stream
  - Cystocele—herniation of the bladder into the vagina (anterior)
  - Urethrocele—bulging of the urethra into the vagina (urethral prolapse)
  - Urinary incontinence—involuntary leakage of urine
- **Gynecologic concerns:**
  - Dyspareunia—pain with or following sexual intercourse
  - Uterine prolapse—herniation of the uterus via the vagina beyond the introitus
  - Vaginal prolapse—herniation of the vaginal apex beyond the introitus
  - Enterocele—herniation of the intestines into the vagina (apical/posterior)
  - Rectocele—herniation of the rectum into the vagina (posterior).
- **Colorectal concerns:**
  - Dyssynergic defecation which is defined as the constipation caused by paradoxical puborectalis

Table 14.2: Types of pelvic floor dysfunction.

Hypertonic PFD	*Hypotonic PFD*
Increased tone or hypertonic pelvic floor muscles	Decrease in the tone of PFM often accompanied by tension in surrounding hip and pelvic muscles such as the piriformis, obturator internus, coccygeus, and hamstrings.
At-risk population: • Gym-goers and weight lifters who statically load their core. • History of holding on urine/feces. • Sympathetic stimulation with stress, fear or anxiety. • Pelvic and abdominal conditions which cause chronic pain can develop tense PFM, e.g., interstitial cystitis, pudendal neuralgia, endometriosis and vulvodynia. • Birth trauma and scar tissue in form of perineal tearing or vaginal tearing.	**At-risk population:** • It is mostly seen after prolonged labor, child birth and in connective tissue disorders like Ehlers-Danlos syndrome. • Associated with stress urinary incontinence, overactive bladder syndrome (urinary urgency, frequency, urgency incontinence and nocturia), pelvic organ prolapse, anal incontinence (gas, liquid, and stool incontinence), constipation, dyspareunia, urgency and pelvic pain.
Signs and symptoms: • Pelvic pain, low back pain, hip pain, coccyx pain • Constipation, incomplete emptying of the bowels, straining when emptying the bladder or bowel • Vulvodynia, painful sex, vaginismus • Urinary incontinence, slow stream, hesitancy of urine stream, urinary urgency and frequency, painful urination	**Signs and symptoms:** The most common clinical presentations for hypotonic PF muscle are: • Pelvic organ prolapse • Stress incontinence • Fecal incontinence

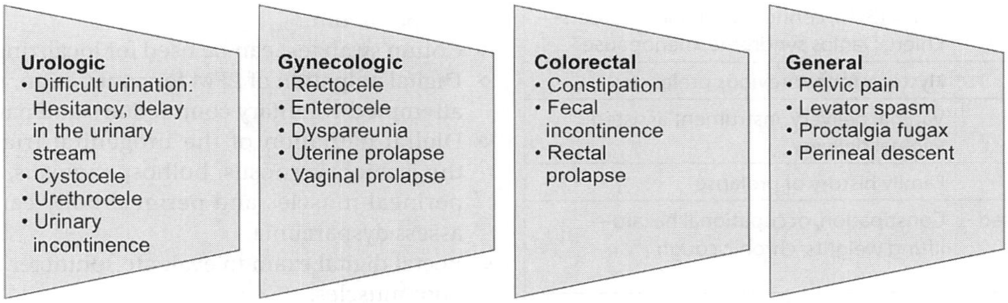

Urologic
- Difficult urination: Hesitancy, delay in the urinary stream
- Cystocele
- Urethrocele
- Urinary incontinence

Gynecologic
- Rectocele
- Enterocele
- Dyspareunia
- Uterine prolapse
- Vaginal prolapse

Colorectal
- Constipation
- Fecal incontinence
- Rectal prolapse

General
- Pelvic pain
- Levator spasm
- Proctalgia fugax
- Perineal descent

Fig. 14.9: Urologic, gynecologic, colorectal, or generic correlates of PFD.

- Contraction or inadequate relaxation of the pelvic floor muscles during attempted defecation
- Fecal incontinence—involuntary leakage of stool
- Rectal prolapse—invagination of the rectum beyond the analverge (procedentia) or proximal to the anus (occult).

❖ **General concerns:**
- Pelvic pain which is lasting more than three to six months, unrelated to other defined conditions
- Levator spasm (levator ani syndrome) because of chronic pelvic pain related to the levator ani muscle
- Proctalgia fugax which is a fleeting spastic pain related to the levator ani muscle
- Perineal descent—herniation of the perineum below the pelvic outlet
- **Pudendal neuralgia:** Irritation/damage to pudendal nerve
- **Coccygodynia:** Pain in coccyx that worsens during and after bowel movements

Pelvic Organ Prolapse

Pelvic organ prolapse (POP) is the herniation of the pelvic organs, including the bladder, bowel, or uterus, to or beyond the vaginal introitus that occurs in up to 50% of parous women.

It is often associated with concomitant pelvic floor disorders, including urinary and fecal incontinence, pelvic pain, voiding, and sexual dysfunctions, which may adversely affect the quality of life.

A prolapse is representative of a defect in support of one or more of the vaginal walls, which are held in place by the integrity of the connective tissues and the pelvic musculature. **Table 14.3** documents some of the common risk factors for POP.

Figure 14.10 describes the pathogenesis of POP in brief.

Types of POP

POP is a PFD, which can also be classified **(Table 14.4)** as:
❖ Anterior: Pertaining to the urethra/bladder
❖ Middle: Affecting the vagina/uterus
❖ Posterior: Related to the anus/rectum

Table 14.3: Common risk factors for POP.

Category	*Risk factors*
General	Parity, advancing age, and body mass index (BMI), connective tissue disorders—Ehlers-Danlos syndrome, menopause
Surgical	Hysterectomy/previous prolapse
Obstetric	Vaginal delivery, instrument assisted vaginal delivery
Hereditary	Family history of prolapse
Prolonged increased intra-abdominal pressure	Constipation, occupational hazard—lifting weights, chronic cough
Ethnic correlation	White and hispanic women

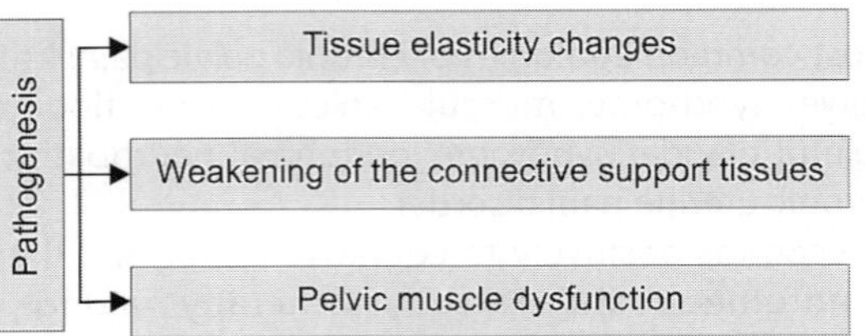

Fig. 14.10: Pathogenesis of POP.

Table 14.4: Types of POP.

Anterior compartment prolapse	**Cystocele**	Anterior vaginal compartment herniates through the vaginal introitus
Posterior compartment prolapse	**Rectocele**	A bulge caused by a herniation of the rectum through the vaginal introitus
	Enterocele	A bulge caused by the small intestines or even sigmoid colon herniating through the vaginal introitus
Apical prolapse		The apex of the vaginal canal descends
Procidentia		All three compartments—anterior, posterior and apical, prolapse simultaneously

Assessment in PFD

Evaluation of patients with PFD is initially focused on their presenting complaints.

As previously mentioned the complaints and concerns often involve multiple systems and hence the evaluation also needs to be multidisciplinary.

History

In view of Urologic, Gynecologic, Colorectal, or Generic correlates of PFD, questions about these domains in history **(Table 14.5)** can help the examiner proceed in a definitive direction.

Diary documentation of voiding, defecation, pain, and diet can be beneficial to assist with the evaluation.

Physical Examination

❖ Visual check-up, for herniation especially with pelvic organ prolapse.
❖ Pelvic floor contraction (to avoid urination), should elevate the perineum.
❖ Cotton swab test can be used for localizing vulvodynia.
❖ Digital palpation of PFM for contraction, relaxation (after attempted voluntary contraction), and pain.
❖ Digital palpation of the urogenital triangle including the ischiocavernosus, bulbospongiosus, and transverse perineal muscles and perineal body can be utilized to assess dyspareunia.
❖ Rectal digital exam to evaluate sphincter tone and pelvic floor muscles.
❖ Anal sensation, i.e., response to touch, and pinprick.

Table 14.5: Domains in history.

General	*Urologic*	*Gynecologic*	*Colorectal*
Pelvic pain/ pressure	• Urinary hesitancy/ frequency/urgency • Dysuria • Bladder pain • Incontinence—urge, and stress	• Dyspareunia (during/ after intercourse) • Sexual arousal • Orgasm • Bulging from the vagina	• Difficult/straining/incomplete evacuation of stool • Bloating • Constipation • Fecal incontinence/leaking • Prolapse/protrusion from anus • Splinting—pressure within the vagina or on the perineum to provide support and assist with voiding or defecation

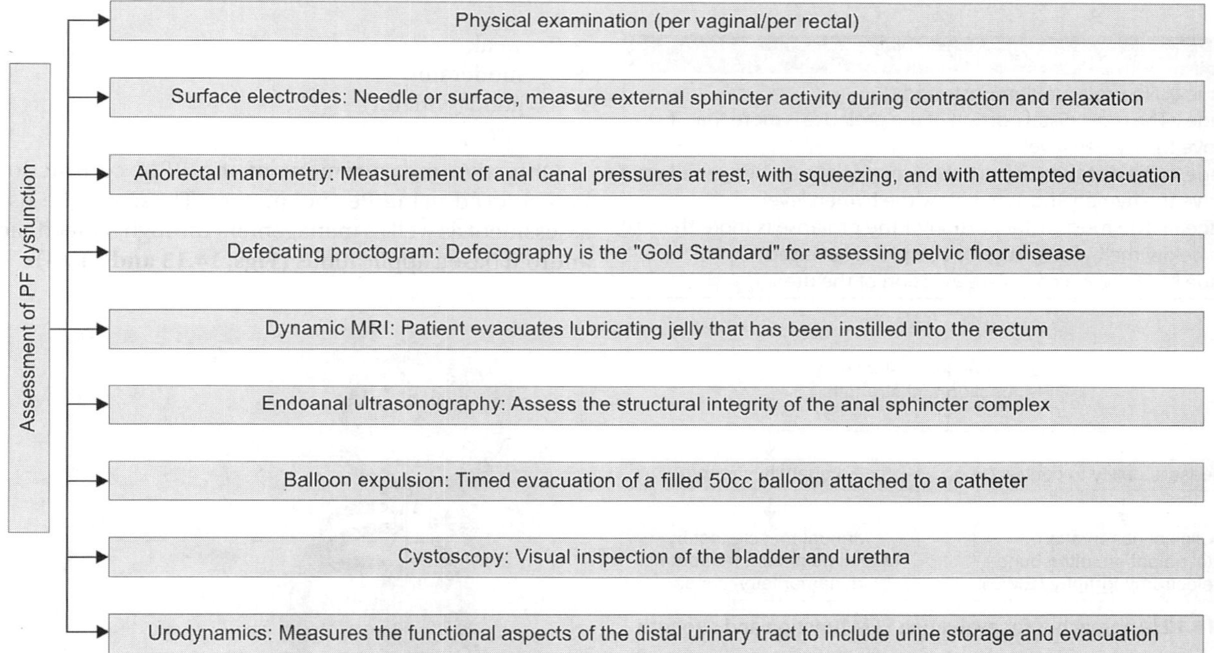

Fig. 14.11: Assessment of PF dysfunction.

- Examination for prolapse with straining/increased intra-abdominal pressure.

Various tests can be incorporated into physical examination to augment the therapist's clinical perception as shown in the **Figure 14.11**. **Table 14.6** describes functional measures that can be used in assessment of POP.

Pelvic Organ Prolapse Quantification (POP-Q)

The International Continence Society defined a system POP-Q, to describe prolapse through a numeric map of the location and extent of the defects. The patient is instructed to perform a Valsalva maneuver which helps display the greatest degree of prolapse and is useful for obtaining Pelvic Organ Prolapse Quantification (POP-Q). The overall stage of the prolapse, at maximum Valsalva effort, ranges from 0 to 4, in ascending degree of severity **(Box 14.2)**.

The vagina is a fibromuscular, flattened, cylindrical tube with three levels of support, as described by DeLancey. The levels of support are shown in **Table 14.7**.

Pelvic Floor Muscle Assessment

PFM examination assesses the ability of the pelvic floor to contract correctly (squeeze and lift) as well as the strength

Table 14.6: Functional measures used in assessment of POP.

Functional measure	*Indication*
Pelvic organ prolapse quantification (POP-Q) system	Describing and staging pelvic support
The pelvic floor distress inventory (PFDI) and PFDI-20	Pelvic floor dysfunction
Female sexual function index (FSFI)	Sexual dysfunction in women
Ultrasound, magnetic resonance imaging (MRI), and X-ray imaging	Image assistance for anatomy of pelvic floor
Bladder and rectum function tests, such as urodynamics, manometry, or defecography	Defecography—radiological study of attempted defecation manometry: Resting pressure and maximum squeeze pressure of puborectalis, external anal sphincter
Neurophysiological testing—pudendal nerve terminal motor latency (PNTML)	Nerve conduction study of pudendal nerve

Table 14.7: The levels of support.

Levels of support	*Structures supported*	*Support provided by*	*Effect of loss of support*
Level 1	Vaginal apex, cervix, and uterus	The uterosacral and cardinal ligaments	Uterine descent or apical prolapse
Level 2	The lateral walls of the vagina	Pubocervical and rectovaginal attachments	Cystocele
Level 3	Distal third of the vagina	Perineal membrane, perineal body, and superficial and deep perineal muscles	Urethral hypermobility—SUI, rectocele, or enterocele

Box 14.2: Stages of pelvic organ prolapse.

- Stage 0: No prolapse demonstrated
- Stage I: The most distal portion of the prolapse is more than 1 cm above the hymen level
- Stage II: The distal-most portion of the prolapse is between 1 cm above the hymen and 1cm below the hymen level
- Stage III: The most distal portion of the prolapse is more than 1 cm below the hymen, but not completely everted
- Stage IV: There is a complete eversion of the uterus

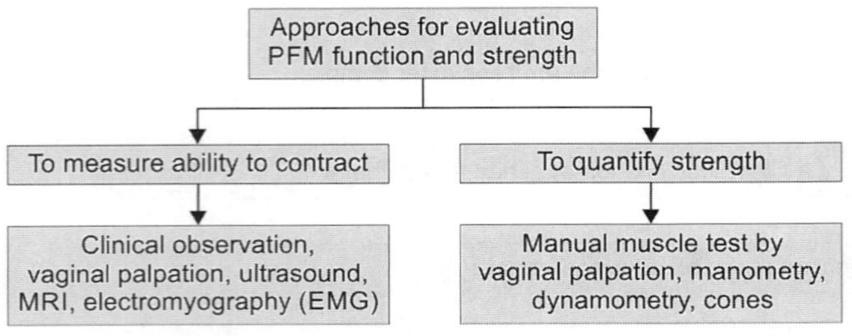

Fig. 14.12: Approaches for evaluating PFM function and strength.

and endurance of the contraction (PFM function). An internal vaginal examination is performed to assess muscle strength, anatomical changes, the symmetry of a contraction, muscle tone as well as any painful areas.

The PERFECT scheme of examination of the pelvic floor muscles developed by Laycock includes following domains:

- **P**ower represents strength of PFM measured as per the Modified Oxford Scale
- **E**ndurance—measure of duration/hold of maximal voluntary contraction (up to 10 seconds)
- **R**epetitions—measure of frequency of maximal voluntary contractions with interspersed rest periods
- **F**ast—measure of total number of 1 second maximal voluntary contractions performed in a row (up to 10)
- **E**levation of the PF
- **C**o-contractions
- **T**iming and co-ordination

Modified Oxford Grading Scale (Laycock): To measure PFM strength using vaginal palpation of the PFM, the following 6-point scale for the strength of PFM contraction is used:

- 0 = no contraction
- 1 = flicker
- 2 = weak
- 3 = moderate
- 4 = good (with lift)
- 5 = strong

Objective measurement of the PFM contraction can be achieved using Perineometers. These can be used for assessment as well as management through biofeedback and android based applications **(Figs. 14.13 and 14.14)**.

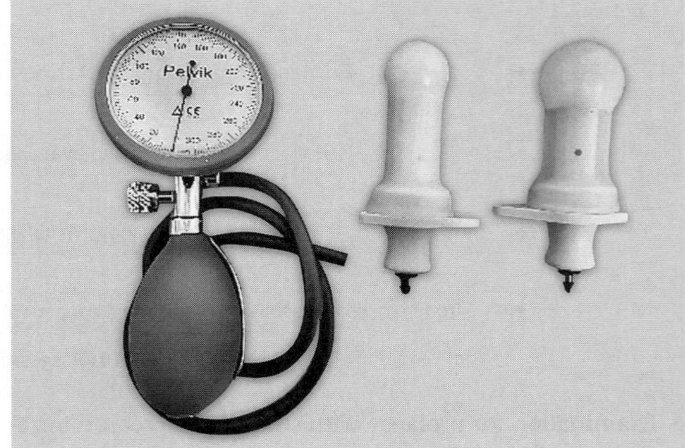

Fig. 14.13: Vaginal squeeze pressure measured with a perineometer and vaginal probe.

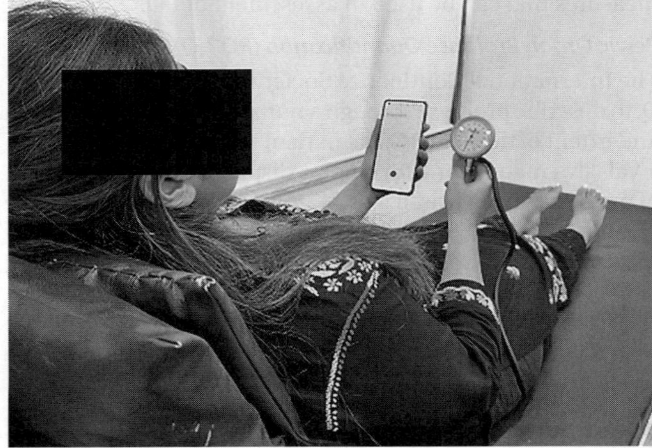

Fig. 14.14: Using android based app for biofeedback along with perineometer.

Table 14.8: Risk factors, biomechanical causes, assessment and management of PFM affections.

Primary causes for PFM reduced function	*Biomechanical causes*	*Biomechanical assessment*	*Restoration of altered biomechanics*
• Age • Childbirth • Genetic • Lifestyle • Neurological • Miscellaneous	• Muscle weakness • Connective tissue concerns: Lax ligaments • Disruption of structures/ avulsions	• Tissue elasticity • Strength of muscles • Motor control strategies	• Medications • Physiotherapy • Complete blood test (CBT) • Surgery • Adjunct therapies

Box 14.3: Differential diagnoses for pelvic pain.

- Myofascial pelvic pain
- Urinary tract infection
- Endometriosis
- Chronic intermittent bowel obstruction
- Chronic constipation
- Irritable bowel syndrome
- Interstitial cystitis
- Ovarian retention syndrome
- Pelvic congestion syndrome
- Vulvodynia
- Diverticular disease
- Inflammatory bowel disease
- Urolithiasis
- Urethral diverticula
- Bladder neoplasm, rectal neoplasm, gynecologic neoplasm, adnexal tumors, uterine leiomyomas
- Prostatitis
- Prostatodynia

Table 14.8 provides a brief summarized quick recall of risk factors, biomechanical causes, assessment and management of PFM affections.

Differential Diagnosis

Pelvic pain is the most frequently encountered symptom in context of PFD. However, it is also the symptom associated with other common etiologies as shown in **Box 14.3**.

Also, urinary incontinence could be caused by excessive urinary volume leading to overflow incontinence. Similarly, retained stool may cause fecal incontinence secondary to encopresis. Hemorrhoid prolapse may often mimic rectal prolapse.

Clinical Pointer

Patients with both hypertonicity and hypotonicity symptoms can obtain some benefit from lifestyle changes, medications, manipulative interventions, and surgical interventions.

PELVIC FLOOR DYSFUNCTION AND ICF

The *International Classification of Impairments, Disabilities, and Handicaps (ICIDH)* which was later upgraded to the *International Classification of Functioning, Disability and Health (ICF)* is a classification system of health and health-related states developed by the World Health Organization (*see* Chapter 7: International Classification of Functioning in Women's Health).

The pelvic floor could function non-optimally or sub-optimally because of various causes including muscle and nerve damage after vaginal birth. ICF considers these as the pathophysiological component. As per ICF, this may lead to impairments in the form of reduced force generation, incorrect timing or lack of coordination while the actual leakage of urine is considered a disability. At an individual level, how it affects the woman's daily activities and quality of life is an activity limitation and restriction in performing fitness activities refer to the participation component.

Pregnancy and Pelvic Floor Dysfunction

During pregnancy, under the influence of relaxin, produced by the placenta, and corpus luteum, there is amplified activity of collagenase, inhibiting collagen synthesis making the ligaments of the pelvic girdle and spine lax. These loose ligaments and the incumbent weight of the pregnant uterus tend to increase lumbar lordosis.

Vaginal Delivery and PFD

Several obstetrical and non-obstetrical factors contribute to the association between vaginal childbirth and PFD.

- Biomechanical modeling has demonstrated that during the second stage of labor, levator ani muscles are stretched more than 200% beyond the threshold for stretch injuries.
- Parity is acknowledged as a leading risk factor in the development of POP.
- The connective tissues supporting the vagina display significant viscoelastic behaviors, indicating that the mechanical properties change based on how much time the tissue has experienced loading. Understanding these time-dependent mechanical properties is important in understanding the contribution of these tissues during events such as gestation, labor, and delivery.
- ***'Operative vaginal delivery' or the 'instrument assisted vaginal delivery'*** are the terms used for traction devices, like forceps and vacuums, to assist uterine contractions and maternal expulsive efforts during the second stage of labor for the delivery of the fetus. Operative vaginal delivery can be considered as a surrogate marker for difficult labor and significantly increase the risk of PFD.

- Episiotomy is an incision on the female perineum done prior to crowning of the fetal head to increase the diameter of pelvic outlet, thus furthering delivery of the fetus. Central episiotomy is known to increase the risk of third- and fourth-degree perineal lacerations.
- Prolonged second stage of labor may cause ischemic necrosis of the pelvic tissues (including nerves and muscles) and stretch injuries, leading to soft tissue injury and neuromuscular damage to the pelvic floor.
- Larger neonatal size (cephalopelvic disproportion) and occiput posterior positions can also increase the risk of perineal injury.

Age and Pelvic Floor

The physiological aging process involves all the connective structures and in case of the pelvic floor, the aging brings about prominent involution in the levator ani muscle.

- Age-related loss of muscle mass and function, sarcopenia, may be caused by multiple mechanisms including the impaired regenerative capacity, attenuated ability to respond to stress, elevated reactive oxygen species production, and low-grade systemic inflammation.
- Sarcopenia of the pelvic floor muscles is of significance in the aging woman as it may underwrite the prolapse of genital organs, and lead to urinary and even anal incontinence especially so in those who suffered from subclinical anal lesions during delivery.

Effect of PFM on Core Muscle Function

As stated in the anatomy section, the superficial pelvic floor or urogenital diaphragm, includes the bulbocavernosus, ischiocavernosus, and transverse perinei. The deep pelvic floor or levator ani includes the puborectalis, pubococcygeus, iliococcygeus, and coccygeus muscle. The piriformis and obturator internus muscles function as the associated muscles, while the deep transversus abdominis, lumbar multifidus, and the diaphragm are functionally considered synergistic muscles.

The maintenance of the function of core stability is a dynamic synergistic conjunction of all these muscles where the PFM are considered as the "floor of the core." The pelvic floor forms the bottom of the abdominal cavity.

- The functions of strong expiration, vocalization, vomiting, and parturition require increased abdominal pressure.
- The pelvic floor plays a vital role in all these motor functions.
- It is probably not a coincidence then that the nucleus retroambiguus, which controls abdominal pressure through its innervation of the abdominal wall muscle motor neurons also innervates Onuf motor neurons to the pelvic floor (S1-S2).

PFD in Spinal Cord Injury Patients

The effects of spinal cord injuries on genitourinary, gastrointestinal, and sexual function are dependent on the specific level and degree of neurologic dysfunction.

- Spinal cord injury (SCI) may lead to either failure to store or failure to empty the bladder.
- Failure to store may be due to detrusor hyperreflexia (or uninhibited bladder contractions) or an areflexic bladder outlet. In comparison, failure to empty may be due to an areflexic bladder or a sphincter that is unable to relax.
- Another common finding in patients with SCIs, is Detrusor-sphincter dyssynergia, wherein the impaired coordination between bladder contraction and sphincter relaxation causes dysfunction.
- Patients with SCI usually present with non-relaxing anal sphincters from an anatomically defined etiology. Bowel dysfunction is one of the most distressing consequences of SCI because it can severely disrupt a person's quality of life and even cause morbidity in extreme cases.
- The puborectalis muscle on contraction lifts the rectum upward forming an angle between the rectum and anus. The external anal sphincter (EAS), internal anal sphincter (IAS), and puborectalis muscle act together to maintain fecal continence. The tonic activity of the IAS maintains continence in the resting state. Normal resting tone is responsible for preserving the approximately 90° angle between the rectum and anal canal.
- However, to prevent incontinence with cough/Valsalva maneuver/increased abdominal pressure, the EAS and puborectalis muscle must contract to prevent accidental passage of formed stool.
- Defecation occurs with easing of the puborectalis muscle and the EAS resulting from the involuntary propulsion of stool into the rectum. This generates a straighter anorectal tunnel for stool to pass, which is supported by peristalsis and increased intra-abdominal pressure.

A neurogenic bowel occurs when there is a dysfunction of the colon due to lack of nervous control. There are two basic types of neurogenic bowel:

1. **Lower motor neuron (LMN) bowel syndrome or areflexic bowel:** Lesion affects the parasympathetic cell bodies in the conus medullaris, the cauda equina, or the pelvic nerve which causes constipation and a significant risk of incontinence due to the lax EAS.
2. **Upper motor neuron (UMN) bowel syndrome or hyperreflexic bowel:** Lesion above the conus medullaris causing disruption of the voluntary control of the EAS and the sphincter remains tight thereby retaining stool. Constipation and fecal retention are features of UMN bowel.

Bowel dysfunction is accompanied by numerous gastrointestinal complications including:

- Ileus
- Gastric ulcers
- Gastroesophageal reflux
- Autonomic dysreflexia
- Pain
- Distention
- Diverticulosis
- Hemorrhoids
- Nausea
- Loss of appetite

- Impaction, constipation, diarrhea, and delayed or unplanned evacuation.

The patients with SCI can accomplish acceptable bowel control with training.

- Using the gastrocolic reflex with increased bowel motility shortly after a meal along with rectal stimulation with either a suppository or enema for reflexive sphincter relaxation can be used to facilitate evacuation.
- This training principle along with an oil-based laxative (mineral oil or Kondremul) can be effectively be used to manage patients with dyssynergic defecation.
- Biofeedback can also be used for relaxation.

Summary

Pelvic floor dysfunction presents with a multitude of symptoms, concerns, and findings related to urologic, gynecologic, and colorectal issues which are often interrelated. Communication and sensitivity are imperative in the evaluation and management of these complex patients. With these tools, patients can be evaluated and monitored in a more consistent manner. Pelvic floor dysfunction is a prime example for healthcare professionals including urologists, gynecologists, urogynecologists, surgeons, and physiotherapists to work in cohesion to provide patient-centered empathetic, efficient, and effective care to patients and enhance the healthcare outcomes.

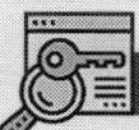

Review Questions

1. Write in detail about the pelvic floor muscles.
2. What are the functions of the pelvic floor muscles?
3. What are the types of the pelvic floor dysfunction?
4. What are the urologic, gynecologic, colorectal, or generic/clinical correlates of the PFD?
5. Write a note on pelvic organ prolapse.
6. Write a note on application of ICF in PFD.

Bibliography

1. Aljuraifani R, Stafford RE, Hall LM, Hodges PW. Task-specific differences in respiration-related activation of deep and superficial pelvic floor muscles. J Appl Physiol (1985). 2019;126(5):1343-52. doi:10.1152/japplphysiol.00017.2019.
2. Bajwa A, Emmanuel A. The physiology of continence and evacuation. Best Pract Res Clin Gastroenterol. 2009;23(4): 477-85. doi:10.1016/j.bpg.2009.04.002.
3. Benson JT. Female pelvic floor disorders: Investigation and management. New York: WW Norton & Company; 1992.
4. Bø K, Berghmans B, Mørkved S, van Kampen M. Evidence-based physical therapy for the pelvic floor. 2nd ed. London: Elsevier; 2007.
5. Cherry D, Rothenberger D. Pelvic floor physiology. Surg Clin North Am. 1988;68(6):1217-30. doi:10.1016/S0039-6109(16)44687-6.
6. DeLancey JO, Morgan DM, Fenner DE, Kearney R, Guire K, Miller JM, et al. Comparison of levator ani muscle defects and function in women with and without pelvic organ prolapse. Obstet Gynecol. 2007;109(2 Pt 1):295-302. doi:10.1097/01. AOG.0000250901.57095.ba.
7. Eickmeyer SM. Anatomy and physiology of the pelvic floor. Phys Med Rehabil Clin N Am. 2017;28(3):455-60. doi:10.1016/j. pmr.2017.03.003.
8. Faubion SS, Shuster LT, Bharucha AE. Recognition and management of nonrelaxing pelvic floor dysfunction. Mayo Clin Proc. 2012;87(2):187-93. doi:10.1016/j.mayocp.2011.09.004.
9. Hall CM, Brody LT. Therapeutic exercise: Moving toward function. Philadelphia: Lippincott Williams & Wilkins; 1999.
10. Islam RM, Oldroyd J, Rana J, Romero L, Karim MN, Hiller JE. Prevalence of symptomatic pelvic floor disorders in community-dwelling women in low- and middle-income countries: A systematic review and meta-analysis. Int Urogynecol J. 2019;30(12):2001-11. doi:10.1007/s00192-019-03992-z.
11. Lien KC, Mooney B, DeLancey JO, Ashton-Miller JA. Levator ani muscle stretch induced by simulated vaginal birth. Obstet Gynecol. 2004;103(1):31-40. doi:10.1097/01.AOG.0000109143.90806.25.
12. Reissing ED, Brown C, Lord MJ, Binik YM, Khalifé S. Pelvic floor muscle functioning in women with vulvar vestibulitis syndrome. J Psychosom Obstet Gynaecol. 2005;26(2):107–13. doi:10.1080/01674820400025041.
13. Rosenbaum TY, Owens A. The role of pelvic floor physical therapy in the treatment of pelvic and genital pain-related sexual dysfunction. J Sex Med. 2008;5(3):513-23; quiz 524–5. doi:10.1111/j.1743-6109.2007.00761.x.
14. Stoker J, Bartram CI, Halligan S. Imaging of the posterior pelvic floor. Eur Radiol. 2002;12(4):779–88. doi:10.1007/s003300101100.
15. Stoker J, Halligan S, Bartram CI. Pelvic floor imaging. Radiology. 2001;218(3):621–41. doi:10.1148/radiology.218.3.r01mr24621.
16. Stoker J. Anorectal and pelvic floor anatomy. Best Pract Res Clin Gastroenterol. 2009;23(4):463-75. doi:10.1016/j.bpg. 2009.04.001.

Multiple Choice Questions (MCQs)

To test your understanding and recall of key concepts.

1. The following structures constitute the pelvic floor muscles________________.

A. Iliococcygeus and pubococcygeus
B. Ischiocavernosus and coccygeus
C. Levator ani and bulbospongiosus
D. All of the above

2. The pelvic floor muscles contain predominantly ______________type of muscle fibers.

A. Fast-twitch fibers (70%)
B. Slow-twitch fibers (70%)
C. Equal proportion of fast- and slow-twitch fibers
D. None of the above

3. Which of the following is *not* a symptom of pelvic floor dysfunction?

A. Chronic pelvic pain
B. Involuntary leakage of stool or urine
C. Herniation of the liver into the thoracic cavity
D. Dyspareunia (pain during intercourse)

4. **The most common clinical presentation of hypotonic pelvic floor muscles is______________.**
   A. Urinary incontinence and pelvic organ prolapse
   B. Pelvic pain and vulvodynia
   C. Constipation with incomplete evacuation
   D. Dyssynergic defecation

5. **Pelvic organ prolapse can involve the herniation of which of the following?**
   A. Bladder
   B. Uterus
   C. Rectum
   D. All of the above

6. **Which stage of pelvic organ prolapse describes complete eversion of the uterus?**
   A. Stage I
   B. Stage II
   C. Stage III
   D. Stage IV

7. **Which test is used to describe and stage pelvic support in pelvic floor dysfunction?**
   A. Modified Oxford Scale
   B. Pelvic Organ Prolapse Quantification (POP-Q)
   C. Perineometer test
   D. Manometry

8. **What is the primary function of the slow-twitch fibers in pelvic floor muscles?**
   A. Quick closure of urethral and anal sphincters
   B. Maintaining resting tone for urinary and fecal continence
   C. Assisting in sexual arousal
   D. Supporting abdominal viscera during childbirth

9. **Which of the following nerves primarily innervates the pelvic floor muscles and external anal sphincter?**
   A. Sacral plexus and obturator nerve
   B. Pudendal nerve and pelvic splanchnic nerves
   C. Vagus nerve and hypogastric plexus
   D. Sciatic nerve and superior gluteal nerve

10. **Which of the following best describes "force closure" in the pelvic floor?**
   A. Stability achieved by the interlocking of bony ridges and grooves
   B. Stability achieved through compressive forces of muscles and fascia
   C. Forceful closure of sphincter during stress
   D. The ability of the urethral sphincter to relax during micturition

11. **What is the primary biomechanical change associated with pelvic organ prolapse (POP)?**
   A. Hypertrophy of pelvic floor muscles leading to tension in connective tissues
   B. Laxity in the pelvic floor due to collagen abnormalities and widening of the levator hiatus
   C. Chronic inflammation of the pelvic ligaments leading to structural instability
   D. Hypertonicity of the puborectalis muscle, causing increased intra-abdominal pressure

ANSWERS

1. D	2. B	3. C	4. A	5. D
6. D	7. B	8. B	9. B	10. B
11. B				

Chapter **15**

Managing the Pelvic Floor

✍ *Kruti Oza Modi*

LEARNING OBJECTIVES

At the end of the chapter, the reader will be able to:

- Describe the ambit of pelvic floor and pelvic floor dysfunction.
- Know the basic types of pelvic floor dysfunction.
- Describe the management of pelvic floor dysfunction using direct and indirect techniques.
- Gain knowledge of the wellness interventions required to treat females with pelvic floor dysfunction.
- Understand bladder irritants in diet, importance of home exercise program and self-management of pain using pelvic trainers, most commonly known as dilators.
- Understand the alternative therapies used to treat females with pelvic floor dysfunction.

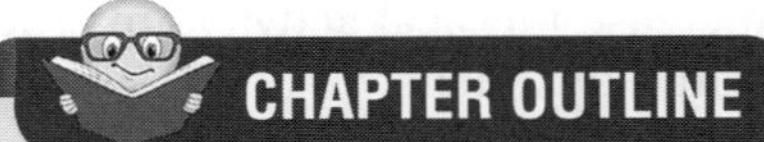

Dedicated to InduBaa and Maa

"Being aware of your pelvic floor and it's intricate connection to your health is essential for your wellbeing"

— Keira W Brown

Let your clinical assessment, anatomical connections guide your treatment. I was once told that no medical field studies musculoskeletal anatomy and its connections like physical therapists do. We all should be proud to offer our expertise to this population.

INTRODUCTION

Pelvic pain is a common problem among women of all ages. Its nature and intensity may fluctuate, and exact causes are unclear. In some cases, no disease is evident. Pelvic pain can be categorized as acute and chronic.

- ***Chronic pelvic pain,*** (CPP) is defined as pelvic and/or lower abdominal pain in a non-cyclic pattern that lasts 6 months or longer in duration in absence of a diagnosis and is associated with poor cognitive, behavioral, sexual and emotional components including symptoms of genitourinary, colorectal or myofascial involvement.
- Pelvic pain can originate in external genitalia or pelvic organs; and can be due to nerve irritation, skeletal/smooth muscle spasm, sexual trauma or psychological.
- ***Acute pelvic pain*** occurs when the body is injured, as in cases of infection, trauma or surgery. Acute pelvic pain conditions include but are not limited to:
  - Ectopic pregnancy
  - Pelvic inflammatory disease
  - Ruptured ovarian cyst
  - Miscarriage
  - Urinary tract infection (UTI)

- Appendicitis
- Acute pelvic floor muscles spasm

An infection treated effectively with antibiotics can resolve acute pain, however, if similar infection returns, chronic pain symptoms such as sleep disturbances, behavioral-emotional-sexual components and musculoskeletal changes may result.

- The spectrum of CPP is broad and in addition to musculoskeletal and physiological pain symptoms patient also experiences comorbidities including depression, sleep disturbances, behavioral and cognitive issues. For example, dyspareunia over a prolonged time may cause distress, depression, pelvic floor muscle tightness and interpersonal distress. **Table 15.1** presents some of common conditions associated with CPP.
- Chronic pelvic pain syndrome (CPPS) is one of the most common healthcare problems in our society and the least discussed. Approximately 25% of women with CPPS may spend 2–3 days in bed each month. More than ½ of women with CPPS cut down on their activities 1 or more days a month and 90% have pain with intercourse. Almost ½ of women feel sad and depressed some of the time. Although CPPS is common among women, it can also occur in men where it is often known as chronic abacterial prostatitis, Type IIIB. In men, pain can manifest in the perineum, rectum, prostate, penis, testicle and abdomen. Chronic pelvic pain impacts people across the gender spectrum including LGBTQ+ and gender non-conforming.

CPPS accounts for 20% gynecological referral, 20% laparoscopic surgery and 12–16% hysterectomy. It has considerable impact on patients' quality of life. It is one of the conditions which has long delays in women getting a diagnosis and accessing adequate care.

In some patients, an underlying structural pelvic pathology can be identified (e.g., endometriosis, adenomyosis, or chronic pelvic inflammatory disease with adhesion or hydrosalpinx) but often pain is idiopathic, meaning it is not due to a visible structural cause (e.g., bladder pain syndrome, irritable bowel syndrome and pain memory). It usually occurs after an episode of acute pain in spite of removal of the painful stimulus. In fact, changes in the brain have been reported in endometriosis patient with CPP but not an asymptomatic woman with endometriosis.

In many cases, the pathology is multifactorial. Follow-up studies have concluded that a surgical intervention is frequently not curative. For instance, for endometriosis 20–28% of patients do not experience a reduction in pain and some require another operation - 25.5% within two years and 40–50% after 5 years.

Table 15.1: Common causes of chronic pelvic pain.

Visceral	*Neuromusculoskeletal*	*Psychological*
• Adenomyosis • PID • Endometriosis • Pelvic adhesions • Vestibulitis • Vulvodynia • Inflammatory bowel disease • Colorectal conditions • IC/PBS • Urethral stricture • Chronic UTI • Post gynecological surgery	• Fibromyalgia • Coccydynia • Spasm of levator ani • Postural imbalance • Dysfunctional abdominal wall musculature due to surgery, injury, scar formation • Neurological pain • Pudendal nerve dysfunction	• Abuse • Depressive disorders • Anxiety disorders • Substance abuse

(PID: pelvic inflammatory disease; IC: interstitial cystitis; PBS: painful bladder syndrome; UTI: urinary tract infection)

Clinical Pointer

CPP is often resistant to surgical and medical treatment and appears to respond better to a multimodal, holistic approach rather than reliance on surgery alone. What is therefore required, is an evidence base for a multidisciplinary approach with a focus on improving the patient's quality of life including self-management and complementary therapies. Like diabetes or hypertension, CPP is chronic, idiopathic and incurable but successfully treatable condition.

Several studies and guidelines have concluded the efficacy of physiotherapy and rehabilitation applications in CPP treatment. Individualized and group exercise programs as well as initiatives to increase physical activity are crucial components of conservative treatment.

Research Pointer

In a study conducted with transvaginal manual therapy in patients with CPP, a significant decrease was observed in pain complaints of 63% of patients.

In another multicenter study, patients with bladder pain syndrome/interstitial cystitis underwent physical therapy including manual therapy and exercise for the pelvic floor and hip muscles, and a significant improvement was observed compared to those treated with global therapeutic massage.

It has been proposed that application of manual therapy to the pelvic floor for 8–12 weeks, twice a week, reduces the pelvic floor hypertonic disorders and significantly improves symptoms.

In one randomized trial, pelvic floor physical therapy and levator ani directed trigger point injections were equally effective in markedly decreasing vaginal pain and sex-related pain.

Complex anatomy and overlapping pathologies such as adductor muscle strain, iliopsoas syndrome, and gluteal tendinopathy make the diagnosis difficult in certain cases. Therefore, comprehensive risk factors should be defined, all kinetic chains should be assessed, and the exercise program should be planned accordingly.

Pelvic floor muscle tenderness is a common finding associated with chronic pelvic pain. Physical therapists use a wide range of manual techniques, modalities and tools tailored to each patient's specific symptoms and clinical findings **(Box 15.1)**.

Common conditions encountered in the clinic are:
- Chronic pelvic pain
- Coccyx pain
- Groin pain
- Vulvar pain
- Vulvar vestibulitis
- Anismus
- Sacroiliac (SI) pain
- Pain with penetration (sexual/gynecological examination)
- Genital pain
- Pudendal neuralgia
- Prostatitis
- Perineal pain
- Proctalgia Fugax

Treatment for pelvic floor dysfunction (PFD), varies based on patient presentation. It is quite unique in the sense that it does not follow specific protocols like total knee replacement (TKR), total hip replacement (THR), biceps tendinosis, spinal decompression, etc. Many different disciplines provide treatment options to pelvic girdle and perineum area including:
- Obstetrics and gynecology
- Urologist
- Proctologist
- Dermatologist
- Colon specialist
- Sexologist
- Physical medicine and rehabilitation (PM and R)
- Occupational therapist (OT)
- Behavioral therapist
- Urogynecologist
- Physical therapist

Our (physical therapist's) unique specialty is the one on one time with our patients which gives us a treatment edge that other disciplines are missing in modern medicine. Physical therapy is usually the last option but it should not be so. Patient presents with frustration, stress, anxiety, hopelessness since no one has validated their complaints and offered any treatment. Being empathetic and validating your patients' symptoms is the first line of treatment, actually in any specialty of the physical therapy profession.

Box 15.1: Techniques and modalities used in physiotherapy.
- Internal and external tissue mobilization
- Myofascial release
- Manipulative therapy to mobilize visceral, urogenital and joint structures
- Biofeedback
- Kegel exercises
- Posture correction
- Core stabilization
- Stretching
- Strengthening
- Flexibility and coordination exercises
- Bladder and bowel retraining
- Pelvic floor muscle stretching
- Active pelvic floor retraining
- Electrical stimulation
- Transcutaneous electrical nerve stimulation
- Electromagnetic chair
- Extracorporeal shockwave therapy
- Acupuncture
- Percutaneous tibial nerve neuromodulation

History of Pelvic Floor Management

Back in the days, many cultures understood pelvic health to be a super important part of overall well-being. In ancient Greece and Rome, there is description by Hippocrates and Gale of pelvic floor exercises practiced in bathhouses. Ancient yogic practice of Ashwini Mudra, connects the breath with the contraction and release of the sphincter muscle.

Today many doctors have a one-word solution to pelvic floor dysfunction—Kegels exercises. Dr Arnold Kegel in the 1940s invented Kegel exercises. In the 1930s, notably before Kegel published his research paper, a physical therapist named Margaret Morris started preaching the importance of breath and pelvic floor muscle training to prevent leaks. Morris was a talented dancer turned holistic healer who found her way into physical therapy after realizing that her dancer's health and posture improved with breathing techniques. Today, many people think of pelvic floor physical therapy as new but the truth is that it has been around for longer than we realize.

Recognition for the need of a physiotherapist (PT) and acknowledgement of women's health status as deserving attention was a direct result of national and international movements in 1960s and 1970s. The name change in 1990s for women's health physical therapy specialty group is reflective of increased visibility and popularity of greater women's health movement to serve all women through their lifespan and to reflect the broader scope of practice (also *see* Chapter 1: Introduction to Physiotherapy in Women's Health).

AMBIT OF PELVIC FLOOR AND PELVIC FLOOR DYSFUNCTION

Refer Chapter 14: Simplifying the Enigma: Pelvic Floor.

MANAGEMENT OF PELVIC FLOOR DYSFUNCTION

APTA position statement on internal physical therapy pelvic examination and intervention is given in **Box 15.2**. Treatment of pelvic floor dysfunction (PFD) can be categorized based on any one of the following:
- Hypertonic vs hypotonic pelvic floor (PF) (types of pelvic floor dysfunction have been described in **Chapter 14:** Simplifying the Enigma: Pelvic Floor in detail)
- PF connections
- PF functions
- Treatment approach

Box 15.2: Position statement on internal physical therapy pelvic examination and intervention (APTA pelvic health)*.

APTA pelvic health, an academy of the American Physical Therapy Association Academy of Pelvic Health Physical Therapy (APTA Pelvic Health) of APTA supports examination and intervention by licensed physical therapists in the management of individuals with pelvic dysfunctions.

Internal vaginal and rectal examination and intervention of pelvic dysfunction, to include external and internal examination of pelvic floor muscles and/or examination of external genitalia specific to diagnoses when those apply, is within the scope of practice of the licensed physical therapist (PT).

In addition, physical therapy assistants (PTAs) may provide internal pelvic floor muscle intervention after the physical therapist performs an internal pelvic floor evaluation examination. PTAs may provide pelvic floor physical therapy interventions: (1) Under general supervision of the PT, (2) under the established PT management plan and plan of care, (3) with documented training and competency and (4) within their state Practice Act. Interventions available for PTA use in the treatment of pelvic floor disorders are listed in APTA Pelvic Health's Position Statement on PTA education, revised in January 2021. Physical therapy students may provide internal pelvic floor physical therapy after they have completed documented training and while working under the supervision of a physical therapist.

Licensed physical therapists, student physical therapists and physical therapy assistants (PTAs) should, at all times know, understand, and adhere to their individual State Practice Acts and any rules/regulations that govern PT and PTA professional licenses as they relate to internal pelvic floor muscle examination and interventions.

APTA pelvic health advises that physical therapy examination of and interventions to the internal pelvic muscles be taught to physical therapists, supervised physical therapy students and PTAs. PTAs may be instructed in examination and interventions of the internal pelvic muscles under the provision that this education is intended for foundational knowledge and that examination of the pelvic dysfunction should remain within the scope of the licensed physical therapist.

APTA pelvic health also recommends the following:

- The supervising PT must have didactic and psychomotor training and experience in pelvic health before mentoring a PTA or PT student.
- Interventions for pelvic dysfunction including, but not limited to, therapeutic exercise, neuromuscular re-education, manual therapy and behavioral retraining may require immediate and continuous examination and evaluation throughout the intervention while at other times may be relatively routine. In routine circumstances, those interventions may be delegated to PTAs and student physical therapists under direct supervision. When immediate and continuous examination and evaluation is necessary, those interventions should be performed only by a licensed physical therapist.
- APTA pelvic health recommends that patient/guardian informed consent be well documented when performing external and internal pelvic muscle examination and intervention. A separate written consent is not recommended since external and internal pelvic muscle examination is within the scope of practice of the physical therapist.
- All clinicians should thoroughly review intake forms and be alert to previous or current sexual abuse that may affect the patient/client's ability to proceed with internal exam. Many patients with a history of trauma will not divulge this information on intake forms but instead verbally share this information with the clinician during the course of treatment.
- APTA pelvic health offers the following recommendations for the examination and intervention of special populations:
  - *Antenatal, peripartum and postpartum:*
    - APTA pelvic health supports internal pelvic muscle examination and intervention in the management of antepartum, peripartum and postpartum women with pelvic dysfunctions.
    - APTA pelvic health recommends internal pelvic muscle examination and intervention be considered for the comprehensive standard musculoskeletal assessment of pelvic dysfunction in antepartum, peripartum and postpartum women.
    - The standard assessment in the antepartum and peripartum population should include external pelvic muscle examination.
    - Caution should be advised when performing internal examination and intervention during the first trimester of pregnancy, during any high-risk antepartum diagnosis, and immediately postpartum prior to medical clearance post delivery. If the licensed physical therapist has concerns regarding such circumstances the academy recommends documenting medical clearance before proceeding with internal pelvic physical therapy.
  - *Pediatric*:
    - The academy of pediatrics' definition of pediatric age ranges are as follows:
      - Infancy: Birth to 2 years
      - Childhood: 2–12 years
      - Adolescence: 12–21 years (Hardin AP, 2017)
    - Patient and parent/guardian's informed consent must be clearly documented.
    - The parent/guardian must be in the room during examination and intervention with a provision for appropriate privacy if requested by the patient.
    - Standard first line examination for a pediatric pelvic patient includes visualization and external surface electrode biofeedback of the external genitalia of the patient.
    - However, APTA pelvic health advises that no internal pelvic examination, either vaginal or rectal, be performed by a physical therapist on a minor or a patient who has not previously had an internal pelvic exam unless there is a written referral from the physician and clear documented consent by the parent/guardian and patient.
    - The physical therapist should be aware of and in compliance with state law in reference to age of consent.
    - APTA pelvic health recommends that the referring physician be contacted with a request for verbal/written referral for a pediatric patient under the age of 16 years or under the legal consent age of 18 years of age.
    - The referring physician should be contacted with any questions, need for clarification of diagnosis, or to be made aware of any questions/concerns regarding the pelvic floor practice by the parent, child, or family member.

Contd...

Contd...

- ♦ Pelvic floor therapy in the pediatric population should be performed only by qualified physical therapists with documented competency and training in pediatric pelvic dysfunction.
- ➢ *Cognitively impaired:* APTA Pelvic Health advises internal pelvic muscle examination and interventions only be performed to individuals who can express clear understanding of the nature of the examination and can provide their informed consent and/or the consent of a guardian.

*Reprinted with written permission by the Academy of Pelvic Health Physical Therapy www.aptapelvichealth.org.

And again, treatment can be focused on function compromised based on the assessment.

PT treatment can be categorized into following components:

- **Direct:** Includes techniques to treat the pelvic floor; which can be internal and external techniques
- **Indirect:** Includes techniques to treat structures related to the pelvic floor and kinetic chain involving pelvic floor
- **Wellness:** Includes strategies to improve overall well-being of the patient

This approach provides opportunity to treat a person's mind body connections, which will provide most successful outcome. It is highly recommended to combine orthopedic and wellness components into treatment as some patients may not be agreeable to internal pelvic floor intervention at first. You can use external and wellness components to begin treatment until patient is agreeable to internal muscle assessment. Area of pelvic health, its language and symptomatology are still taboo in many cultures, no matter what part of the world. Be sensitive towards your patient and use simple medical terminology along with charts to gently ease into treatment approach. On the other side, you may come across patient population who knows what to expect from pelvic floor PT, thanks to Google, and you can assess and treat internally on first session if time allows.

It was previously theorized, that weak pelvic floor muscles cause pelvic floor dysfunction (PFD). Hypertonicity of pelvic floor tissue is a common finding. Pelvic floor muscles and their connective tissue are generally tight and weak and lack coordination with respiratory diaphragm. Pelvic floor muscles form a part of the core system, which comprises (**Fig. 15.1**):

- **Superior:** Respiratory diaphragm
- **Inferior:** Pelvic floor
- **Anterior:** Abdominal wall musculature
- **Posterolateral:** Thoracolumbar fascia and posterior abdominal wall connection

All these components work in conjunction to provide a coordinated movement which is efficient for pressure management and load transfer.

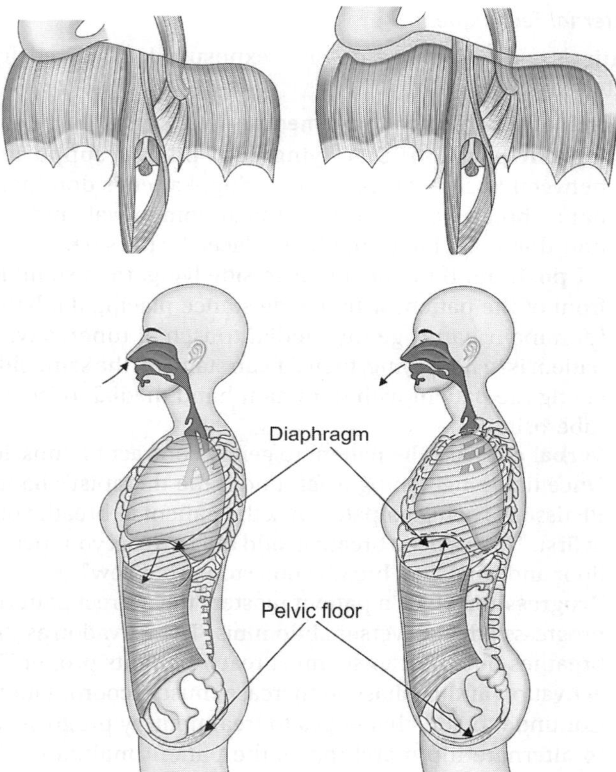

Fig. 15.1: Pelvic floor and respiratory diaphragm *(For color version, see Plate 5).*

Indirect Treatment

It defines treatment based on orthopedic findings including:

- Spinal mobilization
- Nerve mobilization
- Ankle-hip biomechanics correction
- Postural reduction
- Neck pain treatment
- Hip pain (if warranted)

Pelvic floor treatment starts with a concept, which must be learnt by a patient as treatment progression is based on this concept. Pelvic floor and respiratory diaphragm work synergistically to produce a piston like movement as described in **Figure 15.1**. With every inspiration, as respiratory diaphragm contracts and lungs get filled with air it will create pressure on abdominal cavity and lateral chest expansion (360°) which will transfer pressure to pelvic floor and mild bulging of perineum can be visualized. This is pelvic floor relaxation or bulging. During expiration, as pelvic floor contracts into pelvic cavity it will cause respiratory diaphragm to relax, causing it to move superiorly followed by breath-out. This cycle repeats with each breath in and out.

This should be explained using a pelvic model, anatomy pictures or by demonstrating on self. The patient should be asked to verbalize it, practice in supervision of the therapist and repeat at home. As patient continues to progress with the concept, one can add treatment strategies that are most appropriately based on the assessment.

Direct Treatment (Internal and External Techniques)

This approach defines treatment strategies directed to:

- Pelvic diaphragm
- Urogenital diaphragm
- Superficial perineal layer
- Ischiorectal fossa
- Obturator internus
- Visceral mobilization

External Techniques

Patient is dressed and no skin exposure is required for external approach.

Coordinated pelvic floor movement

- **Patient position:** Side lying with pillows supported between knees or supinehook lying. Patient's dominant hand should be placed over the abdomen wall and the non-dominant hand should be placed by the side.
- **PT position:** If the patient is in side lying, then stand in front of the patient with a wide stance placing flat hand (dominant hand) gently medial to ischial tuberosity. If patient is in hook lying, then PT can stand on the same side facing the patient with dominant hand medial to ischial tuberosity.
- **Verbal cue:** Ask the patient to gently contract PF muscle. Once tissue tightening is felt under the therapist's hand, PF tissue is being palpated. Ask the patient to breathe out at first. "Take a deep breath in and bulge/ relax your pelvic floor and when you breathe out, stop urine flow".
- **Progression:** Once a patient masters the correct pattern, progress with transversus abdominis (TA) activation as she breathes out. Therapists must teach patients proper TA activation at this phase to increase muscle coordination. Continue to add challenges to treatment by progressing to alternate hip marching as the patient maintains PF engagement with TA activation. Progress to Quadruped > sitting > standing > lifting.
- **Common substitution pattern:** The therapist may notice excessive gluteal squeeze, adductor activation, abdominal bulging, shoulder elevation, toe curling. Remember, no one can tell if the patient is doing correct PF relaxation and contraction. It is a submaximal and gentle activation.

Educate on pelvic floor activation and relaxation with respiratory diaphragm as discussed above with hand placement for treatment success. These coordination patterns can be difficult for many patients, as they have paradoxical patterns for years which can be challenging to alter in the first few sessions.

Table 15.2 describes various cues to contract and relax the pelvic floor with coordinated breathing.

Table 15.2: Verbal cues to contract and relax the pelvic floor (PF).

PF relaxation with inhalation	*PF contraction with exhalation*
• Relax your buttocks • Widen your hips • Open your vagina • Relax your sit bones • Let go of tension	• Stop urine flow • Stop gas escaping • Close urethra and vagina • Pull perineal body inside pelvic cavity

Elevator concept

It can be utilized to visualize pelvic floor engagement. Have the patient visualize a 3-level building, where the ground floor is relaxed pelvic floor muscles. 3rd floor is contracted pelvic floor muscle and the 2nd floor is resting tone.

Pelvic relaxation and contraction can also be taught with use of a therapy ball. Once a patient is sitting on a therapy ball, place a folded towel under the perineum. Give the patient time to feel the towel and advise to repeat pelvic floor movement with breathing pattern. Towel provides proprioception and can serve as a great tool to connect with the body. Patients tend to squeeze gluteal muscle and abdominal wall which will impair proper pelvic floor activation, therefore excessive activation must be prevented.

Coccyx mobilization

Pelvic floor muscles insert anterior to coccyx. Once you identify hyperflexed coccyx, hyperextended coccyx or left/ right side flexion you can address it with a Drawer stuck test.

Coccyx release and mobilization can provide great relief to patient suffering from:

- Posterior pelvic floor pain
- Painful sitting
- Pudendal neuralgia
- Constipation

Altered pelvic floor muscle tone can also cause deviation of coccyx position from normal.

Technique for coccyx mobilization:

- **Patient position:** High sitting over treatment table with feet supported. Dressed in relaxed and loose clothing.
- **PT position and hand placement:** PT stands behind the patient. Coccyx is located superior to anus. Gently place your flat hand between gluteal fold or in midline at coccyx and ask the patient to gently slump into your hand and have them repeat until you find the tip of coccyx. Slide index finger over coccyx. Coccyx follows lumbar spine movement pattern, meaning with lumbar spine extension, it will extend and with lumbar spine flexion it will flex inside pelvic cavity.
- **Maneuver:** Anchor your index finger gently over the tip of coccyx. Repeat lumbar flexion and extension 2–3 times and towards the last lumbar extension, gently provide traction over coccyx and overlying fascia to remove restriction. Reassess pain and improved coccyx excursion after maneuver.

Abdominal scar mobilization to decrease restriction

Restrictive scar from cesarean section (CS) or abdominal surgeries can cause deeper adhesion leading to restrictions to muscle slide and glide. Also, free nerve endings entrapment can cause sharp pain upon movement and at rest. Most commonly observed is CS scar and appendectomy scar adhesion to ileocecal valve causing lower digestive tract problem along with decreased motility and sharp pain upon turning and lifting.

- **Patient position:** Supine with knees slightly bent with pillows under knees. Expose scars.
- **PT:** Use your index finger and gently sink into the level of restriction and to the patient's comfort. Move your index finger in clockwise and counter clockwise direction, right next to a scar. Repeat over the periphery of the scar. Be sure to read the patient's body language to guide treatment intensity and signs of distress like clenching of jaws, drawing their abdomen inward or curling toes. Decrease your pressure to patients' tolerance.
- **Precaution:** Get physician's clearance, if there is clinical indication for scar mobilization within 6 weeks post-operatively.

Obturator internus—external rotator

- **Patient position:** Side lying with pillow supported between knees. Bottom leg straight. Comfort patient by providing pillow to support head and add folded towel under thoracic spine.
- **PT position for bottom leg treatment:** Behind patient. Gently take tissue slack medial to ischial tuberosity and apply deeper pressure with using 4 fingers. Lift elbow toward ceiling and apply pressure to plinth as tolerated by patient.
- **Patient cues:** Upon identifying trigger point or palpable irregularity, hold steady pressure for 60–90 seconds. Advise patients to relax and contract-relax pelvic floor in coordination with respiratory diaphragm.
- **Treatment variation:** Superior obturator internus can be treated in the same position except hand placement shifted to top leg. Scoop fingers to ceiling with gentle pressure medial and deep to ischial tuberosity.
- **Treatment success:** You will feel muscles softening under your fingers and the patient reports less pain upon the same pressure. Patients may report decreased pelvic pain immediately or in subsequent sessions.

Adductor release

- **Patient position:** Side lying with top leg supported on pillow with hip flexion and bottom leg extended. Comfort patients by providing additional pillows to support head and thoracic curvature.
- **PT position:** Stand behind patient with pillow supported between therapist's body and patient's hip. Gently place the pad of your fingers medial to ischial tuberosity and ask the patient for hip adduction. Upon confirming hand placement, gently friction high adductor tendon at ischiopubic rami. Myofascial release (MFR) on the adductor group starting from the medial knee and following the muscle to proximal attachment to bone can be performed in same position.

Sacrotuberous ligament release

- **Patient position:** Same as above.
- **Therapist position:** PT to stand behind the patient. Gently palpate ischial tuberosity and inferior lateral angle (ILA), of sacrum of the same side. Visualize the sacrotuberous ligament between the two bony landmarks. Gently friction to reduce tension.
- **Indication:** Nerves exiting and entering the spine can get compressed and cause pain symptomatology. Frequently indicated for deep ache hip pain, posterior thigh pain.

Figure 15.2 shows rich and complex ligamentous connection to the bony pelvis.

Side lying gluteal activation

- **Patient position:** Same as above
- **PT position:** PT stands behind patient with one hand over gluteal muscles. Advise patient on isometric glute activation with nonvisual hip extension and muscle tension. Motivate patient on submaximal contraction. Once patient understands movement sequence, allow her to place her own hand to feel proper muscle activation.
- **Indications:** Coccygeal pain, hip tightness, LBP

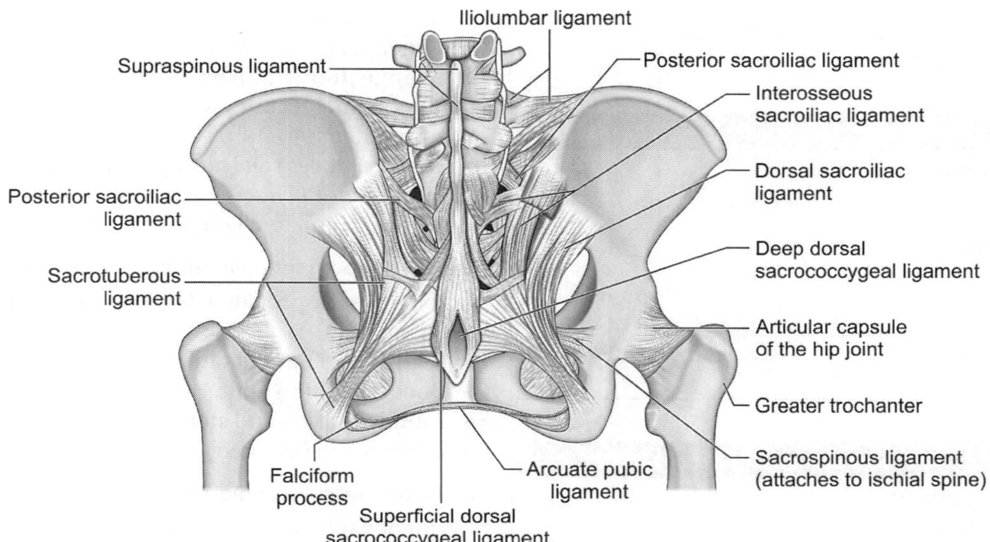

Fig. 15.2: Ligamentous support of bony pelvis *(For color version, see Plate 5)*.

Progress to internal techniques on 1st day or when your patient gives verbal consent.

Clinical Pointer

Ask for consent at each session and multiple times during the session.

Internal Manual Therapy Techniques

APTA defines internal techniques as techniques that are provided utilizing an instrument, dilator or wand, and/or finger directly over perineum, inside vagina or rectum to perform trigger point therapy and treat lack of coordination between soft tissues.

Internal pelvic health treatment includes (recommended pelvic exam by doctor in last 6 months):

- **Perineal techniques:** Covered in chapter (must be practiced prior to direct patient care)
- **Transvaginal techniques:** Covered in chapter (must be practiced prior to direct patient care)
- **Transrectal techniques or anorectal approach:** Beyond scope of current chapter

Pelvic PT is indicated for pelvic pain not related to visceral pathology. Contraindications to internal techniques are described in **Box 15.3**. Precautions with internal techniques should be undertaken in the presence of conditions described in **Box 15.4**.

Manual therapy techniques described are introductory techniques. Physical therapist must practice these techniques under experienced PT before starting patient care.

As a PT we use the term pelvic muscle examination and not pelvic exam, performed by obstetrician-gynecologist with speculum. We complete pelvic floor (PF) muscle exam utilizing index finger with thumb tucked in a fist **(Fig. 15.3)**. Treating therapist must:

- Keep nails short to prevent injury to patient upon manual treatment.
- Perform handwashing prior to treatment.
- Use clean pair of gloves.

Box 15.3: Contraindications to internal techniques.

- Prior to medical exam by gynecologist
- Infection
- Active bleeding
- Immediate postpartum
- Cancer
- Cognitive decline
- Lack of consent
- Severe pelvic pain
- Pediatric patient

Box 15.4: Conditions where precautions should be taken.

- Prior to 6 weeks postpartum
- History of sexual trauma
- Postmenopausal
- Radiated tissue

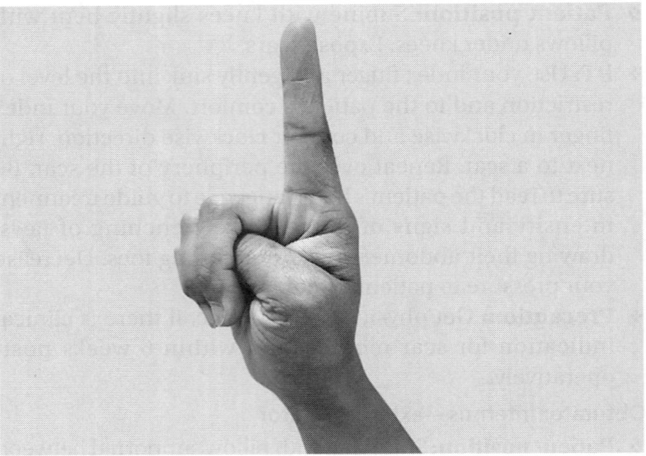

Fig. 15.3: Treating finger.

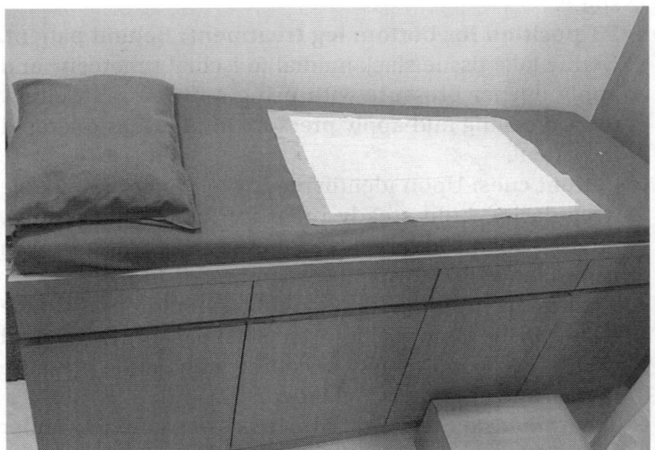

Fig. 15.4: Treatment table set up.

- Lubricate finger for transvaginal and transrectal treatments. You can choose to apply lubrication for perineal techniques if patient appears dry and very sensitive.
- Change hand gloves between perineal techniques, transvaginal techniques and rectal techniques to prevent cross-infection.
- Remove gloves safely using universal techniques.

Professional behavior—professional behavior should be encouraged, and foul language must be avoided.

Treatment room set up for internal treatment (Fig. 15.4)

Patient must be provided with private treatment room. Ideal room includes:

- High-low treatment table
- Documentation table
- Laundry basket and step stool
- Garbage bin (covered)

Tools for internal techniques

Frequently utilized tools for internal techniques are:

- Gown
- Water-based lubricant

- Long cotton Q-tip
- Chux pad
- Box of latex free gloves
- 2 bed sheets—one to spread on table and another to cover patient
- 2–4 pillows for positioning
- Emollient cream for MFR
- Proper lighting in room
- Wipes to clean after treatment

Modalities used are:

- Biofeedback with external and internal sensors
- Electrical stimulator with internal electrodes (same internal sensors as biofeedback)
- Dilator/wand

Treatment set up

Prepare treatment table based on **Figure 15.4** with chux pad directly under perineum to absorb body fluids, if any. Instruct patient on removal of underwear and pants and provide a gown. Once undressed, patient should be positioned on table as per therapist's instruction with a covered sheet. Provide patient 2–5 minute to position. Provide assistance if needed.

Option of a chaperone or a second person in a treatment room should be provided to patient and patient's response must be documented.

Therapist position

Provide sheet to cover pelvic area once in Lithotomy position. Therapist to sit on end of table facing patient **(Fig. 15.5)**. There must be enough lighting to assess skin and allow proper visualization of perineal area.

Treatment introduction phase

Here the therapist can explain the following to the patient—Your subjective complaints and my assessment indicate pelvic floor muscle dysfunction. Once we begin, I will assess and treat external perineal area and deeper pelvic floor muscles via vaginal canal. I will not use any tool and gently insert my gloved lubricated finger deeper in canal as tolerated. I will guide you and cue you as needed. You will be in charge of the whole session and we can stop at any time. Can we proceed?

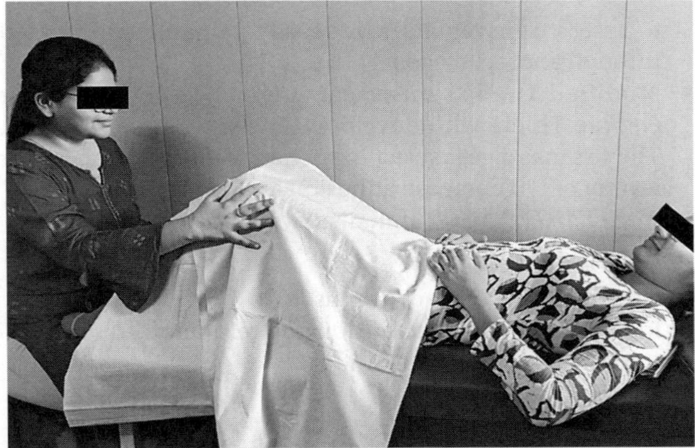

Fig. 15.5: Therapist position.

Pelvic floor coordination

Exposed perineum is a great opportunity to educate the patient on pelvic floor contraction and relaxation. Educate and teach patient on deep breathing and educate on pelvic floor bulging followed by pelvic floor contraction with correct sequence with respiratory diaphragm. Use verbal cues as discussed before. Provide hand-held mirror for patient to visualize, their own body to promote self-awareness and understanding of correct movement pattern.

Pelvic floor preactivation

Educate patient on pressure management when laughing, coughing, sneezing and lifting heavy objects. Correct movement pattern is pelvic floor contractions "closing" rather than bulging. You may find that the patient has a reverse pattern and it could be one of the reasons for urinary symptoms, including incontinence.

Pelvic clock

Understanding pelvic clock is a great way to assess, consistently treat, document involved muscle area and communicate among professionals. As shown in **Figures 15.6A and B**, pelvic floor is numbered like a face of a clock. It is most commonly and widely used among providers. **Figure 15.7** indicates complex pelvic floor anatomy and layers of muscle.

- Center is perineal body
- 12 O'clock is pubic symphysis
- 1 and 11 O'clock are ischiocavernosus muscles of left and right sides respectively
- 2 and 10 O'clock are bulbocavernosus muscles of left and right sides respectively
- 3 and 9 O'clock are superficial transverse perineal muscles of left and right sides respectively
- 4 and 8 O'clock are levator ani—pubococcygeus muscles of left and right sides respectively
- 5 and 7 O'clock are levator ani—Iliococcygeus muscles of left and right sides respectively.

Perineum Techniques

Palpate perineum using clock method for any tenderness. Patient will report burning, dryness and itching sensations most of the times. If pain and/or sensitivity is/are present, apply direct pressure in cephalad direction (deep layer), gently and as tolerated. Hold firm but gentle pressure and allow patient to breathe in coordination with diaphragm as discussed previously in the chapter. Hold for 60–90 seconds and move to next tender spot.

- **Introital stretch:** The index finger is placed between 4 and 8 O'clock **(Fig. 15.7)** 1st knuckle deep into Vaginal canal. A stretch is applied gently for 60–90 seconds. Patient may report dryness, burning and/or symptom reproduction. Complaint improves with sustained stretch.
- **Periurethral release (Fig. 15.8):** Insert finger at 11 O'clock and 1 O'clock position in vaginal opening. Depth of penetration is still 1st knuckle. Once palpable irregularities are identified, hold firm and gentle pressure for 60–90 seconds. Allow patient to breathe and release tension. Avoid pushing on bladder and urethra directly, at 12 O'clock position.

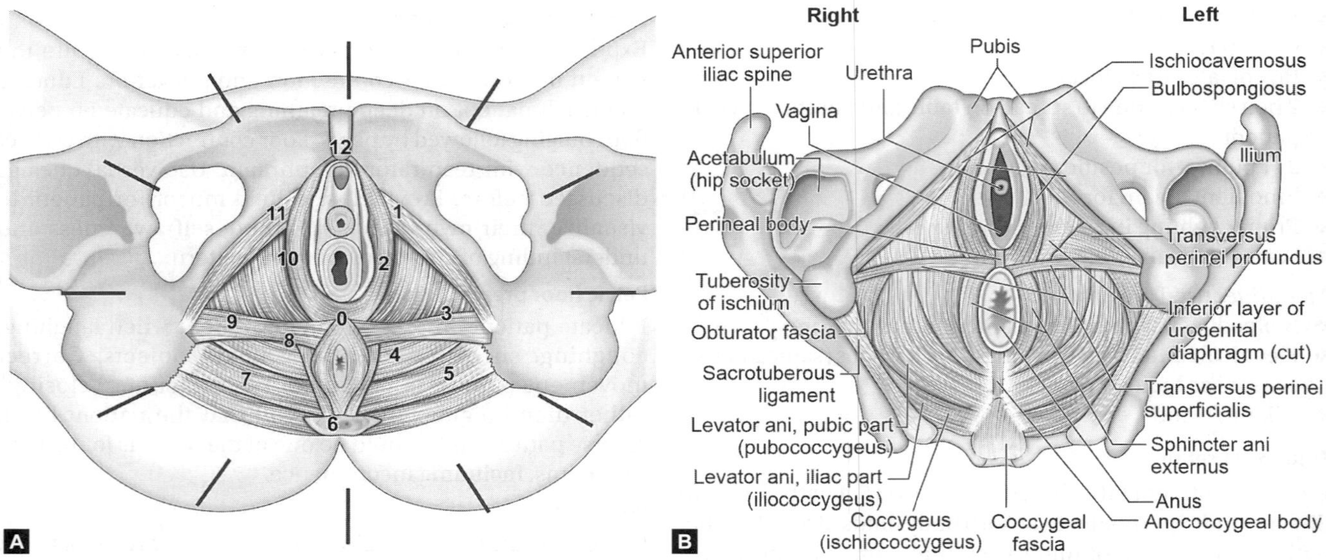

Figs. 15.6A and B: Pelvic clock and muscles *(For color version, see Plate 6).*

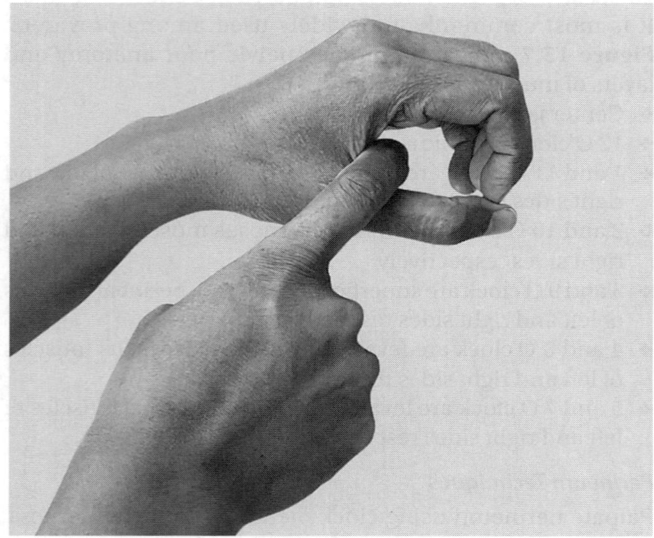

Fig. 15.7: Introital stretch.

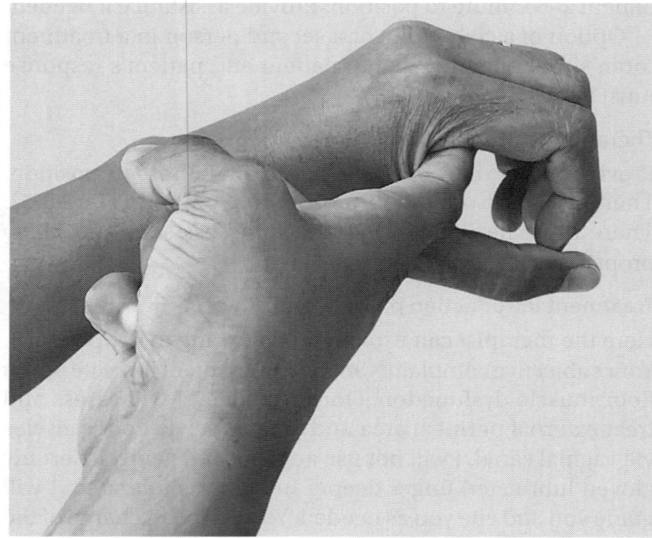

Fig. 15.8: Periurethral release.

- **Levator ani stretch (Figs. 15.9A and B):** Depth of penetration is proximal interphalangeal (PIP) joint of treating finger. Advance the treating finger into vaginal cavity. Finger to curve laterally for pubococcygeus placement and iliococcygeus. If pain/other symptoms or palpable irregularity is present, then apply gentle pressure for muscle release. Hold for 60–90 seconds with breathing techniques.
- **Obturator internus (OI) release (Figs. 15.10A and B):** Treating finger is advanced all the way into pelvic cavity and curved laterally. Confirm location of OI by asking patient to perform isometric hip external rotation.
- **Coccygeus release:** Treating finger is advanced all the way into pelvic cavity. Guide finger toward coccyx and shift just laterally to treat coccygeus. Coccygeus can be difficult to assess transvaginally but easily palpable and treated through anorectal canal.
- **Modified Theile's massage:** Originally named after Dr George Thiele who developed the technique in 1960s. Theile's massage is sweeping action of inserted finger over levator ani to decrease adhesion and tenderness.

Surface EMG *(sEMG)*—unit displayed in **Figure 15.11**.

Indications:

- Down training overactive muscle
- Increase awareness of tension and relaxation
- Improve muscle coordination
- Pediatric population

Glazer protocol for sEMG in chronic pelvic pain: Dr Howard Glazer, developed a method for treating pelvic

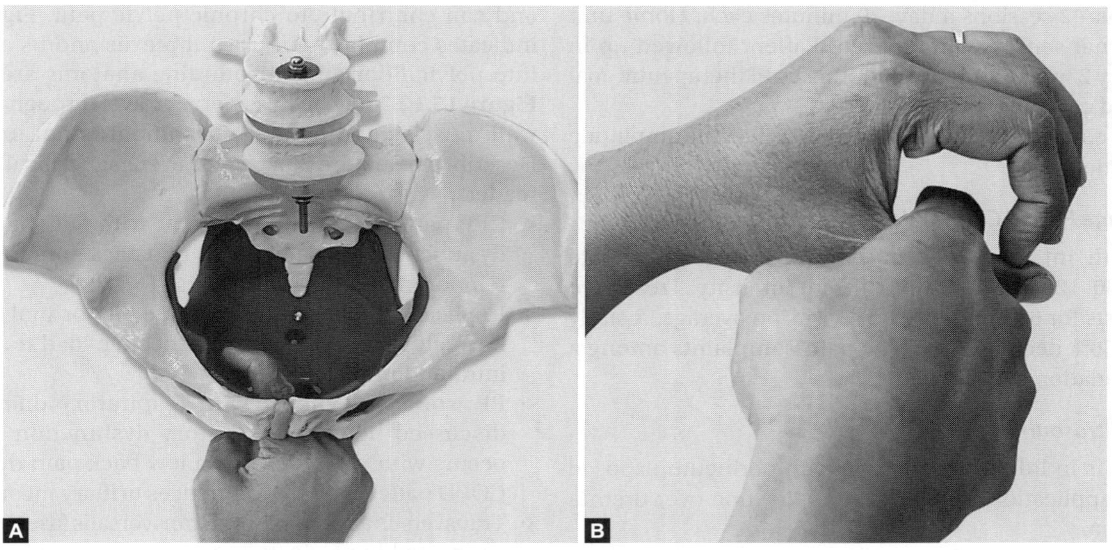

Figs. 15.9A and B: Levator ani stretch.

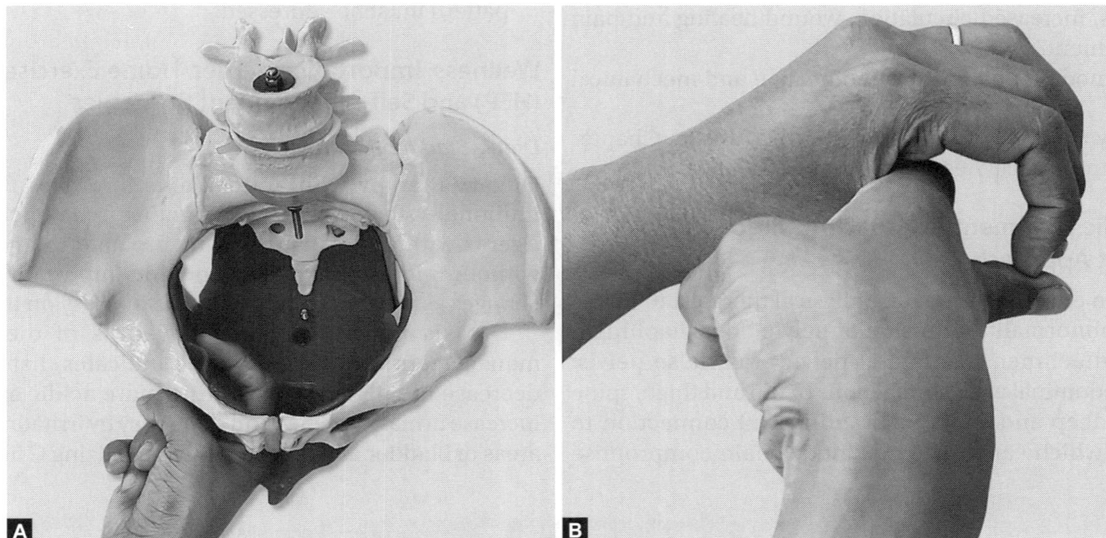

Figs. 15.10A and B: Obturator internus release.

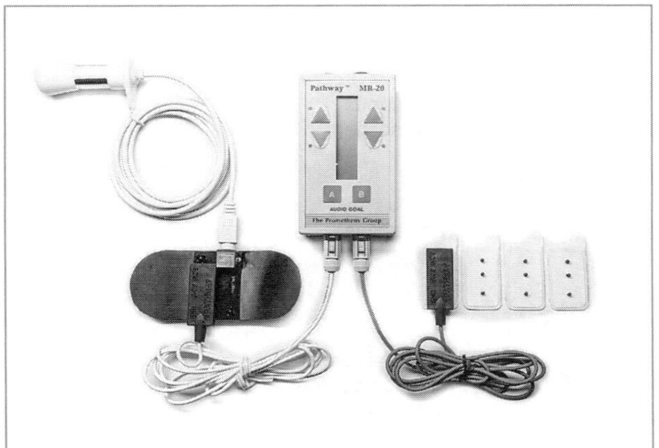

Fig. 15.11: Biofeedback unit with surface electrodes and internal sensors.

pain utilizing biofeedback. Patients who have pelvic pain have demonstrated increased resting tone and increased time to relax after a muscle contraction.

Electrode placement: 3 and 9 O'clock position, just lateral to external anal sphincter. Using gloves, sensors can be placed with patient either in side lying or forward bending position. After placement, patient can be in supine or side lying position.

Check connections and turn on the machine. Parameters used are as follows:

- One minute rest, prebaseline.
- Five rapid contractions with 10 seconds rest in between.
- Five 10 seconds contractions with 10 seconds rest interval between each.
- A single contraction of 60 seconds.
- One minute rest, prebaseline.

Sessions—2 sessions a day, 20 minutes each. Home unit with internal sensors can be used. Patient followed up in clinic every 2 weeks and then monthly until therapeutic goal is achieved or patient plateau.

Muscle coordination is assessed rather than the amplitude of contraction.

High Voltage Pulsed Current (HVPC) for Chronic Pelvic Pain

HVPC with intrarectal Sohn electrode with pulse rate between 80–120 pps and mild current intensity. Treatment session lasts for 60 minutes with 8 visits on average. A study reported 50% decrease in pelvic pain complaints among a study population of 28 patients.

Perineal Ultrasound

- Patient is in lithotomy position with perineum exposed for US application. Avoid direct application over urethra or vagina.
- Frequency: 1 or 3 MHz
- Continuous mode for heating effects to improve elasticity for scars, increased circulation, wound healing and pain management.
- Pulsed mode for edema, wound healing and mechanical effects
- Intensity = 0.5 W/cm^2 as per literature. (Also *see* Chapter 17: Electrophysical Agents in Women's Health).

Orthopedic Treatment Approach/Indirect Treatment Approach

This section encourages treating physical therapist to assess and treat abnormalities outside of pelvic floor diaphragm as it has attachments to lateral pelvic wall, false pelvis, anterior abdominal wall, connections to hip and thigh, spine extensors deep and superficial and fascial connection to GI system which can create biokinetic chain compromise and can contribute to chronic pelvic pain. **Figure 14.1C** indicates complex lumbosacral plexus and its connection into pelvic floor and surrounding anatomy are shown in **Figure 15.12**. Most of these nerves travel through abdominal wall muscles and hence, entrapment is not uncommon. Described below are a few points to engage critical thinking in readers.

- CPP patients generally present with C/O back pain, SI dysfunction, hip pain, upper mid back, thoracic pain and temporomandibular disorders (TMD).
- Implications of pelvic floor tissue on postural correction, form closure, force closure, effective load transfers and intra-abdominal pressure.
- PF works in synergy with respiratory diaphragm as discussed before. Respiratory dysfunction frequently occurs with pelvic floor and low back pain dysfunction. COPD patients often experiences urinary incontinence.
- Transversus abdominis and transversalis fascia are directly connected to pelvic floor muscles and endopelvic fascia, therefore adhesions, weakness and/or poor coordination pattern must be addressed.

Wellness: Importance of Diet, Home Exercise Program (HEP) and Self-management Strategies

Diet—Bladder Irritants

Dietary therapy with antioxidants improves function of immune system and helps in fighting free radical damage. Agents with antioxidant activity are able to improve CPP without undesirable effects and any important metabolic changes associated with hormonal suppression therapy.

Data is not clear on effectiveness of diet for CPP management; however, research indicates that foods that decrease the pH and make urine more acidic are likely to increase urinary urgency and frequency by irritating inflamed areas of bladder and urethra or by sensitizing C fibers.

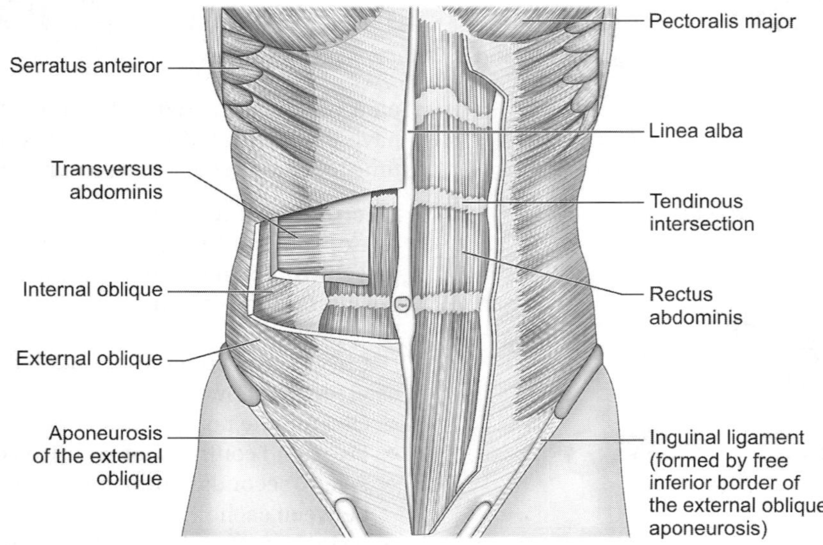

Fig. 15.12: Pelvic floor attachments and connections.

- Most common irritants are alcohol, carbonated beverages and caffeinated beverages.
- Foods that are rich in arylalkylamines may also irritate the bladder. Listings of foods that decrease pH and are high in arylalkylamines are shown in **Box 15.5**.
- Drinking recommended amount of water may help increase urinary pH and dilute effects of specific irritants.
- As CPP patient generally presents with cluster of symptoms possibly urinary frequency and urgency, recommendations on food to avoid can be a useful tool.

Home Exercise Program

Exercise program must be based on assessment and individualized; however, below are some recommended exercises to address chronic pelvic pain.

- **Diaphragmatic breathing in supported child's pose with pelvic floor relaxation:**
  - *Patient position*: Patient in kneeling to supported quadruped position as demonstrated in **Figures 15.13A and B**, with support of cushions and yoga block.

Box 15.5: Foods to avoid.

- Alcoholic beverages
- Apple juice
- Ascorbic acid
- Chili
- Citrus fruits
- Coffee
- Cranberries
- Grapes
- Guava
- Lemons
- Lime
- Nectarine
- Orange
- Pineapple
- Tea
- Vinegar

  - *Instructions*: Relax into the cushion, and sit back on your heels, resting your arms on the ground. Inhale, letting your belly expand, then exhale, and repeat—you should feel your pelvic floor muscles relax and lengthen as you inhale.
- **Deep squat with pelvic floor relaxation (Fig. 15.14):**
  - *Patient position:* Begin in standing position with a stable object like a chair at your side for support. Gradually lower yourself into a deep squat position.
  - *Patient instructions:* Allow your pelvic floor muscles to lengthen and relax. Hold this position then stand up and repeat. Ensure even breathing throughout the exercise to let yourself relax. Stop if exercise is causing worsening of your symptoms or causing any pain.
- **Supine transversus abdominal bracing with pelvic floor contractions (Fig. 15.15):**
  - *Patient position:* Begin lying on your back with your knees bent and feet resting on the floor. Support cervical curvature if excessive tension is present and patient unable to relax.
  - *Patient instructions:* Tighten your abdominal muscle at the same time you contract your pelvic floor muscle as you breathe out. Make sure to remind patient on pelvic floor and respiratory diaphragm coordination pattern.
- **Supine pelvic floor stretches or the happy baby pose (Fig. 15.16):**
  - *Patient position:* Begin lying on your back with your legs bent and feet resting on the ground and gradually lift your legs off the ground with your knees bent and let them fall outwards. Hold on to heels or knees to allow pelvic floor to relax.
  - *Patient instructions:* Inhale letting your belly expand and feel gentle pelvic floor stretch then exhale and repeat.
- **Supine pelvic floor contractions (Fig. 15.17)**:
  - *Patient position:* Begin lying on your back and feet supported.

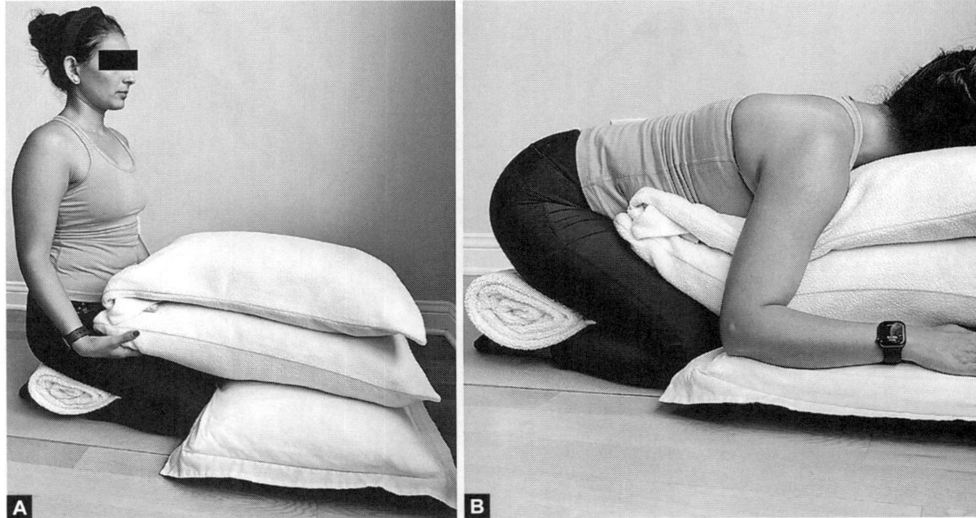

Figs. 15.13A and B: Diaphragmatic breathing in supported child's pose with pelvic floor relaxation.

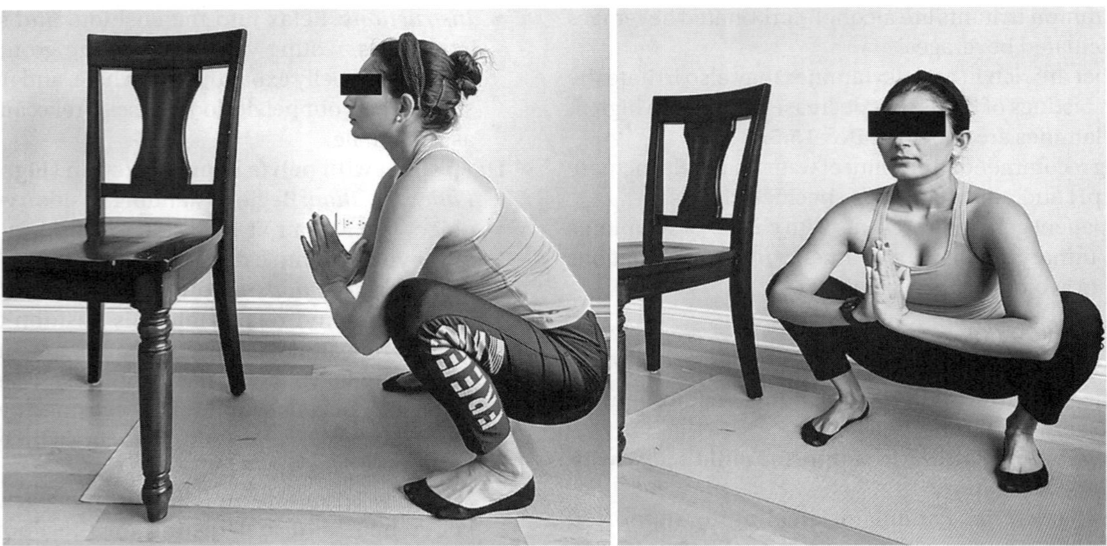

Fig. 15.14: Deep squat with pelvic floor relaxation.

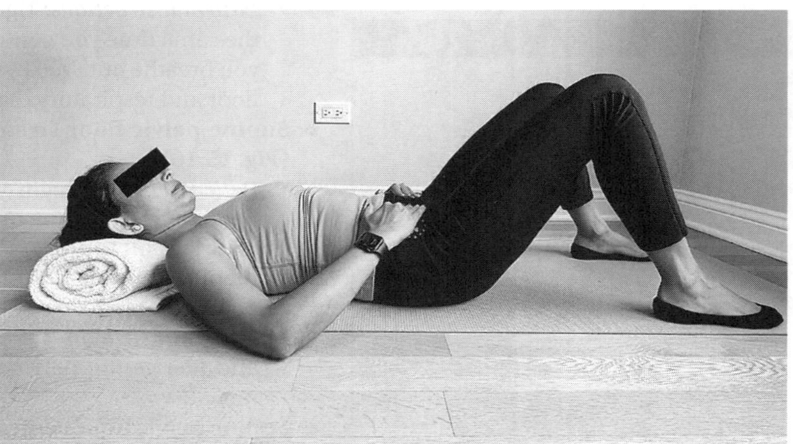

Fig. 15.15: Supine transversus abdominis.

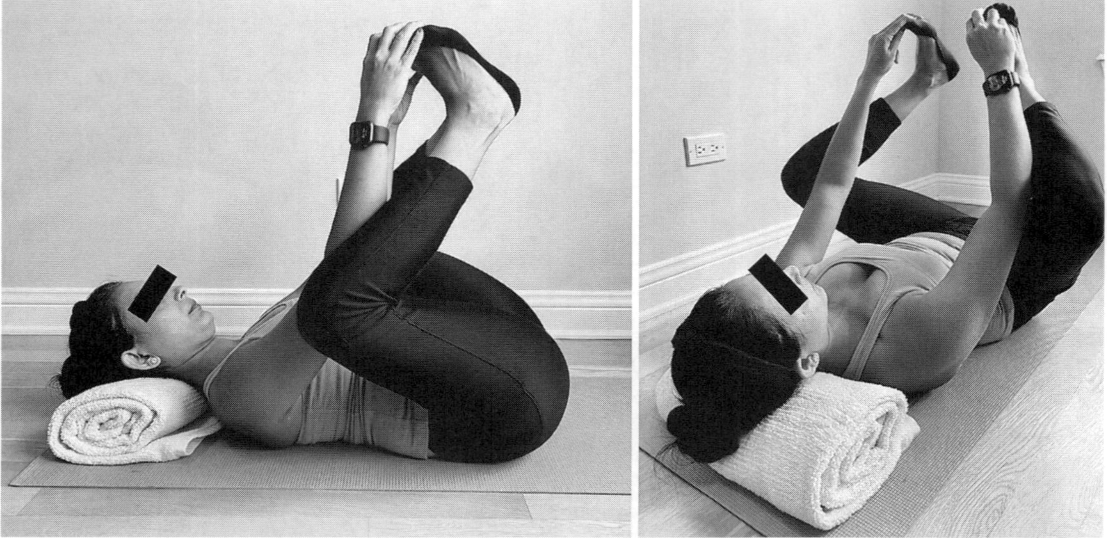

Fig. 15.16: Pelvic floor stretch in supine lying.

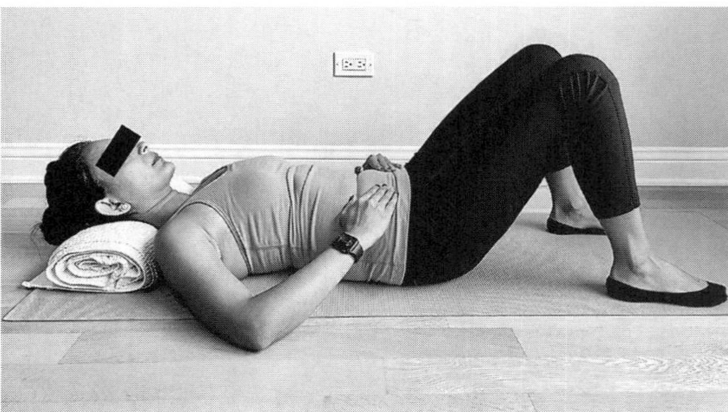

Fig. 15.17: Pelvic floor contraction in supine lying.

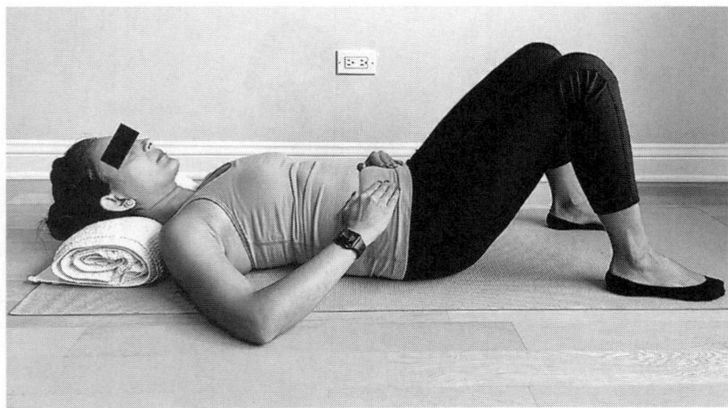

Fig. 15.18: Pelvic clock in supine lying.

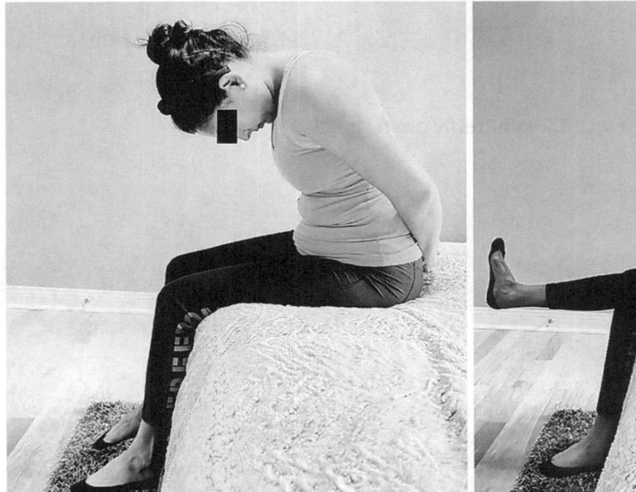

Fig. 15.19: Seated slump neural tensioner.

- *Patient instructions:* Exhale and contract your pelvic floor muscles. Inhale and lengthen your pelvic floor muscles and repeat. Make sure you are focused on pelvic floor muscles keeping hip and thigh muscles relaxed.

❖ **Supine 12-point pelvic clock (Fig. 15.18):**
- *Patient position:* Begin lying on your back with your knees bent, feet flat on the floor and your hands on your hips.
- *Patient instructions:* Imagine pelvis sitting in the middle of clock. Tilt the pelvis forward to 12, come back to center, go to 1, back to the center and so on tilting your pelvis from the center to each hour on the clock. Make sure to focus on pelvic movement.

❖ **Seated slump neural tensioner (Fig. 15.19)**:
- *Patient position:* Begin sitting on edge of the table or bed with both legs hanging off the edge, hands clasped behind your back, and your back slumped forward slightly.
- *Patient instructions:* Straighten one knee, flex foot and bend your head forward at the same time, then lower your foot and bend your head backward at the same time you may feel stretching sensation on back of your thigh. Make sure your leg and head are moving at the same speed at the same time.

❖ **Butterfly groin stretch (Fig. 15.20):**
- *Patient position:* Begin by sitting upright with your knees bent and soles of your feet together.
- *Patient instructions:* Using your arms, gently pull your heel towards your body until you feel a stretch in your groin and hold this position. Ensure that the low back remains straight and is not slouched.

❖ **Supine hip external rotation stretches (Fig. 15.21):**
- *Patient position:* Begin lying on your back with your legs straight.
- *Patient instructions:* Cross one leg over the other, resting your ankle on your opposite knee. Bend the knee of your bottom leg towards your body until you feel a stretch in your hip and hold. Make sure your hip is relaxed and your back flat against the ground.

❖ **Supine bilateral hip internal rotation stretches (Fig. 15.22):**
- *Patient position:* Begin lying on your back with your knees bent and feet flat on the floor, legs shoulder width apart.

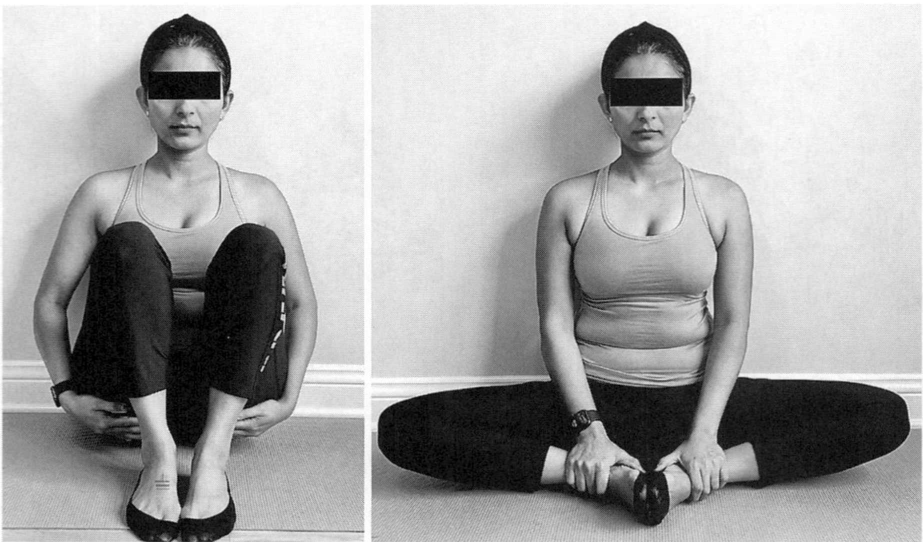

Fig. 15.20: Butterfly groin stretch.

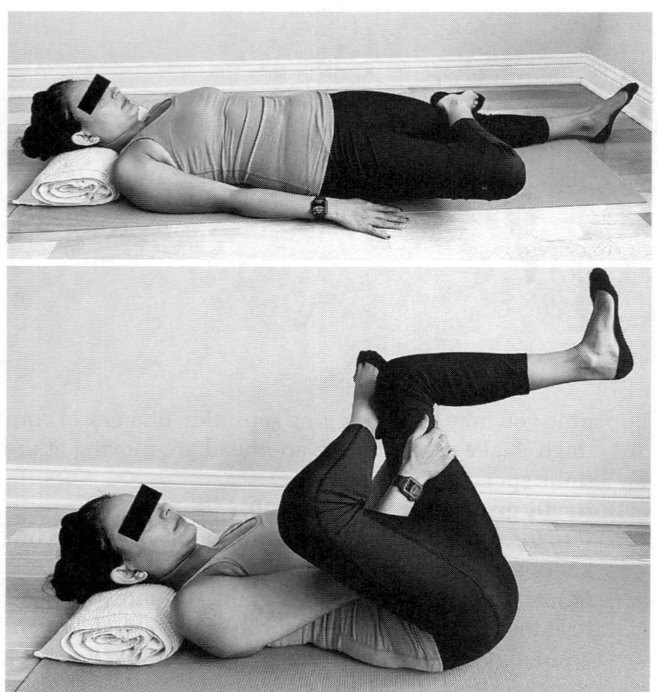

Fig. 15.21: External rotator stretch in supine lying.

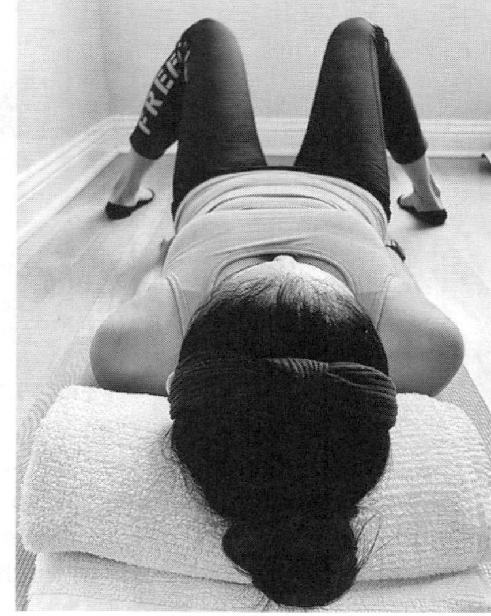

Fig. 15.22: Internal rotator stretch in supine lying.

- *Patient instructions*: Slowly slide your feet outward rotating your knee inward until you feel a stretch on your hip. Make sure to keep your back flat on the floor and do not stretch through pain.

❖ **Side lying thoracic rotation with open book (Fig. 15.23)**:
- *Patient position:* Begin lying on your side with your legs bent at approximately 90° angle with your arms together straight in front of you on the ground.
- *Patient instructions:* Slide your top hand back and forth over your bottom hand five times, rotating your shoulder. Then lift your top arm straight up and over the floor on your other side. Ensure to keep the knees together and rotate only the back and upper arm. Your hips should stay facing forward.

❖ **Inverted hamstring stretches at the wall (Fig. 15.24):**
- *Patient position:* Begin lying on your back with your leg straight and flat against the wall.
- *Patient instruction:* Hold this position. You should feel a stretch at the back of your leg. Increase stretch intensity by flexing your toes towards you. Make sure not to arch the low back during the exercise.

❖ **Inverted piriformis stretches at the wall (Fig. 15.25)**:
- *Patient position:* Begin lying on your back with your leg straight and flat against the wall.
- *Patient instructions*: Cross one leg over the other, resting your ankle on your opposite knee. Bend the knee of your

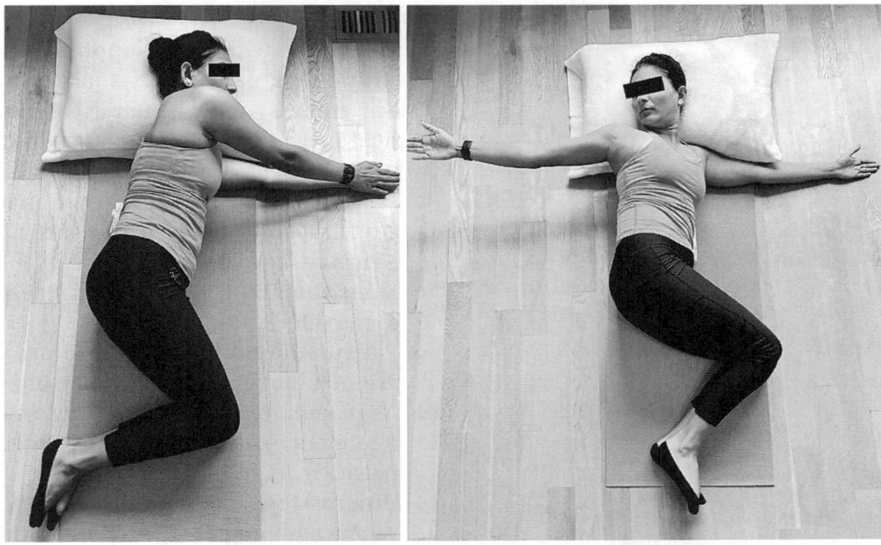

Fig. 15.23: Thoracic rotation in side lying.

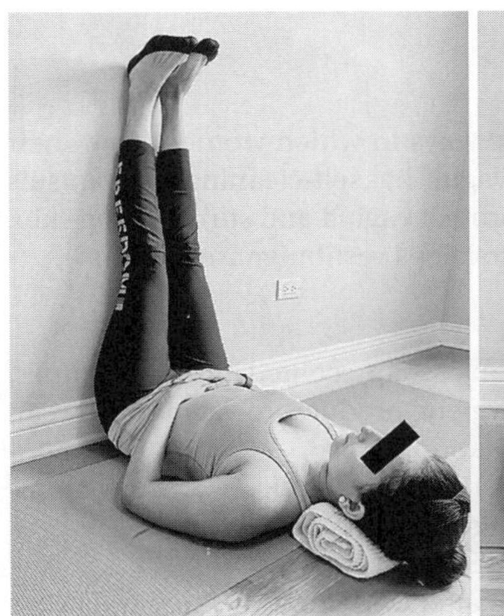

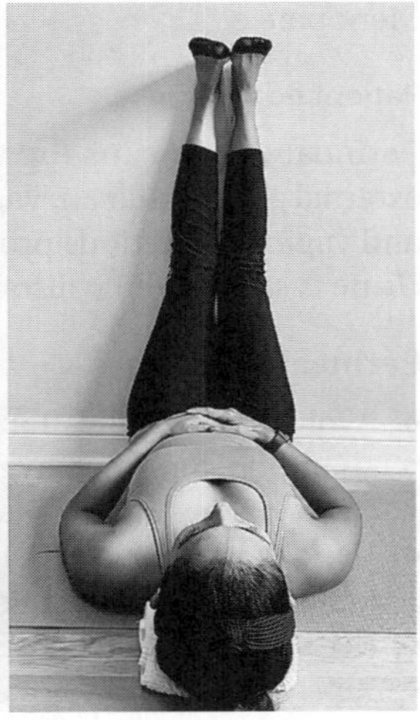

Fig. 15.24: Inverted Hamstrings stretch against wall.

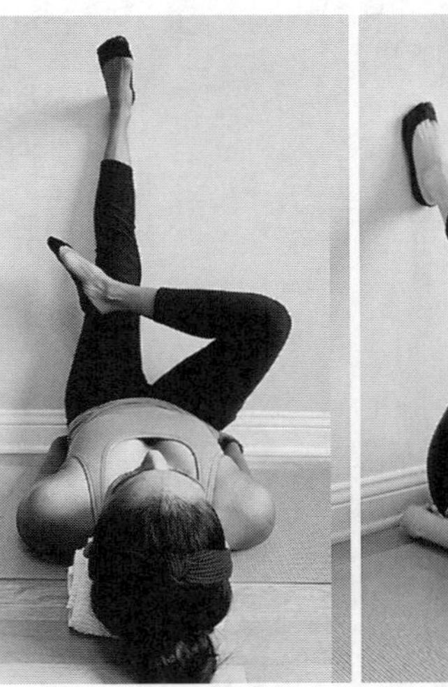

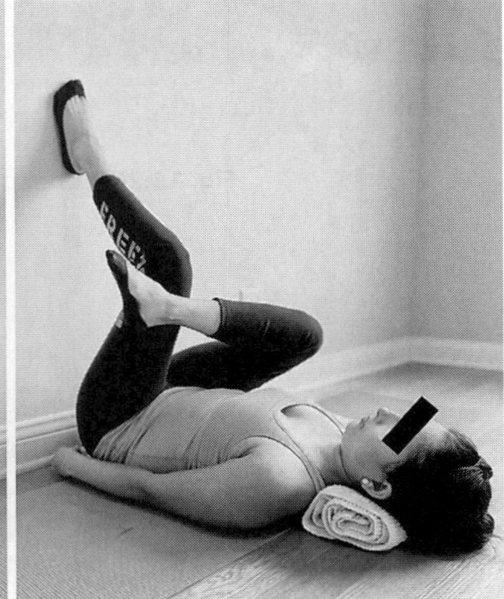

Fig. 15.25: Piriformis stretches against the wall.

bottom leg towards your body until you feel a stretch in your hip and hold. Make sure to keep your low back flat against the ground.

- **Cobra stretch (Fig. 15.26):**
  - *Patient position:* Begin lying on your belly, with your toes pointed and legs straight.
  - *Patient instructions:* Place your hands next to your chest on the floor. Push your hands into the floor and lift your chest off the floor and straighten your elbows. Keep your pubic bone on the floor. Look forward and return to lying on your belly and repeat. Make sure your shoulders are engaged downward to keep your neck long.
- **Cat and cow stretch (Fig. 15.27):**
  - *Patient position:* Begin on all fours with your arms directly under your shoulder and knees bent to 90°.
  - *Patient instructions:* Slowly round your back up towards the ceiling, then let it sag down to the floor eyes looking up and repeat. Make sure to use your entire back for the motion and keep your moment slow and controlled.

Self-management Strategies

Self-management using dilators

Pelvic trainer is an umbrella term including dilators, pelvic wand, pelvic weights, cones, anal dilators, rehab vibrators, Kegel trainers. We will be discussing only Dilator in this chapter. Dilators come in different sizes as shown in **Figure 9.6** and are made up of mostly plastic and silicone material. Vaginal dilators are effective:

- To help patient desensitize
- For gradual stretching to decrease fear of penetration
- To serve purpose of maintenance and progressive stretching by self

Patient should practice inserting dilator with PT prior to beginning as home regime. Dexterity must be present to allow safe insertion. Patient should be advised to purchase water-based lubricant for insertion.

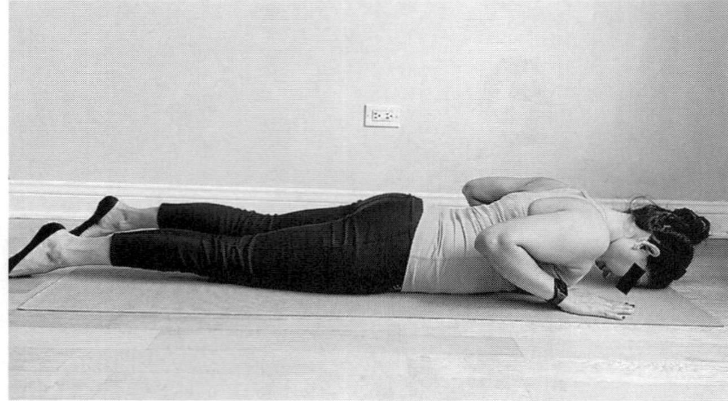

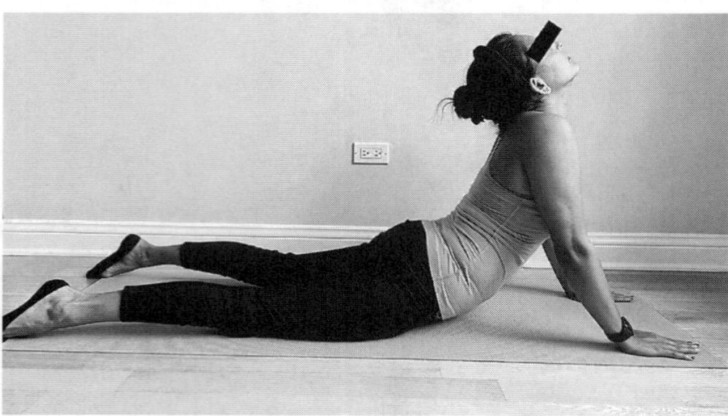

Fig. 15.26: Cobra pose.

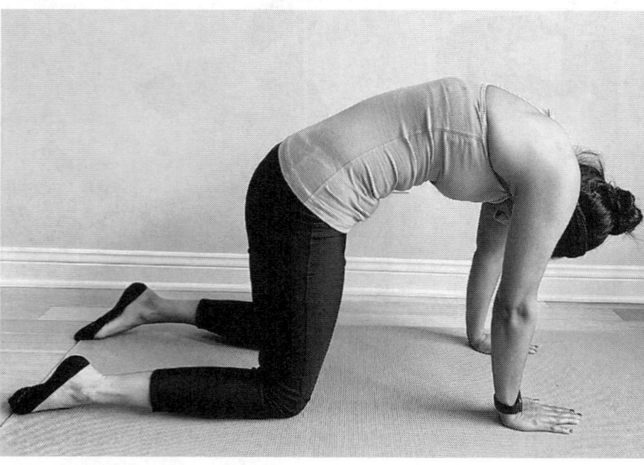

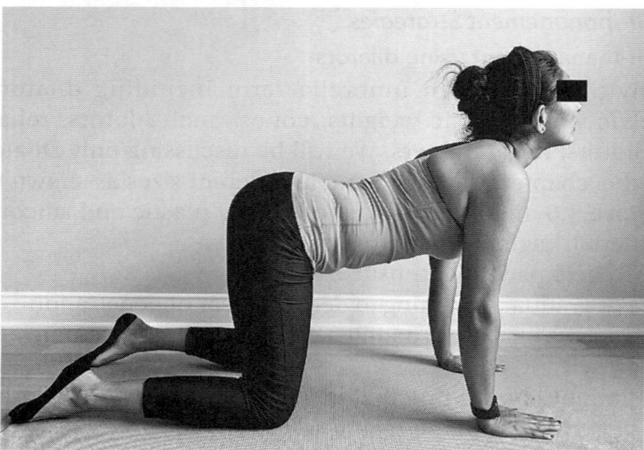

Fig. 15.27: Cat and cow exercise.

Patient position

Semireclined with head support with knee bent to allow insertion. Ask patient to visualize vulva using mirror for self-awareness. Apply generous amount of lubrication over vaginal area and dilator. Ask patient to gradually insert dilator when PF muscles are relaxed, during inhalation.

- Patient is advised on slow insertion up to 1 inch and hold/stretch at different pelvic clock positions, starting 6 O'clock as it is easily tolerated.
- Stretch hold 60–90 seconds and repeat × 5 and then progress to next clock position.
- Patient should be advised to use dilators daily 15–20 minutes along with relaxation to maximize outcome.
- As patient becomes more comfortable with self-guided treatment, patient can insert the device up to 3 inches in pelvic cavity.
- **Progression:** Repetitive movement of dilator in and out of vagina and progress to increase width.

Therapist must follow up with the patient if they have any concerns with on-going application. Also *see* Chapter 9: Menopause.

Patient education

Perineal care means the ways in which women keep their external genitalia clean. Vagina has self-cleaning mechanisms and vaginal secretions protect vagina and surrounding skin. Urine is sterile which also keeps vestibular area clean.

Perineal hygiene

- Avoid direct application of soap, scented lotion, perfumes, shampoo, feminine hygiene products to vagina. They can cause dryness and irritation.
- Use clean water and hands for vestibule area. Mons pubis, labia majora can be washed with gentle soap.
- Use soft white unscented toilet paper.
- Rinse vulva with water after urination.
- Avoid daily use of panty liners and use of cotton undergarment should be made as much as possible. Change undergarment frequently to prevent redness.
- Use cotton menstrual pads and tampons.
- Wipe front to back to prevent spread of fecal material into vagina.
- Urinate before and after sex to prevent possibility of infections.
- If urine color is dark yellow it is a sign of dehydration. Hydrate with 2 to 3 L of water every day.
- Maintain normal urinary frequency during daytime is 5 to 8 and at night 0–1.
- Use water-based lubricant for sexual penetration.
- Do not use bleach or harsh chemicals on undergarments.

Understanding norms

- Sexual intercourse should not be painful.
- Stool consistency should be well formed with sausage shape. Consistently very soft or very hard stools are not normal.

- Defecation frequency 3 × day to 3 × week.
- Deep squats like Indian toilet or use of raised platform for feet to relax PF muscle can be useful.

Yoga

Research has indicated that after 8 weeks of yoga therapy, CPP subjects had lesser intensity of pain as shown by significantly reduced pain scores and improved quality of life (QOL) with significant increase in physiological, psychological and social well-being. Better pain management using yoga can help reduce dependence on NSAIDs and its associated side effects. Studies indicate deep breathing, OM chanting, Pranayama and relaxation for 5× week for 8 weeks help patients with CPP. Yoga poses including cat, cobra and fish have demonstrated reduced pain from dysmenorrhea. Further use of Yoga for women is described in Chapter 34: Yoga in Women's Health.

Mindfulness and relaxation techniques

Relaxation and mindfulness training have documented positive physiological and functional effects. Mindfulness exercises decrease urinary urgency and CPP.

Cognitive behavioral therapy

Although pelvic pain may be due to an inciting event, the chronicity of pain predisposes patient to depression, anxiety and social isolation. Depression leads to worsening of quality of life for women with chronic pelvic pain. It is essential to not waste time in determining what the primary condition may be and rather focus on treating both conditions with equal urgency. Cognitive behavioral therapy is a goal-oriented therapy and, when used in conjunction with medical and physical therapy, has the advantage of addressing the effects of depression and pain on relationships and other aspects of well-being.

Patients learn modulation of their thoughts and manipulation of their environment to lessen their pain perception and improve coping skills. Emotional well-being should be assessed at every visit and professional counseling should be considered and offered to every patient with chronic pelvic pain. It is critical that the patient understands that the referral does not mean that the pain is psychosomatic or any less real. Instead, counseling enables patient to opt in support in parallel with the other treatments being recommended to address the chronic pain generators.

Sex therapy

Although there may be a myofascial component to genito-pelvic pain, this condition may require the additional expertise of individual counseling, couple therapy or sex therapy to overcome the specific psychosocial barriers to recovery. Sex therapy can be a useful adjunctive treatment to physical therapy to assist couples in the return to normal, pain-free intercourse. Female orgasmic disorder and genito-pelvic pain have shown to improve by sex therapy.

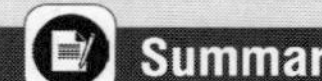

Summary

Chapter focuses on introductory manual therapy techniques to treat painful, overactive, hypertonic pelvic floor muscles. Pelvic floor coordination with respiratory diaphragm is discussed as a key concept to pelvic floor rehabilitation. Readers are strongly encouraged to practice techniques prior to applying to patient population. Room set up, language around patient care and norms have been discussed for wellness purpose. Author motivates its readers to assess and treat musculoskeletal conditions outside of true pelvis and treat the patient as a whole for optimal patient satisfaction. Anorectal treatment techniques, visceral mobilization are direct form of manual therapy approaches but outside the scope of current chapter.

CLINICAL EXAMPLE

History

A 24-year-old female G0P0 presented to PT with complaints of generalized pelvic pain, neck pain, left foot pain. Patient had imperforated hymen which was corrected surgically almost 10 years ago. Patient reported that she had sharp pain which gets worse with insertion of tampon and with sexually activity. Patient reports constant but mild burning in perineal area. Pain in neck and foot is mostly achy and present throughout the day, denied any history of trauma or injury. Patient reports that she is newly married and wanting to have painfree sex life as she is planning to become pregnant and to have a family. Reports husband is supportive and willing to wait and follow therapy guidelines. She also reports frequent sleep disturbances and is in counseling for depression. Patient is a fitness instructor and currently virtually training clients. She does intense work out 5 × week, 30–45 min session.

Medical diagnosis: Chronic pelvic pain s/p Hymenectomy.

Medication: Vaginal valium depository 1 × night. Over the counter Ibuprofen 200 mg as needed for neck pain. Multivitamin daily

Postural observation: Bilateral ankle toe in pattern with hip in internal rotation. Forward head posture with increased tension in SCM. Excessive abdominal muscle engagement, draw in present. Rib flare present. No antalgic gait pattern observed.

Pain evaluation: Neck pain and ankle pain varies 2– 4/10 and mostly achy feeling.

A/C increase pain= sitting in front of computer, post work out, morning. A/C decrease pain hot packs, stretches but pain returns.

Pelvic pain: Mostly sharp 8–9/10 during and after sexual intercourse. Pain present superficially and deep. Unable to complete intercourse due to pain. No orgasm.

Flexibility: Tightness in B/L hamstring, adductor, iliopsoas, calf, pectorals group.

Joint mobility: Decrease sacral springing, decrease Cx joint play in A<>P direction. Decrease hip P>A glides and decrease in hip ER.

Strength: B/L lower extremity measures WNL except hip flexors 4/5 and hip rotators 4-/5 in available ROM. Deep neck flexor 2/5, poor activation pattern. Levator Ani 6 contraction at 2/5 muscle strength with 3 sec hold each followed by 4 fast contractions 2/3/6//4 PERFECT score.

Palpation: Decrease muscle rolling of abdominal wall. Palpable irregularity and tenderness over adductor group, obturator internus and posterior neck muscles.

Pelvic floor palpation of superficial layer: Perineal body elevated. No movement of pelvic floor with breathing. Pain at 2,3,4,5,7,8,9,10 location.

Pelvic floor levator ani palpation: Able to tolerate after educating on correct breathing pattern. Hypertonicity of Levator ani and obturator internus present on left and tenderness.

Bladder: No reporting of urge incontinence or stress incontinence

Bowel: Occasional constipation but managed with stool softener.

Intervention

PT frequency = 1 × week for 4 weeks and then every 2 weeks, in addition to home exercise program, to assess progression and to make adjustment into self-care.

Patient education on pelvic floor coordination with respiratory diaphragm breathing.

Pelvic floor relaxation exercises as a home protocol to manage musculoskeletal abnormalities.

Hip and abdominal wall stretching to allow normal biomechanics.

Postural re-education to decrease excessive abdominals engagement and improve neck alignment.

To teach patient dilator use as a daily self-management protocol and must do prior to sexual intercourse to decrease pain.

Manual therapy: Abdominal skin rolling, adductor and glut STR to allow soft tissue gliding and to allow ability correct posture and improve optimal muscle function.

Trigger point release: Introitus stretch, TPR in clock direction to decrease tension. Levator ani, obturator internus trigger point release to decrease pain complains upon penetration as described above.

Hip and ankle biomechanics correction to decrease constant strain on core pelvic musculature.

Outcome

At end of 6 sessions, over a period of 2 months, patient reported decrease in neck pain and foot pain to intermittent and 0–2/10, after prolonged use of computer. Pelvic pain at 2–4/10 and able to have full penetration and deep thrusting. Patient stated that she can relax and breathe correctly now during sexual activity which has helped a lot. Patient reported no need for vaginal valium which is a huge improvement for her and her doctor. Patient at dilator size 4 and progressing towards next size. Patient demonstrated good pelvic floor coordination but still having delayed relaxation. Patient is aware of pelvic floor tension and home exercises program to manage it. Pelvic pain tenderness still present but patient able to tolerate more pressure and able to hold longer duration.

Patient reported that she is very grateful and hopeful after PT that her symptoms will continue to resolve over period year. Patient scheduled follow-up after 6 months or come in sooner in case of flare up. Patient have good understanding of home exercises program, pain management and is aware of postural correction techniques.

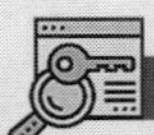

Review Questions

1. Explain acute and chronic pelvic pain in brief.
2. Explain types of pelvic floor in detail.
3. Describe the indirect and direct methods of pelvic floor treatment.
4. Write short notes on:
   a. Role of patient education in pelvic floor dysfunction.
   b. Yoga for pelvic floor.
   c. Cognitive behavioral therapy for pelvic floor dysfunction.
   d. Sex education for pelvic floor dysfunction.

Bibliography

1. Ahangari A. Prevalence of chronic pelvic pain among women: An updated review. Pain Physician. 2014;17(2):E141-7. PMID:24658485.
2. American College of Obstetricians and Gynecologists. Committee Opinion No. 673: Persistent vulvar pain. Obstet Gynecol. 2016;128(5):e78-84. doi:10.1097/AOG.0000000000001766. PMID:27776071.
3. American College of Obstetricians and Gynecologists. Practice Bulletin No. 218: Chronic pelvic pain. Obstet Gynecol. 2020;135(3):e98-e109. doi:10.1097/AOG.0000000000003709.
4. American Physical Therapy Association, Section on Pelvic Health. Position statement on internal physical therapy pelvic examinations and interventions [Internet]. 2021 [cited 2025 Jan 11]. Available from: https://aptapelvichealth.org/wp-content/uploads/2021/01/Position-Statement-on-Internal-Physical-Therapy-Pelvic-Examinations-and-Interventions-Updated-1-11-2021-1.pdf
5. Anderson RU, Wise D, Sawyer T, Nathanson BH, Smith JN. Equal improvement in men and women in treatment of urologic chronic pelvic pain syndrome using a multimodal protocol with internal myofascial trigger point wand. Appl Psychophysiol Biofeedback. 2016;41(2):215-24. doi:10.1007/s10484-016-9333-0. PMID:27059819.
6. Ayorinde AA, Bhattacharya S, Druce KL, Jones GT, Macfarlane GJ. Chronic pelvic pain in women of reproductive and postmenopausal age: A population-based study. Eur J Pain. 2017;21(3):445-55. doi:10.1002/ejp.947. PMID:27734598.

7. Ball E, Khan KS. Recent advances in understanding and managing chronic pelvic pain in women with special consideration to endometriosis. F1000Res. 2020;9:F1000 Faculty Rev-83. doi:10.12688/f1000research.20750.1. PMID:32089831; PMCID:PMC7001750.
8. Bergeron S, Likes WM, Steban M. Psychosexual aspects of vulvovaginal pain. Best Pract Res Clin Obstet Gynaecol. 2014;28(7):991-9. doi:10.1016/j.bpobgyn.2014.07.002. PMID:25108498.
9. Continence Foundation of Australia. The hypertonic pelvic floor [Internet]. [cited 2025 Jan 11]. Available from: https://www.continence.org.au/pages/the-hypertonic-pelvic-floor.html
10. Faubion SS, Shuster LT, Bharucha AE. Recognition and management of nonrelaxing pelvic floor dysfunction. Mayo Clin Proc. 2012;87(2):187-93. doi:10.1016/j.mayocp.2011.09.004. PMID:22305030; PMCID:PMC3498251.
11. FitzGerald MP, Anderson RU, Potts J, et al. Randomized multicentre feasibility trial of myofascial physical therapy for the treatment of urological chronic pelvic pain syndromes. J Urol. 2009;182(2):570-80. doi:10.1016/j.juro.2009.04.022. PMID:19535099; PMCID:PMC2872169.
12. FitzGerald MP, Kotarinos R. Rehabilitation of the short pelvic floor. II: Treatment of the patient with the short pelvic floor. Int Urogynecol J Pelvic Floor Dysfunct. 2003;14(4):269-75; discussion 275. doi:10.1007/s00192-003-1050-7. PMID: 14530840.
13. Glazer HI, Marinoff HC. The treatment of vulvovaginal pain disorder with surface electromyography-assisted pelvic floor therapy [Internet]. Available from: https://www.hcp.obgyn.net
14. Grant SR, Salvati EP, Rubin RJ. Levator syndrome: An analysis of 316 cases. Dis Colon Rectum. 1975;18(2):161-3. doi:10.1007/BF02586774. PMID:1121146.
15. International Pelvic Pain Society. Education resources [Internet]. Available from: http://www.pelvicpain.org/education
16. Learman LA, Gregorich SM, Jacob A, Jackson RA, Kupperman M. Symptom resolution after hysterectomy and alternative treatment for chronic pelvic pain: Does depression make a difference? American Journal of Obstetrics and Gynecology. 2011; 204 (3): 269.
17. Miller J-JR, Sand PK. Kegel Exercises, Dietary and Behavioral Modifications: Simple Strategies for Getting Started. In: Culligan PJ, Goldberg RP, editors. Urogynecology in Primary Care. London: Springer; 2007. p. 60-6. doi:10.1007/978-1-84628-167-9_6.
18. Pereira VM, Arias-Carrion O, Machado S, Nardi AE, Silva AC. Sex therapy for female sexual dysfunction. Int Arch Med. 2013;6:37. doi:10.1186/1755-7682-6-37. PMID:24082842; PMCID:PMC 3848652.
19. Polpeta NC, Giraldo PC, Juliato CRT, Gomes do Amaral RL, Linhares IL, et al. Clinical and therapeutic aspects of vulvodynia: The importance of physical therapy. Minerva Ginecol. 2012;64(5): 437-45. PMID:23044764.
20. Rakhshaee Z. Effect of three yoga poses (cobra, cat, and fish) in women with primary dysmenorrhea: A randomized clinical trial. J Pediatr Adolesc Gynecol. 2011;24(4):192-6. doi:10.1016/j.jpag.2011.01.059. PMID:21514190.
21. Scholz J. Mechanisms of chronic pain. Mol Pain. 2014;10(Suppl 1):O15. doi:10.1186/1744-8069-10-S1-O15. PMCID:PMC4304360.
22. Sharma N, Rekha K, Srinivasan JK. Efficacy of transcutaneous electrical stimulation in treatment of chronic pelvic pain. J Midlife Health. 2017; 8(2):76-80. doi:10.4103/jmh.JMH_19_17. PMCID:PMC5533507.
23. Simons DG, Travell JG, Simons LS. Travell & Simons' myofascial pain and dysfunction: The trigger point manual, 2nd edition. Baltimore: Williams & Wilkins; 1999.
24. Sohn N, Weinstein MA, Robbins RD. The levator ani syndrome and its treatment with high-voltage electrogalvanic stimulation. Dis Colon Rectum. 1982;25(7):653-6. doi:10.1007/BF02553969. PMID:7125100.
25. Speax by Thinx. A history of pelvic health: Who invented Kegels? [Internet]. [cited 2025 Jan 11]. Available from: https://www.speax.com/blogs/learn/who-invented-kegels
26. Thiel GH. Coccydynia: Cause and treatment. Dis Colon Rectum. 1963;6:422-36. doi:10.1007/BF02616691. PMID:13987361.
27. Vural M. Pelvic pain rehabilitation. Turk J Phys Med Rehabil. 2018;64(4):291-9. doi:10.5606/tftrd.2018.3616. PMID:31453525; PMCID:PMC6648037.
28. Williams AC, Eccleston C, Morley S. Psychological therapies for management of chronic pain in adults. Cochrane Database Syst Rev. 2012;11:CD007407. doi:10.1002/14651858.CD007407.pub3. PMID:23152245.
29. Zoorab D, South M, Karam M, Sroga J, Maxwell R, Shah A. A pilot randomized trial of levator ani injections versus physical therapy treatment for pelvic floor myalgia and sexual pain. Int Urogynecol J. 2015;26(6):845-52. doi:10.1007/s00192-014-2580-0. PMID:25236856.

Multiple Choice Questions (MCQs)

To test your understanding and recall of key concepts.

1. **A 32-year-old female patient presents with chronic pelvic pain (CPP) and reports sharp pain during tampon insertion and intercourse. On examination, levator ani and obturator internus muscles are found to have increased tone. Which initial intervention is *most* appropriate to reduce her symptoms?**
   A. Strengthening exercises for the pelvic floor muscles
   B. Transcutaneous electrical nerve stimulation (TENS) for pain management
   C. Trigger point release combined with diaphragmatic breathing
   D. Progressive pelvic floor contractions using biofeedback

2. **A patient undergoing treatment for CPP reports persistent burning and dryness during vaginal penetration due to perineal muscle tension. Which therapeutic approach is *most* appropriate?**
   A. Pelvic floor strengthening exercises
   B. Periurethral release with coordinated breathing techniques
   C. Sacroiliac joint mobilization
   D. Supine transversus abdominal bracing exercises

3. **A 40-year-old woman with CPP experiences pain despite pharmacological treatment. Her clinical history includes dyspareunia, urinary urgency, and mild depression. Which of the following is the *best* combination of interventions to address her symptoms holistically?**

A. Biofeedback, levator ani strengthening, and yoga therapy
B. Manual therapy, cognitive-behavioral therapy, and dietary modifications
C. Electrical stimulation, sacral nerve block, and Kegel exercises
D. Surgery, physical therapy, and mindfulness training

4. **A postpartum female with hypertonic pelvic floor muscles and pelvic girdle pain is unable to tolerate internal manual therapy. Which approach would be the *most* effective starting point for her?**
A. Internal techniques using pelvic wan
B. Indirect techniques such as postural correction and hip mobilization
C. Direct stretching exercises for the pelvic floor
D. Electromagnetic stimulation for deep muscle activation

5. **A clinical trial comparing pelvic floor physical therapy with levator ani trigger point injections for CPP found equal effectiveness in reducing vaginal and sex-related pain. Which factor should *most* influence a clinician's choice of intervention?**
A. The patient's preference and comfort level with invasive procedures
B. The cost-effectiveness of trigger point injections over therapy
C. The time required for each intervention to show results
D. The availability of skilled providers and resources in the clinical setting

6. **According to APTA, the treatment techniques that are provided directly over perineum, inside vagina or rectum are called as the________________.**
A. Internal techniques B. External techniques
C. Wellness techniques D. Accessory techniques

7. **Which of the following is *not* true in relation to the pelvic clock:**
A. Center is perineal body
B. 12 O'clock is pubic symphysis
C. 11 O'clock is the right ischiocavernosus muscle
D. 10 O'clock is the right iliococcygeous muscles

ANSWERS

1. C	2. B	3. B	4. B	5. A
6. A	7. D			

Chapter 16

Psychosexual Dimensions of Women's Health

Komal Shah, Priyasingh Rangey

LEARNING OBJECTIVES

At the end of the chapter, the reader will be able to:

- Learn about psychosexual dimensions of women's health.
- Know the psychosexual disorders in females.
- Understand the classification of psychosexual disorders.
- Gain knowledge about evaluation and management of various psychosexual disorders in females.
- Understand the psychological and sexual problems faced by women during early adulthood, pregnancy, postpartum, at workplace and menopause.
- Know the role of physiotherapy in various psychosexual disorders in females.

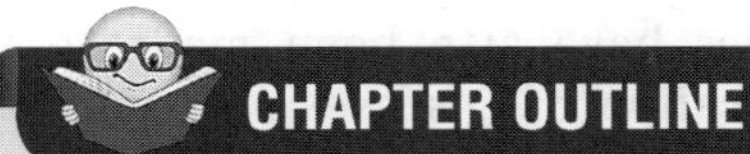

- Introduction
- Etiology
- Classification of psychosexual disorders
- Female sexual interest/arousal disorder (SIAD)
- Female orgasmic disorder
- Genitopelvic pain/penetration disorder
- Psychological and sexual issues during puberty, adolescence and early adulthood
  - Management
- Psychological and sexual issues during and after pregnancy
  - Physical aspects of sexuality during pregnancy
  - Factors that inhibit sexual activity during pregnancy
  - Psychological aspects of sexuality in pregnancy
  - Psychosexual problems in the postpartum period
  - Management
- Psychological and sexual problems at workplace
- Psychosexual problems during menopause
  - Management
- Management strategies
  - Cognitive behavior therapy (CBT)
  - Mindfulness based cognitive therapy (MBCT)
  - Sex therapy
  - Dilators and insertion techniques
  - Electrical stimulation
  - Manual therapy

INTRODUCTION

Human psychology and sexuality are complex and relate to a lot of other dimensions like anatomical, physiological, social and cultural aspects. With women, this becomes even more complex due to changing hormonal levels throughout the month and throughout life.

Psychosexual disorders are sexual disorders that occur due to psychological problems and have no associated pathological disorder. Occasionally, one component may predominate the other or result in to the other, e.g., hypoactive sexual disorder arising due to depression. These disorders may arise due to physical, environmental or psychological factors like fear, anxiety, trauma, rape, distorted body image, etc. A superimposition of misinformation, ignorance, improper sexual education and cultural factors further worsens the condition. Symptoms of psychosexual disorders vary between individuals and occasionally may not even conform to the categories defined by the literature. They may manifest as paraphilia, sexual dysfunction or even gender identity disorder. Psychosexual disorders are a multidimensional complex problem involving biological, cultural, psychological and social factors; it is required that these problems are a manifestation of mental and emotional factors, there should not be involvement of any physical problem or medical illnesses and therapeutic drugs.

Epidemiological studies related to psychosexual disorders are limited in India but the few studies that have been conducted have concluded that the prevalence of male sexual disorders ranges from 10–52% whereas, that of female sexual disorders is around 14% (as per a limited population study conducted in South India). The reasons behind these psychosexual disorders in Indian population are varied—lack of sex education, misinformation, perception of sex being culturally, socially and religiously inappropriate, performance anxiety, superstitions, unpleasant past experiences and even somatic disorders like back pain or hip pain.

The World Health Organization (WHO) considers psychosexual health to be a significant component of general health and well-being. As physiotherapists treat female subjects for various disorders, including gynecological and obstetric conditions, they should possess knowledge about sexual health in order to help their clients in the best possible way.

ETIOLOGY

The etiology mainly comprises mental and emotional factors including the following:
- Anxiety
- Body image negativity
- Depression
- Guilt
- Improper sex education
- Stress, superstition or sexual trauma
- Phobia towards sexual activities
- Job-related problems
- Family disputes
- Marriage-related issues
- Emotional relationship with the partner
- General emotional well-being
- Concerns about safety (risks of unwanted pregnancy or sexually transmitted diseases)
- Sexual health of the partner
- Negative past sexual experiences
- Low levels of testosterone

CLASSIFICATION OF PSYCHOSEXUAL DISORDERS

Earlier human sexual response was described in four phases—excitement, plateau, orgasm and resolution. Later, it was modified into a triphasic model by Kaplan—desire, arousal and orgasm. Based on this classification, sexual disorders can be classified into problems of desire, arousal and orgasm.

The Diagnostic and Statistical Manual of Mental Disorders V (DSM-V) classifies sexual dysfunctions into various categories as shown in **Table 16.1** and **Figure 16.1**. Along with those described in **Table 16.1**, the DSM-V classification also includes substance/medication induced sexual dysfunction, other specified sexual dysfunction, and unspecified sexual dysfunction. Gender identity disorders were modified to include gender dysphorias.

Table 16.1: Classification of sexual disorders.

Type of disorder	*Males*	*Females*
Desire	Male hypoactive sexual desire disorder	Female sexual interest/arousal disorder
Arousal	Erectile disorder	Female sexual arousal disorder
Orgasm	Delayed ejaculation Early ejaculation	Female orgasmic disorder
Pain	Genitopelvic pain (scrotodynia, penodynia)	Genitopelvic pain/penetration disorder (vaginismus, vulvodynia, dyspareunia)

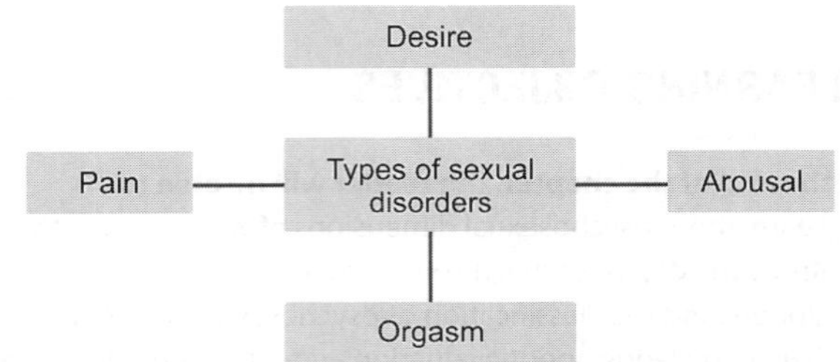

Fig. 16.1: Types of sexual disorders.

Substantial changes have also been made to the International Classification of Diseases – 11 (ICD-11) compared to ICD-10 which classified sexual dysfunctions into "organic" and "inorganic" dysfunctions.

According to guidelines proposed in the ICD-11, a diagnosis of sexual dysfunction can only be considered:
- If the condition has been persistent or recurrent over a period of several months
- If the condition is frequent, though may fluctuate in severity
- If the condition is associated with clinically significant distress

The duration requirement can be discarded in case of an immediate acute cause of the dysfunction, e.g., spinal cord injury or breast cancer and subsequent treatment.

Box 16.1 describes the sexual disorders in brief. Most of these conditions are out of the scope of physiotherapy, hence only some conditions have been described here.

FEMALE SEXUAL INTEREST/AROUSAL DISORDER

Female sexual interest/arousal disorder (SIAD) is defined as reduced or low level of sexual desire, sexual fantasies/thoughts, initiation or reception of sexual activities, desire triggered by sexual stimuli, sexual pleasure and/or genital or nongenital sensations, persisting or recurring since a minimum period of six months. Based on this definition, a community prevalence of 0.6% has been determined. Low sexual desire is one of the most common complaints amongst women across the life cycle.

Box 16.1: Brief description of sexual disorders.

- **Delayed ejaculation:** It is inability to ejaculate or marked delay in ejaculation despite adequate sexual stimulation and the man's desire to ejaculate.
- **Premature/early ejaculation:** It is ejaculation occurring prior to or shortly after vaginal penetration.
- **Erectile disorder:** It is the inability to achieve or maintain an erection during sexual activity with a partner. The problem should be at least 6 months old and should occur in at least 75% of the sexual occasions.
- **Male hypoactive sexual desire disorder:** A persistent or recurrent absence or deficiency of sexual desire and sexual/erotic fantasies or thoughts in males persisting for at least six months.
- **Female orgasmic disorder:** It is difficulty in experiencing orgasms or a marked reduction in the intensity of orgasm. To be diagnosed as a disorder, the problem should have lasted at least 6 months and should occur on all or almost all (75–100%) sexual occasions.
- **Female sexual interest/arousal disorder:** To be diagnosed as having female sexual interest/arousal disorder, the woman should have at least three of the six indicators—reduced or absent sexual interest, reduced or absent sexual/erotic thoughts or fantasies, reduced or absent initiation of sexual activity and being unreceptive to initiations by the partner, reduced or absent sexual excitement during all or almost all sexual encounters, reduced or absent sexual interest/arousal in response to any external or internal sexual cues, reduced or absent genital or nongenital sensations during all or almost all sexual encounters. These symptoms should persist for at least six months.
- **Genitopelvic pain or penetration disorder:** This involves persistent or recurrent difficulties in vaginal penetration during intercourse, marked vulvovaginal or pelvic pain during vaginal intercourse or attempt at vaginal penetration, marked anxiety or fear towards vaginal penetration about vulvovaginal or pelvic pain, marked tightening or tensing of pelvic floor muscles during vaginal penetration for at least six months.

SIAD may arise due to a multitude of reasons:
- Sexual abuse
- Childhood trauma
- Low estrogen levels
- Increasing age
- Neuroendocrine changes
- Perceived stress, distraction and body image
- Partner's sexual dysfunction
- Familial obligations
- Conflicts with the partner or family
- Cultural, social and religious values

Evaluation

The evaluation begins with comprehensive history taking that also focuses on psychosocial factors that may affect a person's sexual desire. The woman may complain of absent or decreased vaginal lubrication or decreased genital warmth secondary to increased blood flow that occurs with sexual stimulation. Medical conditions like hypertension, diabetes and hyperlipidemia have been linked to low arousal states. Relevant drug history also needs to be noted as there are certain drugs that may reduce one's sexual desire **(Table 16.2)**. It should be deduced from the history whether the condition is acquired or lifelong, situational or generalizable. Investigations should include determination of:

- Estradiol (E2)
- Sex-hormone binding globulin (SHBG)
- Total testosterone (TT)
- Calculated free testosterone (cFT)
- Prolactin
- Thyroid stimulating hormone (TSH)

Table 16.2: Drugs affecting female sexual arousal/interest.

Class	*Examples*
Psychological/ neurological	• Selective serotonin reuptake inhibitors • Lithium • Benzodiazepines • Phenytoin • Antipsychotics
Hormonal	• Contraceptives • Antiandrogens • Aromatase inhibitors • Tamoxifen • Ketoconazole
Cardiovascular	• Digoxin • Spironolactone • Beta blockers • Methyldopa • Clonidine
Pain	• Opioids • Indomethacin • Tricyclic antidepressants

Management

Medical management for acquired, generalized female SIAD in premenopausal women includes administration of Flibanserin in the United States. A trial of testosterone therapy for 3–6 months in postmenopausal females with low androgen levels has been recommended by the Endocrine Society. Hormone replacement therapy improves sexual desire in postmenopausal women. Phosphodiesterase inhibitors have been recommended to improve genital blood flow which in turn improves sexual arousal.

Sexual difficulties may be associated with cognitive distraction during sexual activity. This may be caused due to anxiety or depression, which distract the subject's mind away from the sensations generated in their body and dissuade them from feeling sexual pleasure. Management strategies should, hence, be focused on reducing this distraction to allow the subject to fully comprehend the situation, be attentive to their bodily reactions to sexual stimuli and take pleasure.

- Counseling focusing on the woman's relationship with their partner, self-awareness about their body and psychosexual beliefs can be tried.
- Several studies have reported reduction in the proportion of women complaining of such difficulties after administration of cognitive behavior therapy (CBT). Studies have reported

more improvement using CBT compared to drug therapy for reduced arousal.

- Mindfulness-based cognitive therapy (MBCT) has been proven to be effective in improving sexual desire, improving overall sexual function and reducing sex-related distress. MBCT helps the female become more aware of the physical changes being experienced by them during sexual activity or in anticipation of it. This enhances and maintains their sexual arousal and desire and thereby integrates their physiological and psychological experience.
- Early researches have talked about the role of pelvic floor muscle exercises in improving the sexual arousal and intensity of orgasmic response. A positive correlation has been established between strength of female pelvic floor muscles and the intensity of the orgasm.

FEMALE ORGASMIC DISORDER

Female orgasmic disorder is persistent or recurrent delay, difficulty or absence of attaining orgasm following adequate sexual stimulation and arousal, causing distress for at least six months.

Evaluation

Similar to SIAD, for women complaining of distress due to difficult, delayed or absent orgasms, a thorough history focusing on medical and psychosocial factors is important. It is imperative to deduce whether the problem is acquired or lifelong, situational or generalized. Female orgasmic disorder is most often associated with other sexual dysfunction disorders like arousal disorder or sexual pain. Physical examination should include vulvoscopy and clitoral and vaginal examination. Some subjects may exhibit clitoral phimosis which may or may not be related to an underlying pathology. Screening and examination for genital mutilation should also be performed.

Management

Management of female orgasmic disorder is difficult but should involve a multidisciplinary approach:

- If there is any physical trauma associated with the disorder, it should be managed by a gynecologist or other medical care provider.
- Studies have reported benefits with MBCT, Yoga, use of sex toys and sex therapy.
- For females having lifelong anorgasmia, directed masturbation has been found helpful. CBT helps in improving attitude, causes sexually-relevant thought changes and reduces anxiety. Strategies like sensate focus, systematic desensitization techniques, sex education, Kegel exercises and communication skill training help.

GENITOPELVIC PAIN/PENETRATION DISORDER

Genitopelvic pain/penetration disorder (GPPPD) involves significant clinical distress since six months due to persistent or recurrent difficulties with:

- Vaginal penetration during sexual activities
- Severe vulvovaginal/pelvic pain during sexual activity or penetration attempts
- Severe tightening of pelvic floor muscles during vaginal penetration attempts
- Marked fear or anxiety related to vaginal penetration or attempt at penetration.

GPPPD affects around 14–34% premenopausal and 6.5–45% postmenopausal women. It may be associated with female sexual interest/arousal disorder and/or female orgasmic disorder. There may be presence of other pain disorders like fibromyalgia, interstitial cystitis or irritable bowel syndrome as well. Genitopelvic pain can be provoked or spontaneous; may be related to sexual intercourse or may occur during urination; may be burning, throbbing, cutting or shooting in character; may be lifelong or acquired. It is important to consider some other factors—relationship factors (discrepancy in desire for sexual activity or communication problems), partner factors (partner's sexual health), psychiatric factors (any associated psychiatric comorbidities like depression or anxiety, negative body image, history of sexual abuse), cultural or religious factors (attitudes towards sexuality) and medical factors.

Pain can be:

- Superficial, i.e., vulvovaginal or occurring during penetration (levator ani syndrome or vaginismus).
- Deep, i.e., pelvic or occurring only with deeper penetration (dyspareunia).
- Localized over the vestibule (provoked vestibulodynia).

However, sometimes vaginismus may be secondary to dyspareunia. Hence, the DSM-V classifies all these under the same category of GPPPD.

Evaluation

Assessment of GPPPD, like other sexual dysfunctions includes comprehensive history taking and genitopelvic examination that involves measurement of vaginal pH, 'pain mapping' and evaluation of pelvic floor tonus. These are usually done by the gynecologist.

Management

Box 16.2 presents some goals of management of GPPPD.

- If there is any specific etiological diagnosis, treatment should be focused on that first.
- CBT works best for vestibulodynia. Cognitive behavioral psychotherapy can be performed on individuals, couples or groups. The main targets here are emotional dysregulation, cognitive distortions and maladaptive behaviors that lead to symptoms related to GPPPD and disrupt the woman's sexual life.

Box 16.2: Some realistic goals of management of GPPPD.

- Reduction of pain from severe to moderate or mild
- Reduction in the pelvic floor muscle tone
- Positive coping
- Reduction in negative thoughts or feelings
- Improvement in sexual function

- Psychoeducation of the couple should be the foremost approach. It should be emphasized that neither the patient nor their partner should have a passive role.
  - Education involves making the couple understand the problem, teaching about female anatomy (using a mirror so that the patient visualizes herself) and challenging myths. They should be educated about the biopsychosocial aspect of GPPPD and the role of marital issues and psychological issues as triggers and persistence factors. Behavioral strategies should be taught to the couple to improve pain **(Table 16.3)**.
  - Psychoeducation should also incorporate strategies to reduce anxiety. It is commonly seen that the couple is stuck in an avoidance circle. They avoid sexual activity as it may result in pain. They avoid discussion of personal problems, intimacy and a search for solution. Hence, it is very likely that they may feel anxious when they approach someone for help. In such case, positive reinforcement should be provided in the form of assurance that they have sought help. It should be explained that the therapy focuses on improving the couple's desire, intimacy and excitement rather than focusing on the frequency of sexual activity.
  - Cognitive distortions commonly faced by such women—hypervigilance and catastrophic pain, should be challenged. Use of sexual fantasies should be encouraged to increase desire and arousal and ultimately, improve lubrication which reduces pain.
  - Display of physical affection and emotions should be encouraged. Attempts should be made to uncouple physical affection and anticipation of genitopelvic pain. Sensate focus is a technique which forbids penetration in the earlier phases of therapy and gently moves from nongenital touch to genital touch and later, ultimately penetration. Forbiddance of penetration reduces the patient's anxiety and allows her to focus on the pleasant sexual sensations.
  - In cases of vaginismus, systemic desensitization should be encouraged, where progressively larger vaginal dilators are used along with physiotherapy techniques to relax the tensed muscles.

Table 16.3: Behavioral strategies for reduction of pain.

Condition	***Behavioral strategies***
Sexual activity	• Use of water-based lubricants • Exploring different sexual positions • Use of Sitz bath **(Fig. 16.2)** or ice packs after sexual activity • Urinate immediately after sexual activity
Physical activity	• Avoiding exercises that put pressure or produce friction in the vulvar area (e.g., cycling) • Avoiding saunas/steam baths and swimming pools
Clothing	• Avoiding tight lower body clothing • Removing wet clothing as soon as possible immediately after an activity • Avoiding synthetic fabric underwear; using cotton underwear • Washing clothes with hypoallergenic products
Personal hygiene	• Avoiding shaving the vulvar area • Avoiding washing the genital area more than once daily • Avoiding scented products

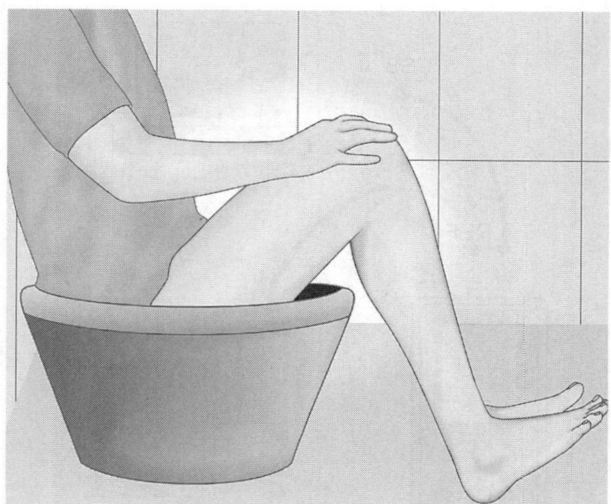

Fig. 16.2: Use of Sitz bath.

- Medical management involves use of topical anesthetics and corticosteroids to reduce pain in dyspareunia and vulvodynia; low doses of anticonvulsants and tricyclic antidepressants for vulvodynia. Use of botulinum toxin injections and topical corticosteroids and anesthetics is done to treat vaginismus but the evidence supporting it is modest and hence they are not recommended as first-line treatment. Lubricants can be used to reduce sexual pain. Hormonal therapy with systemic or topical estrogen may help in postmenopausal women.
- Surgical management includes vestibulectomy for localized vulvodynia, when other options fail. It has been reported that a combination of physical therapy and psychosexual therapy works as effectively as surgery in provoked vestibulodynia. Vulvodynia can be treated using systemic analgesic drugs or electroanalgesia and ganglion impar blocks for local effect in postmenopausal women. Surgical interventions also include laparoscopic uterosacral nerve ablation.
- EMG biofeedback **(Fig. 16.3)** has proved a successful treatment strategy for GPPPD. An EMG sensor providing information about the degree of pelvic floor muscle contraction, is inserted into the vagina of the woman. The woman is then asked to relax the pelvic floor muscles using the EMG sensor information as feedback. EMG biofeedback used along with CBT works well for vaginismus. EMG biofeedback in combination with electrical stimulation also provides benefits.
- Pelvic floor muscle exercises and electrostimulation have shown benefits in both, dyspareunia and vaginismus. Use of high voltage galvanic stimulation has been studied for levator ani syndrome. EMG biofeedback, electrostimulation and pelvic floor muscle exercises are all aimed towards:

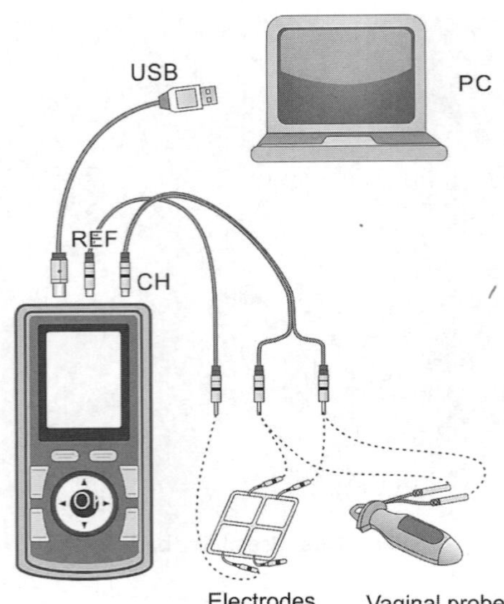

Fig. 16.3: EMG biofeedback device for pelvic floor.

- Directing the woman's attention towards the pelvic floor muscles and controlling them
- Reducing the pelvic floor muscle tone at rest
- Increasing elasticity of the vaginal introitus
- Allowing the woman exposure to penetration and making them comfortable about it

❖ Postpartum dyspareunia occurs due to vaginal dryness, reduced lubrication and lowered libido secondary to fatigue, lactation and hormonal disturbances. Along with this, factors like painful or adhesive scar tissue due to spontaneous tearing or episiotomy also contribute. Use of therapeutic ultrasound for deep heating of the tissues in perineal laceration in cases of postpartum dyspareunia has been reported.

 **Clinical Pointer**

Physiotherapy management of GPPPD involves:
- Education
- CBT—particularly using vaginal dilators
- Rehabilitative approaches—PFM strengthening and relaxation using electrical stimulation and biofeedback
- Palliative treatment methods to improve tissue mobility and reduce pain
- Manual therapy techniques—soft-tissue and bony mobilization, massage and stretching

PSYCHOLOGICAL AND SEXUAL ISSUES DURING PUBERTY, ADOLESCENCE AND EARLY ADULTHOOD

Adolescence is the age from 10–19 years. It can be divided into—early (10–13), middle (14–16) and late (17–19). Puberty occurs during adolescence. Females are likely to achieve puberty 12–18 months before males. Girls are more likely to have negative health outcomes during adolescence than males.

Onset of menstruation, development of secondary sexual characteristics, attitudes of the family and society and cultural influence on these matters, affect the psychological health of the girl. Lack of proper sex education leads to unprotected sex, sexually transmitted diseases, unwanted pregnancy and a resultant poor reproductive health.

Early or 'precocious' puberty is when a girl achieves puberty at an early age. This causes the girl to have a negative body self-image, a feeling of her being different than others, at a time when a child wants to fit in the most. This results in depression, substance abuse, early sexual behavior, eating disorders and disruptive behavior disorders.

The prevalence of mental disorders has been found at least 20% in the general population of 18–24 year olds.

Management

Physiotherapy management of psychological and sexual problems seen during adolescence focusses on improving the sexual health and mental health. Most of the strategies have been discussed in Chapter 8: Adolescence, Puberty and Menarche. Some of the strategies have been discussed here.

Body-based Awareness Therapy

Use of body-based awareness therapy (BBAT) has been studied in young girls. It is a resource-oriented and holistic 'body-mind' physiotherapeutic technique aimed to strengthen and restore essential functions of the physical self.

Principles of BBAT:
- ❖ To improve stability and balance
- ❖ To facilitate grounding
- ❖ To facilitate flow of movement
- ❖ To improve breathing
- ❖ To improve mental/cognitive awareness and embodied presence

It works on principles similar to mindfulness techniques. It makes the subject become aware of their body movements and bodily presence and helps them rediscover bodily resources and abilities. The physiotherapist helps the subject to explore, experience and integrate affective and sensory dimensions of the body, thereby facilitating verbal expression of bodily experiences.

Postural Training

There is considerable bone growth during puberty and adolescence. Young adolescent girls develop incorrect postures under societal and cultural influences which persist with time, leading to multiple musculoskeletal issues in the future. Discomfort with changing body image, especially due to development of breasts is a huge factor playing role in the affection of posture. Physical and sexual abuse or depression can also lead to postural changes.

Postural training can help deal with these poor posture complaints. Stretching and strengthening of relevant structures helps in improving the posture. Getting involved in sports activities can help improve the posture as well as improve the mental health of the girl. A good posture can develop a positive body image which enhances the confidence of the girl and removes any negative impressions in her mind.

PSYCHOLOGICAL AND SEXUAL ISSUES DURING AND AFTER PREGNANCY

A review of the literature reveals that many women experience decreased sexual desire and frequency of intercourse due to a variety of, often unspoken, physical and psychological factors.

Physical Aspects of Sexuality During Pregnancy

- Physical changes occur during pregnancy, but the connection between these changes and sexuality often is not clear. Normal physiology during pregnancy becomes a source of numerous deterrents to sexual activities.
- Various pregnancy related symptoms like nausea, vomiting, fatigue, heartburn and urinary frequency and urgency can make sexual expression awkward and uncomfortable.
- The breasts are especially tender in early pregnancy, in response to both hormonal and vascular alterations. If not anticipated, the milk let-down associated with orgasm, which often occurs later in pregnancy, can be very distressing to both the woman and her sexual partner.
- The amount of vaginal secretions normally increases in pregnancy and is further augmented during sexual arousal. The cervix is more likely to bleed during pregnancy because of direct trauma from penile thrusting. An uninformed couple can be alarmed by unexpected postcoital bleeding. The normal engorgement of genitalia during pregnancy is further exacerbated during sexual arousal. Vasocongestion is not well relieved, even after orgasm, and the residual sensation of fullness in the pelvic organs may be uncomfortable enough to cause a woman to avoid coital activity. Orgasm may be accompanied by cramping or muscle spasms.
- Alterations in the endocrine environment during pregnancy cause vaginal discomfort for some women particularly in the first and third trimesters of pregnancy.
- Diminished androgen levels in women have been proposed to contribute to the sexual dysfunction common during pregnancy.

Factors that Inhibit Sexual Activity During Pregnancy

- Awkwardness of having coitus
- Fear of injury to fetus
- Breast tenderness
- Genital vasocongestion
- Reduced libido
- Negative body image
- Dyspareunia
- Physical discomfort
- Fatigue
- Urinary frequency and urgency

Psychological Aspects of Sexuality in Pregnancy

- Desire for sex and sexual functioning are affected by many environmental, interpersonal, and intrapersonal considerations. Sexual performance can be inhibited by lack of knowledge or by anger, fear, and other potentially negative attitudes.
- Prenatal counseling can reassure couples that their problems are no different than those of any other couple during pregnancy.
- The background to these psychological factors is the unspoken fear of both partners that penile penetration can cause injury to the fetus.

Psychosexual Problems in the Postpartum Period

- The postpartum period is a vulnerable and stressful period in a woman's life. It is also influenced by different cultural backgrounds. Nearly 40–45% women exhibit reduced sexual desire and lack of satisfaction during this period.
- There are certain psychological factors like feeling less attractive, stresses of motherhood, fatigue and lack of sleep that can affect sexual activities.
- There are certain physical factors like nipple tenderness, milk leakage, uncomfortable coital position, episiotomy sutures and pelvic floor muscle weakness which may lead to painful sexual activities.
- Postpartum depression can adversely affect a woman's sexuality and desire for intercourse.
- Biological changes too occur in the postpartum period. One of the main events following birth is hormone withdrawal with a steep decrease in estrogen and progesterone. Prolactin increases during lactation and the breasts change their outer appearance, often becoming tender and engorged. At the same time the size of the uterus diminishes and the vaginal discharge returns to normal. These changes also lead to decreased sexual desire and sexual dysfunction.

Management

- Prevention—counseling
- Specific—sex education
- Marriage and relationship counseling
- Cognitive behavior therapy (CBT)

PSYCHOLOGICAL AND SEXUAL PROBLEMS AT WORKPLACE

- Workplace abuse and stress related to poorer mental health can lead to several psychological disorders like sleep disorder, depression, anxiety, post-traumatic stress disorder and psychological distress.
- Workplace stress has also been associated with increased musculoskeletal injuries and disorders and also cardiovascular risk.
- It should be the duty of the management to collect regular feedbacks from their employees and try to create and maintain an employee-friendly environment. Employees should be provided paid psychological counseling sessions if needed, paid vacation days may also be provided to improve their mental health.

- The employees should also try to balance their personal and professional lives so that both remain separated and stress-free. Problems should be communicated well with the higher authorities. Help should be sought whenever needed.

PSYCHOSEXUAL PROBLEMS DURING MENOPAUSE

Menopause is a natural phenomenon in the life of a woman. Most females pass through this without any difficulty but some may face physical, psychosexual or psychosocial problems. These problems are especially seen in females undergoing sudden menopause, e.g., in case of hysterectomy.

Physical manifestations of menopause may lead to psychological issues like anxiety, depression and cognitive disturbances. The woman may feel abandoned by her family, which may give rise to psychosocial issues. There may be vaginal dryness and atrophy and decreased libido. This may result in decreased sexual arousal or interest or painful intercourse. **Table 16.4** presents some factors associated with psychosexual problems in menopause.

During menopause, a reduction in estrogen causes a decrease in the lactobacilli residing in the vagina. This causes the vaginal environment to become basic, leading to a change in the vaginal flora and causing vaginal dryness, ultimately resulting in vulvovaginal atrophy. Almost 45% of postmenopausal females are affected with symptomatic vulvovaginal atrophy. This is also associated with reduced secretions from sebaceous glands and decreased vaginal lubrication during sexual stimulation. Secondary to all these changes, the woman exhibits a decline in sexual interest, avoidance of sexual activity or pain during intercourse.

Management

- Psychological counseling of the woman alone or with her partner can be done.

Table 16.4: Factors associated with psychosexual issues in menopause.

Domain	Factors
Physical	• Aging • Menstrual problems or irregular menses • Dysmenorrhea • Spotting between menses • Premenstrual tension • Estrogen depletion • Surgical menopause • Medical illness
Psychological	• Psychological well-being • Stressors and personality factors • Negative attitude towards menopause
Psychosocial	• Quality of personal relationships • Social class • Past sexual function • Education and employment • Sociocultural environment

- Sexual therapy of the woman alone or with the partner also helps.
- Behavioral exercises can be used to reduce anxiety associated with sexual dysfunction.
- Studies have reported no increase of libido or sexual function with hormone therapy using estrogen. Evidence does not support the use of estrogen alone or combination of estrogen and progesterone to treat sexual arousal or sexual interest disorder in menopause. Hormone therapy may help women with vulvovaginal atrophy by increasing vaginal lubrication and decreasing dyspareunia.
- Several randomized controlled trials have reported improvement in sexual function and desire following treatment using testosterone in menopausal women. However, such treatment regimes should be continued at least for 4–16 weeks to get benefits. Testosterone therapy has its own share of adverse effects like increase in levels of triglycerides and low-density lipoproteins.
- A systematic review found that PFM exercises were the most commonly used intervention for postmenopausal women and they improved sexual function significantly. One of the studies reported improvement in females with genitourinary syndrome whereas another reported improvement in females with dyspareunia.
- Mind-body exercises like Yoga or Rusie Dutton Thai Yoga **(Figs. 16.4A to O)** have also reported improvements in sexual domains of quality of life in postmenopausal women.
- Aerobic and resistance training help in improving mental health in peri- and postmenopausal women and thereby help in improving sexual health as psychological factors can also lead to sexual dysfunction.

MANAGEMENT STRATEGIES

The physiotherapy approach to treatment of women with complaints of inability to have intercourse, or painful intercourse, includes taking a detailed history, performing a physical examination, and providing a treatment plan consistent with the goals of the patient. Treatment tools utilized by the physiotherapist include:

- Education, i.e., providing anatomical and physiological information
- Cognitive behavioral therapy, particularly with vaginal dilators
- Rehabilitative approaches, such as PFM strengthening
- Relaxation with tools, such as biofeedback
- Palliative treatment methods to decrease pain and improve tissue mobility
- Manual techniques including massage, stretching, and soft-tissue and bony mobilizations.

The physiotherapy intervention generally consists of evaluation and treatment with education and cognitive behavioral therapy, exercises, manual therapy techniques, and modalities including pelvic floor biofeedback and electrical stimulation.

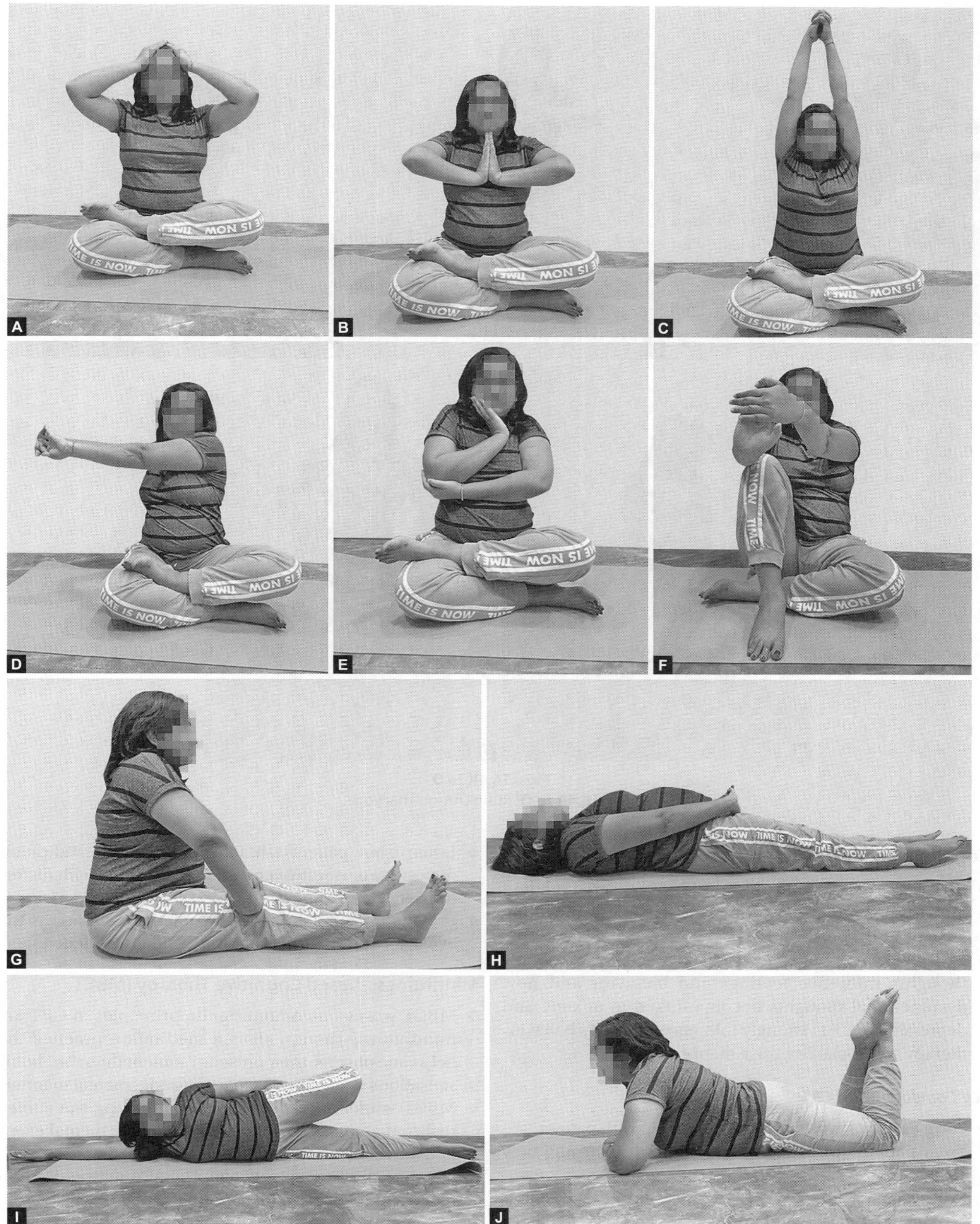

Figs. 16.4A to J

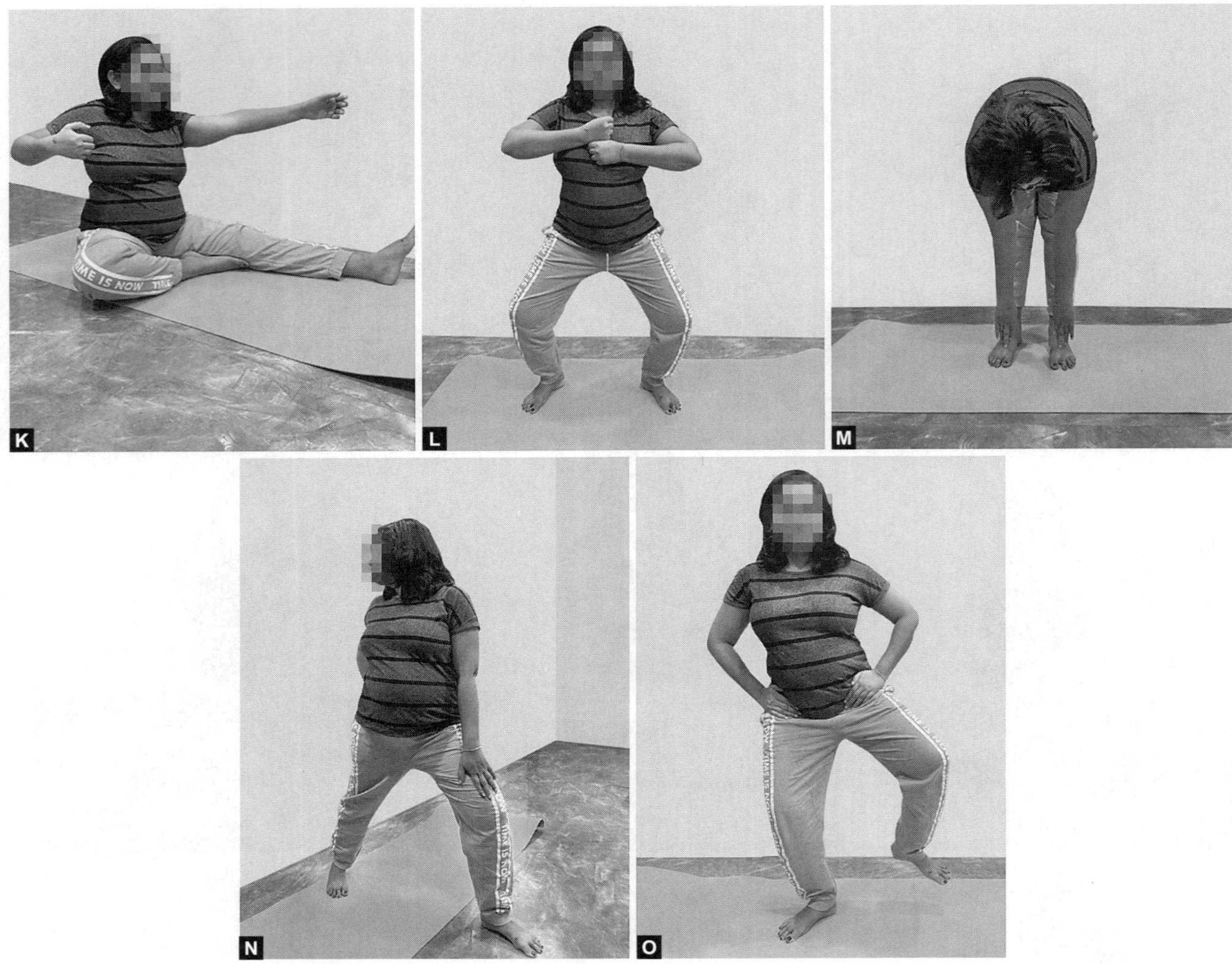

Figs. 16.4K to O

Figs. 16.4A to O: Rusie Dutton Thai yoga.

Cognitive Behavior Therapy (CBT)

- CBT is a widely practiced, empirically validated method for treating common psychological disorders, including anxiety and depression.
- CBT focuses on helping patients become aware of how thoughts influence feelings and behavior and how dysfunctional thoughts become linked to anxiety and depression. CBT is strongly influenced both by behavior therapy and social cognitive theory.

Key Components of CBT

- Form a supportive, working relationship with patient.
- Treat patients as active collaborators in learning new skills.
- Promote self-efficacy by helping patients develop capabilities and self-confidence.
- Be aware of how thoughts, behavior and emotions interact to affect motivation, learning and retention.
- Listen to how patients talk about themselves for indications of positive or negative cognitions associated with distress (anxiety, depression, stress).
- Provide encouragement and support in situations that evoke unwarranted anxiety and avoidant tendencies.

Mindfulness-based Cognitive Therapy (MBCT)

- MBCT works on combining the principles of CBT and mindfulness therapy. It is a meditation practice that helps one observe their present-moment thoughts, bodily sensations and emotions in a non-judgemental manner.
- MBCT works on decentering, i.e., making the subject realize that thoughts and feelings are only mental events and not reality or truth about oneself.
- It helps in reducing the symptoms of depression and recurrence of depression.
- The main components of MBCT include mindfulness techniques like gentle mindful yogic exercises, body scans and sitting meditation.

Sex Therapy

- Sex therapy involves sensate focus exercises, i.e., a series of planned progressive nondemand pleasuring exercises whereby each partner takes turns giving and receiving sensual and later on, sexual touches, caresses, etc.
- Guiding verbally and nonverbally as to what feels most pleasurable is encouraged.
- Usually each session lasts 15–20 minutes and two or preferably three sessions occur each week for 3–6 weeks.
- As sessions are planned, touches may often be sensual rather than specifically sexual. However, when sexual touches are wanted, oral and manual genital stimulation or the use of a vibrator can be considered.

Dilators and Insertion Techniques

- The use of vaginal dilators can help women with dyspareunia to control their fear of pain and promote pelvic floor relaxation during insertion.
- The dilators also might prove beneficial to elongate shortened PFMs and improve flexibility and tissue viscoelastic properties.

Electrical Stimulation

- Electrical stimulation **(Fig. 16.5)** is a therapeutic modality widely used in physical therapy and, based on the parameters used, it can act on pain through several mechanisms, including the improvement of muscle proprioception, the increase in local blood circulation.
- Electrical stimulation can be a worthwhile component of treatment.

Manual Therapy

- It includes stretching, massage, and myofascial techniques and is typically considered the cornerstone of physical therapy interventions. The reader can *refer* Chapter 15: Managing the Pelvic Floor for details.

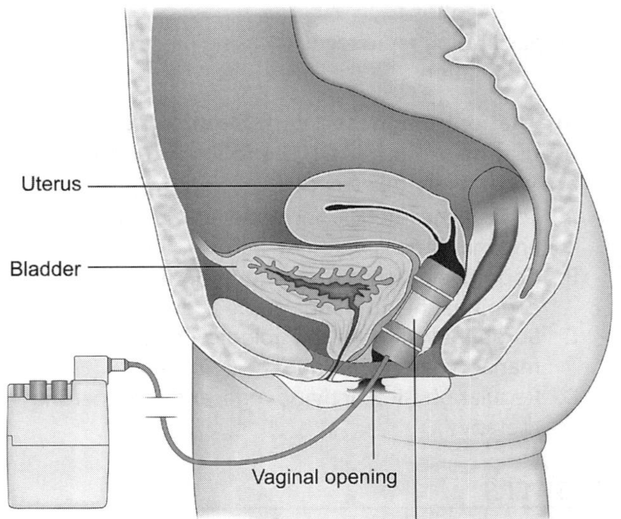

Fig. 16.5: Pelvic floor electrical stimulation device.

- It aims to facilitate muscle relaxation, release tensions and trigger points, improve blood circulation and mobility in the pelvic-perineal region, adjust postural imbalances, and increase the vaginal opening and desensitize the area.

Summary

Psychosexual disorders are very prevalent in the modern world, especially among females. The DSM-V classifies these disorders in various categories—female sexual interest/arousal disorder, female orgasmic disorder and genitopelvic pain/penetration disorder. Females may face some or the other psychological or sexual issues throughout their lifespan. Psychosexual disorders usually stem from problems with the partner or the family, cultural or religious background, past experiences or social problems. It is the role of the physiotherapist to understand such problems and help the woman in the required manner.

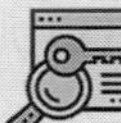

Review Questions

1. What are psychosexual disorders?
2. What are the causes of psychosexual disorders?
3. Explain the classification of psychosexual disorders.
4. What are the psychosexual problems faced during pregnancy?
5. What are the psychosexual problems faced during menopause?
6. Explain management strategies for psychosexual disorders.

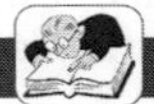

Bibliography

1. American Psychiatric Association. The diagnostic and statistical manual of mental disorders, 5th edition. Washington, DC. American Psychiatric Association; 2013.
2. Backman H, Widenbrant M, Bohm-Starke N, Dahlof LG. Combined physical and psychosexual therapy for provoked vestibulodynian evaluation of a multidisciplinary treatment model. J Sex Res. 2008;45(04):378-85.
3. Berghmans B. Physiotherapy for pelvic pain and female sexual dysfunction: an untapped resource. Int Urogynecol J. 2018;29(5):631-38. doi: 10.1007/s00192-017-3536-8. Epub 2018 Jan 9. PMID: 29318334; PMCID: PMC5913379.
4. Bornstein J, Goldstein AT, Stockdale CK, et al. Consensus vulvar pain terminology committee of the International Society for the Study of Vulvovaginal Disease (ISSVD). International Society for the Study of Women's Sexual Health (ISSWSH). International Pelvic Pain Society (IPPS). 2015 ISSVD, ISSWSH, and IPPS.
5. Britnell SJ, Cole JV, Isherwood L, Stan MM, Britnell N, Burgi S, et al. Postural Health in Women: The Role of Physiotherapy. J Obstet Gynecol Can. 2005;27(5):493-500.
6. Carcelén-Fraile MDC, Aibar-Almazán A, Martínez-Amat A, Cruz-Díaz D, Díaz-Mohedo E, Redecillas-Peiró MT, et al. Effects of physical exercise on sexual function and quality of sexual life related to menopausal symptoms in peri- and postmenopausal

women: A systematic review. Int J Environ Res Public Health. 2020;17(8):2680. doi: 10.3390/ijerph17082680. PMID: 32295114; PMCID: PMC7215442.
7. Dias-Amaral A, Marques-Pinto A. Female genitopelvic pain/penetration disorder: Review of the related factors and overall approach. Rev Bras Gynecol Obstet. 2018;40(12). https://doi.org/10.1055/s-0038-1675805.
8. Domoney C. Psychosexual disorders. Obstet Gynecol Reprod Med. 2018;28(10):22-27.
9. Goldstein AT, Pukall CF, Brown C, Bergeron S, Stein A, Kellogg-Spadt S. Vulvodynia: Assessment and treatment. J Sex Med. 2016;13(04):572-90. Doi:10.1016/j.jsxm.2016.01.020.
10. Kar SK, Choudhury A, Singh AP. Understanding normal development of adolescent sexuality: A bumpy ride. J Hum Reprod Sci. 2015;8(2):70-4. doi: 10.4103/0974-1208.158594. PMID: 26157296; PMCID: PMC4477452.
11. Krakowsky Y, Grober ED. A practical guide to female sexual dysfunction: An evidence-based review for physicians in Canada. Can Urol Assoc J. 2018;12(6):211-16. doi: 10.5489/cuaj.4907. Epub 2018 Feb 23. PMID: 29485038; PMCID: PMC5994984.
12. Meston CM, Hull E, Levin RJ, et al. Disorders of orgasm in women. J Sex Med. 2004;1:66-8.
13. Narang T, Garima, Singh SM. Psychosexual disorders and dermatologists. Indian Dermatol Online J. 2016;7(3):149-58. https://doi.org/10.4103/2229-5178.182349.
14. Paterson LQP, Handy AB, Brotto LA. A pilot study of eight-session mindfulness-based cognitive therapy adapted for women's sexual interest/arousal disorder. J Sex Res. 2017;54(7):850-61.
15. Rani S. The psychosexual implications of menopause. Br J Nurs (Mark Allen Publishing). 2009;18(6):370-3.
16. Reed GM, Drescher J, Krueger RB, Atalla E, Cochrane SD, First MB, et al. Disorders related to sexuality and gender identity in the ICD-11: revising the ICD-10 classification based on current scientific evidence, best clinical practices, and human rights considerations. World Psychiatry: official journal of the World Psychiatric Association (WPA). 2016;15(3):205-21. https://doi.org/10.1002/wps.20354.
17. Rosenbaum TY. The role of physical therapy in female sexual dysfunction. Curr Sex Health Rep. 2008;5:97-101. https://doi.org/10.1007/s11930-008-0017-6.
18. Rosenbaum TY. The role of physiotherapy in sexual health: Is it evidence-based? J Assoc Chartr Phys Women's Health. 2006:99.
19. Sathyanarayana Rao TS, Darshan MS, Tandon A. An epidemiological study of sexual disorders in south Indian rural population. Indian J Psychiatry. 2015;57:150-7.
20. Shirotsuki K, Noda S. Cognitive Behavior Therapy and Mindfulness-based Intervention for Social Anxiety Disorder. In: Kocabaşoğlu N, Çağlayan RHB, (eds). Anxiety Disorders - From Childhood to Adulthood [Internet]. London: IntechOpen; 2018 [cited 2022 Jul 29]. Available from: https://www.intechopen.com/chapters/62344 doi: 10.5772/intechopen.79345
21. Strömbäck M, Malmgren-Olsson EB, Wiklund M. Girls need to strengthen each other as a group: experiences from a gender-sensitive stress management intervention by youth-friendly Swedish health services – a qualitative study. BMC Public Health. 2013;13:907. https://doi.org/10.1186/1471-2458-13-907.
22. Strömbäck M, Wiklund M, Renberg ES, Malmgren-Olsson E. Gender-sensitive and youth-friendly physiotherapy: Steps toward a stress management intervention for girls and young women. Physiother Theory Pract. 2016;32(1):20-33.
23. Thornton K, Chervenak J, Neal-Perry G. Menopause and Sexuality. Endocrinol Metab Clin North Am. 2015;44(3):649-61. doi: 10.1016/j.ecl.2015.05.009. PMID: 26316248; PMCID: PMC5994393.

Multiple Choice Questions (MCQs)

To test your understanding and recall of key concepts.

1. What are the categories of sexual disorders according to DSM V?

A. Pain, arousal, desire, and orgasm
B. Desire, excitement, arousal, and plateau
C. Plateau, resolution, and climax
D. Excitement, desire, and resolution

2. Which psychological factors are most likely to contribute to psychosexual disorders?

A. Low levels of testosterone and poor blood circulation
B. Anxiety, body image negativity, and improper sex education
C. Physical injury and chronic infections
D. High stress and regular physical activity

3. Which of the following is *not* a characteristic feature of genitopelvic pain/penetration disorder (GPPPD)?

A. Persistent or recurrent difficulties with vaginal penetration during intercourse
B. Marked vulvovaginal or pelvic pain during vaginal intercourse
C. Marked fear or anxiety about vulvovaginal or pelvic pain in anticipation
D. Chronic infections

4. A physiotherapist is treating a patient with dyspareunia using manual therapy and mindfulness-based cognitive therapy (MBCT). This treatment approach is reflective of following principle_____________.

A. Enhancing muscular strength to prevent prolapse
B. Reducing anxiety and increasing awareness of bodily sensations
C. Restoring hormonal balance through external interventions
D. Facilitating rapid recovery using electrical stimulation

5. In a patient diagnosed with female sexual interest/arousal disorder (SIAD), the following interventions are most likely be effective_____________.

A. Topical anesthetics, hormone replacement therapy, and mindfulness exercises
B. Cognitive behavioral therapy, mindfulness-based cognitive therapy, and couple's counseling
C. Surgery to alleviate physiological barriers and stress management techniques
D. Regular physical activity, yoga, and testosterone therapy

ANSWERS

1. A	2. B	3. D	4. B	5. B

Chapter 17

Electrophysical Agents in Women's Health

Shivani Sheth, Megha Sandeep Sheth, Priyasingh Rangey

LEARNING OBJECTIVES

At the end of the chapter, the reader will be able to:

- Understand the various impairments in women that can be treated by electrophysical agents.
- Learn about the use of electrophysical agents in impairments and conditions related to female health.
- Learn the precautions and dosage of various commonly used and safe electrotherapeutic agents.

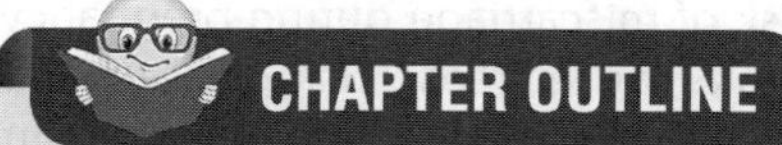

CHAPTER OUTLINE

- Introduction
- Role of electrotherapy
- Electrophysical agents
  - Thermotherapy
  - Transcutaneous electrical nerve stimulation
  - Neuromuscular electrical stimulation
  - Interferential current
  - Diadynamic currents
  - Low level laser therapy
  - Pulsed electromagnetic field
  - Therapeutic ultrasound
  - Intermittent pneumatic compression
  - Hydrotherapy
  - Biofeedback

INTRODUCTION

The history of use of electrotherapy in women's health dates to the late 1800s. Since the 1900s electric currents have been used for amenorrhea, dysmenorrhea, and endometriosis. Electrotherapy can be useful in various stages of a woman's life. Beginning with relief of pain during dysmenorrhea, continuing with pain relief during labor to management of incontinence in the later stages, electrotherapy plays a role in various life stages of a woman along with exercises. It is important to keep in mind precautions that need to be taken and electrotherapy should be used in adjunct to exercise therapy for best results.

ROLE OF ELECTROTHERAPY

Electrotherapy in women, may be used for the following impairments:

- Pain
- Dysesthesias—tingling, numbness
- Muscle weakness
- Swelling

During pregnancy, electrotherapy can be used in place of strong medications that can cross the placental barrier and affect the fetus. Electrotherapy has been found useful in the following conditions in women:

- Primary dysmenorrhea
- Lumbopelvic pain
- Pelvic pain
- Carpal tunnel syndrome
- Varicose veins
- Labor
- Incontinence
- Bruised perineum: This is seen following normal or prolonged labor. It can also be seen following road traffic accidents. It is a painful condition which may be associated with incontinence.

Clinical Pointer

Pregnancy is generally a contraindication (red flag) or should be considered with precaution (yellow flag) for the application of any physical agent if it can have effects on the fetus. Most of the effects of electrophysical agents on the fetus are not known.

Stimulation of the abdomen, lumbar, or pelvic region may increase hemorrhage during menstruation.

ELECTROPHYSICAL AGENTS

Electrophysical agents (EPAs) should be used based on findings of a proper assessment and appropriate clinical decision-making skills.

Clinical Pointer

The EPA should be indicated, safe to use, all contraindications should be ruled out and necessary precautions should be taken. Select the most appropriate EPA, technique and dosage parameters. The precautions and contraindications should be considered before using any electrotherapeutic modality in women.

Appropriate precautions should be taken before using any electrical modality. Clinical judgement must be made reasonably with consent of patient and gynecologist in females who have had history of:

- Miscarriage or abortion
- Epilepsy
- Irritable uterus
- Pacemaker or defibrillator
- History of malignancy

Safe Practice

For safe practice of electrotherapy always:

- Check sensations
- Inspect skin area
- Rule out red flags
- Take consent and ask for a chaperone when using invasive electrodes

Modalities that may, be used to reduce impairments in women are described in the following pages.

Thermotherapy

- **Superficial heat therapy** has been used for relieving thigh pain and lower abdominal pain of ***primary dysmenorrhea.*** Research has suggested that low-level topical heat therapy (in the form of heat pads or heat patch) has been as effective as ibuprofen for the treatment of dysmenorrhea. A 180 cm^2 heat patch capable of supplying 38.9°C heat for 12 hours per day for 3 days can be used.
- **Microwave diathermy** has also been reported to be efficacious in pain relief caused by ***dysmenorrhea.*** The suggested dosage has been intensity set to the level that the patient feels moderate heat sensation. With the patient lying in the supine position, a reflector can be directed toward the lower abdomen, kept 5 cm away from the skin surface and held for 20 min.
- **Contrast bath and cryotherapy** are often safe and suggested management approaches for symptomatic relief of ***carpal tunnel syndrome*** **(Fig. 17.1)**.
- **Warm baths, heat or cold packs, hydrotherapy** may be used for ***pelvic girdle pain***.
- **Infrared therapy** has been used to treat ***sore perineum*** and ***postoperative wounds***.
- **Cryotherapy** can be given with no harmful effects for relief of ***musculoskeletal symptoms*** during ***pregnancy***.

Clinical Pointer

Heat can increase the body's core temperature and can sometimes pose a risk of miscarriage during pregnancy. Maternal hyperthermia can increase risk of abnormal development of fetus including growth retardation, microencephaly, neural tube defects, etc. Full body immersion like hydrotherapy should be avoided. Superficial heat to small areas of the body can be safely given.

Precautions when Using Heating Pads

The following precautions should be taken when using or advising heating pads or heat wraps during pregnancy:

- Heating pads should not be used for more than 15 minutes at a time
- The temperature should not be more than 100°C
- The lady should not go to sleep during the treatment session
- The wire connections should be checked
- Do not use over the abdomen or when leaking amniotic fluid or bleeding is present

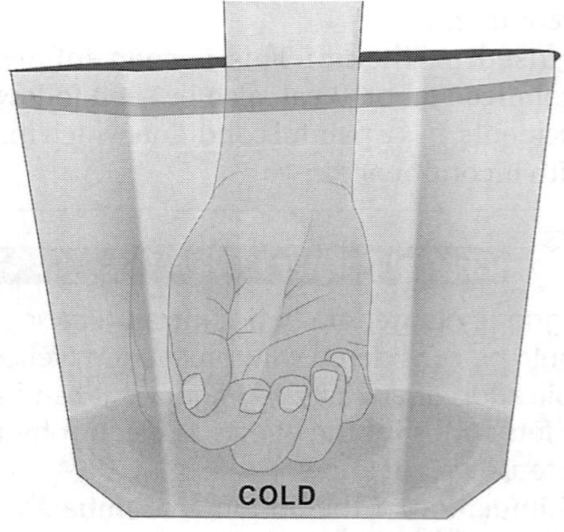

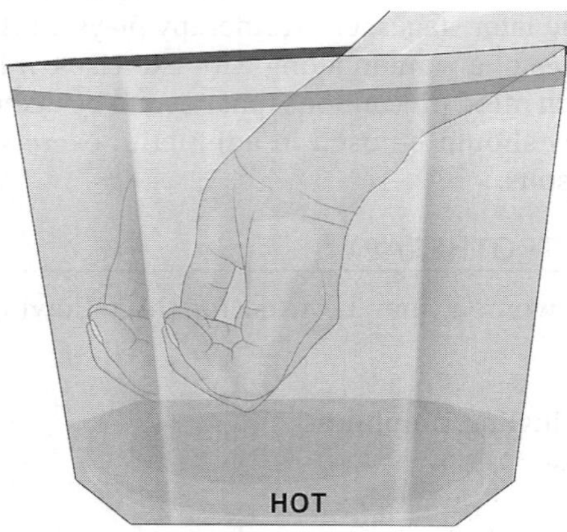

Fig. 17.1: Contrast bath for carpal tunnel syndrome.

Research Pointer

- Recent literature has reported NO association between use of short-wave diathermy (SWD) in pregnant women and spontaneous abortion, prematurity, stillbirth or reduced fertility.
- Center for disease control and prevention (CDC), USA has stated evidence which suggests that pregnancies exposed to shortwave diathermy did not appear to be at increased risk of miscarriage. Though prolonged static exposure of SWD or MWD (as is possible in a working clinical physiotherapist or technician) can lead to low birthweight and/or congenital malformations in the fetus.
- Some guidelines however suggest that thermal and non-thermal SWD should not be applied during pregnancy, over testes in men, and over pelvic regions in menstruating women.

Transcutaneous Electrical Nerve Stimulation

Transcutaneous electrical nerve stimulation (TENS) is a low-voltage electrical current used to activate descending inhibitory systems in the central nervous system to relieve pain. TENS has been used during pregnancy without any side effects seen for either the mother or the child. TENS enhances the blood flow to the placenta. Recently there have been discussions about risk to the fetus by the electrical field produced by the TENS unit.

Indications

- Persistent low back pain, pelvic girdle pain including symphysis pubis dysfunction
- Placental insufficiency to increase placental blood flow.

Uses

- TENS has been reported to provide excellent subjective pain relief and significantly reduced menstrual flow, and clot formation in dysmenorrhea. Conventional TENS with a frequency of 120 Hz and pulse duration of 100 μ second can be applied for a total of 20 minutes daily in ***primary dysmenorrhea***. Analgesia following application of TENS in dysmenorrhea may be a result of reduction of myometrial ischemia which may be seen due to local increase in blood flow or a decrease in oxygen consumption.
- TENS has been used for ***pregnant*** women experiencing ***back pain, sacroiliac joint dysfunction (SIJD) pain, and pelvic girdle pain*** for more than a decade. Exercise therapy should always remain the first choice of treatment for these musculoskeletal problems, but for a pain which does not respond sufficiently to exercise therapy, TENS can be added in the treatment plan. It has been found safe for use in pregnancy and is also found to increase placental blood flow. The suggested dosage for low back pain is continuous waves of stimulation at a frequency of 120 Hz and pulse duration of 100 microseconds, intensity can be as per tolerance threshold. Four, 5-centimeter square surface electrodes can be placed over the painful region. This dosage is suggested for twice weekly sessions for up to 3 weeks, in females who have had no previous diagnosed back pathology or any history of miscarriage nor abortion.
- The European guidelines for diagnosis and treatment of pelvic girdle pain suggest there is no evidence to recommend use of electrotherapy.

Clinical Pointer

In pregnancy the electrodes of TENS should not be placed suprapubically if the mother is thin, i.e. likely to have less than 2.54 cm (one inch) of fat, and the fetus is occiput posterior (OP) in presentation. The treatment for pelvic girdle and spinal pains may be more effective if the electrodes are placed posteriorly over the lumbosacral nerve roots.

- TENS has been found to be safe and effective when given during ***labor***. It is found to be helpful in relieving labor pain and to shorten the duration of the active stage of labor. It has the advantages that:
  - It is non-invasive
  - The mother has a level of control
  - The mother remains fully alert during the birth
  - It has no side-effects.

Use of TENS can be introduced during antenatal classes. A portable TENS device can be given to mother for use during labor. Two electrodes are placed over spinal roots at T10-L1 and the other two electrodes are placed over spinal roots at S2–S4 **(Fig. 17.2)**. Such an arrangement is used, as these roots carry painful information coming from the uterus, cervix and perineal structures. The type of TENS used is a combination of conventional and burst TENS—conventional output being used during the contraction and burst output being used between contractions. Frequency and intensity can be varied by the woman. However, newer reviews suggest that TENS

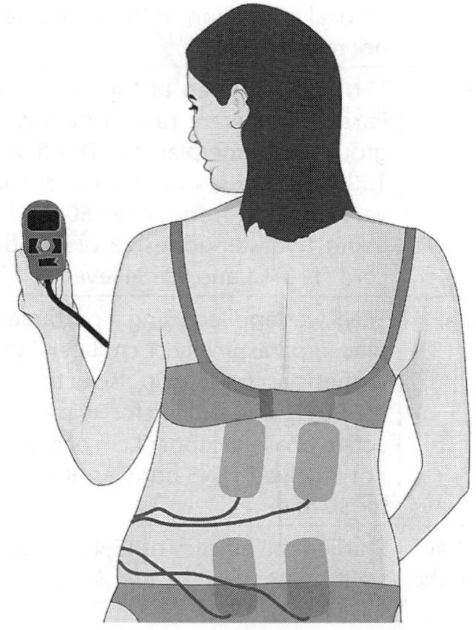

Fig. 17.2: Electrode placement for labor.

is not helpful in reducing labor pain and it has no impact on other outcomes for the mother or the child. **Table 17.1** presents some evidences regarding use of labor TENS.

- TENS is helpful in ***postnatal uterine contraction pain*** and can be given in breastfeeding women. The suggested dosage for this has been a frequency of 100 Hz, a pulse duration of 75 μs and amplitude adjusted to produce a strong and tolerable sensation for 40 min.
- Intravaginal TENS has been recommended for the management of postpartum dyspareunia and vulvar pain in women after vaginal deliveries.

Possible Areas of Concern

- In pregnant women, induction of uterine contractions may occur if TENS is used over certain acupuncture points and labor may be induced. The contractions stop once stimulation is stopped and no teratogenic effects have been seen.

Clinical Pointer

Acupuncture TENS during pregnancy, should be used with caution as it may induce uterine contractions. The machine should be switched off if contractions are induced.

- Induction of changes in development of fetus have not been seen when TENS has been given to patients with placental insufficiency.
- Effects on electrical conduction of fetal heart have not been studied sufficiently.

Clinical Pointer

TENS in pregnancy

The points to keep in mind for safe use of TENS during pregnancy are:

- The depth of fat layer under the electrodes
- Density of the current at the skin (which will decrease by the time it reaches the uterus)
- The position of the baby in utero

Neuromuscular Electrical Stimulation

Some authors suggest that neuromuscular electrical stimulation (NMES) is contraindicated "anywhere" for pregnant women however without evidence and so it may be safe to use if indicated.

Electrical stimulation has been an integral part of pelvic rehabilitation in postnatal women to regain strength and tone of pelvic floor muscles.

Table 17.1: Evidence for labor TENS.

Study details	*Intervention*	*Conclusion*
Samadzadeh et al. (2017)	Pregnant females in the age group of 20–40 years were treated with TENS or Entonox or a combination of both during the first phase of labor.	At cervical dilations of 4–6 and 6–8 cm, the pain was less severe in the combination group. Duration of the first phase of labor was longer in TENS group than the other two groups.
Maryam Rezaeyan et al. (2017)	Pregnant females were randomly divided into two groups—TENS and lidocaine. All participants received 5 cc of local infiltration of 1% lidocaine before episiotomy, and TENS electrodes were placed over acupressure points during the crowning of fetal head for blinding. The TENS group received TENS (100 Hz; 250 μs) from first stage of labor till the completion of episiotomy. The lidocaine group received 10 cc of local infiltration of 1% lidocaine before episiotomy repair and did not receive TENS.	TENS and lidocaine were equally effective in reducing pain at episiotomy cutting and start and end of episiotomy repair. However, lidocaine provided better pain relief during episiotomy repair. TENS provided better pain relief after episiotomy repair and was also better at reducing edema.
Báez-Suárez et al. (2018)	TENS was applied at the beginning of the active phase of labor. Participants were randomly divided into two groups—two TENS groups and one placebo. The first TENS group received TENS using 100-Hz, 100-μs, whereas the second group received TENS using a varying high-frequency (80–100 Hz), 350 μs. TENS was applied using two self-adhesive electrodes placed parallel to the spinal cord (T10–L1 and S2–S4 levels).	The second TENS group showed improvement in pain scores. Participants of both TENS groups were more satisfied than the placebo group. High frequency and high pulse width TENS is effective for relieving labor pain.
Santana LS et al. (2016)	TENS was applied using a portable unit. Two pairs of electrodes were placed paraspinally (1 cm laterally) at T10–L1 and S2–S4. A modified biphasic asymmetric pulse with pulse width of 100 μs and frequency of 100 Hz was applied for 30 minutes starting at the beginning of the active phase of labor (4 cm of cervical dilation). The control group did not received TENS but was attended to by the principal investigator for 30 minutes.	TENS produced a significant decrease in pain during labor and also postponed the need for pharmacological analgesia for pain relief in the postnatal period.
Thuvarakan et al. (2020) (systematic review)	Studied the efficacy of TENS for labor pain control compared to other treatments.	TENS showed significant efficacy in the reduction of labor pain intensity. However, better quality studies using better methods need to be performed.

- **Electrical stimulation** *(ES)* of pelvic floor muscles is commonly used for management of ***urinary incontinence***.
- **Low intensity electrical stimulation** has been useful in cases of ***postpartum incontinence*** for stimulation of the pudendal nerve. Patient position- side lying. Indifferent electrode is placed over lumbosacral region. Vaginal or rectal electrode is lubricated with sterile jelly and inserted into vagina or rectum. If these are unavailable a large button electrode is placed over the urogenital region or the anal region. Select a suitable duration and frequency of surge to obtain a good contraction of the muscles. Slowly increase the intensity to obtain a strong contraction. The muscles of the pelvic floor are thin and fatigue easily. So the treatment time is kept short up to 15–20 contractions at a time
- ES is useful in urinary incontinence as it increases the strength of pelvic muscle fibers with rapid contraction. ES can be given using transvaginal or transrectal (males) application, depending on gender. **Transvaginal electrical stimulation** (TVES) is commonly used for management of urinary incontinence in females **(Fig. 17.3)**. It is an invasive application of electrical current using a sensor with electrodes placed in the vagina to directly stimulate the pelvic floor muscles to contract and relax. Stimulation may help strengthen the muscles and ease ***stress urinary incontinence*** (SUI) and can also help control urgency by acting on the nerves and decreasing bladder irritability. Recommended dosage is 20–50 Hz for SUI. ES can be given transvaginally daily for 15–30 min at the maximum intensity individually tolerated for a variable period of 4–12 weeks.
- Neuromuscular electrical stimulation (NMES) can increase peak flow velocity in popliteal vein, improve blood flow, decrease venous stasis and assist in improving symptoms and quality of life in women with postpartum ***varicose veins***.

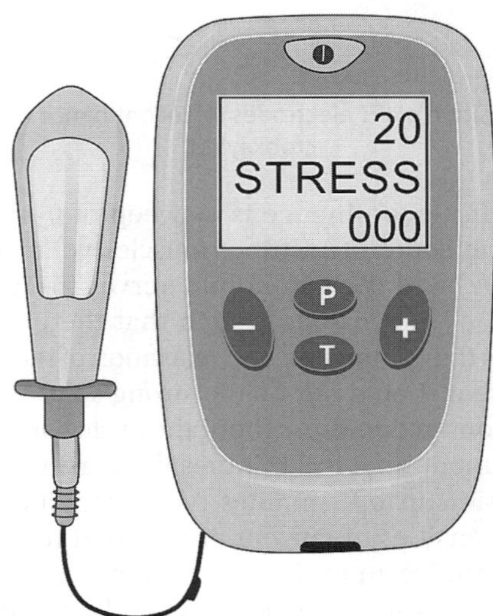

Fig. 17.3: Electrical stimulator with transvaginal electrode for stress urinary incontinence.

- **Percutaneous tibial nerve stimulation** (PTNS) has shown to decrease pain and improve quality of life in women with ***chronic pelvic pain***. It is a minimally invasive technique.
- **Electropuncture** can be also used for ***chronic pelvic pain***.
- **Sacral nerve stimulation** (SNS) and percutaneous tibial nerve stimulation can be used for ***fecal incontinence***. Studies show SNS is better than PTNS to improve functional outcomes and quality of life. Adverse events included pain at site of the implanted pulse generator, tingling in vaginal region, wound infection, hematoma, and urological events.
- Newer technological advancements have resulted in the development of a **medical chair device** that can be used for non-invasive electromagnetic ***stimulation of the pelvic floor muscles*** and is being used to treat urinary incontinence in both males and females **(Figs. 17.4A and B)**. It tightens the pelvic floor muscles and improves blood flow. It is also helpful in improving sexual dysfunction in males and females. The chair provides approximately 12,000 supramaximal pelvic floor contractions in 28 minutes. A typical treatment session lasts for 30 minutes and the regime lasts for 6 sessions, scheduled twice a week. The advantage is that a large number of contractions can be obtained in a short time and there is no invasion of privacy of the patient as they sit fully clothed on the chair. The chair uses high-intensity focused electromagnetic (HIFEM) technology to produce contraction of the pelvic floor muscles. It differs from regular Kegel exercises in the frequency of contractions. The frequency is so high that it provides less time to the muscles to relax and thereby strengthens them more. Performing regular Kegel exercises can be rather boring for the patient, thereby reducing the compliance, which is not a problem with the medical chair device.

Clinical Pointer

Electrical stimulation

- Avoid any kind of electrical stimulation over the back, abdomen or pelvis during pregnancy especially over acupuncture points.
- Stimulation near reproductive organs or genitalia needs special training and should otherwise be avoided.
- ES should be avoided over swollen or infected areas in the presence of varicose veins, phlebitis.

Interferential Current

Interferential current (IFC) or interferential therapy (IFT) is a medium frequency current that leads to pain relief, stimulation of skeletal and smooth muscles and stimulation of sympathetic and parasympathetic nerves.

- IFT has been found to be effective in relieving symptoms of ***primary dysmenorrhea*** such as low back pain and referred lower limb pain. Menstrual pain lasting 24–48 hours is found to be reduced in duration and intensity. The suggested dosage for IFC is frequencies of 0–100 Hz and 90–100 pulses/second (10 minutes each), to increase

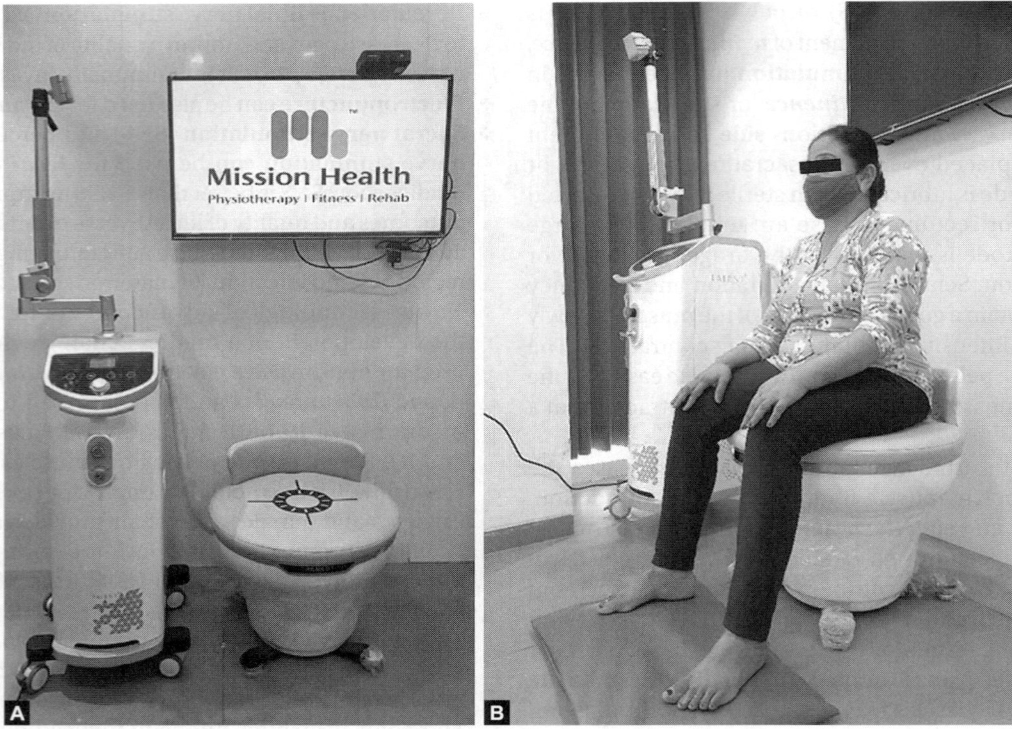

Figs. 17.4A and B: Chair device for pelvic floor stimulation. (*Courtesy:* Mission Health).

circulation (0–100 pulses/second) and to have a sedative effect respectively.

- People having ***urge incontinence, overactive bladder syndrome*** are often treated with Interferential Current therapy (IFC). The frequency needs to be progressively increased over the first six sessions (twice a week), starting with a frequency of 5,500 Hz and finally at the frequency of 7,500 Hz. This treatment dosage has been found to be effective in reducing feelings of incomplete bladder voiding, feeling of urgency and nocturia.
- Patient is treated in the crook lying position **(Fig. 17.5)**. Elderly patients can be treated seated in a wheel chair itself. Vacuum electrodes are used. If unavailable, plate electrodes can be used. Electrodes are placed - 2 on the lower abdomen just above the outer half of the inguinal ligament; the other two electrodes are placed on the upper part of the inner aspect of the thigh, close to the origin of hip adductors **(Fig. 17.5)**. The crossing of the current should take place at the urethral sphincter.
- IFT and ES are useful in incontinence with sphincter weakness, but not for anatomical (unrepaired injuries) or psychological (nocturnal enuresis) causes. IFT stimulates the unstriped muscles. **Table 17.2** shows the differences between use of SF and IFT for incontinence.
- IFT can also be used to treat ***fecal incontinence.*** To stimulate the anal sphincter, the lower electrodes are placed more anteriorly and the upper electrodes are placed over the sacroiliac joints. The crossing of the currents thus takes place in the posterior part of the pelvic floor.

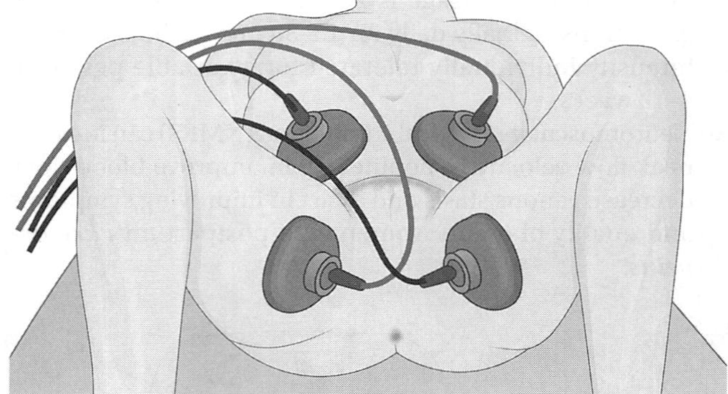

Fig. 17.5: Position of IFT electrodes for incontinence with patient in crook lying.

- **Dosage** for incontinence is a sweep of 0–100 Hz. This allows stimulation of unstriped muscles, voluntary muscles (10–50 Hz) and the autonomic nerves (5–100 Hz). The intensity of the current is such that the patient barely perceives the contraction and relaxation of the pelvic floor. The current should not be too strong so as to produce a tetanic contraction throughout the cycle. On the first day the treatment time is 8 minutes, increasing a minute in each session up to 15 minutes. As the condition improves, lower intensities of current are needed to produce the contraction. Treatment is given 2–3 times/week, otherwise it leads to fatigue. 12 sessions should be sufficient. Older patients may need a second course of sessions after an interval of 2–4 weeks.

Table 17.2: Differences between use of SF and IFT for incontinence.

Surged Faradic (SF) or electrical stimulation (ES)	***Interferential therapy***
Treatment uses low frequency current	Treatment uses medium frequency currents to produce a low frequency current
Sensation may be uncomfortable	Sensation is comfortable
Direct stimulation of pelvic floor muscles	Electrodes are placed over the abdomen and on thighs, so that low frequency current is produced by interference over the pelvic floor
Treatment is with fixed number of contractions per day—10–15 stimulations per session; can be treated on daily basis	Treatment is for a fixed time and so may cause fatigue of the muscles; patient is called on alternate days with a rest day in between
The treatment needs active participation of the patient for re-education purposes to contract the muscles along with stimulation	**Advantage:** Does not require the patient to contract the muscles during treatment. Thus, the treatment is effective even when the patient is unwilling to perform any voluntary exercises—especially if painful
Influences the sphincter indirectly by stimulation of striped muscles of the pelvic floor	Influences both, the unstriped and striped muscles directly

- IFT can be initiated as soon as difficulty in continence is experienced postpartum. It also helps increase circulation and healing and so can be used for ***bruised perineum***. The position of patient and electrodes is same as above. But since patient has pain, a 10 minute constant 130 Hz treatment is given. This can be followed by a 10 minute sweep of 50–100 Hz working up to 10–100 Hz to decrease the swelling. Treatment for bruising is given daily.

Clinical Pointer

The advantage of IFT is that the electrodes are placed at a place away from the perineum.
- This reduces likelihood of pain or infection.
- The presence of sutures or clips at the site do not come in the way of treatment.
- The patient can wear normal protective clothing or pad during treatment.

IFT can also be given for incontinence in males, following prostatectomy and for relief of non-specific prostatitis.

Diadynamic Currents

Recent literature suggests that diadynamic currents are often more effective in pain-relief for ***primary dysmenorrhea*** and are found to improve the quality of life, by reduction in menstrual cramps, back pain and fatigue. The diadynamic currents can be given for a duration of 20 mins, for a frequency of 50–100 Hz and the pulse duration of 10 milliseconds for 5 days during the menstruation.

Low Level Laser Therapy

Low level laser therapy—LLLT has been found to be effective in relieving pain and symptoms of paresthesia of ***carpal tunnel syndrome*** during pregnancy.

Clinical Pointer

Avoid LLLT over the pelvis, low back and abdomen during first 35 weeks of pregnancy and the testes in men.

Pulsed Electromagnetic Field

Pulsed electromagnetic field (PEMF) has been suggested as an adjunct or complementary therapy for the management of ***chronic pelvic pain*** due to interstitial cystitis/bladder pain syndrome. However, further research is still ongoing to conclude any effects.

Therapeutic Ultrasound

- Ultrasound (US) can be used in pregnant women with ***carpal tunnel syndrome***, but care should be taken about the placement of the hand being treated, i.e., the affected hand should be placed away from the womb and ultrasound should be given with proper precautions or avoided if in doubt of putting the woman at risk.
- Therapeutic ultrasound decreases pain and swelling post vaginal delivery and can improve the ***healing of the pelvic floor***. Ultrasound leads to improvement in pain and quality of life in postpartum dyspareunia.
- Therapeutic ultrasound can also relieve symptoms related to ***chronic pelvic pain*** and ***adhesions due to endometriosis***. Recommended dosage parameters are: frequency 1 MHz; mode—continuous; intensity—1.5 W/cm^2; at each site. Therapeutic ultrasound increases the subcutaneous tissue temperature, decreases the nerve conduction velocity, activates the pain gate mechanism, acts as a proinflammatory agent, improves local blood flow, increases extensibility of collagen bands and breaks down adhesions.

Clinical Pointer

Ultrasound
- Pregnancy—continuous or pulsed US should not be used over back, abdomen, pelvis or uterus. High intensity—low frequency waves in continuous mode are potentially most harmful because of their depth of penetration and heating effect
- Reproductive organs—continuous or pulsed US should not be used directly over reproductive organs

Intermittent Pneumatic Compression

Intermittent pneumatic compression (IPC) is recommended for management of ***varicose veins*** and its associated symptoms such as leg cramps, edema, pain, feeling of heaviness in leg and paresthesia. External pneumatic compression appears to reduce ankle swelling. A suggested dosage of 30 minutes of IPC for 2 weeks has been reported to reduce edema and produce a reduction in feeling of heaviness and visible varicosities (*refer* **Fig. 29.8**).

Hydrotherapy

- Hydrotherapy uses water temperature to cause positive effects. It can be used as ice, heat or contrast methods.
- Hydrotherapy is suggested in postpartum women to promote ***relaxation***, reduce pain and muscle spasm.

Biofeedback

Biofeedback and electrical stimulation have been found to be helpful to train pelvic floor muscles in the postnatal phase.

- **Surface electromyographic (sEMG) assisted biofeedback training** is a highly recommended management strategy for ***incontinence***. Biofeedback is useful to promote correct control of contraction and visualization, because many women cannot at first contract their pelvic floor muscles and require some type of motivation. Extensive patient education is required prior to initiating biofeedback.
- ***Obstetrical anal sphincter injuries*** (OASI), formerly referred to as "complete" or "incomplete" perineal tears, are a frequent complication in postnatal women. Intra-anal electromyographic biofeedback therapy has been suggested to improve continence and quality of life in women with altered fecal continence after delivery. The electrical stimulation of the anal sphincter can be done as per tolerance of the patient.
- EMG biofeedback along with the Kegel perineometer can be used to provide feedback to relax the pelvic floor muscles to relieve pain for ***hypertonic pelvic floor***.

Table 17.3 provides evidences for electrophysical agents in women's health.

Table 17.3: Evidence for electrophysical agents in women's health.

Modality	*Study details*	*Intervention*	*Conclusion*
Ultrasound	Dan Wang et al. (2013)	Participants in the experimental group received low-intensity ultrasound therapy for 30 min/day, daily for 3 consecutive days after cesarean section. The control group received no particular treatments.	Ultrasound group showed greater descent of the uterine fundus with higher rate of vaginal bleeding cessation than the control group at 30 days postpartum. The ratio of incomplete uterine involution was significantly lesser in the ultrasound group than in the control group.
TENS	Mehendale P et al. (2018)	Subjects received either acupuncture TENS (frequency 2 Hz) or conventional TENS (frequency 120 Hz) twice a day for 15 minutes each post-LSCS (lower segment cesarean section). Four electrodes were placed in crossed pattern—two above and two below suture site. The control group received no TENS.	TENS is better than no treatment and both—acupuncture and conventional TENS, are equally effective in reducing post LSCS incision pain.
ES	Stewart F et al. (2017)	Systemic review about electrical stimulation (ES) with non-implanted devices to improve pelvic floor muscle function and reduce involuntary urine loss.	Electrical stimulation is probably more effective than no active or sham treatment for stress urinary incontinence. It improves quality of life of subjects with incontinence.
ES	Bae et al. (2019)	Low frequency intravaginal electrical stimulation was given as home-care treatment to women suffering from urinary incontinence for 12-minute sessions, twice daily for 8 weeks. Along with ES, hyperthermic conditions of 35°C to 40°C and microvibrations were administered.	8 weeks of treatment significantly improved the quality of life, health and incontinence.
ES	Xu Han et al. (2022)	Systemic review about studies evaluating the effect of ES on urinary incontinence.	ES provides short-term reduction in urine leakage and long-term reduction in frequency of incontinence episodes.
Biofeedback with Faradic electrical stimulation	Elshatby et al. (2021)	The patients were randomly divided into three groups. Group I received biofeedback-assisted pelvic floor muscle training and faradic electrical stimulation, group II received posterior tibial neuromodulation, and group III received anogenital neuromodulation.	All three techniques are equally effective in treatment of mixed urinary incontinence.

Contd...

Contd...

Modality	*Study details*	*Intervention*	*Conclusion*
IFT	Patitapaban et al. (2020)	Females having stress urinary incontinence were divided randomly into two groups. Group 1 received Kegel exercises, interferential therapy (output intensity 0–90 mA, frequency channel I 4,000–4,250 Hz, channel II 4,000 Hz constant, base 0–100 Hz, Spectrum 0–150 Hz) and transversus abdominis strengthening; Group 2 received Kegel exercise and transversus abdominis strengthening for 5 days/week for 4 weeks.	Both groups showed significant improvement in stress urinary incontinence.
ES	Constantinos Similli et al. (2018)	Systematic review and meta-analysis studying literature on sacral nerve stimulation versus percutaneous tibial nerve stimulation for fecal incontinence.	Sacral nerve stimulation results in significantly improved functional outcomes and quality of life compared to percutaneous tibial nerve stimulation.
TENS	Arik M et al. (2022)	Systematic review and meta-analysis studying literature on effect of TENS for pain relief in women with primary dysmenorrhea.	TENS is effective for relieving pain in primary dysmenorrhea.
Heat therapy	Junyoung J et al. (2018)	Systematic review and meta-analysis studying literature on effect of heat therapy for pain relief in primary dysmenorrhea.	Heat therapy is effective in reducing pain in primary dysmenorrhea compared to placebo and analgesic drugs.
Medical chair for urinary incontinence	Józef Babecka (2021)	Six HIFEM sessions (two per week) were given for 28 minutes each.	HIFEM significantly improved incontinence symptoms.
Medical chair for urinary incontinence	Hailparn T (2020)	Females with vulvovaginal issues were treated with radiofrequency for 3 sessions 4–6 weeks apart.	It improved female sexual health, urinary symptoms, dryness and associated pain, and cosmetic concerns.

(ES: electrical stimulation; IFT: interferential therapy; LSCS: lower segment cesarean section; SNS: sacral nerve stimulation; PTNS: percutaneous tibial nerve stimulation; PD: primary dysmenorrhea; HIFEM: high performance fossilized electromagnetic field)

Summary

The role of electrotherapy in women is immense, when applied along with therapeutic exercises. Precautions have to be taken while making decisions about the electrophysical agents. Factors to be considered while deciding the electrotherapy modality are—the history of the case—if the female has had any abortion, miscarriage, preterm deliveries, strength and condition of the pelvic floor muscles should be examined properly before applying any form of treatment. When using invasive application of electrodes (such as intravaginal, intrarectal) patient should be properly informed, if possible signed consent should be taken and treatment should be given in the presence of a chaperone.

CLINICAL EXAMPLE

History and Assessment

R is a 37-year-old, mother of two, who reports to a physiotherapy clinic with complaints of a small amount of urine leak, while laughing, running up the stairs and while lifting her 2-year-old. She had assumed the urine leak would go away, following the birth of her child, but the issue has remained, and she wishes to go back to her routine of running 4–8 km thrice a week.

The chief complaints suggest the diagnosis of stress urinary incontinence.

Examination of pelvic floor muscles after taking consent was done and revealed weak muscles. Along with that poor posture and tight back extensors were also documented.

Suggested Management

- Conventional exercise therapy for strengthening pelvic floor muscles and correcting posture
- Patient was told to bring a chaperone with her for electrotherapy management. Options of treatment were explained and transvaginal electrical stimulation was given for 4 weeks daily.
- As the bladder diary showed no episode of urine leak for the last 5 days, electrotherapy was discontinued gradually.

Review Questions

1. Enlist the electrophysical agents that can be used in primary dysmenorrhea.
2. Describe the prenatal impairments and the electrical modalities useful in the management.
3. Explain the role of electrotherapy in postpartum women.
4. Enlist the electrical modalities contraindicated in pregnant women.

Bibliography

1. Arik MI, Kiloatar H, Aslan B, Icelli M. The effect of TENS for pain relief in women with primary dysmenorrhea: A systematic review and meta-analysis. Explore (NY). 2022;18(1):108-13. doi: 10.1016/j.explore.2020.08.005. Epub 2020 Aug 29. PMID: 32917532.
2. Baez-Suarez A, Martin-Castillo E, Garcia-Andujar J, Garcia-Hernandez JA, Quintana-Montesdeoca MP, Loro-Ferrer JF. Evaluation of different doses of transcutaneous nerve stimulation for pain relief during labor: a randomized controlled trial. Trials. 2018;19(1):652. doi: 10.1186/s13063-018-3036-2. PMID: 30477529; PMCID: PMC6258317.
3. Batten M, Stevenson E, Zimmermann D, Isaacs C. Implementation of a hydrotherapy protocol to improve postpartum pain management. J Midwifery Women's Health. 2017;62(5):210-214. DOI:10.1111/jmwh.12580
4. Bedwell C, Dowswell T, Neilson JP, Lavender T. The use of transcutaneous electrical nerve stimulation (TENS) for pain relief in labor: a review of the evidence. Midwifery. 2011;27(5):e141-e148.
5. Brenda S. Interferential Therapy. Wolfe Publishing Limited. London. First Published 1984. Reprinted 1990. ISBN 0723418314.
6. Cameron M. Physical Agents in Rehabilitation. Saunders Elsevier. Publisher Linda Duncan; 2009.
7. Dowswell T, Bedwell C, Lavender T, Neilson JP. Transcutaneous electrical nerve stimulation (TENS) for pain management in labor. Cochrane Database of Systematic Reviews. 2009, Issue 2. Art. No.: CD007214. DOI: 10.1002/14651858.CD007214.pub2. Accessed 21 June 2022.
8. Elshatby NM, Imam MH, Shoukry MS, et al. Pelvic floor rehabilitation in the treatment of mixed urinary incontinence among women. Egypt Rheumatol Rehabil. 2021;48:41. https://doi.org/10.1186/s43166-021-00087-w
9. Gokyildiz S, Kizilkaya Beji N, Yalcin O, Istek A. Effects of percutaneous tibial nerve stimulation therapy on chronic pelvic pain. Gynecol Obstet Invest. 2012;73(2):99-105. doi: 10.1159/000328447. Epub 2012 Jan 20. PMID: 22269443.
10. Han X, Shen H, Chen J, et al. Correction to: Efficacy and safety of electrical stimulation for stress urinary incontinence in women: a systematic review and meta-analysis. Int Urogynecol J. 2022;33:1363. https://doi.org/10.1007/s00192-022-05142-4
11. Hay-Smith EJ. Therapeutic ultrasound for postpartum perineal pain and dyspareunia. Cochrane Database Syst Rev. 2000;1998(2):CD000495. doi: 10.1002/14651858.CD000495. PMID: 10796210; PMCID: PMC7043270.
12. Jo J, Lee SH. Heat therapy for primary dysmenorrhea: A systematic review and meta-analysis of its effects on pain relief and quality of life. Sci Rep. 2018;8:16252. https://doi.org/10.1038/s41598-018-34303-z.
13. Lopez-Liria R, Torres-Alamo L, Vega-Ramirez FA, Garcia-Luengo AV, Aguilar-Parra JM, Trigueros-Ramos R, et al. Efficacy of physiotherapy treatment in primary dysmenorrhea: A systematic review and meta-analysis. Int J Environ Res Public Health.2021;18(15):7832.https://doi.org/10.3390/ijerph18157832.
14. Njogu A, Qin S, Chen Y, et al. The effects of transcutaneous electrical nerve stimulation during the first stage of labor: a randomized controlled trial. BMC Pregnancy Childbirth. 2021;21:164. https://doi.org/10.1186/s12884-021-03625
15. Schreiner L, Santos TG, Souza AB. Nygaard, CC, Silva Filho IG. Electrical stimulation for urinary incontinence in women: A systematic review. Int Braz J Urol. 2013;39:454-64.
16. Simillis C, Lal N, Qiu S, Kontovounisios C, Rasheed S, Tan E, Tekkis PP. Sacral nerve stimulation versus percutaneous tibial nerve stimulation for faecal incontinence: a systematic review and meta-analysis. Int J Colorectal Dis. 2018;33(5):645-48. doi: 10.1007/s00384-018-2976-z. Epub 2018 Feb 22. PMID: 29470730.
17. Starkey C. Therapeutic modalities. FA Davis Company. 4th edition; 2004.
18. Stewart F, Berghmans B, Bo K, Glazener CMA. Electrical stimulation with non-implanted devices for stress urinary incontinence in women. Cochrane Database of Systematic Reviews. 2017;12. Art. No.: CD012390. DOI: 10.1002/14651858.CD012390.pub2. Accessed 28 June 2022.
19. Taskinen H, Kyyronen P, Hemminki K. Effects of ultrasound, short waves, and physical exertion on pregnancy outcome in physiotherapists. J Epidemiol Community Health. 1990;44(3):196-201. doi: 10.1136/jech.44.3.196. PMID: 2273355; PMCID: PMC106064
20. Terlikowski R, Dobrzycka B, Kinalski, M. et al. Transvaginal electrical stimulation with surface—EMG biofeedback in managing stress urinary incontinence in women of premenopausal age: a double blind, placebo-controlled, randomized clinical trial. Int Urogynecol J. 2013;24:1631-38. https://doi.org/10.1007/s00192-013-2071-5.
21. Thaha MA, Abukar AA, Thin NN, Ramsanahie A, Knowles CH. Sacral nerve stimulation for faecal incontinence and constipation in adults. Cochrane Database Syst Rev. 2015;(8):CD004464. doi: 10.1002/14651858.CD004464.pub3. PMID: 26299888.
22. Thuvarakan K, Zimmermann H, Mikkelsen MK, Gazerani P. Transcutaneous Electrical Nerve Stimulation As A Pain-Relieving Approach in Labor Pain: A Systematic Review and Meta-Analysis of Randomized Controlled Trials. Neuromodulation: Technology at the Neural Interface. 2020. doi:10.1111/ner.13221
23. Walling HW. Some of the Uses of Electricity in Gynaecology, Am Gynecol Obstet J. 1901;18:122-28.
24. Walsh DM, McAdams ET. TENS: Clinical Applications and Related Theory. Churchill Livingstone; 1997.

Multiple Choice Questions (MCQs)

To test your understanding and recall of key concepts.

1. Which condition is *not* an indication for the use of electrophysical agents in women's health?

A. Primary dysmenorrhea B. Pelvic pain
C. Chronic hypertension D. Incontinence

2. TENS is considered as a safe electrical modality for management of certain conditions during pregnancy because_____________.

A. It stimulates fetal growth and development
B. It bypasses systemic effects and avoids harm to the fetus
C. It eliminates the need for exercise therapy
D. It permanently cures all musculoskeletal issues

3. A postpartum woman complains of dyspareunia and mild incontinence. Which electrophysical agent would most likely be prescribed as part of her treatment plan?

A. Interferential current therapy
B. Therapeutic ultrasound
C. Transvaginal electrical stimulation
D. Pulsed electromagnetic field therapy

4. **TENS differs from interferential therapy (IFT) in the management of pain and incontinence because_____.**
   A. TENS uses high-frequency currents while IFT uses medium frequency currents
   B. TENS targets localized superficial tissues, while IFT can penetrate deeper tissues
   C. IFT is invasive, while TENS is strictly non-invasive
   D. TENS has no harmful effects, whereas IFT has side effects

5. **A clinician decides against using short-wave diathermy (SWD) in a pregnant woman with pelvic girdle pain. Which of the following most justifies this decision?**
   A. SWD's heating effects may lead to fetal hyperthermia and developmental defects
   B. SWD is less effective than conventional TENS in managing musculoskeletal pain
   C. SWD is a very expensive modality
   D. SWD is contraindicated for all gynecological complaints

5. **While designing an electrotherapy protocol for a post-menopausal woman with mixed urinary incontinence, which combination of modalities and techniques would be best suited to address her condition?**
   A. TENS for pelvic floor strengthening, biofeedback for muscle retraining, and therapeutic ultrasound for pain relief
   B. Neuromuscular electrical stimulation (NMES) to improve pelvic floor tone, IFT for sphincter stimulation, and biofeedback to monitor progress
   C. Pulsed electromagnetic therapy for bladder irritability, infrared heat therapy for relaxation, and sacral nerve stimulation for urgency control
   D. Transvaginal laser therapy for muscle contractility, diadynamic currents for pain reduction, and cryotherapy for muscle relaxation

ANSWERS

1. C	2. B	3. C	4. B	5. B

Chapter 18

Barriers in Health Seeking Behavior Among Women

Daxa Mishra

LEARNING OBJECTIVES

At the end of the chapter, the reader will be able to:
- Understand the importance of the role of women in society and her health.
- Understand the influence of gender difference on health.
- Know the various factors influencing women's health.
- Know the structural, financial and sociocultural barriers affecting women's health.
- Know the possible measures to be taken for promoting health of women.

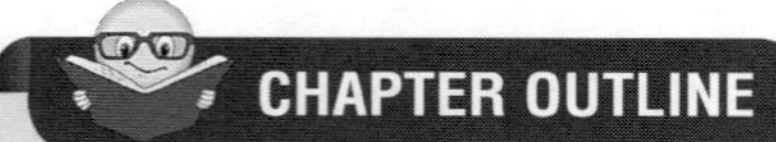

INTRODUCTION

Women's health is important as it determines the health of future generation. When we compare women's health with that of men, there is a paradox as there are significant physiological and behavioral differences between these two sexes that affect the overall health. There is a major gap found in the way disease and illness affect women and women's health trends. This is because of biological difference and influence of hormones amongst them.

Though a woman lives few years more as compared to her male counterpart, she visits a doctor more frequently, spends more days with disability (more disability days), has higher number of illnesses and procures more use of health services. This is not merely due to her biology but lot many other factors which influence her health either directly or indirectly such as society, the culture and the environment in which she lives, social values and attitude, economic status, participation in occupation, policies, family support and interaction with healthcare system.

This illustrates that women's health is achieved not merely by treating disease, but also through advocacy and action at the individual, community, state, national and international levels.

BARRIERS FACED BY WOMEN

Unfortunately, for long, women's health has been linked to problems related to motherhood. Maternal mortality is considered as a parameter of her problem and in countries like India it was the indicator of country's development. In spite of larger efforts from the government side towards pregnancy related issues, the utility of this care is lagging behind. It has been found that low proportion of women are utilizing the benefits of the government schemes and services. This may be because of low literacy, lack of awareness and inability to identify the dangers related to pregnancy and delay in making a decision regarding when to seek treatment. This may lead to increase in maternal morbidity and mortality. Malnutrition during younger age and during child-bearing age also increase the mortality and most women do not have knowledge about it. Moreover it has been found that very few women are recommended the antenatal care visits by the medical practitioners. Unfortunately, for long, very little attention was given to gynecological problems in non-pregnant women, even though the reproductive morbidities occur far more frequently and affects woman's life. In India, almost 39% of currently married women report at least one reproductive health problem related to infertility, vaginal discharge, and sexual problems like dyspareunia apart from menstrual problems. In medical practice also, most of the time women's health was considered as synonymous to her reproductive health.

Over time, due to increase in life expectancy, the leading cause of mortality has shifted away from infectious conditions to chronic conditions like cardiac diseases, cancer, diabetes, stroke, and other lifestyle disorders (noncommunicable diseases). Though these conditions are common in men and women, women will have different experiences.

RURAL-URBAN DIVIDE IN HEALTH SEEKING BEHAVIOR

Rural Women

- In spite of a positive move in women's health issues like improvement in access to care, improved surveillance, education and equal right opportunities, their role is overlooked especially in rural regions and they are still viewed as an economic burden. Though India is emerging as a developing country, majority of its population lives in villages and women in rural India often prioritize family roles over personal health. This dynamic interplay of social and environmental factors has profound and multifaceted societal implications on women's health.
- In India, still literacy rate of women is lower as compared to men but if it comes to working population, large percentage of women work in India but they are paid less. This is mainly seen in rural India or in urban slum regions of India. In rural India, 89.5% of labour force is contributed by females **(Fig. 18.1)**.
- Economic disadvantage has a strong association with health disadvantage. Due to widening of economic gap between men and women, more women are living in poverty and face frequent illness due to malnutrition, poor living conditions, high level of stress etc. If they lose their job due to sickness, vicious cycle sets in **(Fig. 18.2)**. Rural women still have little autonomy and they live under the control of their fathers initially, then their husbands and finally their sons.

Urban Women

- In urban India, women participation in paid workforce is impressive in numbers. Women of urban India, though comparatively less in number, legally have equal rights with men and enjoy parity with their male counterparts in terms of wages and roles, but working women are not adequately protected from exploitation. Insecurity has compelled majority of them to accept an inferior status.

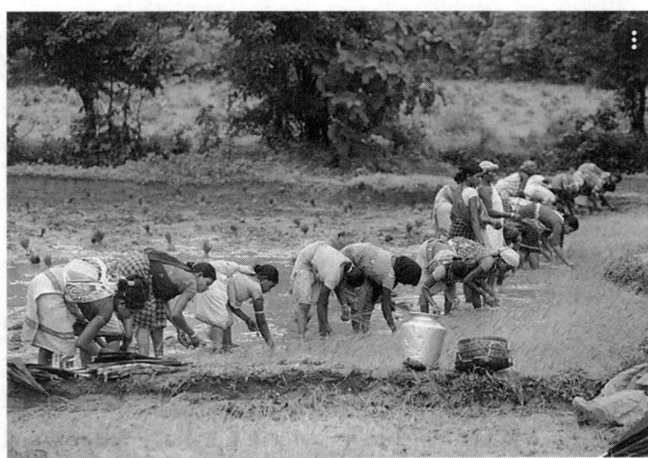

Fig. 18.1: Females involved in labor work.

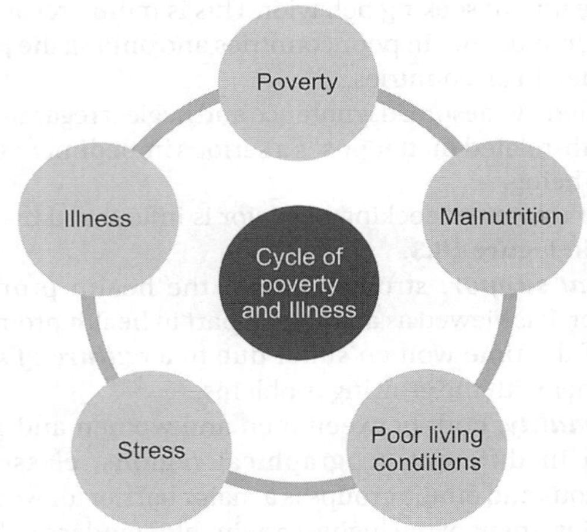

Fig. 18.2: Cycle of poverty and illness.

- Women's equality in terms of education, employment and power is still an individual rather than a Universal achievement.
- As the average life expectancy of women across the globe has increased, it is essential to provide them with good quality of life without much disability. It is important, therefore, that a comprehensive healthcare plan be implemented to alleviate the symptoms and associated morbidities.

HEALTH/TREATMENT SEEKING BEHAVIOR

In the real picture, the health issues which are major impediments to advancing women's health are not even considered and most of them especially gynecological health issues remain under-represented.

- Few of the issues may not be a life threat, but they may cause shame, discomfort and make women lose their self-confidence. Most of the time women may not talk about these problems openly and they keep suffering in silence till the symptoms become severe or life-threatening.

- In routine practice, awareness is lacking among many healthcare professionals and because of that they do not refer them to the concerned health provider. For example, pelvic floor muscle strengthening exercise is the most preferred and first approach in treatment of urinary incontinence, but studies quote that medical practitioners were ignorant about the role of pelvic floor muscle exercise in urinary incontinence.

In addition to this, society's expectation from the women and its negative and dependent behavior towards women, leads to negative mental health and depression.

- Though the society has progressed considerably over past two decades and the Indian constitution has granted equal rights to women, she is still caged in strong patriarchal traditions and customs which persist in many societal parts and is creating a big barrier in their health seeking or treatment seeking behavior. This is more prevalent not only in India but in poor countries and among the poorest women in all countries.
- Women's widespread ignorance and neglect regarding their health-related matter poses a serious impediment to their well-being.

Their treatment seeking behavior is influenced by factors shown in **Figure 18.3**.

Social support strongly affects the health promoting behavior. It is viewed as an integral part in health promotion. Most of the time women suffer due to a ***culture of silence*** within her with the growing problems.

Inequality, both between men and women and among women in different geographical regions, classes and indigenous and ethnic groups is a major barrier for women to the achievement of the highest attainable standard of health. Because of these, health and well-being elude the majority of women.

Barriers also exist because of many ***existing taboos, myths and beliefs*** about sexual and gynecological health which do not allow most of the women to seek treatment. This silence makes delay in diagnosis and sometimes makes their life difficult by hampering their quality of life to a great extent. They are hesitant to undergo internal pelvic examination as they have a feeling of personal intrusion. Non-married women feel it as a violation of their virginity. For procedures like perineometry which is used to assess the strength of pelvic floor muscle, same reluctance is faced because of similar misconception. They feel that they may not be able to conceive, it will affect sexual life or it may lead to permanent damage inside. Lot of guilt, embarrassment and fear are associated with this.

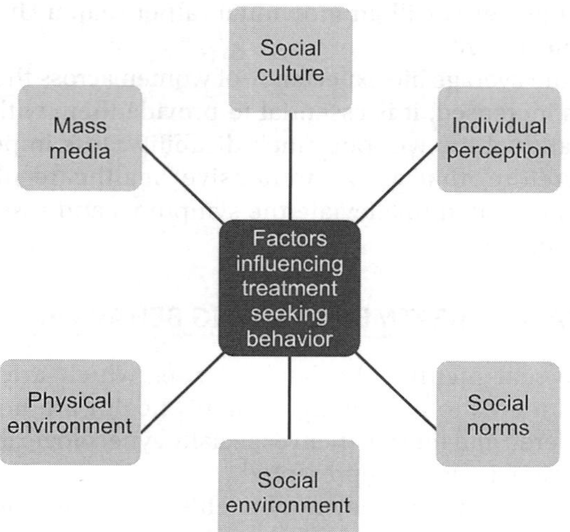

Fig. 18.3: Factors influencing treatment seeking behavior.

Females consider that vaginal discharge, incontinence or abdominal pain is simply because of their fate and so it will not change by seeking any medical help. Being a woman they have to accept it as part of their life. As they do not consider it as a problem, they are ignorant about its remedy.

Even if they seek any treatment most of the time it is from the quack or unqualified persons.

Women are reluctant enough to share or talk about the same even to female members in the family specially to their daughter in law and even to their husband, making them totally ignorant about their health status. However it has been found that villages where the village health workers are available, women prefer to share their problem with them as they are very close to them and regularly communicating regarding their health issues as part of their work task through home visits. They feel comfortable with them for sharing their problems.

Gender issue still exists in consultation. They do not prefer to discuss their problem with male consultants. Examination by them is big 'NO'. Many times it is not only the stigma around the disease but lack of awareness about that condition and accepting it as part of their life, being a woman or due to aging, prevents them from seeking treatment.

Many times, they face non-supportive nature of family members. They have to seek permission from their husband or mother in law for taking any decision. Many women whether they are literate or illiterate do not get time to think about or to take care of their problems. Priority for household chores and lack of time due to household activities are also the reasons for not seeking treatment. Earning for self and family is priority over health.

With regard to their physical fitness, women feel that there is no need to put in extra effort to keep themselves fit as their involvement in household chores is exercise in itself. While doing that if they feel some aches and pain, they take some rest and that is enough. Many women attend fitness center or do regular exercise/yoga at home, but their motto is to look well figured and beautiful to make their presence felt. They are highly influenced by the Bollywood or TV actresses to look good. To attain this look, women especially young women adopt crash dieting without any consultation which affects their health directly. Women who can afford the maids, are busy involved in watching TV shows and social media. They can afford to go to gym but avoid it if they do not find company or feel lazy.

MEASURES TO IMPROVE HEALTH SEEKING BEHAVIOR

Lack of priority towards health, ignorance and inability to protest for their rights, neglect about self and blaming destiny as the cause for the problem are observed. Stigma, myths, misconceptions and various cultural beliefs associated with gynecological problems impose a big hurdle in seeking health care and aggravate the existing condition and forces women to suffer in misery.

To alleviate these issues some measures must be taken at local level as well as centrally. As discussed above, one may conclude that health seeking behavior is actually interplay of ignorance, lack of awareness, motivation as well as sociocultural factors. To meet the unmet needs of good health the women require continuous motivation and multi factorial interventions. But to understand the need, more community-based qualitative research should be conducted to get a deeper insight of health issues, the perceptions about it, existing myths amongst women, especially in rural regions and those who are underprivileged.

Recommendations

- Village health workers should be intensely trained for health education as they are generally successful in changing behavior of family and community. This will help in going a long way in improving health status of rural women.
- The graduates of healthcare profession will have to develop a skill whereby they will include in their routine history-taking of women who are at risk for developing health problems, after gaining sufficient confidence and at the same time maintaining her dignity. This will make them aware about ease of preventing the unbearable suffering.
- Social, medical, cultural and political efforts are required for overall improvement of living as well as literate state of women. Improved literacy level of women has a positive impact on health seeking behavior.
- Their awareness needs to be increased in a culturally appropriate way regarding their health issues, its consequences and its remedies. Primary prevention can be achieved by promoting awareness and education. Efforts should start from their adolescent age during schooling. Middle-aged women can become the source and force for their daughters to incorporate healthy lifestyle changes thereby contributing to making a healthy society.

Till now we have crossed many milestones in promoting good health for women but we have not reached the final destination yet. So, let us join hands in achieving this goal. We being healthcare professionals have to work at all levels and if required we have to approach them at their doorsteps.

'If they don't reach to you, go where they are'

Summary

Women's health is important not only for their sake but also for building a strong society. There is a gender-wise difference in health of women and men due to physiological and hormonal influences which affect their response to any pathology and outcome of its treatment.

Apart from the physiology, the factors like social, cultural, environmental and financial factors have direct impact on the health and its outcomes in women. In low and middle income and developing countries health may get affected due to availability of health centers, the quality of care provided or the distance to be traveled to reach such centers. Low finance and low level of literacy are closely linked to poor health and health seeking behavior in women. In rural villages and in traditionally patriarchal society they do not have the power to take decisions on their own even for their own health.

They feel shy in sharing their problems especially related to reproductive issues and many of them accept it as their fate.

There is a strong need to take a step ahead through conducting more qualitative research and understand the depth of these issues and design and apply appropriate measures to alleviate these issues and provide healthy and respectful life to women.

CLINICAL EXAMPLE

A 34-year-old lady residing in a village has complaint of constant low back pain. She also has white vaginal discharge since 1 month. She lives in a joint family with her husband, two children and her in-laws. Because of her poor financial condition and her illiteracy she has to work in the farm as a laborer to support her family. She feels shy in sharing her discharge problem and has accepted back ache as fate but she feels low and remains irritated because of her problem. After she feels the pain is unbearable she approaches a physiotherapist.

- What will be the approach to help in alleviating her problems?
- Discuss a strategic plan keeping the ICF-based physical and functional diagnosis.

Suggested Management Approach

- While taking initial history from her, one must ensure about her preference of therapist (male/female) and privacy, build up rapport, and take care of her sociocultural background and belief aspect.
- Educate her regarding her problem and its possible correlation with the existing symptoms. Also alleviate any associated stigma. Educate her regarding available management and its benefits.
- Examine her using appropriate steps to differentiate the causative pathology (organic/chemical/mechanical).

- While preparing ICF, apart from impairments and activity limitations due to back pain, contextual factors such as barriers and/or facilitators are important to mention as the effectiveness of treatment and overall health outcome depends on it. For example illiteracy, family support, financial constraints, low self-esteem are barriers, for which educating about health condition and its management, making aware about government policy benefits, building confidence can be attended to.
- For back pain due to musculoskeletal problem, any pain relieving modality with core stability, endurance building and mobility exercises can be prescribed.
- Explain the benefit of modality, its safe use and exercise along with ergonomic care at home and workplace.
- The therapist needs to refer the female to the gynecologist for her vaginal discharge problem after educating her and later along with medication appropriate modality can be used at physiotherapy unit.

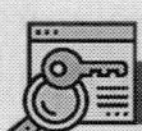

Review Questions

1. Write a brief note on various factors influencing women's health.
2. Enlist the various barriers affecting the health/treatment seeking behaviors in woman. Explain any two in detail.
3. Which are the various approaches we can adopt to improve the health seeking behavior in women?

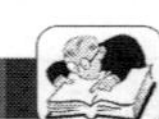

Bibliography

1. Bhanderi MN, Kannan S. Untreated reproductive morbidities among ever married women of slums of Rajkot City, Gujarat: the role of class, distance, provider attitudes, and perceived quality of care. J Urban Health. 2010;87(2):254-63.
2. Gopalakrishnan S, Eashwar VA, Muthulakshmi M. Health-seeking behavior among antenatal and postnatal rural women in Kancheepuram District of Tamil Nadu: A cross-sectional study. J Family Med Prim Care. 2019;8(3):1035.
3. Ismail SA, McCullough A, Guo S, Sharkey A, Harma S, Rutter P. Gender-related differences in care-seeking behavior for newborns: A systematic review of the evidence in South Asia. BMJ Global Health. 2019;4(3):e001309.
4. Kamalapur SM, Reddy S. Women health in India: An analysis. Int Res J Soc Sci. 2013;2(10):11-5.
5. Karne M. Health Seeking Behavior of Women in Urban Areas: Findings from Primary Data.
6. Mishra D, Raithaththa S, Pathak A, Vaishnav S. Treatment Seeking Behavior in Women with Urinary Incontinence: Our Experience in Rural Gujarat, India.
7. Mishra GD, Kumar D, Pathak GA, Vaishnav BS. Challenges encountered in community-based physiotherapy interventions for urinary incontinence among women in rural areas of Anand District of Gujarat, India. Indian J Public Health.2020;64(1):17.
8. Reddy PM, Rineetha T, Sreeharshika D, Jothula KY. Health care seeking behavior among rural women in Telangana: A cross sectional study. J Family Med Prim Care. 2020;9(9):4778.
9. Sajedinejad S, Majdzadeh R, Vedadhir A, Tabatabaei M, Mohammad K. Maternal mortality: a cross-sectional study in global health. Glob Health. 2015;11(1):4.
10. Shaikh BT, Hatcher J. Health seeking behavior and health service utilization in Pakistan: challenging the policymakers. J Public Health. 2005;27(1):49-54.
11. Singh N, Shinde M, Dafal H, Trivedi A, Chouhan Y. Age at natural menopause and factors affecting menopausal age: A cross sectional study among postmenopausal female attendees of obstetrics and gynecology outpatient department. Int J Med Sci Public Health. 2018;7:994-1000.
12. World Health Organization, editor. Women and health: today's evidence tomorrow's agenda. Geneva: World Health Organization. 2009:91.
13. Yadav R, Zaman K, Mishra A, Reddy MM, Shankar P, Yadav P, et al. Health seeking behavior and healthcare utilization in a rural cohort of North India. In Healthcare. 2022;10(5):757. MDPI.

Multiple Choice Questions (MCQs)

To test your understanding and recall of key concepts.

1. Following is identified as a common barrier to health-seeking behavior among women in rural areas_______.

A. High literacy rates
B. Lack of awareness and societal stigma
C. Gender-neutral healthcare policies
D. Proactive family support

2. Economic disadvantage influences a woman's health-seeking behavior because________________.

A. It creates better healthcare opportunities through targeted government schemes
B. It discourages women from prioritizing health due to financial constraints and malnutrition
C. It has no significant impact on health-seeking behavior
D. It promotes independence in seeking medical advice

3. In a rural setting, healthcare professionals identify low literacy and societal norms as barrier for village women to report health issues. They can address these barriers most effectively by________.

A. Offering generalized health education programs for the entire community
B. Ensuring one-on-one counseling with culturally sensitive explanations
C. Referring her to a male gynecologist in the nearest urban clinic
D. Emphasizing the importance of seeking permission from family members

4. In a rural setting, healthcare professionals observe that rural women attribute their chronic pelvic pain to fate and refuse treatment. Which of the following reflects the underlying cause of their behavior?

A. Limited access to healthcare facilities
B. Deep-rooted cultural beliefs and lack of awareness about medical interventions
C. Overdependence on traditional medicine
D. Economic constraints preventing access to healthcare

5. **A community health program identifies that despite free medical camps, attendance of rural women remains low. This could be attributed to_______________.**
   A. Poor quality of services provided at the camps
   B. Irrelevance of the offered treatments to community health needs
   C. Women's lack of autonomy and decision-making power in their families
   D. Excessive travel time to the camp locations

6. **An optimum community-based intervention program to improve health-seeking behavior among women in rural region would include____________.**
   A. Training village health workers, organizing mobile health clinics, and addressing cultural taboos through education
   B. Deploying advanced diagnostic tools, building urban hospitals, and enforcing mandatory health check-ups
   C. Increasing healthcare fees to improve service quality, focusing on individual treatments, and promoting herbal remedies
   D. Distributing health pamphlets, relying on male community leaders, and reducing healthcare staff salaries

ANSWERS

1. B	2. B	3. B	4. B	5. C
6. A				

Section 4

Mother and Childcare

Section Outline

Chapter 19

Pregnancy—Clinical

Pushpa Yadava, Priyasingh Rangey

LEARNING OBJECTIVES

At the end of the chapter, the reader will be able to:

- Understand the physiological changes occurring during pregnancy.
- Gain knowledge regarding the diagnosis of pregnancy.
- Gain knowledge regarding high-risk pregnancy.
- Learn about normal labor and its management.
- Know various types of instrument-assisted deliveries.
- Discuss normal puerperium and its management.
- Describe physiology of lactation.
- Know the role of a physiotherapist during pregnancy and after delivery.

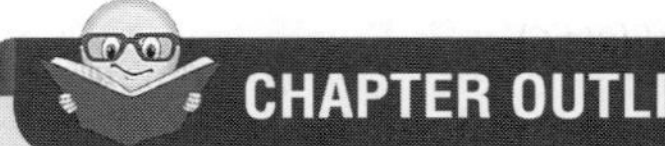

INTRODUCTION

Medicine is an ever-evolving science. Evidence-based obstetrics is the new norm but the foundation pillars of obstetrics such as maternal anatomy and physiology, scheduled antenatal care, labor, delivery and puerperium have had minor changes over the years.

Preconceptional counseling and various imaging techniques have brought the second patient in obstetrics—**the fetus**—in fore front as its well-being can now be detailed in-utero.

The almost 9 months of antenatal period and further 6 weeks of puerperium is a phase of immense changes in women—be it the physical appearance which is outwardly visible or the mental health. Internally majority of organs undergo various changes: anatomical and physiological. Majority of these changes revert back almost to normal once childbirth has occurred.

Even though a physiotherapist's involvement throughout antenatal period is a well-accepted fact in Western world, it still has not permeated deeply here in India. Physiotherapy has a valuable role throughout the antenatal, intranatal and postpartum periods.

Pelvic organ prolapse, urinary incontinence have lifetime risk of requiring surgery of 11%, almost 1/3rd require re-operation, thus a huge number of women suffer

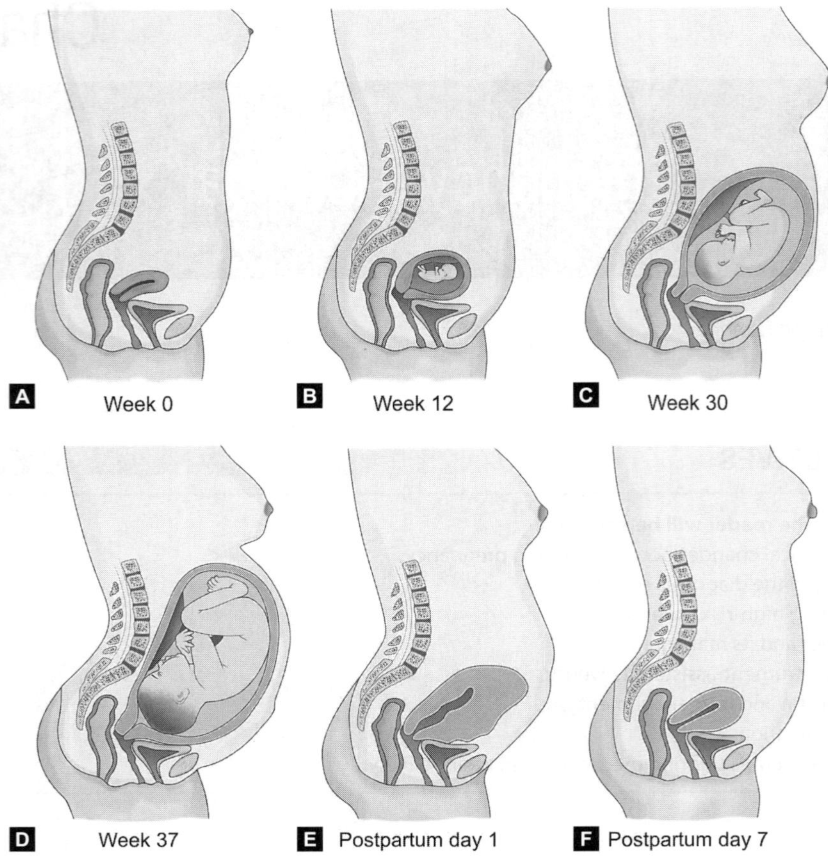

Figs. 19.1A to F: Physical changes with pregnancy *(For color version, see Plate 6)*.

silently with these and other similar conditions, which are not life-threatening but definitely affect quality of life. Majority of women with urinary incontinence benefit from physiotherapy, and show significant recovery especially if detected and targeted in early stages.

PHYSIOLOGICAL CHANGES IN PREGNANCY

Physical changes during pregnancy are shown in **Figures 19.1A to F**. Changes in the height of the fundus of the uterus at different weeks of gestation are shown in **Figure 19.2**. During pregnancy, women need to bring about postural adaptations to maintain balance as the center of gravity shifts. This depends and varies from person to person as there is difference in muscle strength, joint range, fatiguability, etc. Nearly half of pregnant women report backache. A systematic review of 10 trials recommended aerobic exercises during pregnancy and concluded that regular aerobic exercises improved physical fitness.

In the last trimester due to increased water retention and pedal edema, range of movement is considerably reduced. Fluid retention and increased pressure in the carpal tunnel can lead to carpal tunnel syndrome. Changes in musculoskeletal system both before, during and after pregnancy need physiotherapists. Due to massive changes in body structure a pre-pregnant healthy woman adapts better to these changes, physiotherapists can best judge, assess and advise on physical health before, during and after pregnancy. Women with comorbidities need closer supervision, e.g., diabetic mother needs close monitoring with changes in drugs schedule and well-prepared exercising schedule.

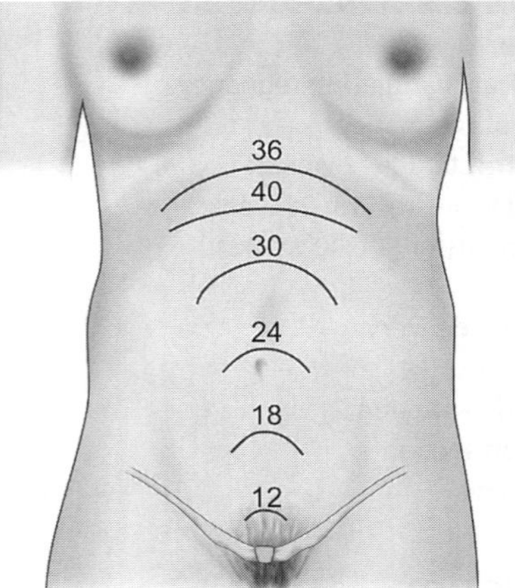

Fig. 19.2: Height of fundus at different weeks of gestation.

The changes occurring in pregnancy are mainly due to interplay of four factors:

1. The changes occurring in collagen and involuntary muscles under hormonal regulation
2. Increased blood flow to uterus and kidney as a result of increase in total blood volume

3. The increase in size and displacement from pelvis of the uterus to accommodate growing fetus
4. The changes in center of gravity and posture due to increasing weight during pregnancy.

 **Research Pointer**

Recent studies throw light on effect of exercise during pregnancy. It is advocated that mild to moderate exercise helps maintain physical well-being. The pregnant woman should not do strenuous exercise and supine position should be avoided after 16 weeks of pregnancy. When the pregnant woman assumes supine position, the inferior vena cava is compressed by the gravid uterus, resulting in decreased venous return centrally. This is termed as supine hypotension syndrome or inferior vena cava compression syndrome.

Cardiovascular System

The following changes are seen:

- There is an increase in the ventricular wall mass, cardiac compliance and myocardial contractility. Heart rate and stroke volume increase leading to a 30–50% increase in cardiac output. Most of these changes occur early in the pregnancy. 75% of these changes occur by end of the first trimester. Cardiac output plateaus during 28–32 weeks of pregnancy. The increased cardiac output during the third trimester is due to increase in heart rate.
- Uterine blood flow increases 10-fold whereas renal blood flow increases by 50%. No significant changes occur in the blood flow to the liver or brain.
- With rise in cardiac output, there is decrease in systemic and pulmonary vascular resistances. A decline in blood pressure also occurs early in the pregnancy due to vasodilatory effects of progesterone, prostaglandins and nitric oxide. It rises again later in the pregnancy.
- During second trimester women can feel faint on standing for a long time or on getting up suddenly from lying position which can lead to falls.
- In latter half of pregnancy, uterine weight can compress aorta and inferior vena cava against lumbar spine, may enhance chances of dizziness and unconsciousness.
- A new area of interest is exercising in water but it is important to know about physiological effects of immersion—the different muscle groups that are used and effect on cardiovascular system.

Table 19.1 summarizes the effects of pregnancy on cardiovascular system.

These cardiovascular changes start very early in pregnancy so a physiotherapist who is preparing an exercise program should be aware that similar amount of exercise will produce greater increase in cardiac output in pregnant woman than in non-pregnant one.

Table 19.1: Effects of pregnancy on cardiovascular system.

Variable	*Change*
Heart rate	Increase
Stroke volume	Increase
Cardiac output	Increase (30–50%)
Pulmonary and systemic vascular resistance	Decrease
Colloid osmotic pressure	Decrease
Pulmonary capillary wedge pressure	No significant change
Hemoglobin concentration	Decrease

Respiratory System

- Under the influence of estrogen, the respiratory system undergoes changes like increased vascularity and edema of the upper respiratory mucosa, explaining the increased incidence of epistaxis and rhinitis during pregnancy.
- There is a 30–50% increase in tidal volume, starting early in the pregnancy. No change in respiratory rate occurs, however, the minute ventilation increases by 30–50%. These changes occur due to the influence of progesterone.
- The enlarged uterus and rising fluid levels increase the intra-abdominal pressure, pushing the diaphragm 4–5 cm upwards, resulting in basilar atelectasis, bibasilar alveolar collapse and a 10–20% decrease in functional residual capacity and total lung capacity.
- There is a decline in expiratory reserve volumes and an increase in inspiratory reserve volumes, thereby keeping the vital capacity unchanged.
- The arterial partial pressure of oxygen (PaO_2) increases to 101–105 mm Hg and the partial pressure of carbon dioxide ($PaCO_2$) decreases to 28–31 mm Hg. This occurs due to the increase in minute ventilation.

Gastrointestinal System

The gastrointestinal system is affected during pregnancy.

- Nausea and vomiting need not necessarily be only in morning as its name "morning sickness" suggests, nor be self-limiting by 15–16 weeks of pregnancy. They can lead to maternal dehydration, malnutrition and weight loss leading to high-risk for fetal growth retardation (FGR) and possibly fetal anomalies also.
- Severe, persistent nausea and vomiting during pregnancy is termed as hyperemesis gravidarum (HG) and often requires hospitalization. If left untreated, it may lead to maternal and fetal morbidity.
- Though the exact pathophysiology behind nausea and vomiting is unknown, it is stipulated that it results from metabolic and endocrine factors of placental origin. Higher human chorionic gonadotropin (hCG) levels lead to increased risk of nausea and vomiting. Ovarian hormones—estrogen and progesterone, are also thought to be associated with it.
- There is reduced gastric emptying time, slackness of cardiac sphincter due to hormones.
- The changes in position of stomach and increased intra-abdominal pressure due to increased uterine size may cause gastric reflux.
- Rise in progesterone levels during pregnancy delays gastric emptying and prolongs the small intestine transition time

by 30–50%. This, along with pressure from the gravid uterus and reduced gastric muscle tone of lower esophageal sphincter, results in gastroesophageal reflux.

- Rise in estrogen causes increase in levels of serum cholesterol, thyroid binding globulin, ceruloplasmin, cortisol binding globulin, fibrinogen and other clotting factors.

Nervous System

Water retention may put unusual pressure on nerves especially those enclosed in bony canals or fibrous tissue (e.g., carpal tunnel) ending in neuropraxia. This can be tackled with splints. Some women complain of paresthesia of hand due to increase in the weight of arms secondary to retention of water.

Urinary System

- As pregnancy advances, the bladder becomes an abdominal organ instead of a pelvic organ.
- The urethrovesical angle changes, the smooth muscles of urethra are slightly hypotonic, the supporting fascia and ligaments of the tract and pelvic floor get laxer. These changes lead to urge and stress incontinence.
- Delivery can cause damage to micturition process by damaging sphincter, and can also damage pudendal nerve. Cesarean section does not render full protection.
- There is dilatation of urinary collecting systems, causing urinary stasis (more evident on the right side due to dextrorotation of uterus and right ovarian vein) and making the pregnant female prone to urinary tract infections.
- Renal blood flow and glomerular filtration rate (due to vasodilation of afferent and efferent arterioles) increase by 50%.

Endocrine System

From a physiotherapist perspective, the interplay of progesterone, estrogens and relaxin hormones is of utmost importance as there is increase in joint laxity during pregnancy.

- Amongst the effects of progesterone on different organs its major effect is uterine quiescence, i.e., keeping uterus relaxed.
- Estrogen probably primes receptor sites for relaxin apart from other effect.
- Relaxin causes gradual remodelled modified collagen to be replaced at pelvic joints, joint capsules, cervix, etc., which increases the extensibility and pliability.
- The myometrial activity is inhibited till 28 weeks when Braxton Hicks contractions can be felt by women. This helps in uterine distension, development of additional connective tissue for the muscle fibers.

Other changes include:

- Decreased plasma iodide concentrations lead to enlargement of the thyroid gland in about 15% of the women.
- Due to upregulation of thyroid binding globulin, there is increase in production of thyroid hormones also during pregnancy, resulting in increase in T3 and T4 levels. However, there is a decline in thyroid stimulating hormone (TSH) levels in the first half of pregnancy.

Musculoskeletal System

The joints become lax and joint range changes under hormonal influence. This happens by replacing old collagen fibers with newer ones which have higher water content thus are more pliable. The pregnant woman needs to change her posture as her center of gravity changes. The theory that an increased lumbar lordosis is a result of increase in pelvic tilt has been challenged. Increasing body weight puts more pressure on spine and more torsional strain in joints. These changes increase the chances of tripping, falling and injuries in women.

The abdominal wall distends to accommodate an enlarging uterus. Muscle fibers stretch but the collagen under hormonal influence gives the extra distensibility. Unless a woman uses her hips and knees when picking up things, weight gain in pregnancy will cause difficulty in doing so. Water retention in latter half of pregnancy causes edema in ankles and joints restricting joint movements, as well as causing pressure on nerves. Therefore, the women need to be fit before, during and after pregnancy.

Musculoskeletal disorders during pregnancy

Major anatomical changes during pregnancy occur at pelvic girdle:

- Sacrum is attached to the innominates by strong interosseous and posterior sacroiliac ligaments which stabilize the pelvic girdle. The ventral sacroiliac ligament is not so strong and sustains tears during child birth frequently.
- Upper sacrum has iliolumbar ligament attached to 4th and 5th lumbar vertebra whereas lower sacrum by sacrospinous and sacrotuberous ligament attaches to posterior iliac spines and ischial tuberosities.
- Weight of upper limb and trunk (upper body) is transmitted via sacrum through individual movements by pushing sacral prominence downward and forwards which causes the sacrum to rotate around a transverse axis.
- This causes the ligaments to tighten, bringing the surfaces of ilia closer to sacrum, often this is accelerated by lumbar lordosis as in pregnancy with few adaptations, i.e., the hip and knee get flexed, thoracic kyphosis occurs along with extension of chin causing cervical extension.
- The sacrum slides on the ilia to produce lumbar lordosis. The pelvis as a whole does not cause forward tilt and this altered pelvic tilt may persist if postural adaptations are not corrected postpartum **(Fig. 19.3)**.

During pregnancy the increased levels of estrogen, progesterone and relaxin increase the relaxation at pelvic girdle joints. Breastfeeding lengthens the time taken for the hormones to reach normal levels. In 3–4 months after birth the pelvic girdle returns to pre-pregnancy state. External stabilization may be needed during this period.

Sonography and X-ray reveal various changes of pelvic girdle.

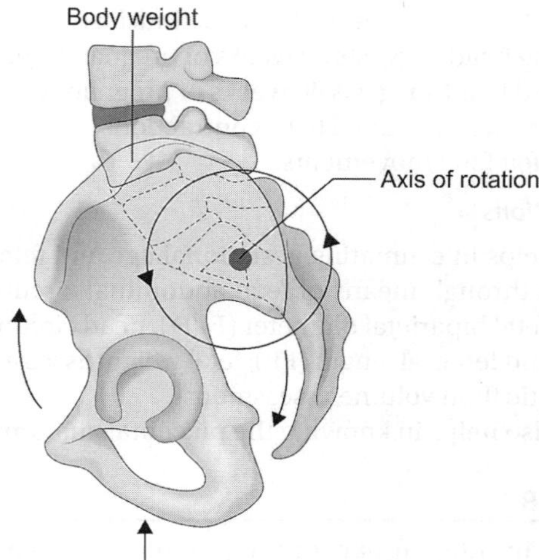

Fig. 19.3: Movement of pelvis.

- Symphysis width of up to 6.3 mm with vertical change of up to 1.8 mm is commonly attained by 35 weeks of pregnancy. Change of up to 1 cm is considered normal. Separation greater than this is thought to be partial or complete rupture, may be up to 12 cm. The gliding of sacrum and ilia give the advantage of increasing pelvic diameter for smooth delivery of baby.
- This occurs to greater extent on squatting, when the area of outlet is increased by almost 28%.

Integumentary System

Hyperpigmentation is seen among 85–90% women, particularly during the second half of pregnancy. The exact mechanism is not understood but it can be attributed to a combination of hormonal influences, genetic factors and ultraviolet exposure. Generalized hyperpigmentation can occur, but the more commonly affected areas include, areolas, nipples, inner thigh, axillae, genitalia and periumbilical area. Darkening of linea alba (linea nigra) occurs. Rare phenomena like Voigt or Futcher lines and Melasma may also occur.

Breast

Breast changes are most significant in primigravida.

Following changes occur in the breast:
- Hyperpigmentation of the areola and nipple
- Enlargement and tenderness of the breast
- Increased prominence of the veins of breast
- Erectile nipples
- Nipple sensitivity
- Enlargement of Montgomery glands
- Occasionally, pregnancy-associated hyperkeratosis of the nipple and areola
- Axillary tail may become enlarged and painful
- Development of secondary areola (outer zone of less marked and irregular pigmented area) usually in the second trimester.

Sticky secretion can be oozed out from the nipples at 12th week, which becomes thick and yellow by 16th week. Colostrum may be expressed in latter months.

DIAGNOSIS OF PREGNANCY

First Trimester (0–12 Weeks)

Subjective Symptoms

- Amenorrhea—cyclic bleeding may occur up to 12 weeks
- Morning sickness—occurs immediately following missed period and may continue up to 16 weeks
- Increased frequency of micturition
- Breast discomfort—feeling of fullness and prickling sensation
- Fatigue.

Objective Signs

- Breast changes—enlargement of breasts with vascular engorgement; nipple and areola become more pigmented. Montgomery's tubercles become prominent and thick yellowish discharge (colostrum) occurs from nipples.
- Uterus may be felt as a suprapubic bulge
- Positive Chadwick's sign—dusky hue of anterior vaginal wall and vestibule at about 8th week of pregnancy due to vascular congestion
- Vaginal signs—softening of vaginal walls, non-irritating mucoid discharge in copious amount occurring at 6th week
- Osiander's sign—increased pulsation felt at the vaginal walls at about 8th week of pregnancy
- Goodell's sign—softening of the cervix occurring at about 6th week
- Uterine signs—enlargement of uterus; pregnant uterus feels soft and elastic
- Hegar's sign—on bimanual examination, the abdominal and vaginal fingers appose below the body of the uterus
- Palmer's sign—bimanual examination elicits regular and rhythmic uterine contraction.

Investigations

Table 19.2 shows the investigations that can be done in the first trimester to confirm pregnancy.

False positive tests may result in women having heterophile antibodies in serum, those getting exogenous hCG injections, having delayed hCG clearance due to renal failure and neoplasms producing hCG.

Table 19.2: Pregnancy tests.

Test	*Inference*
Agglutination inhibition test (Latex test)	Positive if shows no agglutination 2 days after missed period
Direct agglutination test (hCG direct test)	Positive if shows agglutination 2–3 days after missed period
Enzyme-linked immunosorbent assay (ELISA)	Color bands in control and test window Five days before first day of missed period
Fluoroimmunoassay (FIA)	First day of missed period
Radioimmunoassay (RIA)	Detects pregnancy as early as 8–9 days after ovulation

(hCG: human chorionic gonadotropin)

Ultrasonography (USG) can identify the gestational sac as early as 29–35 days of gestation.

Second Trimester (13–28 Weeks)

Subjective Symptoms

- Nausea, vomiting and frequency of micturition subside.
- Quickening—perception of active fetal movements by the pregnant woman; usually felt by 18th week in primigravida and by 16th week in multipara
- Progressive enlargement of lower abdomen.

Objective Signs

- Chloasma—pigmentation over cheeks and forehead
- Breast changes—further enlargement of breasts with veins becoming more prominent beneath the skin; demarcation of secondary areola in primigravidae at around 20th week; Montgomery's tubercles may extend to secondary areola
- Linea nigra becomes visible by 20th week
- Striae gravidarum become visible in the lower abdomen and more towards the flank
- Fundal height is increased—height of uterus is midway between symphysis pubis and umbilicus at 16th week, at the umbilicus at 24th week and at junction of upper 2/3rd and lower 1/3rd of distance between umbilicus and ensiform cartilage at 28th week
- Uterus becomes ovoid in shape and feels soft and elastic
- Braxton Hicks contractions become evident
- Active fetal movements can be felt on palpation by 20th week
- Fetal heart sound (FHS) can be auscultated using ordinary stethoscope between 18–20 weeks (fetal heart rate may vary between 110–160 beats/minute)
- Bluish discoloration of vagina, vulva and cervix becomes even more evident.

Investigations

- Ultrasonography—gestational age can be determined using biparietal diameter (BPD), abdominal circumference (AC), head circumference (HC) and femur length (FL); fetal viability is determined using real-time ultrasound; fetal organ anatomy is also surveyed for any malformation
- Magnetic resonance imaging—used to survey fetal anatomy, biometry and complex malformation.

Third Trimester (29–40 Weeks)

Subjective Symptoms

- Progressive enlargement of abdomen which may cause mechanical discomfort such as palpitation or dyspnea on exertion
- Lightening—relief occurs from the pressure symptoms at around 38 weeks as engagement of presenting part occurs
- Increased frequency of micturition
- More pronounced fetal movements.

Objective Signs

- Cutaneous changes more prominent due to increased pigmentation and striation
- Uterus becomes spherical from cylindrical
- Floating head suggests 32 weeks of pregnancy whereas an engaged head suggests 40 weeks of pregnancy
- More evident Braxton Hicks contractions
- Easily felt fetal movements.

Investigations

- USG helps in estimating gestational age and fetal growth profile through means of fetal abdominal circumference (AC), fetal biparietal diameter (FPD), head circumference (HC) and femoral length (FL); fetal weight assessment and amniotic fluid volume assessment
- USG also helps in knowing the placental anatomy.

LABOR

Labor is an integral part of the pregnancy process which starts at conception and completes after puerperium. In the latter half of pregnancy between 37 to 42 weeks, labor ensues and is completed on delivery of fetus.

Labor has three stages as described in Chapter 21: Labor and Childbirth. Prelabor is a stage where the preparation for labor begins.

- Cervical softening and position of fetus (in 97% it is head down or cephalic) impact the smooth process of labor.
- Labor gets established with rhythmic, gradually intensifying contractions along with cervical dilatation and effacement. Signs of labor include:
  - *Mucoid 'show'* often pinkish in color passed per vaginum. This mucus plug prevents ascending infections whereas its passage at the time of labor indicates its establishment.
  - *Ruptured membranes*: The amniotic sac ruptures with gradual loss of amniotic fluid. If the quantity is more, it requires medical attention as it could lead to umbilical cord prolapse and compression leading to fetal jeopardy.
  - *Contractions*: 'Braxton Hicks' are painless contractions felt in later half of pregnancy and are forerunners to establishing labor contractions.

Labor is said to be triggered due to combination of various factors:

- **Rise in oxytocin levels:** The growing fetus probably stimulates neurogenic reflex from the cervix resulting in release of increased levels of oxytocin from posterior pituitary.
- **Prostaglandin production:** The uterine muscles produce prostaglandins which are metabolized quickly, therefore have predominantly local effects. These contribute to establishment of labor.
- **Fetal adrenal hormone:** These hormones increase prior to labor, cause reduction in progesterone while increasing estrogen production. Rise in estradiol increases prostaglandin production in placenta.
  - Uterine contractions begin at cornual ends of fallopian tubes, spread along fundus and then down towards the isthmus which stretches to form the lower uterine segment.

- The woman coming to labor room undergoes systemic examination and obstetric examination including per vaginum examination. She is carefully monitored along with fetal monitoring for progress of labor with minimal vaginal examination to prevent chances of infections through vagina.
- As fetus descends, it dilates the vagina, stretches the perineum while separating and displacing levator ani muscles. The stretching and thinning of pelvic floor and perineum especially when instruments are used (e.g., forceps and vacuum) can cause pudendal nerve damage resulting in fecal and urinary incontinence.
- Fascia might be overstretched and muscle fibers are torn. Studies have shown that episiotomy does not result in lesser trauma.

Clinical Pointer

- **First stage** of labor is for monitoring maternal and fetal well-being, relief of pain, maintaining fluid balance, etc.
- **Second stage** of labor mandates caring for mother and fetus till delivery of fetus.
- **Third stage** of labor is equally important as delivering placenta correctly ensures that many of the complications of 3rd stage of labor do not occur.

INSTRUMENTAL DELIVERY

Also *see* Chapter 21: Labor and Childbirth.

Forceps

Forceps application may be needed if:
- Progress is slow
- There is fetal jeopardy
- There is a maternal illness or exhaustion
- To deliver a preterm or breech delivery for the after-coming head.

Forceps application requires certain conditions to be fulfilled. It can be done with local, pudendal, spinal or epidural anesthesia.

Forceps can be:
- High cavity forceps (Kielland's)—usually for deep transverse arrest
- Mid cavity and low forceps (Wrigley's)—when head is on perineum.

Vacuum Extraction

Indications for vacuum extraction are same as those of forceps. Instead of metallic blades as in case of forceps a suction cap, now silicon made, is applied on fetal scalp. Vacuum is created to assist in pulling the head along with forceps and uterine contraction. No difference in complications is seen, with either forceps or vacuum extraction.

Cesarean Section

Cesarean section is delivery of fetus through abdominal route. It has low morbidity and mortality as compared to previous years. It has been found that miscarriage, placenta previa and placenta accreta and ectopic pregnancy increase in subsequent pregnancies following cesarean section. Cesarean section is described in more detail in Chapter 23: Cesarean Section.

EPISIOTOMY

Episiotomy involves making a controlled incision in the perineum and posterior vaginal wall to enlarge the vaginal orifice and facilitate difficult deliveries. It reduces the chances of third- and fourth-degree perineal tears **(Table 19.3)** during delivery. It is usually done in the second stage of labor. Also *see* Chapter 21: Labor and Childbirth. Perineal tears is described in more detail in the Chapter 13: Gynecological Conditions: Clinical and Physiotherapy—Part II.

Types of Episiotomies
- Midline
- Modified-median
- Mediolateral
- J-shaped
- Lateral
- Anterior
- Radical

Indications
- In case of rigid perineum
- When perineal tear is anticipated, e.g., large baby, breech delivery or shoulder dystocia
- For operative delivery, e.g., forceps or ventouse delivery
- In case of previous perineal surgery like pelvic floor repair or perineal reconstructive surgery.

Advantages
- Straightens the birth canal
- Facilitates intravaginal manipulation and forceps delivery
- Minimizes compression of fetal head

Complications

Immediate complications:
- Extension of incision to involve the rectum
- Vulval hematoma
- Infection
- Wound dehiscence

Remote complications:
- Dyspareunia
- Perineal lacerations
- Scar endometriosis

Table 19.3: Classification of perineal tears.

Degree	*Tissues involved*
First degree	Vaginal mucosa and perineal skin with no underlying tissue involvement
Second degree	Vaginal mucosa and perineal skin with underlying subcutaneous tissue and perineal muscles
Third degree	Injury to perineum with involvement of anal sphincter musculature
Fourth degree	Extending through the rectal muscle into rectal mucosa

ANTENATAL, INTRANATAL AND POSTNATAL COMPLICATIONS

Table 19.4 shows a list of complications that can occur during pregnancy.

Ectopic Pregnancy

Ectopic pregnancy results due to implantation of an embryo outside the uterus, mostly in the fallopian tubes. Other possible sites include—myometrium, cervix, ovaries, uterine cornea, abdominal cavity, etc. It can lead to rupture of the fallopian tube, causing major internal bleeding. It is associated with a high rate of morbidity and mortality.

Risk factors

- Previous ectopic pregnancy
- History of pelvic inflammatory disease, tubal ligation or any other obstruction leading to fallopian tube damage
- Known history of management of infertility.

Clinical features

- Pelvic pain/discomfort
- Abdominal pain/discomfort
- Nausea
- Vomiting
- Syncope
- Lightheadedness
- Vaginal bleeding

Investigations

- Transvaginal ultrasound imaging
- Serum hCG level measurements
- Diagnostic laparoscopy

Management

- Administration of intramuscular methotrexate—single or double dose depending on the hCG levels.
- Salpingostomy or salpingectomy to remove the ectopic pregnancy surgically.

Anemia

- Hemoglobin (Hb) level below 11 g/dL is labeled as anemia, while it is severe anemia if it lands below 6 g/dL.

Table 19.4: List of complications.

Antenatal	*Intranatal*	*Postnatal*
Early • Ectopic pregnancy • Vesicular mole **Late** • Anemia • Antepartum hemorrhage • Multiple gestations • Pregnancy-induced hypertension • Gestational diabetes	• Cardiac disease • Multiple gestations • Breech presentation • Gestational diabetes • Pregnancy induced hypertension • Cardiac disease • Breech presentation	• Anemia • Cardiac disease • Postpartum hemorrhage • Retained placenta • Inversion of uterus • Gestational diabetes • Pregnancy-induced hypertension • Cardiac disease

- It is the most prevalent disorder in women in reproductive age group.
- Iron deficiency is the commonest though thalassemia, sickle cell anemia and megaloblastic anemia also need to be ruled out.
- Improved nutrition and oral iron preparations normally correct iron deficiency anemia. Some non-compliant patients or those with intolerance to oral iron require parenteral therapy.
- Anemia causes fatigue, breathlessness, increased susceptibility to infections in the mother, intrauterine growth retardation, intrauterine death, abruptio placentae, etc., in the fetus. The intrapartum and postpartum complications also increase due to anemia.
- According to World Health Organization (WHO) and American College of Obstetricians and Gynecologists (ACOG) guidelines, anemia during pregnancy is defined as:
  - First trimester: Hb <11 g/dL
  - Second trimester: Hb <10.5 g/dL
  - Third trimester: Hb <10.5–11 g/dL.

Physiologic anemia of pregnancy

- Physiologic (dilutional) anemia occurs during pregnancy as the plasma volume increases more rapidly than the red blood cell mass.
- It is the commonest cause of anemia in pregnancy but is non-pathologic in nature.
- The hemoglobin values are usually above 10 g/dL.

Antepartum Hemorrhage

Bleeding from genital tract between 24 weeks till birth is antepartum hemorrhage. This can endanger both mother and fetus.

- *Placenta previa* occurs when placenta is implanted in the lower segment near the internal os of the cervix, contractions of the uterus cause separation of placenta resulting in bleeding. If it is self-contained, pregnancy can be carried to term taking care to replace the amount of loss of blood.
- *Abruptio placentae* is more serious and requires termination at any stage of gestation. A normally situated placenta separates, often resulting in fatal consequences for the mother and fetus. Delivery of the fetus is the only way to stop further morbidity and mortality for the mother. Pregnancy-induced hypertension (PIH) and anemia contribute to this complication, though exact cause is still not known.

Multiple Gestations

This is a high-risk pregnancy as there is increased physical and emotional strain on the mother.

- A likelihood of complications like anemia, PIH, eclampsia, fetal growth retardation also increases.
- With the advent of ultrasonography (USG), distinction between monochorionic and dichorionic twins can be made early in pregnancy as the outcome, management, and complications that can occur are totally different, apart from a few common ones. Monochorionic twins

additionally have increased chances of twin-to-twin syndrome, acardiac twins, etc.

Pregnancy-induced Hypertension (PIH)

The rise in blood pressure beyond 140/90 mm Hg after 20 weeks is still the demarcation of PIH. PIH can be broadly classified into—gestational hypertension, preeclampsia and eclampsia. Primary features of PIH are—hypertension, proteinuria and pathologic edema. In about 1 in 1000 deliveries preeclampsia can progress to eclampsia; the pathognomic feature being convulsions. Incidence is 10% of all pregnancies. Definitive cause is yet not known. Among other causes, it is more common in:

- Lower socioeconomic groups
- Primigravidae especially in extremes of age
- Twin pregnancy

Figure 19.4 explains the pathophysiology of PIH.

Preeclampsia affects multiple systems like:

- Kidneys
- Liver
- Brain
- Coagulation system

Delivery of the fetus is the only definitive treatment. Early onset PIH has major effects on mother and fetus. Damage can occur to kidneys, cerebral hemorrhage, and even maternal death. Fetus can have retarded growth, apart from increased chances of intrauterine death.

Management includes:

- Early detection of increase in blood pressure with USG to serially monitor fetal growth
- Medications to optimize blood pressure
- Regular monitored antenatal visits.

Diabetes Mellitus

Women develop impaired glucose tolerance during pregnancy. Mild hyperglycemia of the mother if not treated appropriately with drugs and insulin can affect the fetal outcome. In case of women with family history or a bad obstetric history, diabetic monitoring should start before conception as poor glycemic control in the first trimester has led to congenital anomalies in the fetus.

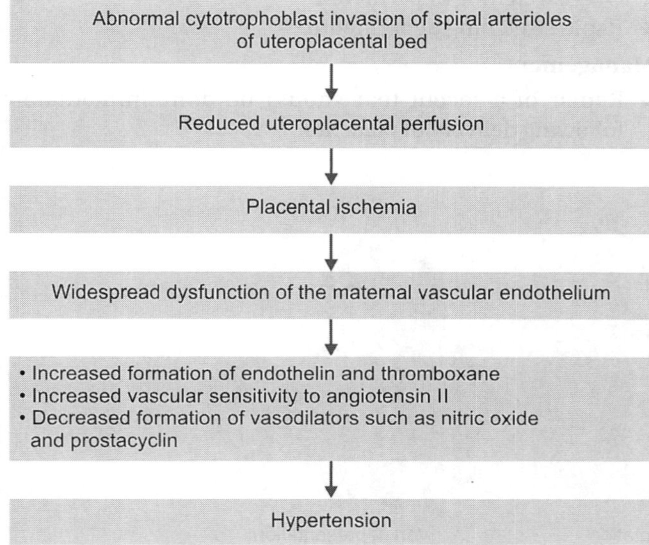

Fig. 19.4: Pathophysiology of PIH.

Gestational diabetes mellitus

Gestational diabetes mellitus (GDM) is severe de novo carbohydrate intolerance during pregnancy. It usually occurs in the second or third trimester.

Risk factors include:

- Family history of diabetes
- Previous birth of overweight child of 4 kg or more
- Previous stillbirth
- Persistent glycosuria
- Age >30 years
- Obesity
- Polyhydramnios or recurrent vaginal candidiasis.

Management:

- Diet with 2,000–2,500 kcal/day for normal weight pregnant female and 1,200–1,800 kcal/day for overweight pregnant female
- Preference of complex carbohydrates over simple carbohydrates
- Self-blood glucose monitoring
- Exercise

Breech

This is the position a fetus may acquire during pregnancy but during the late third trimester, majority of them are in cephalic position. If breech position persists, it may be due to oligohydramnios, fibroids, placenta previa, uterine anomaly, etc.

External cephalic version can be tried between 34–36 weeks but with due consent of the mother. Primigravidae are usually advised cesarean section while multigravida after due assessment can be delivered vaginally. **Box 19.1** lists some other types of fetal presentations.

Apart from these conditions which add risk to pregnancy, few intranatal complications can also occur.

Postpartum Hemorrhage (PPH)

Though few patients are predisposed to PPH and it can be anticipated in certain conditions like—twin pregnancy, elderly primigravidae, grand multipara, polyhydramnios and oxytocin infusion for long time to augment labor. Many a times PPH occurs without warning and tests the preparedness of labor room as well as the promptness and skill of the doctors and nursing staff. The earliest it is handled, especially with blood transfusion, the better is the outcome. Once shock sets in, with various metabolic disturbances, it becomes difficult to reverse the changes.

Retained Placenta

Normally placenta is delivered within 15 minutes of birth of fetus. One can wait till 30 minutes for the delivery of placenta. If signs of placental separation (fresh bleeding and apparent lengthening of umbilical cord) are not seen after 30 minutes

Box 19.1: Types of fetal presentations.

- **Cephalic:** Normal fetal presentation where the head leads **(Fig. 19.5):**
  - *Vertex/crown:* The crown appears first
  - *Sinciput:* Forehead appears first
  - *Brow:* Eyebrows appear first
  - *Face:* Face appears first
  - *Chin:* The chin appears first
- **Shoulder:**
  - Arm
  - Shoulder
  - Trunk
- **Breech (Fig. 19.6):**
  - *Complete/flexed breech:* Fetal legs are flexed at hips and knees and fetus appears to be sitting cross legged
  - *Frank/extended breech:* Fetal legs are up near the abdomen, knees are extended and feet lie close to the ears; most common type of breech presentation
  - *Footling breech:* Feet appear first
  - *Kneeling breech:* Knees appear first
  - *Compound:* When any other body part accompanies the head

then patient should be prepared and shifted to the operation theatre for manual removal of placenta under deep general anesthesia. This procedure requires experts—anesthetists and obstetricians.

Inversion of Uterus

This is again a complication that can occur post fetal delivery. If the umbilical cord is pulled prior to separation of placenta, the uterus is inverted and comes in the vagina, this can cause neurogenic shock as well as hemorrhagic shock.

Immediate replacement and correction of uterus can be done. The same can be tried in 24 hours. But if time lapses more than this period it requires operative intervention to correct inversion. Sometimes surgery is delayed for 2–3 months, so that complete involution of uterus occurs prior to surgery. This predisposes the inner uterine surface to infection as it lies exposed in the vagina. Both morbidity and mortality are increased in all these complications which are definitely avoidable if the third stage of labor is properly managed.

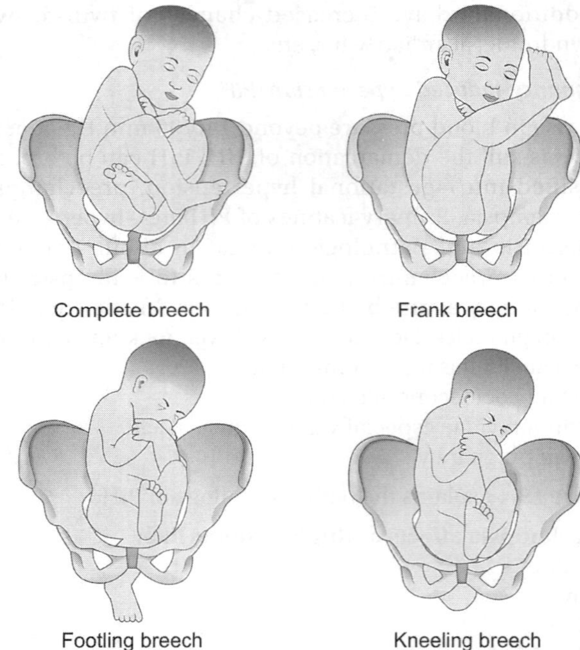

Fig. 19.6: Types of breech presentation.

Maternal Obstetric Injuries

Vulval injuries

Lacerations can occur in the vulva posteriorly and paraurethral tear on the inner aspect of labia minora may be associated with brisk hemorrhage. It should be repaired immediately using sutures after placing urethral catheter to prevent injury to the urethra.

Perineal injuries

Minor injuries (first and second degree) are common during first delivery. Major injuries (third and fourth degrees) occur due to mismanagement of second stage of labor.

Causes

- Over-stretching of perineum
- Rapid stretching of perineum

Management

- Repair of a recent tear should be done immediately following delivery of placenta.

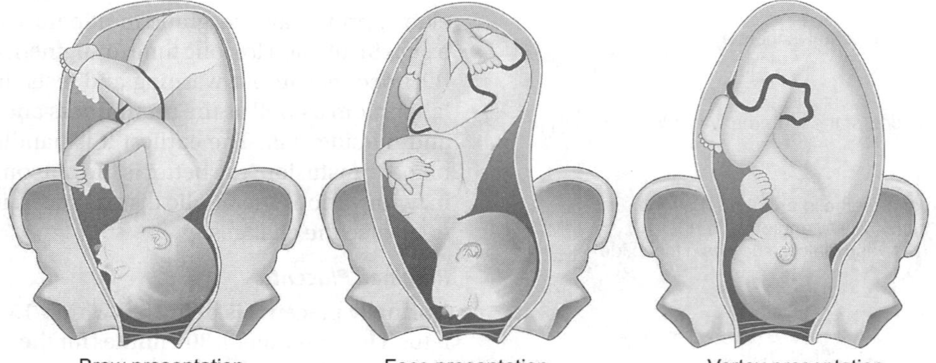

Fig. 19.5: Types of cephalic presentation.

- In case of a delayed tear (beyond 24 hours), repair should be withheld and antibiotics should be administered.
- A delayed complete tear should be repaired after 3 months.

Vaginal injuries

Vaginal injuries are usually associated with instrumented or manipulative delivery. The tears are extensive and associated with brisk hemorrhage. Management involves exploration under general anesthesia and repair by interrupted or continuous catgut sutures.

Cervical injuries

Small cervical lacerations may occur during the first delivery and usually heal spontaneously. However, an extensive tear may lead to postpartum hemorrhage.

Causes:

- Iatrogenic
- Rigid cervix
- Strong uterine contractions
- Detachment of cervix

Complications:

- Severe postpartum hemorrhage
- Pelvic cellulitis
- Thrombophlebitis
- Broad ligament hematoma
- Cervical incompetence with resultant mid-trimester abortion.

Management

Repair is required only for deep cervical tears with bleeding.

Urinary bladder injuries

Causes

- Instrumental vaginal delivery
- Cesarean section
- Sloughing fistula—obstructed labor leading to prolonged compression of bladder between fetal head and symphysis pubis.

Management involves immediate local repair.

Uterine rupture

Uterine rupture is termed as discontinuation in all the uterine layers—endometrium, myometrium and serosa, any time beyond 28 weeks of pregnancy.

Table 19.5 enlists the causes of uterine rupture.

Management

- Resuscitation if required
- Hysterectomy, repair alone or repair with sterilization.

HIGH-RISK PREGNANCY

High-risk pregnancy involves complications in pregnancy due to factor/s adversely affecting maternal and/or perinatal outcomes. All pregnancies and deliveries are potentially high risk but especially those where the mother, fetus or neonate is in a jeopardized state. Such pregnancies require extra care.

Table 19.5: Causes of uterine rupture.

Spontaneous rupture	• Multiparity • Congenital malformation of uterus • Abruptio placentae • Placenta percreta • Perforating mole • Following obstructed labor • Pelvic tumor
Iatrogenic rupture	• Injudicious administration of oxytocin • Fall or blow on abdomen • Forcible external version • Use of prostaglandins for induction of labor or abortion • Internal podalic version • Manual removal of placenta
Scar rupture	• Classical cesarean section or hysterectomy scar • Previous manual removal or dilatation and curettage • Cornual resection of ectopic pregnancy

Screening of High-risk Cases

History

- Maternal age <16 years or >30 years
- Pregnancy following a prolonged period of infertility, after induction of ovulation
- Reproductive history of two or more miscarriages or previous-induced abortion, previous stillbirth, neonatal death or child with congenital anomalies, previous preterm labor, child with intrauterine growth retardation or macrosomy, grand multiparity, previous cesarean section or hysterotomy, previous abnormalities in the third stage of labor.
- History of medical disorders like tuberculosis, renal diseases, thyroid disorders, psychiatric illness, cardiac illness, epilepsy, eclampsia and preeclampsia, viral hepatitis, anemia and infections during pregnancy.
- History of previous surgeries like myomectomy, repair of complete perineal tear, stress incontinence or vesicovaginal fistula.
- Family history of diabetes, hypertension, congenital malformation or multiple pregnancies.
- History of alcohol or drug abuse.
- History of exposure to radiation.

Examination

- Height below 150 cm or 145 cm in India
- Overweight or underweight mother
- High blood pressure
- Anemia
- Orthopedic or cardiopulmonary disorders
- Disproportionately small or large uterus
- Genital prolapse
- Pelvic inadequacy
- Associated tumors
- Cervical dilatation or laceration
- Presence of preeclampsia, anemia, high fever, Rh isoimmunization, hemorrhage, lack of uterine growth, diabetes mellitus, post-maturity or abnormal presentation.

Complications of Labor

- Delivery under general anesthesia
- Difficult forceps or breech delivery
- Failed forceps delivery
- Intrapartum fetal distress
- Postpartum hemorrhage or retained placenta
- Delay from diagnosis of fetal distress to delivery.

Postpartum Complications

- Apgar score <7
- Birth weight <2,500 g or >4 kg
- Hypoglycemia
- Fetal infection
- Anemia
- Jaundice
- Convulsions
- Congenital anomalies
- Hemorrhagic diathesis
- Respiratory distress syndrome
- Persistent cyanosis

Management

- Regular provision of obstetric service
- Folic acid therapy
- Advice regarding proper diet, rest, activities and medications
- Antepartum fetal and maternal monitoring if required
- Close monitoring during labor and postpartum.

Box 19.2 describes pregnancy in special conditions.

DILATATION AND EVACUATION

Dilatation and evacuation (D&E) is the standard surgical technique used for abortion after about 12 weeks.

Procedure

- There is a greater volume of fetal tissue in second trimester compared to the first trimester. So preoperative cervical dilatation is needed to allow for safe, appropriate instrumentation.
- Cervical preparation with osmotic dilators can be achieved after several hours or by placement the day prior. The most used dilators are small tents of dried and sterilized seaweed.
- By gently opening the cervix over several hours, the osmotic dilators reduce the risk of uterine perforation and cervical injury. Another strategy for cervical preparation is the administration of misoprostol, a prostaglandin.
- Surgeons use a combination of suction and uterine forceps to remove fetal and decidual tissue. In some cases, intraoperative ultrasound guidance may assist the surgeon during D&E. Inspection to identify expected fetal tissues and the placenta confirms a complete procedure.

Indications

D&E is recommended during the late first trimester and second trimester of pregnancy. It is also recommended when:

- The mother is in the second trimester and is diagnosed with the fetus having severe developmental abnormalities.
- There is an incomplete medical abortion.
- There is fatality of the embryo (spontaneous abortion) due to any reason.
- A woman does not realize that she is pregnant until the second trimester and needs termination.

Risks

- It is a comparatively safe procedure.
- The common complications are bleeding, infection, uterine perforation, and damage to surrounding organs or tissues.
- The risk of infection is decreased by using antibiotics.
- Rare risks of D&E include uterine perforation, retained products of conception, and rare risk of hysterectomy.
- There is no evidence that surgical abortion causes an increase in infertility or adverse outcomes in subsequent pregnancies.

Box 19.3 gives conditions where special care may need to be provided to the mother undergoing D&E.

IMPORTANCE OF PHYSIOTHERAPY IN CHILDBIRTH

While taking due care during antenatal period is getting well established, preconception care is also gaining importance. The role of physiotherapist is important as they can inform the woman regarding safe exercises during pregnancy, assessing and treating back problems, physiological changes in ligament, urinary disorders (stress incontinence, urgency, etc.) and pelvic floor and abdominal muscle exercises.

Box 19.2: Pregnancy in special conditions.

Cardiac Disease

Nowadays women with various cardiac problems can become pregnant and hope to have a live fetus. With improved monitoring of cardiac status, operative interventions as in case of mitral stenosis, and cohesive intervention by obstetricians and cardiologist, women with cardiac problems can think of carrying a pregnancy till term. These are high-risk cases and need integrated antenatal care of highest degree. Cardiac output increases by 30–50% during pregnancy therefore chances of cardiac decompensation especially at 8 months of amenorrhea, during labor and in 4 days following delivery are highest. Those women with prosthetic valve would also require management of anticoagulation therapy with timely switches between warfarin and heparin.

Pregnancies in women with spinal cord injuries and systemic lupus erythematosus are also managed well now.

Box 19.3: Health conditions that may necessitate special care during D&E.

- Anemia
- Alcohol and/or drug abuse by mother
- Asthma
- Blood clotting disorders
- Diabetes
- Hypertension
- Uterine abnormalities
- Heart diseases
- Previous hysterectomy
- Morbid obesity
- Seizures

- Pelvic floor muscle (PFM) contractions if taught early on during pregnancy and if diligently practiced result in lesser chances of urinary incontinence during postpartum.
- Maintaining good posture and pelvic tilting while sitting on chair helps in maintaining abdominal muscle strength. It corrects posture and reduces backache.
- Frequent foot and ankle exercises are must for women in sedentary jobs. Ankle dorsiflexion, plantarflexion and foot circling for even 30 seconds or so regularly improves blood circulation. Calf stretches, avoiding sitting for long time reduces calf muscle cramps.
- Various methods have been developed for advocating stress-free techniques.
- The Mitchell method of physiological relaxation developed by Laura Mitchell for hunched shoulders
- Contrast method—Edmund Jacobson
- Visualization and imagery—Payne encouraged pleasant imagining and warm environment
- Breathing exercises—slow easy rhythmic breathing is taught. This also helps during labor process.

Antenatal Exercises

The physiological changes during pregnancy are benefited if women do exercises. The maternal and fetal risks should be evaluated before beginning. Swimming, yoga and walking are popularly advocated during pregnancy instead of aerobics and strenuous exercise. The role of physiotherapists starts early on in pregnancy. The techniques can be taught to prevent backache, reasons for which can be different at different times of pregnancy. Easy techniques to roll over while getting up from lying down position and in reverse while lying down. The height of the chair should be such that feet are flat on ground with a lumbar roll for back support. Women should be encouraged to get up and move after some time and not sit for long. Positioning of a woman for stability as well as comfort is needed. Standing may need support of wall and supine lying will require lateral tilt. Pregnancy associated osteoporosis (PAO) normally affects women beyond 27 years of age. As backache is common during pregnancy, osteoporosis can be missed.

Physiotherapy is important especially for physical as well as mental fitness of the patient. This is essential to enhance the ability to cope with stress of pregnancy as more and more nuclear families with both partners working till the end of pregnancy is becoming commoner rather than the previous norm of joint families where the elderly ladies could guide and take care of the pregnant lady. Importance of knowing how to minimize backache and prevent any urinary and back problems later on after delivery thus gains prominence.

Summary

Pregnancy is a crucial period in the life of a woman. Though most of the changes occurring during this period are normal, some pregnancies may become difficult due to various risk factors. Regular antenatal and postnatal obstetric care form the cornerstone of a healthy pregnancy. High-risk pregnancies should be dealt with utmost care in order to improve outcomes.

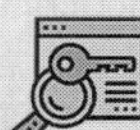

Review Questions

1. What are the normal physiological changes occurring during pregnancy?
2. Discuss clinical features and investigations used in the diagnosis of pregnancy.
3. Explain the process of labor in detail.
4. What is high-risk pregnancy and how to screen for it?
5. Write short notes on:
   a. Lactation
   b. Instrument assisted delivery
   c. Role of physiotherapist during antenatal and postnatal period
   d. Complications of pregnancy and childbirth

Bibliography

1. Braunthal S, Brateanu A. Hypertension in pregnancy: Pathophysiology and treatment. SAGE Open Med. 2019;7: 2050312119843700. doi: 10.1177/2050312119843700. PMID: 31007914; PMCID: PMC6458675.
2. Constantine MM. Physiologic and pharmacokinetic changes in pregnancy. Front Pharmacol. Sec. Obstetric and Pediatric Pharmacology. 2014l. https://doi.org/10.3389/fphar.2014.00065.
3. Gandhi MH, Gupta V. Physiology, Maternal Blood. In: StatPearls [Internet]. Treasure Island (FL): StatPearls Publishing. 2022. [Updated 2022Apr 28]. Available from: https://www.ncbi.nlm.nih.gov/books/NBK557783/.
4. Giugliani ERJ. Common problems during lactation and their management. J Pediatr. 2004;80(5 Suppl):S147-S154.
5. Granger JP, Alexander BT, Bennett WA, Khalil RA. Pathophysiology of pregnancy-induced hypertension. Am J Hypertens. 2001; 14(6 Pt 2):178S-85S. doi: 10.1016/s0895-7061(01)02086-6. PMID: 11411754.
6. Gudeta TA, Regassa TM. Pregnancy induced hypertension and associated factors among women attending delivery service at Mizan-Tepi University Teaching Hospital, Tepi General Hospital and Gebretsadik Shawo Hospital, Southwest, Ethiopia. Ethiop J Health Sci. 2019;29(1):831-40. doi: 10.4314/ejhs.v29i1.4. PMID: 30700950; PMCID: PMC6341446.
7. Horowitz KM, Ingardia CJ, Borgida AF. Anemia in pregnancy. Clin Lab Med. 2013;33(2):281-91. doi: 10.1016/j.cll.2013.03.016. Epub 2013 Apr 19. PMID: 23702118.
8. Kim DR, Wang E. Prevention of supine hypotensive syndrome in pregnant women treated with transcranial magnetic stimulation. Psychiatry Res. 2014;218(1-2):247-8. doi: 10.1016/j.psychres.2014.04.001. Epub 2014 Apr 12. PMID: 24768354; PMCID: PMC4057965.
9. Konar H. DC Dutta's Textbook of Obstetrics. 9th edn, New Delhi. Jaypee Brothers Medical Publishers Ltd. India; 2018.
10. Lee NM, Saha S. Nausea and vomiting of pregnancy. Gastroenterol Clin North Am. 2011;40(2):309-34, vii. doi: 10.1016/j.gtc.2011.03.009. PMID: 21601782; PMCID: PMC3676933.
11. Motosko CC, Bieber AK, Pomeranz MK, Stein JA, Martires KJ. Physiologic changes of pregnancy: A review of the literature. Int J Womens Dermatol. 2017;3(4):219-24. doi: 10.1016/j.ijwd.2017.09.003. PMID: 29234716; PMCID: PMC5715231.
12. Mummert T, Gnugnoli DM. Ectopic Pregnancy. In: StatPearls [Internet]. Treasure Island (FL): StatPearls Publishing; 2022.

[Updated 2022 Jun 21]. Available from: https://www.ncbi.nlm.nih.gov/books/NBK539860/.
13. Pillay J, Davis TJ. Physiology, Lactation. In: StatPearls [Internet]. Treasure Island (FL): StatPearls Publishing. 2022. [Updated 2022 Jul 18]. Available from: https://www.ncbi.nlm.nih.gov/books/NBK499981/.

Multiple Choice Questions (MCQs)

To test your understanding and recall of key concepts.

1. **Which hormone is responsible for maintaining uterine quiescence during pregnancy?**
   A. Estrogen B. Progesterone
   C. Relaxin D. Oxytocin
2. **What is the term for the bluish discoloration of the vaginal wall during pregnancy?**
   A. Goodell's sign
   B. Chadwick's sign
   C. Hegar's sign
   D. Palmer's sign
3. **Pregnant females are advised to avoid supine position after 16 weeks of gestation because ________.**
   A. It causes gastrointestinal discomfort
   B. It results in compression of the aorta by the gravid uterus
   C. It leads to inferior vena cava compression, decreasing venous return
   D. It induces uterine contractions
4. **A pregnant female in her third trimester complains of tingling and numbness in her radial two and a half fingers. Which of the following should be advised to her?**
   A. Relaxation exercises for the pelvic floor
   B. Splinting to relieve carpal tunnel syndrome
   C. Core stability exercises
   D. Postural correction exercises
5. **A patient with gestational hypertension is in her third trimester and has been prescribed Physiotherapy. Her Physiotherapy program, along with breathing exercises to reduce stress, must include________.**
   A. Avoid activities that elevate blood pressure and focus on gentle physical activity
   B. Engage in moderate to high-intensity resistance training to enhance vascular resistance
   C. Prioritize supine exercises to improve circulation
   D. Recommend prolonged rest to prevent hypertensive episodes
6. **A pregnant patient at 28 weeks of gestation complains of severe pelvic pain, particularly when walking or climbing stairs and has been diagnosed with pubic symphysis dysfunction. The physiotherapy intervention most suitable for her includes________________.**
   A. Aerobic exercise, pelvic floor training, and kinesiology taping
   B. Pelvic support belt, gentle stabilization exercises, and activity modification
   C. Weightlifting, jogging, and cold therapy
   D. High-intensity resistance training and squats to strengthen the pelvis
7. **A pregnant woman in her second trimester reports back pain exacerbated by prolonged standing and static unsupported postures. Which of the following best addresses her complaints, integrating physiological changes of pregnancy?**
   A. Lumbar support braces and avoidance of physical activity
   B. Core stabilization exercises, pelvic tilts, and education on proper ergonomics
   C. Complete avoidance of weight-bearing activities until symptoms subside
   D. High-intensity core training and lumbar extension exercises
8. **A woman is diagnosed with gestational diabetes mellitus (GDM) at 30 weeks of gestation. She complains of fatigue and difficulty maintaining blood sugar levels. Which integrated approach should the physiotherapist employ?**
   A. Educate on seated resistance exercises and focus on improving glycemic control through diet alone
   B. Develop a moderate-intensity walking plan and coordinate care with the obstetrician and nutritionist
   C. Prescribe high-intensity interval training to boost insulin sensitivity
   D. Recommend complete bed rest to avoid hypoglycemia during activity
9. **A 28-year-old pregnant woman at 32 weeks of gestation presents with persistent headaches, blurred vision, and swelling in her hands and feet. Her blood pressure is 150/95 mm Hg, and proteinuria is detected. Based on these findings, which is the most appropriate immediate course of action?**
   A. Start antihypertensive medication and advise moderate intensity exercise
   B. Refer to a high-risk obstetric unit for monitoring and potential delivery
   C. Recommend a low-sodium diet and schedule follow-up in 2 weeks
   D. Prescribe a physiotherapy regimen focusing on aerobic exercises

ANSWERS

1. B	2. B	3. C	4. B	5. A
6. B	7. B	8. B	9. B	

Chapter 20

Physiotherapy in Pregnancy

✍ *Nupur Shah*

LEARNING OBJECTIVES

At the end of the chapter, the reader will be able to:
- Describe the physiotherapy management for pregnant women.
- Understand the common complications during pregnancy.
- Discuss the physiotherapy management for the complications of pregnancy.
- Conduct antenatal classes effectively.
- Gain knowledge on labor preparation.

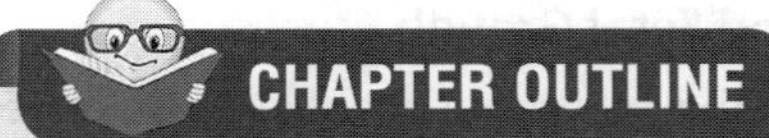

INTRODUCTION

Pregnancy is the phase when numerous changes happen within the body. The entire female body naturally changes during pregnancy. There is no other time that produces the same bodily transformations. The pregnant body works for 40 weeks for the proper growth and development of the fetus during which there is a constant natural effort to balance all the organs and systems. Due to all these changes that occur in a pregnant woman, exercise has to be given special importance for the overall well-being.

COMPLICATIONS AND PROBLEMS REPORTED DURING PREGNANCY

- **Low back pain:** It is commonly reported among pregnant women due to postural changes, stretching of abdominal muscles, and forward shift of the center of gravity (COG) (**Fig. 20.1**).
- **Pelvic girdle pain:** The pain is between the posterior iliac crest and gluteal fold, especially around the sacroiliac (SI) joint. In some patients, pain may radiate towards the posterior thigh and the symphysis pubis. Due to this the ability to walk, stand and sit reduces. Standard treatment includes an exercise program, use of a pelvic belt, and patient education.
- **Gestational diabetes:** Glucose/carbohydrate intolerance with onset or first detection during pregnancy; uncontrolled gestational diabetes (GDM) can cause macrosomia (ACOG 2019).
- **Anxiety:** Mainly seen during the first pregnancy of a woman.
- **Mood swings**
- **Depression:** Exercise has a positive effect on treating prenatal depression.
- **Morning sickness**
- **Preeclampsia**
- **Muscle cramps:** Most common in the calf muscles. Adequate hydration and regular stretching of these muscles can help in relieving muscle cramps.

EFFECTS OF PHYSIOTHERAPY ON MATERNAL AND FETAL HEALTH/BENEFITS OF EXERCISE DURING PREGNANCY

Box 20.1 lists the potential benefits of exercise during pregnancy.

Exercise and Weight Gain

- Adequate weight gain during pregnancy is necessary for the growth and development of maternal and fetal tissues.
- Excessive weight gain can lead to many health adversities for the mother and her offspring.

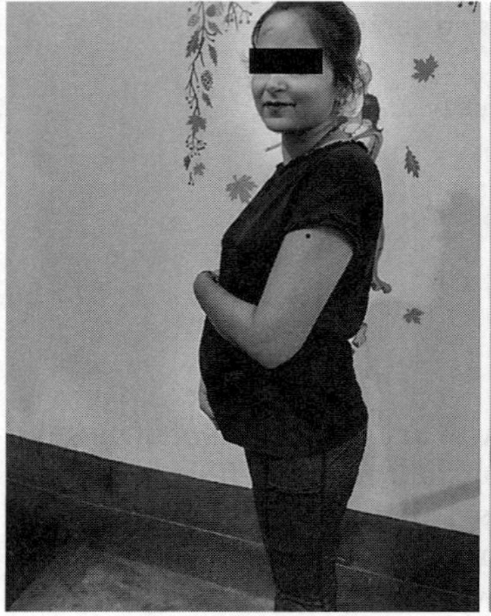
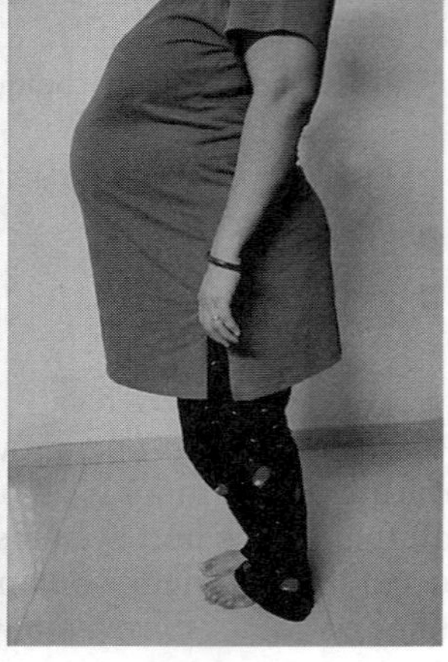

Fig. 20.1: Postural changes during pregnancy.

Box 20.1: Benefits of exercise in pregnancy.

- Higher chance of normal delivery
- Lower incidence of:
  - Preterm birth
  - Cesarean birth
  - Low birth weight
  - Gestational diabetes
  - Preeclampsia
  - Excessive gestational weight gain

- Complications like preterm birth are more likely to occur. Women end up having more chances of cesarean delivery, and preeclampsia and end up retaining excess weight after delivery.
- Regular exercises during pregnancy reduce the risk of excess weight gain during pregnancy.

Exercise and Psychological Well-being

- During pregnancy, various neuroendocrine and biological changes occur in the body that results in profound psychological effects.
- Women who follow a pregnancy fitness regime cope better with the emotional and physiological strains of pregnancy. It helps in building better body image and self-esteem and also treats antenatal depression.

Maternal Exercise and Fetal Growth

- Studies have shown the positive effect of exercise on fetal growth in low-risk prenatal patients. For women who undergo low to moderate-intensity exercise on a regular basis, the birth-weights are about 100 grams higher as compared to non-exercisers. With higher exercises, the birthweight increments have been found to be 300 grams.
- Other benefits to the fetus include:
  - Decreased fetal heart rate
  - Increased level of amniotic fluid
  - Improvement in the viability of the placenta
- It also helps in endothelium-dependent vasodilation and reduces the chances of preeclampsia.
- Offspring of women practicing aerobic maternal exercise program show:
  - Improved insulin sensitivity
  - Decreased body fat
  - Better cardiac autonomic nervous system control in offspring
  - Increased lean mass
  - Improved vascular endothelial and smooth muscle function

COMMON PROBLEMS SEEN DURING PREGNANCY

Physiotherapy plays a major role in reducing several complications and even helps in preventing them. It includes exercise therapy which improves strength, endurance, and flexibility. Therapists also provide ergonomic advice, postural exercise, and a home exercise program. If necessary the use of modalities is done such as the application of ice/

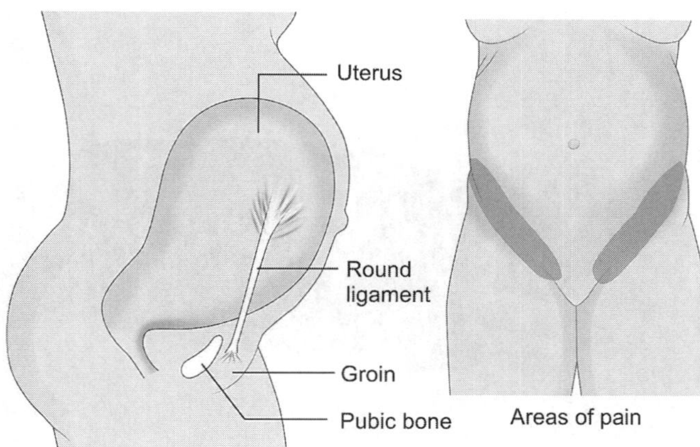

Fig. 20.2: Round ligament pain.

hot packs or electrical stimulation to reduce pain, swelling/stiffness. Physiotherapy also works in reducing obstetric comorbidities.

Uterine Ligament Pain (Round Ligament Pain)

- This is seen due to the rapidly growing uterus and even due to the remodeling of skeletal ligaments and collagenous connective tissue.
- The quality of the pain is sharp, sudden, and stabbing in the area of the lower abdomen, mostly unilateral **(Fig. 20.2)**.
- Usually experienced in the second trimester.
- Light massaging or stroking at the site of pain or a cold pack can help.

Fatigue

- Fatigue is experienced in the first and the third trimester and it is not noticeable in the second trimester.
- Expectant women, family members, and employers should be prepared for the possible reduction in their working capacity. Sometimes the pregnant female may even experience evening sickness.
- Relaxation strategies and the knowledge that this will pass are helpful.

Costal Margin Pain (Rib Pain) and Intercostal Neuralgia

- The woman experiences pain over the anterior part of the lower ribs in the third trimester, sometimes accompanied by unilateral thoracic pain over the back.
- As the uterus grows, it presses the rib cage in the outward direction on both sides resulting in the stretching of costal interarticular tissues. This flare can increase the diameter of the chest by 10 to 15 cm. If the pain is intermittent, it is termed '*intercostal neuralgia*', it radiates around the chest and lateral abdomen.
- Rib lifting techniques **(Fig. 20.3)** such as raising both the arms (clasp) overhead or side flexion (arm raised away from the painful side) will provide relief. A cold pack can be applied directly to the painful site.

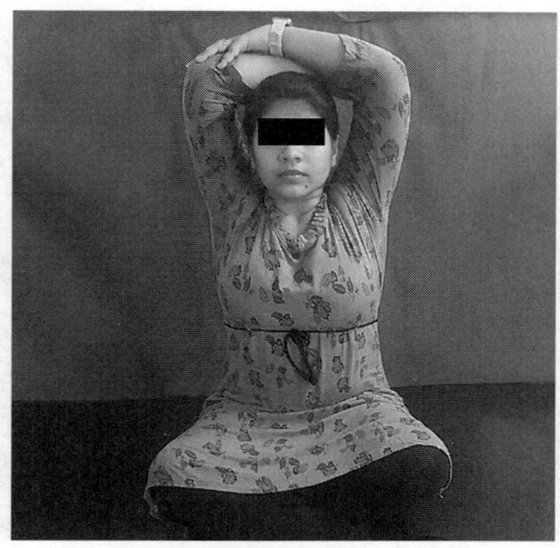

Fig. 20.3: Rib lifting.

Varicose Veins

- It occurs due to hormone-induced hypotonia of the walls of the veins and raised intra-abdominal pressure **(Fig. 20.4)**.
- It is usually seen during the first trimester and in repeated pregnancies.

Intervention

- Focusing on leg circulation is important. Standing for long periods, cross-legged sitting, and leg-dependent positions while sitting should be avoided. Regular ankle-toe movements can improve circulation (30 seconds at a time). Sitting with feet raised, and raising the bed on bricks (leg side) can be useful.
- Exercises should be prescribed in the non-dependent position as much as possible to avoid discomfort.
- External support such as elastic stockings can be prescribed. It provides counter pressure against distended veins and support.
- The patients should be instructed to keep their legs elevated.

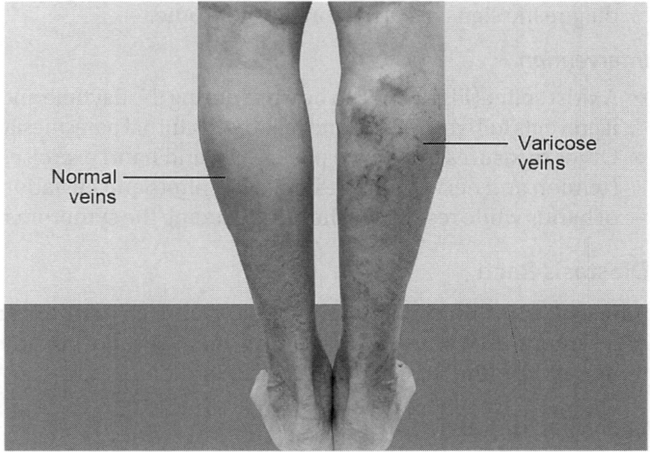

Fig. 20.4: Varicose veins.

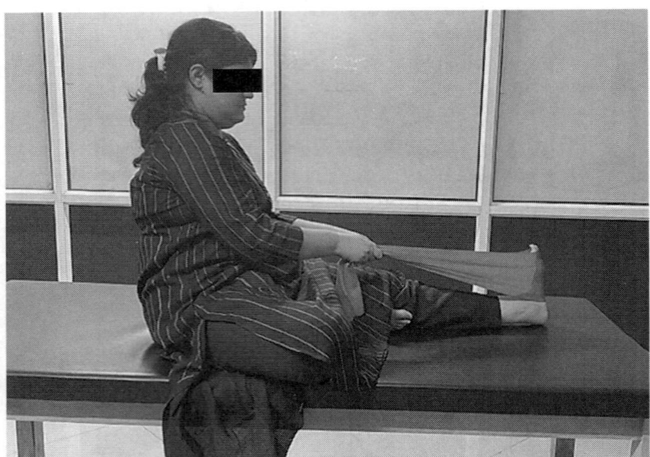

Fig. 20.5: Calf stretch.

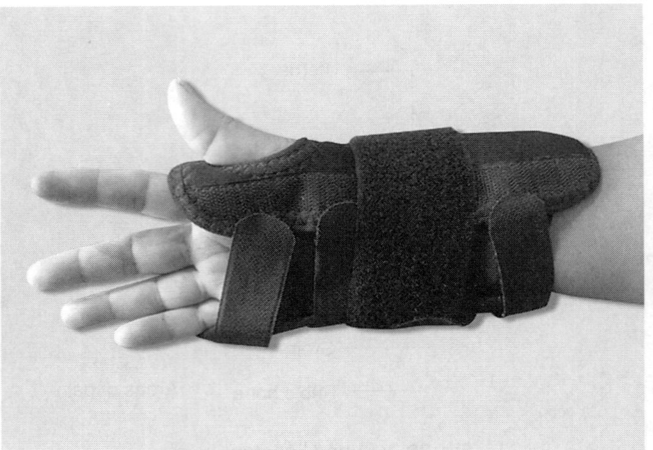

Fig. 20.6: Wrist splint.

Cramps

- Many women suffer from cramps during pregnancy.
- Calf muscles are the most common site of cramps.
- It can occur due to increased fluid retention or decreased level of mobility in the evenings. It is always triggered by plantar flexion stretch.
- Dorsiflexion stretch **(Fig. 20.5)** is applied to get relief. Walking before going to bed, a warm bath, and foot exercises can help to reduce the symptoms.

Carpal Tunnel Syndrome

- It is the nerve compression syndrome occurring during pregnancy and usually, its symptoms subside after delivery. The causes are postural changes, fluid retention, hormonal changes, or circulatory compromise.
- Clinically, it is recognized as sensory and sometimes motor nerve function impairment caused due to the compression of the median nerve under the flexor retinaculum. Women having general edema have more chances to get this condition in the third trimester.
- Patients complain of pain and paresthesia which is experienced at night and often the sleep is disturbed. Phalen's test and sensory impairment in hand are the diagnostic signs of carpal tunnel syndrome.

Intervention

- A wrist splint **(Fig. 20.6)** can be worn during the daytime and it prevents full wrist flexion and relieves nocturnal paresthesia.
- Other measures like an ice pack, wrist and hand exercises (tendon and nerve gliding exercises), splints and elevation of hands while resting will help in reducing the symptoms.

Diastasis Recti

Assessment of diastasis recti can be found in Chapter 4: Assessment in Women's Health and management for the same can be found in Chapter 22: Postnatal Care.

Sacroiliac or Pelvic Girdle Pain

- Pain is felt in the posterior pelvis and it is described as stabbing pain that radiates down to the buttocks/posterior side of the thigh or knee and even on lateral leg in the distribution of L5/S1 nerve roots.
- It is felt during walking, sitting, standing, stair climbing, and turning in bed, unilateral standing, or rotational activities.

External Stabilization

Use of external stabilization such as corsets or belts designed for pregnancy should done while walking.

Exercises

- Hip stabilization exercises
- Trunk stabilization exercises
- Patients should be educated to activate the pelvic floor muscles and abdominal muscles during transitional activities to stabilize the trunk and pelvis.

 **Clinical Pointer**

Exercises to be avoided during pelvic girdle pain:
- One leg standing
- Excessive hip abduction
- Excessive hip extension
- Fire hydrant exercise **(Fig. 20.7)**

 **Clinical Pointer**

Activity modification during ADL:
- Log roll instead of segmental roll
- While getting into the car, sit down and then rotate into the car
- In a side-lying position, place a pillow under the abdomen and between the knees
- During climbing stairs, use one step at a time
- Avoid cross-leg sitting

Low Back Pain

- Low back pain occurs due to postural changes during pregnancy, increased laxity of the joints, hormonal influences, reduced abdominal muscle function, and anterior shift of COG.

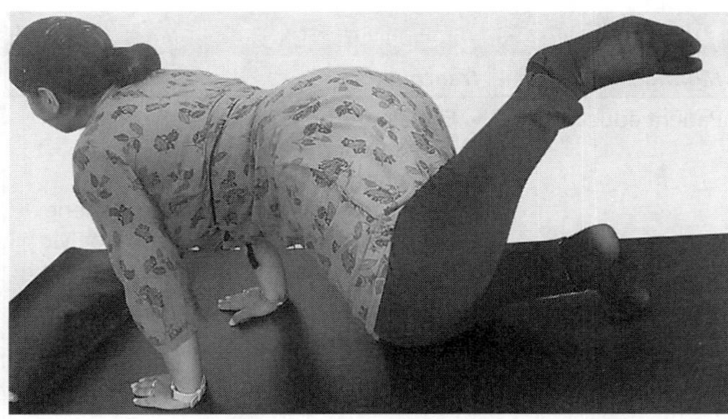

Fig. 20.7: Fire hydrant exercise (to be avoided in case of pelvic girdle pain).

- Around 50–80% of pregnant women report back pain at some point during pregnancy. This can lead to reduced quality of life, decreased functional ability, and lost workdays.
- Women who are physically fit and have good abdominal tone and core strength have fewer chances of low back pain. In a few cases, the pain is felt during the postpartum period for as long as one year.
- The symptoms worsen as the day progresses due to muscle fatigue. It can be reduced by rest, change of position, and prenatal physiotherapy.

Interventions

- Low back pain symptoms can be treated effectively by basic exercises, proper ergonomics, posture correction, and superficial modalities.
- The use of traction and electrical stimulation/heating modalities is contraindicated.

Basic exercises for low back pain:
- Cat and cow stretch **(Figs. 20.8 and 20.9)**
- Spinal stretch (sitting/standing) **(Fig. 20.10)**
- Butterfly pose holds with an anterior pelvic tilt **(Fig. 20.11)**
- Spine twist (rotation of the back while sitting)
- Tadasana
- Pelvic bridging **(Fig. 20.12)**

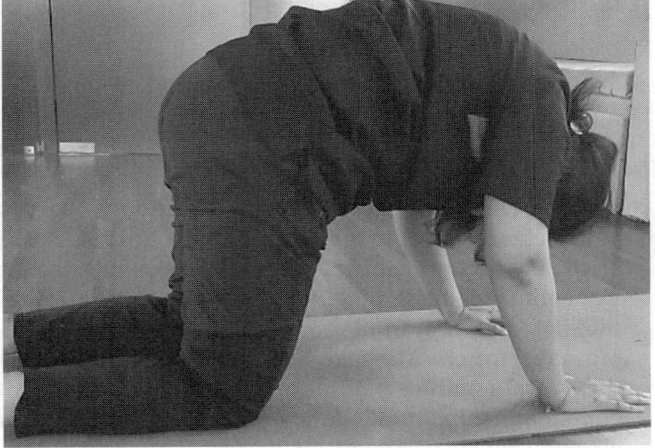

Fig. 20.8: Cow pose.

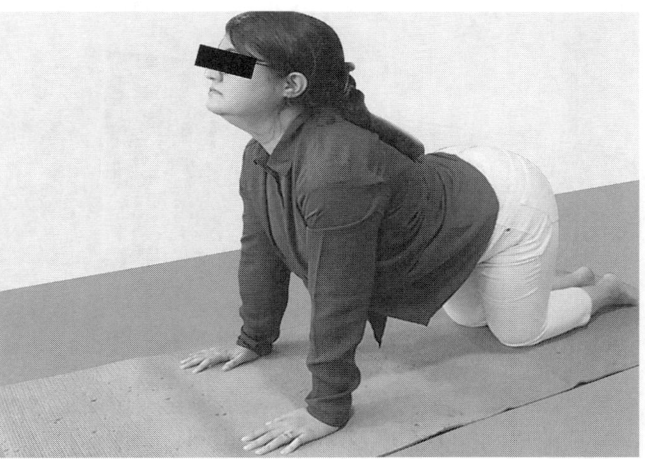

Fig. 20.9: Cat pose.

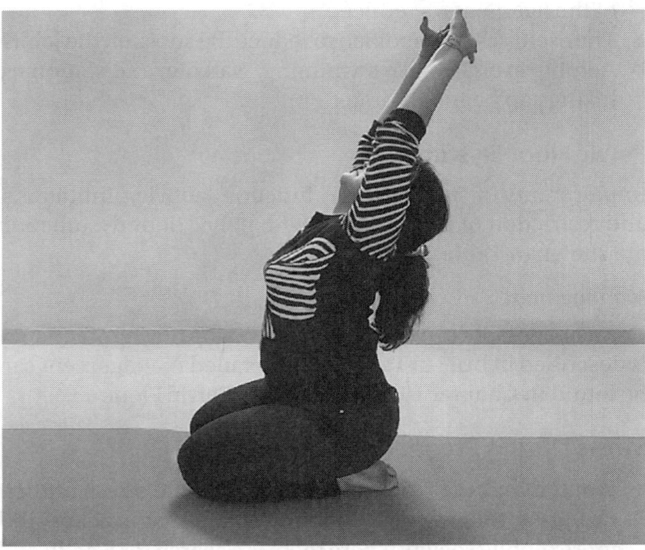

Fig. 20.10: Spinal stretch.

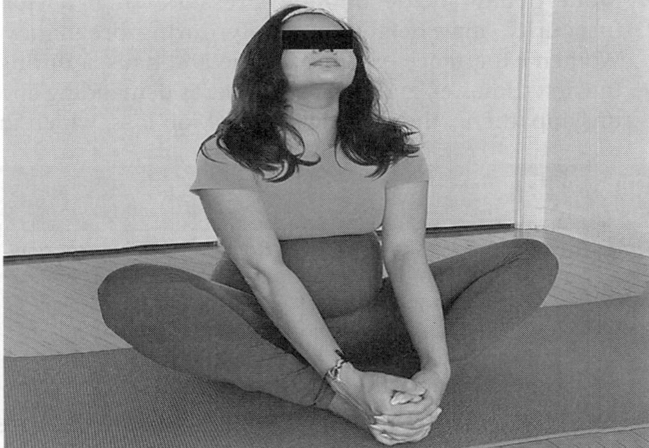

Fig. 20.11: Butterfly pose hold (with anterior pelvic tilt).

Laxity of Joints

- Joint laxity occurs due to the release of the hormone 'Relaxin'. There is a high-risk of injuries if the woman is

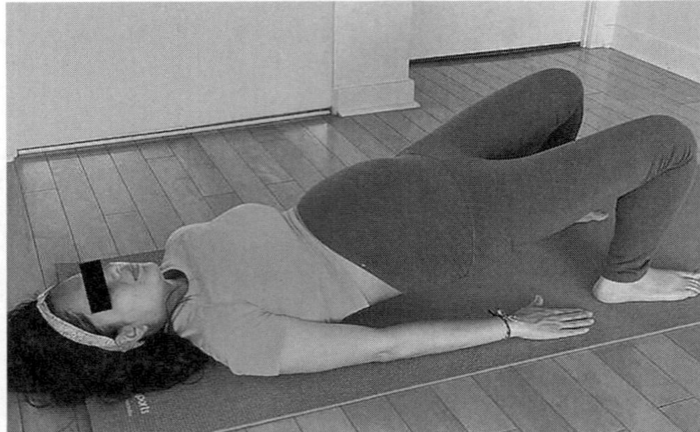

Fig. 20.12: Pelvic bridging.

not aware of joint protection strategies. The tensile quality of the ligaments is reduced.

- The exercises are modified to reduce the stress on the joints.
- Aerobic exercises like swimming, walking, and stationary biking can be incorporated.

Pelvic Floor Dysfunction

Impairments of structure and function, activity limitations, and restriction of participation with pelvic floor dysfunction are shown in **Table 20.1**.

Management

The management of pelvic floor dysfunction during pregnancy is described in brief in **Table 20.2**. Detailed management can be found in Chapter 15: Managing the Pelvic Floor.

Table 20.2: Management of pelvic floor dysfunction.

Management plan	***Treatment***
Patient education	• Explain the anatomy and physiology of pelvic floor muscles • Explain the treatment of their impairments and maintaining hygiene • Educate about the risk factors of pelvic floor impairments (constipation/obesity)
Discuss the treatment with other health professionals	• Consult the physician for medicines and further investigations • Consult the dietitian for a professional diet chart • Refer for internal pelvic floor assessment as required
Educate on self-management	• Discuss recommended fluid intake and bladder irritants • Make use of a voiding diary • Record daily exercises • Teach pain management and self-care techniques • **Urge suppression techniques:** ➢ Distract the mind ➢ Remain still for one minute (standing/sitting) ➢ Do not rush to the toilet ➢ Use pelvic floor contraction ➢ Remain calm
Teach the awareness of pelvic floor muscle control in the activities of daily living (ADL)	• The activation and relaxation of pelvic floor muscles have to be done with ADL. • **Neuromuscular pelvic floor activation:** ➢ Useful for disuse atrophy and proprioceptive deficits of the pelvic floor muscles ➢ Manual stretch of levator ani (at vaginal/anal orifice) ➢ Teach isolated contraction of pelvic floor muscles by palpating the perineal body for correct activation ➢ The awareness of positioning

Stress During Pregnancy

- Women and their partners experience the stress of their changing role while sustaining in this materialistic and more mobile society where there is a search for wealth and possessions and a loss of family support.
- Modern day socioeconomic stressors, such as job insecurity, may heighten anxiety during pregnancy. Women experience extreme fatigue and nausea during the first trimester, and if the employer is demanding and unsympathetic, there are chances of job loss, which in turn leads to financial anxiety. Obstetric physiotherapists play a vital role to educate the patient on the physiological effects of stress, becoming aware of it, to self-manage and dissipate it.

Table 20.1: Impairments, activity limitations and participation restriction due to pelvic floor dysfunction.

Impairments	• Weakness of pelvic floor, soft tissue disruption • Poor proprioception and dystrophy of pelvic floor muscles • Lack of knowledge of pelvic floor muscle function • Overactive pelvic floor muscles • Pain during voiding
Activity limitations	• Incontinence due to poor sphincter control • Difficulty in voiding
Participation restriction	Reduced participation in work or community activities due to poor control of the sphincter/pain/discomfort/skin issues/improper hygiene

Relaxation

- **Contrast method:** The contrast method of Jacobson involves contracting and relaxing the muscles alternately. It is done on various muscles of the body to recognize the difference between tension and relaxation.
- **Mitchell's method of physiological relaxation:** One group of muscles relaxes and the other group contracts. This is also known as the reciprocal method. For example, ask the woman to pull the shoulders towards the feet. STOP. Feel the shoulders away from your ears.
- **Massage/touch:** Massage and touch especially from the partner induce relaxation and create a sense of companionship. Stroking, effleurage, and kneading on essential areas cause a person to relax.

- **Breathing exercises:**
  - Expiration provides a sense of relaxation as it releases the tension and provides relief.
  - Rhythmic, slow and easy breathing induces calmness. The position of the mother should be comfortable. She is positioned lying, side-lying, or sitting. Diaphragmatic breathing is taught.
  - During late pregnancy, the supine position should be avoided to prevent hypotension.

GUIDELINES FOR MANAGING THE PREGNANT WOMAN

Antenatal assessment has been described in Chapter 4: Assessment in Women's Health.

Box 20.2 lists potential impairments during pregnancy and **Table 20.3** provides some intervention strategies to be used during pregnancy.

Box 20.2: Potential impairments of pregnancy.

- **Potential impairments of structure and function:**
  - Muscle imbalances and musculoskeletal pain
  - Lower limb swelling and discomfort
  - Poor body mechanics due to changing body size and shape
- **Pelvic floor impairments:**
  - Incontinence
  - Overactive pelvic floor
  - Poor proprioception
  - Prolapse of organs

Table 20.3: Intervention strategies to be used during pregnancy.

Management plan	*Treatment*
Educate about posture during pregnancy	Strengthen, stretch and train the main muscles maintaining the posture
Teach safe body mechanics	• Transitions such as sitting to stand, turning, lying, lifting, sitting, and standing • Position of labor and delivery
Improve the strength of the upper limb as preparation for childcare	Resisted exercises of the upper limb
Improve the strength of lower limb muscles to fulfill the demands of weight-bearing and circulation	• Resisted exercises of the lower limb • Elastic stockings, and stretching techniques
Relaxation should be incorporated	Teach relaxation exercises along with breathing exercises
Prepare physically for labor, delivery, and postpartum	Strengthen the muscles needed during labor
Improve cardiovascular fitness	Prescribe safe aerobic exercises
Educate about diastasis recti	• Prevent and monitor diastasis recti • Exercises for diastasis recti and abdominal strengthening are taught

- Educate the client about uterine cramping. If it ceases after moderate activity, it is acceptable but when it does not stop after activity, it is not acceptable and a medical professional should be contacted.
- **Education on positioning:** Supine position for a long time is avoided after the first trimester as it can compress the vena cava due to the enlargement of the uterus. A small wedge or a towel is placed under the hip of the right side to reduce the effects of vena cava compression as it turns the patient slightly towards the left side.

  The transitions should be done slowly to avoid the effect of orthostatic hypotension.

  Encourage the woman to empty her bladder completely before starting prenatal exercises.
- Hip opening exercises like deep squatting (Indian toilet sitting), duck walking, and butterfly pose hold (*see* **Fig. 20.13**) are incorporated on a regular basis from the 36th week of pregnancy for increasing chances of normal delivery.

Canadian guidelines for physical activity throughout pregnancy (2019):

- Women are advised to be physically active throughout their pregnancy after all the contraindications are ruled out.
- 150 minutes of moderate-intensity physical activities every week are recommended to reduce the occurrence of complications and achieve meaningful health benefits.
- Various resisted exercises and aerobic exercises should be incorporated to achieve greater health benefits.
- Pelvic floor muscle training (e.g., Kegels exercises) is advised to be done daily in order to prevent urinary incontinence.
- If the supine position is uncomfortable during exercising, it should be avoided and exercises should be performed in alternative positions.

ANTENATAL TEAM

The antenatal team comprises the following members:

- Obstetricians
- General practitioners
- Midwives
- Obstetric physiotherapists
- Dieticians
- Dentists
- Laboratory professionals
- Health visitors
- Radiologists/ultrasound operators
- Pediatricians

ANTENATAL CLASSES

The classes are designed to fulfill the needs of parenthood. Antenatal education is effective only if everyone from the class contributes and avoids the teacher/student image.

- Couples are educated on physiological changes of the body during pregnancy, labor, and puerperium.
- The methods of coping with physical discomforts during pregnancy are taught.

- Tool kit of coping strategies should be assembled.
- Couples are educated on necessary lifestyle changes and emotional maturity.
- They are encouraged to talk about their problems and seek solutions.

EXERCISE PRESCRIPTION

General Instructions/Safety Precautions

- Exercise should be avoided in humid climates/during excessive heat and choose a thermoneutral environment.
- Avoid contact activities or activities that have risk of falling. Examples are football, baseball, ice hockey, horse riding, and racquet sports.
- Avoid scuba diving.
- Women who reside at low altitudes, should avoid physical activity in high altitudes (>2,500 m).
- Women considering athletic competition or exercising with high intensity should consult the obstetric care provider in order to get knowledge of the impact of such physical activities on maternal and fetal outcomes.
- Maintain adequate nutritional level and hydration.
- Women should educate themselves about the warning signs of exercise.
- Avoid Valsalva maneuver during exercise.
- Metabolic demand increases by 300 kilocalories per day so women should increase their caloric intake to meet the demand of pregnancy and exercise.

FITT Recommendation

- **Frequency:** 3/more days per week for aerobic exercises and 2 to 3 non-consecutive days per week for resistance exercises.
- **Intensity:** Moderate intensity for aerobic activities. Women can use the 'Talk Test' (able to talk comfortably while exercising) to keep the intensity in check during their workout. Initially, the exercises should be of low weights with multiple repetitions. **Table 20.4** presents the recommended upper limit of heart rate range during exercise for various age groups. Exercises should not increase the heart rate beyond these values.
- **Time:** Moderate-intensity physical activities of 15 min/day initially, progressing to 30 min/day and gradually increasing to 150 minutes per week.
- **Type:** Exercises have to be dynamic, rhythmic physical activities making use of large muscle groups. For example, walking and cycling.

Table 20.4: Heart rate range.

Age (years)	*Heart rate range (beats/min)*
<20	140–155
20–29	135–150
30–39	130–145
>40	125–140

Clinical Pointer

Exercise prescription and progression for twin pregnancies remains same as that for single pregnancy.

Table 20.5 presents a standard treatment protocol for physiotherapy during the second/third trimester

Table 20.5: Standard physiotherapy protocol during second/third trimester.

Warm-up	Active movements of head/neck, shoulder, wrist, ankles, hip, knee, and lumbar region
Exercises in sitting	• Chest toning exercises • Postural exercises: Scapula retraction • Side stretch • Butterfly stretch **(Fig. 20.11)** • Long hip adductors stretch • Spine twist • Breast lifting exercises • Hip opening exercises on Swiss ball **(Fig. 20.13)**
Exercises in standing	• Hip rotation and abduction • Squats • Calf raise **(Fig. 20.20)** • Toe raise with shoulder elevation • Sidewalk
Exercises in supine lying	• Pelvic bridging • Elbow against the floor • Pelvic clock exercise • Hip adductors isometrics • Butterfly hold • Unilateral straight leg raise (SLR)
Exercises in side-lying	• 90° leg stretch • Clamp exercise • Active hip abduction • Multiple angle isometrics of hip abductors
Exercises in a quadruped position	• Cat and camel stretch **(Figs. 20.8 and 20.9)** • Alternate arm and leg raise • Modified child pose with Swiss ball **(Fig. 20.14)**
Lower limb strengthening (weight cuff of 0.5 kg or 1 kg)	• **With weight cuff:** ➢ Hip flexion–extension ➢ Hip abduction ➢ Pelvic rotation ➢ Knee flexion and extension • **Without weight cuff:** ➢ Mini squats ➢ Supported lunges ➢ Calf raises ➢ Heel drop exercises
Low-impact cardio exercises (0.5/1 kg dumbbell)	• Shoulder—flexion and extension ➢ Internal and external rotation ➢ Abduction and adduction • Elbow—flexion and extension • Wrist—flexion and extension ➢ Radial/ulnar deviation ➢ Circumduction
Cool down	• Calf stretch **(Fig. 20.5)** • Modified knee to chest stretch • **Breathing exercises:** Pursed lip breathing, diaphragmatic breathing **(Fig. 20.15)**

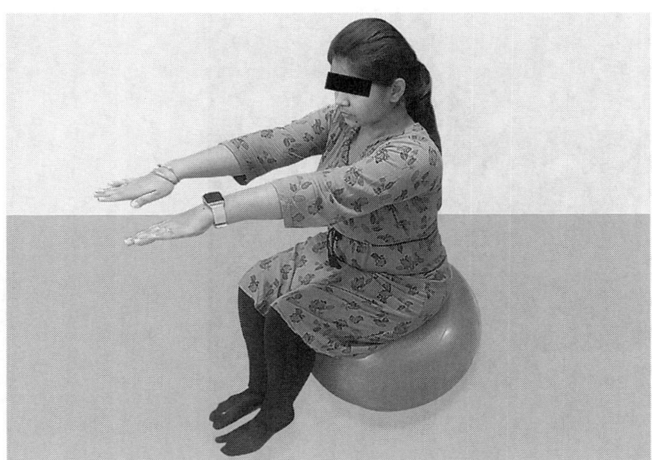

Fig. 20.13: Circling on the ball (hip opening exercise).

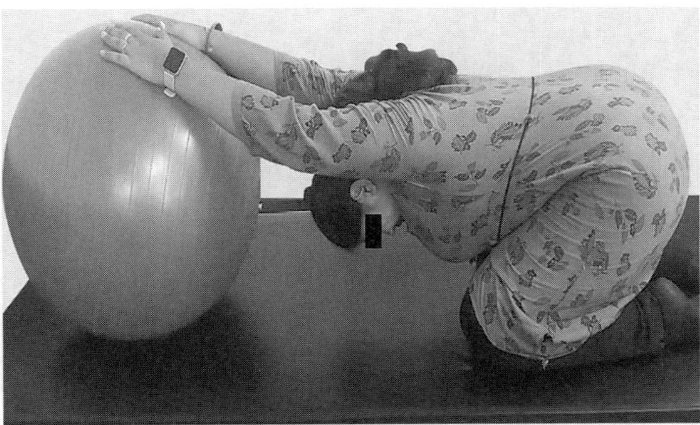

Fig. 20.14: Modified child pose with Swiss ball.

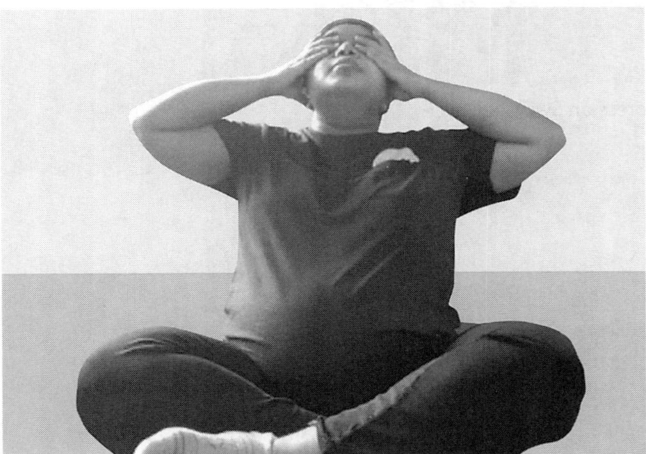

Fig. 20.15: Breathing exercise (Bhramari pranayama).

of pregnancy. The exercises should be started after a thorough antenatal assessment. The client should be given information on warning signs of exercises. Low-impact cardio exercises for the upper and lower limbs can be added. Props such as pillows, towels, dumbbells, and Thera bands can be used.

Clinical Pointer

Pregnant women who have a sedentary lifestyle or have a medical condition should gradually increase their physical activity to meet the levels mentioned above.

After the first trimester, exercises in the supine position are reduced.

Clinical Pointer

Pregnant women who are obese or have gestational diabetes mellitus or hypertension should get permission from the physician in order to begin the exercises. Their exercise prescriptions should be adjusted with their medicines, symptoms, and functional level.

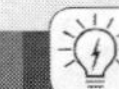

Clinical Pointer

All exercises in the antenatal period should be strictly done under the supervision and guidance of a trained and experienced physiotherapist.

Figures 20.16 to 20.22 show some exercises done during an antenatal class in standing position and while sitting on Swiss ball.

Aquatic Exercises and Swimming during Pregnancy

Swimming is among the safest recommended exercises during pregnancy. Non-swimmers can do the exercises in the pool and undergo a relaxation program in the pool. The buoyancy of the water supports the lady's body weight which enables her to tone her body and develop strength. It helps in improving overall physical fitness and endurance and creates a sense of well-being.

The regular swimmers can continue it throughout her pregnancy. The strokes and distance can be modified and she should be warned to listen to her body and take breaks or reduce the intensity when needed. Non-swimmers can do water walking and suitable exercises for arms, trunks, and legs. Warm-up and cool-down are necessary.

The session of relaxation aided by the buoyancy of water can be helpful, especially in the last trimester. Care should be taken regarding the temperature of the water so that the core body temperature does not rise a lot.

Yoga

Yoga can be practiced during pregnancy under the supervision of trained professionals. The emphasis is placed on stretches and mobility. Proper assessment is needed before any form of yoga is practiced. Further reading is suggested from Chapter 34: Yoga for Women's Health.

After the onset of COVID-19, many online yoga sessions have commenced **(Fig. 20.23)**.

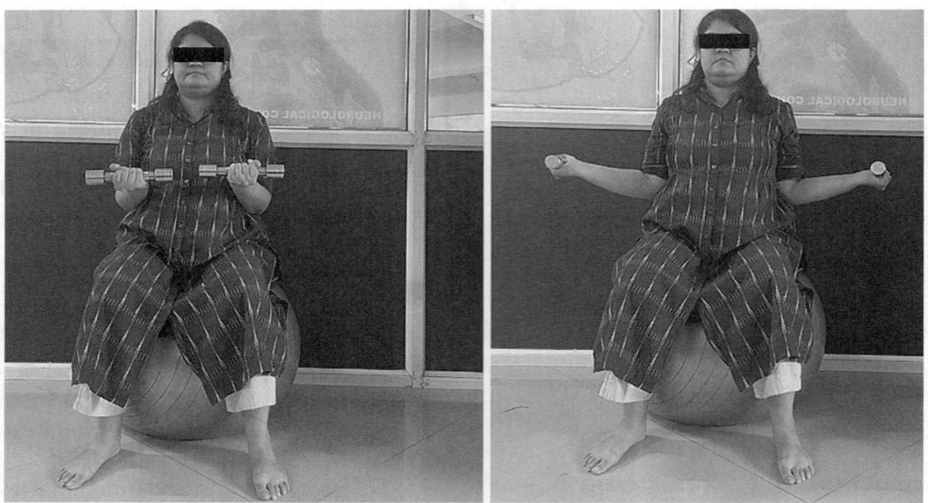

Fig. 20.16: Strengthening of shoulder rotators on Swiss ball.

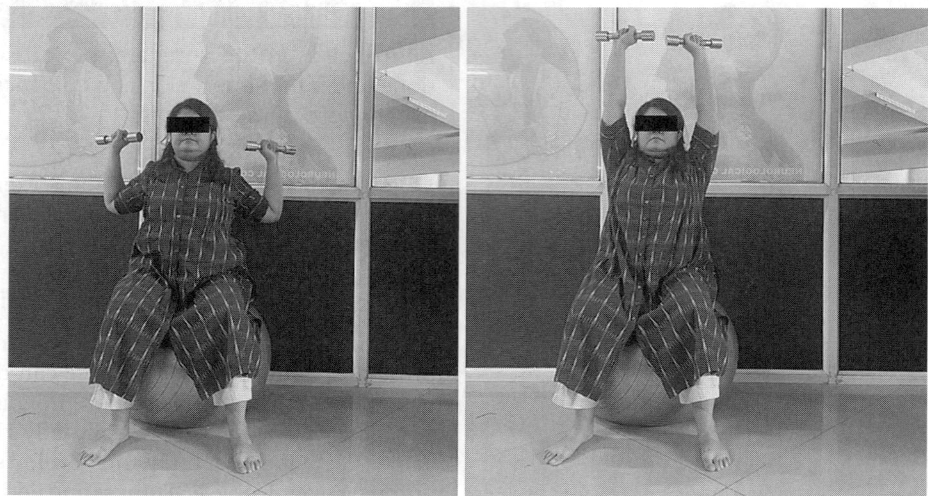

Fig. 20.17: Dumbbell press on Swiss ball.

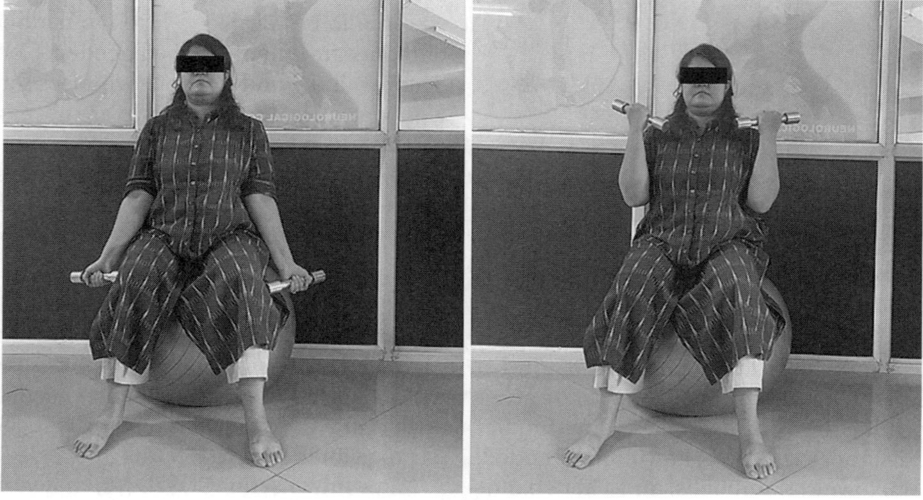

Fig. 20.18: Strengthening of biceps on Swiss ball.

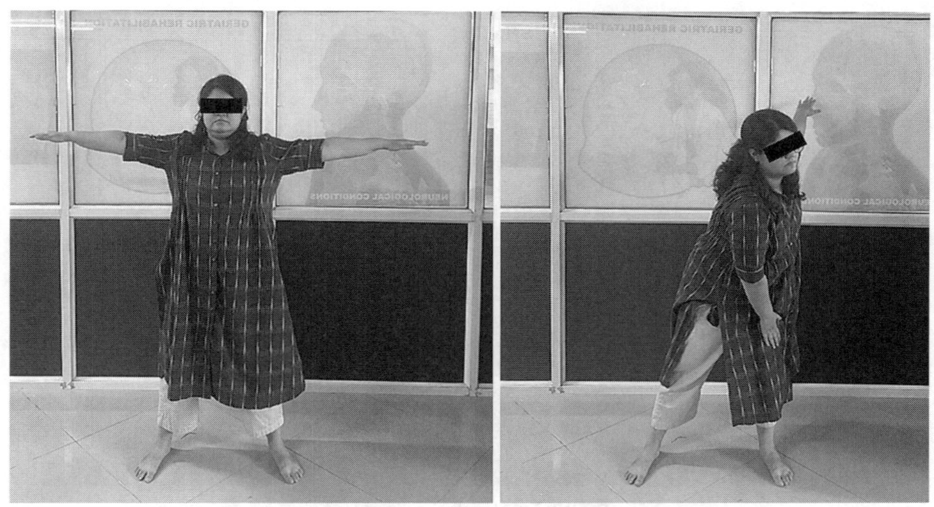

Fig. 20.19: Alternate toe touch in standing.

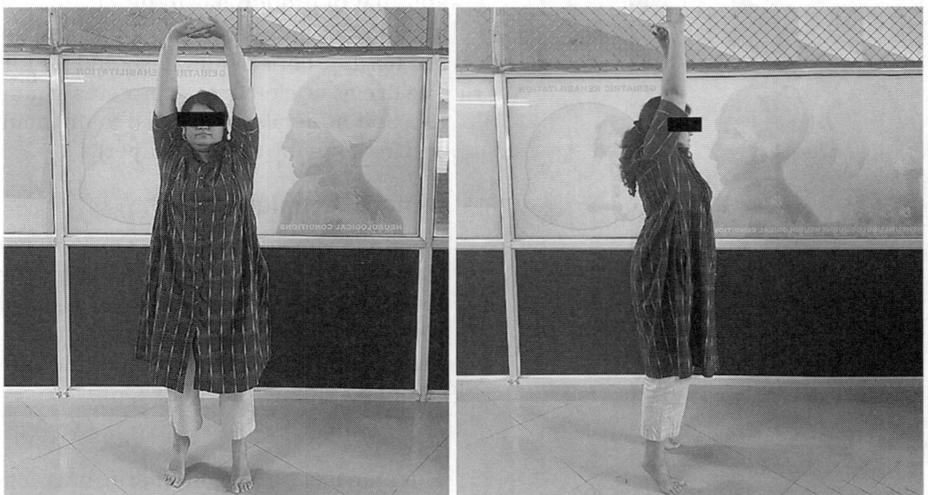

Fig. 20.20: Heel raise in standing (should be done with care).

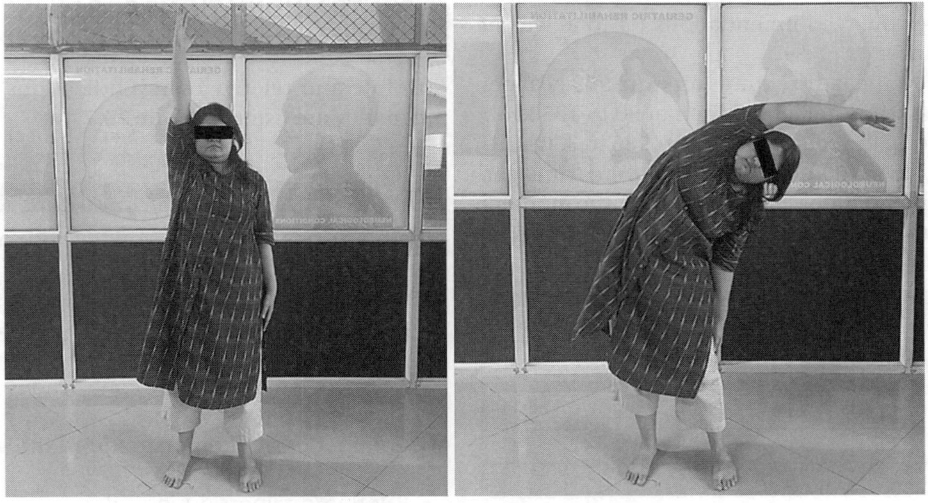

Fig. 20.21: Trunk side bending in standing.

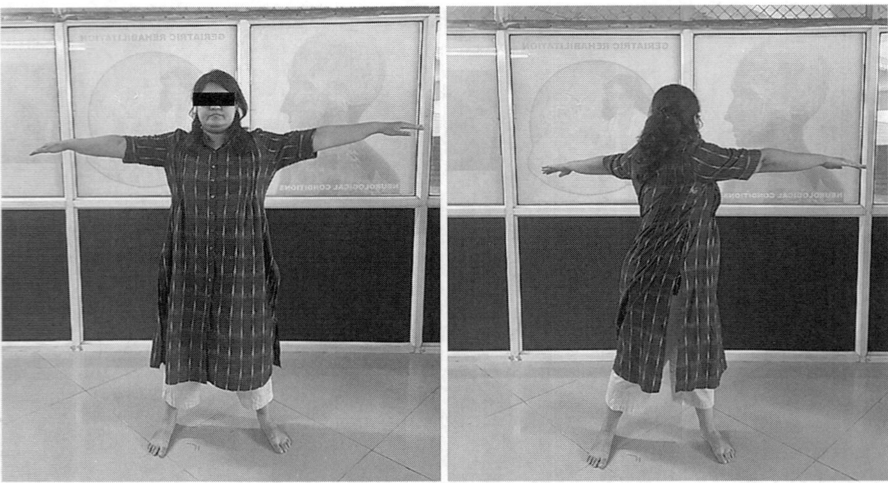

Fig. 20.22: Trunk rotation in standing.

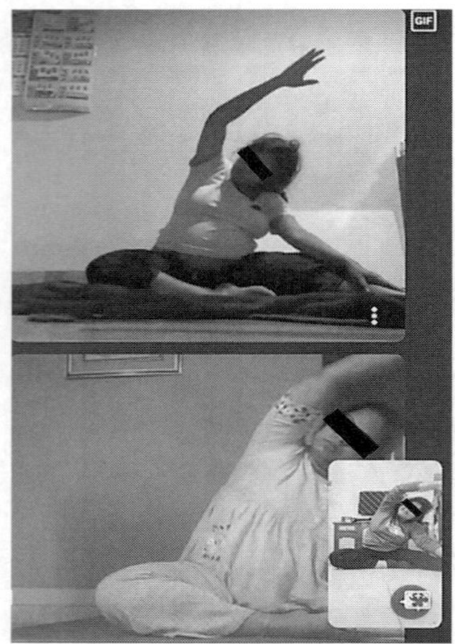

Fig. 20.23: Virtual prenatal physiotherapy session.

Weight Gain and Diet During Pregnancy

Table 20.6 describes the recommendations for total weight gain during pregnancy.

During pregnancy, the lady requires an extra 239 kcal per day. During the first trimester, an additional 90 to 125 kcal/day is required, during the second trimester 286 to 350 kcal/day is required, and 466 to 500 kcal/day in the third trimester. As per WHO recommendations, all women, from the moment they begin trying to conceive until 12 weeks of gestation, should take a folic acid supplement (400 μg folic acid daily) and that of protein has to be 71 g/day. The recommended intake of carbohydrates is 175 g/day and that of iodine is 220 μg/day. For calcium, it should be 1,000 to 2000 mg/day. The five basic elements as proteins, vitamins, carbohydrates, fats, and minerals are needed to maintain a mother's health and for her baby to grow properly.

Table 20.6: Recommendations for total weight gain during pregnancy.

Pregnancy BMI	*Range in kgs*
Underweight (<18.5)	12.5–18
Normal weight	11.5–16
Overweight	7–11.5
Obese	5–9

(BMI: Body mass index)

Lamaze Technique

It was developed by French Obstetrician Fernand Lamaze. It is a psychophysical technique that emphasizes controlled breathing and relaxation rather than pain elimination. It helps women to recognize their innate abilities and cope successfully during labor. This technique is practiced during labor and prenatal sessions.

Benefits

- It manages pain without drug interaction.
- Women feel more confident about labor after taking Lamaze classes.

CONTRAINDICATIONS FOR EXERCISING DURING PREGNANCY

Absolute and relative contraindications of exercise during pregnancy are listed in **Table 20.7**.

Clinical Pointer

Warning signs to stop the workout and contact the medical professional:

- Excessive shortness of breath that does not reduce even on rest
- Unbearable chest pain
- Repeated painful uterine contractions
- Bleeding from the vagina
- Continuous fluid discharge from the vagina, indicating rupture of membranes
- Fainting/dizziness during exercise

Table 20.7: Contraindications of exercise during pregnancy.

Absolute contra-indications	• Restrictive lung disease • Incompetent cervix • Ruptured membranes • Multiple gestations at risk of premature labor • Hemodynamically significant heart disease • Placenta previa after 26 weeks of gestation • Persistent second or third trimester bleeding • Pregnancy-induced hypertension • Premature labor during the current pregnancy
Relative contra-indications	• Severe anemia • Chronic bronchitis • Uncontrolled diabetes mellitus • Extreme morbid obesity • Extreme underweight • History of sedentary lifestyle (extreme) • Uncontrolled hypertension • Orthopedic limitations • Poorly controlled thyroid level • Heavy smoker • Intrauterine growth restriction in present pregnancy • Unevaluated maternal cardiac dysrhythmia

PREPARATION FOR LABOR

The woman should be taught relaxation techniques in order to manage stress during labor. It is important that the woman should relax and allow the natural physiologic process to take place without creating excessive tension in the unrelated muscles.

Guided Imagery Technique (Visual Imagery)

- Soothing music and verbal commands are used.
- Ask her to imagine her favorite vacation spot or any of her most desirable destinations. The same image is focused on throughout her pregnancy so that image can be called up to a conscious level during labor.
- This technique has proven to reduce stress/anxiety and various pain conditions.

Isometric Exercises

- The position should be comfortable and preferably lying.
- She is asked to contract and relax her gluteal muscles, pelvic floor, and quadriceps muscles. Slowly the proximal muscles are focused on, such as the trunk, upper extremity, facial and neck muscles.
- She should be awake during the process of labor and focus on softening the muscles as it progresses along with slow-deep breathing.

Selective Tension and Relaxation

- Contraction should be done on one part of the body and the other part should be relaxed simultaneously. For example, when the lady is contracting her legs and feet, the upper extremities should be relaxed. The ability to control both the sensations is reinforced (tension and relaxation).
- The partner can shake the extremity which is relaxed to further reduce the tension if any.

Breathing Exercises

- Slow and deep breathing is very effective during labor. The relaxation of the abdomen is taught while inhalation when it feels like the ribs are moving laterally and the abdomen is filling up.
- During expiration, the abdominal cavity becomes small and active contraction is not necessary. Slow breathing is important to prevent hyperventilation.

Relaxation during labor is described in Chapter 21: Labor and Childbirth.

Clinical Pointer

Breath-hold needs to be avoided otherwise tension will increase in the pelvic floor and if the Valsalva maneuver occurs it causes an adverse effect on the cardiovascular system.

Summary

Physiotherapists play a vital role during the journey of pregnancy. Many complications can be prevented and managed adequately via physiotherapy. Women can be taught physiological changes, self-exercise programs, and stress management. The knowledge of effective weight gain and the guidance of diet can be given. Advice on lifestyle modifications will be helpful to cope up with the hormonal changes during pregnancy.

CLINICAL EXAMPLE

Examination

A 30-year-old lady who was in her second trimester (16 weeks) enrolled for the prenatal physiotherapy sessions. She was a school teacher working for 5 to 6 hours daily. The general assessment was taken such as her last menstrual period, expected due date, weight before conception, and current weight and posture examination. Ultrasound and blood reports were examined to check the position of the placenta, length of the cervix, and development of the baby. The patient complained of moderate low back pain at the end of the day. The blood report was normal.

Suggested Management

Pregnancy exercises were commenced with a special focus on lower back strengthening. Other exercises such as breast lifting, upper/lower limb strengthening, and low impact cardio exercises were also done in the class. In between, relaxation is prescribed for example Jacobson's technique of relaxation or just diaphragmatic breathing to avoid exceeding the heart rate above moderate intensity. The duration of the session was 1 hour, 3 days a week. The patient was advised to walk for 30 minutes daily. After 36 weeks of pregnancy, hip opening exercises like duck walk, deep squatting, and physio ball exercises were carried out. The patient reported that her overall well-being and fitness had improved due to the prenatal exercise program. The lower back also got much relief. She was able to deliver normally during her 42nd week of gestation.

Review Questions

1. Write a note on antenatal classes.
2. Write a note on measures taken by a physiotherapist to prevent and treat low back pain during pregnancy.
3. Describe preparation of labor.
4. Describe common complications of pregnancy and the role of physiotherapist to manage them.
5. What is gestational diabetes? Discuss the fetal outcomes of untreated gestational diabetes.
6. Describe hip-opening exercises which are done when the expected due date is nearby.

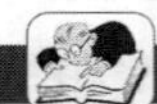

Bibliography

1. Acharry N, Kutty RK. Abdominal exercise with bracing, a therapeutic efficacy in reducing diastasis-recti among postpartal females. Int J Physiother Res. 2015;3(2):999-1005.
2. Bulgakov AV, Babieva NS, Levanova EA, Gridyaeva LN, Erofeeva MA, Sokolovskaya IE, et al. Specific features of psycho-emotional states of working women during pregnancy. Elect J General Med. 2018;15(6).
3. Donovan EL. Getting mothers moving: maternal exercise during pregnancy and long-term offspring health benefits. Exercise and Sport Sciences Reviews. 2015;43(4):179-80.
4. Harris ST, Liu J, Wilcox S, Moran R, Gallagher A. Exercise during pregnancy and its association with gestational weight gain. Matern Child Health J. 2015;19(3):528-37.
5. Hatch MC, Shu XO, McLean DE, Levin B, Begg M, Reuss L, et al. Maternal exercise during pregnancy, physical fitness, and fetal growth. Am J Epidemiol. 1993;137(10):1105-14.
6. https://my.clevelandclinic.org/health/articles/15586-labor-without-medication-coping-skills
7. Jallo N, Ruiz RJ, Elswick RK, French E. Guided imagery for stress and symptom management in pregnant African American women. Evidence-based Complementary and Alternative Medicine. 2014.
8. James P, Morgant R, Merviel P, Saraux A, Giroux-Metges MA, Guillodo Y, et al. How to promote physical activity during pregnancy: A systematic review. J Gyneco Obstet Hum Reprod. 2020;49(9):101864.
9. Kumari S. The role of physiotherapy in women health. International Journal of Yogic, Human Movement and Sports Sciences. 2018;3(1):199-201.
10. Mottola MF, Davenport MH, Ruchat SM, Davies GA, Poitras VJ, Gray CE, et al. 2019 Canadian guideline for physical activity throughout pregnancy. Br J Sports Med. 2018;52(21):1339-46.
11. Nahabedian MY. Management strategies for diastasis recti. In Seminars in Plastic Surgery. 2018;32(03):147-54.
12. Perales M, Nagpal TS, Barakat R. Physiological changes during pregnancy: main adaptations, discomforts, and implications for physical activity and exercise. In Exercise and Sporting Activity During Pregnancy. 2019:45-56.
13. Rasmussen KM, Yaktine AL. Weight gain during pregnancy: re-examining the guidelines.
14. Riebe D, Ehrman JK, Liguori G, Magal M, American College of Sports Medicine, (Eds). ACSM's Guidelines for Exercise Testing and Prescription. Wolters Kluwer; 2018.
15. Wedenberg K, Moen B, Norling Å. A prospective randomized study comparing acupuncture with physiotherapy for low-back and pelvic pain in pregnancy. Acta Obstetricia et Gynecologica Scandinavica. 2000;79(5):331-5.
16. Welch L, Miller L. Emotional and educational components of pregnancy. Glob. Libr. Women's Med. 2008:1-8.

Multiple Choice Questions (MCQs)

To test your understanding and recall of key concepts.

1. Swimming is considered as one of the best exercises during pregnancy because______________.

A. It increases cardiovascular fitness while reducing joint stress
B. It strengthens the pelvic floor exclusively
C. It promotes rapid weight loss during pregnancy
D. It requires minimal caloric expenditure

2. Which physiotherapy intervention is most appropriate for a pregnant patient who presents with low back pain due to postural changes?

A. Traction and electrical stimulation
B. Core strengthening exercises and posture correction
C. High-impact aerobics to improve overall fitness
D. Prolonged bed rest to alleviate symptoms

3. A patient in her third trimester reports muscle cramps in her calves. What should the physiotherapist recommend?

A. Walking before bed and dorsiflexion stretches
B. Ice pack application and complete rest
C. Strengthening exercises for the hamstrings
D. Massage therapy with essential oils

4. A pregnant female in her third trimester, complains of rib pain and difficulty breathing. What is her probable diagnosis?

A. Round ligament pain
B. Intercostal neuralgia
C. Diastasis recti
D. Gestational diabetes

5. The purpose of pelvic belts in managing sacroiliac pain during pregnancy is__________________.

A. Support the lumbar spine
B. Stabilize the pelvis during weight-bearing activities
C. Reduce intra-abdominal pressure
D. Prevent venous pooling in the legs

6. A prenatal physiotherapy class for women in their second trimester should include______________.

A. Posture correction, low-impact cardio, and relaxation techniques
B. Dietary restrictions, supine exercises, and high-intensity workouts
C. Stress management, Valsalva maneuvers, and weight loss
D. Sedentary lifestyle tips and pharmacological pain management

7. A pregnant female in her 3rd trimester complains of paresthesia in her hands, especially at night. What is the most likely diagnosis and preferred intervention?

A. Gestational diabetes; recommend blood sugar monitoring
B. Carpal tunnel syndrome; provide a wrist splint and hand exercises
C. Peripheral neuropathy; suggest complete rest and vitamin B supplements
D. Sacroiliac dysfunction; initiate trunk stabilization exercises

8. A pregnant female in her 3rd trimester complains of pelvic girdle pain seeks guidance for daily activities. The physiotherapist should advice her to__________.

A. Avoid all physical activities until delivery
B. Perform unilateral weight-bearing activities
C. Use a pillow between the knees while lying and avoid cross-legged sitting
D. Focus on vigorous intensity exercises for pain relief

ANSWERS

1. A	2. B	3. A	4. B	5. B
6. A	7. B	8. C		

Chapter 21

Labor and Childbirth

Manisha A Rathi

LEARNING OBJECTIVES

At the end of the chapter, the reader will be able to:
- Understand what is labor and childbirth.
- Identify causes of spontaneous labor and indications of induction of labor.
- Describe stages of normal labor.
- Understand types of delivery.
- Describe complications of normal labor and assisted delivery.
- Describe and discuss the role of physiotherapist during labor and use of various interventions for reducing pain during labor.

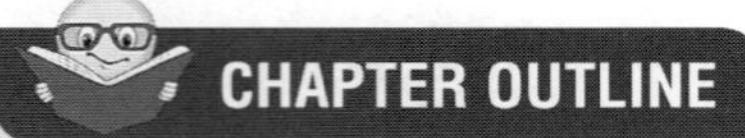

- Introduction
- Signs of labor
  - Prodromal (pre-labor) stage
  - Onset of labor
- Induction of labor
  - Contraindications to the induction of labor
- Physiological changes in mother and fetus during labor
  - Stages of normal labor
- Types of delivery
  - Vaginal delivery
  - Cesarean section
- Complications of labor
- Role of physiotherapist in labor

INTRODUCTION

It is very important for the physiotherapist to have a sound knowledge about labor so that they can appropriately take care of women during labor. The information delivered to the women should be accurate and realistic otherwise it may lead to disappointment about the experience of labor.

Labor is a series of events that occurs in the genital organs in an effort to expel the viable products of conception out of the womb through the birth canal into the outer world. Normally in between 37–42 weeks of gestation, labor commences resulting in the delivery of the fetus. Delivery means expulsion/extraction of the fetus out of the womb.

Labor is normal if it has:
- ❖ Delivery of a single baby
- ❖ Delivers vaginally
- ❖ By vertex presentation
- ❖ With spontaneous onset and at or near the term
- ❖ Entire process gets over within 24 hours
- ❖ Leaving behind a healthy mother and a healthy fetus
- ❖ With minimal intervention

Box 21.1 presents the causes of onset of spontaneous labor.

SIGNS OF LABOR

Prodromal (Pre-labor) Stage

Term is the end of normal gestation in humans and normally the range for this is 37–42 weeks. Even though the estimated date of delivery (EDD) is 280 days from the first day of the last menstruation period, but only 3–5% of women deliver on their EDD. Most common events that occur in the last weeks of pregnancy are:
- ❖ **Lightening:** As there is the descent of the fundal level followed by engagement of the head, female may feel

Box 21.1: Causes of onset of spontaneous labor.

Precise cause of spontaneous labor is unknown but following can be factors responsible for the same:
- **Estrogen theory:** Rising estrogen levels as the pregnancy progresses, leading to the stimulation of myometrial sensitivity to oxytocin and prostaglandin synthesis.
- **Progesterone withdrawal theory:** Prior to labor there is significant drop in the progesterone synthesis leading to predominance of the excitatory action of estrogen.
- **Prostaglandins theory:** Release of prostaglandins from the myometrium, decidua membranes, triggered by the rising estrogen levels.
- **Oxytocin theory:** Even though oxytocin is a strong stimulator of uterine contraction, its natural role is not clear. The secretion of oxytocinase enzyme from the placenta is decreased near term due to placental ischemia leading to predominance of oxytocin's action.
- **Fetal cortisol theory:** Increased cortisol production from the fetal adrenal gland before the onset of labor may influence its onset by increasing estrogen production from the placenta.

relief from abdominal pressure symptoms like dyspnea and dyspepsia.
- **Shelfing:** As the head of fetus gets engaged in the pelvic inlet, it makes the upper abdomen look like a shelf in the standing position.
- **Pelvic pressure symptoms:** Due to the engagement of the head in the pelvic cavity, pressure in that region leads to increase in the frequency of micturition and difficulty in walking. There may be increase in vaginal discharge.
- **Pelvic pain:** Pelvic pain may develop mainly false pain which is irregular, short duration, not progressive in nature.

Onset of Labor

- **True labor pain:** It is characterized by true pelvic pain due to uterine contractions which are regular, rhythmic, progressively increasing in intensity and frequency. It is associated with effacement and dilatation of cervix.
- **Mucoid discharge and show:** The show is an expulsion of cervical mucus plug with blood stains resulting from separation of membrane from the lower uterine segment. Labor generally lasts for several hours to few days after show.
- **Spontaneous rupture of membrane:** As the stretching of the lower uterine segment occurs, the membranes are detached easily due to their loose attachments with the poorly formed deciduas. This often occurs after labor has begun and the mucoid plug can be released unnoticed.
- **Dilatation of the cervix:** It is a reliable sign of the commencement of labor.

Figure 21.1 shows the signs of labor.

INDUCTION OF LABOR

Induction of labor is bringing about onset of labor by artificial means. Gestation of 40–41 weeks with a well-applied fetal head and effaced cervix are favorable conditions when

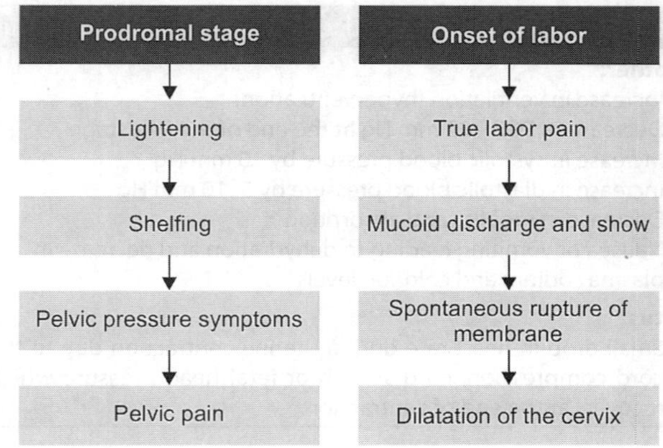

Fig. 21.1: Signs of labor.

Box 21.2: Conditions where induction of labor is advised.
- Preeclampsia
- Prolonged pregnancy
- Intrauterine growth retardation (IUGR)
- Hypertension
- Diabetes mellitus
- Intrauterine fetal death (IUFD)
- Fetal malformations

induction of labor can be initiated. If conditions shown in **Box 21.2** are present then induction of labor is advised.

Contraindications to the Induction of Labor

Some contraindications of the induction of labor are:
- Cephalopelvic disproportions
- Abnormal presentations
- Unstable lie
- Fetal distress when urgent cesarean section is needed
- Prolapsed umbilical cord

Induction of labor can be done by artificial rupture of membrane by stretching of the cervix and stripping the membrane from the lower uterine segment, administration of oxytocin through intravenous infusion and administration of prostaglandins by high vaginal insertion although it can be given orally or intravenously. Sometimes combination of two methods may be required for better results.

PHYSIOLOGICAL CHANGES IN MOTHER AND FETUS DURING LABOR

During the entire labor, some physiological changes seen in mother and fetus are listed in **Box 21.3**.

Stages of Normal Labor

There are overall four stages of labor observed during the entire labor process **(Fig. 21.2)**.

First Stage of Labor

First stage is the stage of cervical dilatation and effacement. It starts from onset of true labor pain and ends with full dilatation of the cervix and it takes about 12–16 hours in primigravidae and 6–8 hours in multigravidae.

Box 21.3: Physiological changes during labor in the mother and fetus.

Mother:
- Increase in ventilation (hyperventilation)
- Decrease in PCO_2, 22 mm Hg at the end of the first stage
- Increase in systolic blood pressure by 10 mm Hg
- Increase in diastolic blood pressure by 5–10 mm Hg
- Decrease in motility and absorption
- Nausea or vomiting leading to dehydration and decrease in plasma sodium and chloride levels

Fetus:
- Small drop in heart rate during uterine contraction due to the cord compression, cord stretch or fetal head pressure which recovers at the end of contraction

There are two subphases of this stage: Latent phase and active phase.

- During the latent phase, cervix is effaced to less than 0.5 cm and dilates from closed to 3–4 cm dilatation **(Fig. 21.3)**. Duration of this latent phase is 3–8 hours in primigravidae and it may be shorter than this in multigravidae.
- *Active phase* starts with further dilatation of cervix up to full dilatation, i.e., 10 cm and the duration of this phase is variable **(Fig. 21.4)**.

There is also formation of lower uterine segment where demarcation of active upper and relatively passive lower segment is seen. These two segments are demarcated by a ring called physiological retraction ring. Upper segment contracts to the maximum whereas lower segment relaxes which enables the expulsion of fetus by the formation of complete birth canal with the fully dilated cervix. Cesarean section is performed through lower segment.

Management

Management of this stage of labor consists of:
- Noninterference with watchful expectancy
- Woman is given encouragement, emotional support and adequate pain relief during the entire course of labor
- Careful monitoring of the progress of labor, maternal condition and fetal behavior so as to detect any deviation from normal
- Partograph is recorded where pulse, blood pressure, temperature, urine output, and any drug when given is recorded.

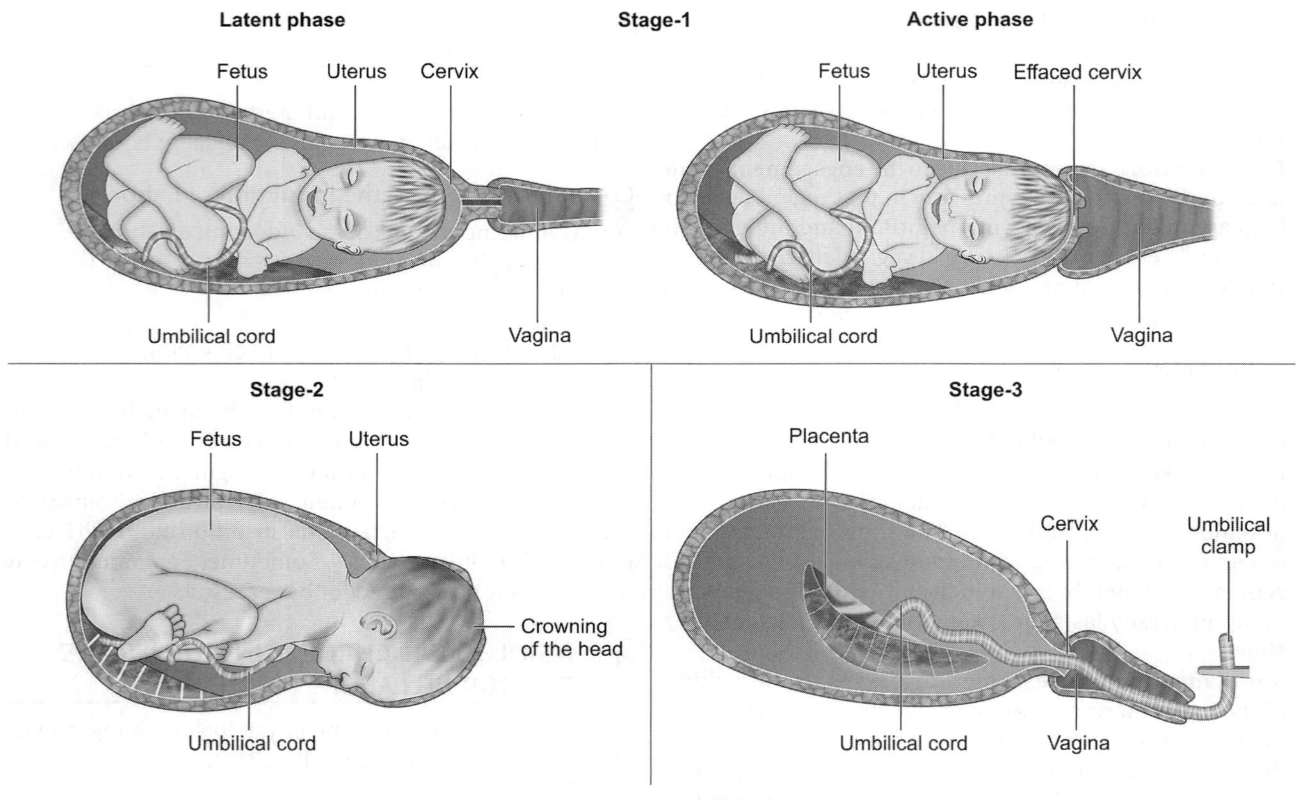

Fig. 21.2: Stages of labor.

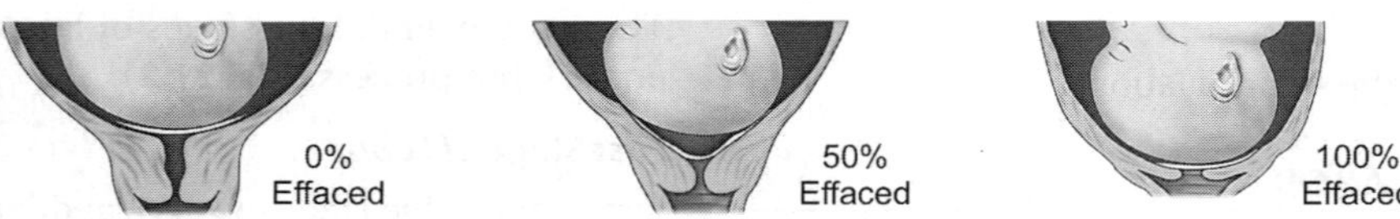

Fig. 21.3: Cervical effacement and dilatation *(For color version, see Plate 7)*.

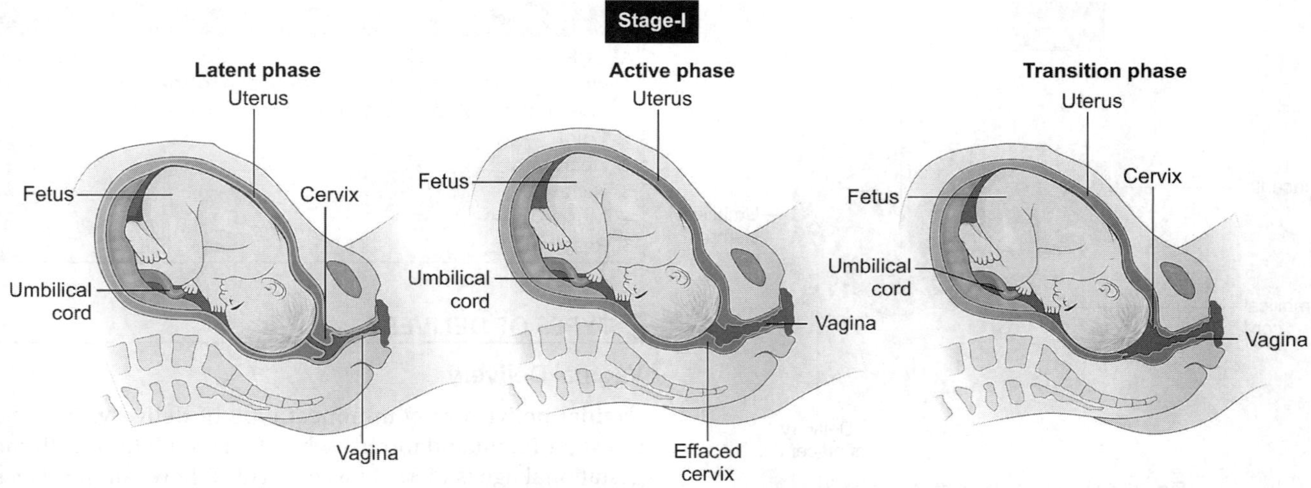

Fig. 21.4: Events in first stage of labor.

Second Stage of Labor

Second stage is the stage of expulsion which starts from complete dilatation of cervix to the expulsion of fetus from vagina and it takes about 2–4 hours in primigravidae and 30 minutes to 1 hour in multigravidae. There are two subphases:

An initial passive phase known as propulsive phase and a later phase known as expulsive phase.

- The propulsive phase (also known as phase of descent) is an extension of the first phase where the presenting part touches the pelvic floor. When cervix is fully dilated, the membrane usually ruptures and some amount of amniotic fluid escapes. Hence the uterine cavity reduces. At the same time, uterine contraction and retraction become stronger. When uterine contraction occurs, uterus elongates, while anteroposterior and transverse diameter reduces.
- *Expulsive phase* starts when active maternal pushing occurs. Delivery of the fetus is generally accompanied by the downward thrust caused by uterine contraction (power of retraction) which is enhanced by voluntary contraction of abdominal muscle (bearing down efforts) against the resistance offered by the bony and soft tissues including vagina and pelvic floor muscles **(Fig. 21.5)**. Mother may show features of exhaustion. With the maternal efforts supported by external force, delivery of baby occurs.

Management

The principles in the management are:

- To assist in the natural expulsion of the fetus slowly and steadily.
- **To prevent perineal injuries:** During the conduction of delivery, the head is delivered slowly in between contractions. Flexion is maintained so that smaller diameter of the head stretches the perineum. Thus, timely performed episiotomy prevents perineal laceration. Shoulders are delivered slowly with next contraction. Immediate care of the newborn is taken including caring of the air passage and eyes, clamping and ligaturing of the umbilical cord and APGAR scoring.

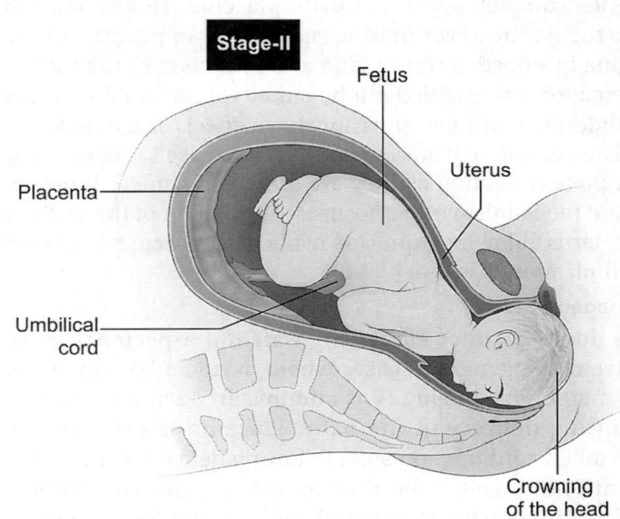

Fig. 21.5: Events in second stage of labor.

Third Stage of Labor

Third stage is the stage of expulsion of placenta and membranes. It starts from the delivery of fetus to the delivery of placenta and membranes and it takes about 15 minutes in both primigravidae and multigravidae. This comprises the phase of placental separation, its descent to the lower segment and finally the expulsion of placenta with the membrane. The plane of separation of the placenta runs through the deep spongy layer of decidua basalis **(Fig. 21.6)**.

Marked retraction of uterus effectively reduces the surface area of the placental site to about its half which was 20 cm at the beginning of the labor. There are two ways of separation of placenta:

1. Central separation
2. Marginal separation

This is followed by separation of membrane which is facilitated partly by uterine contraction and weight of the placenta as it descends down from the active part.

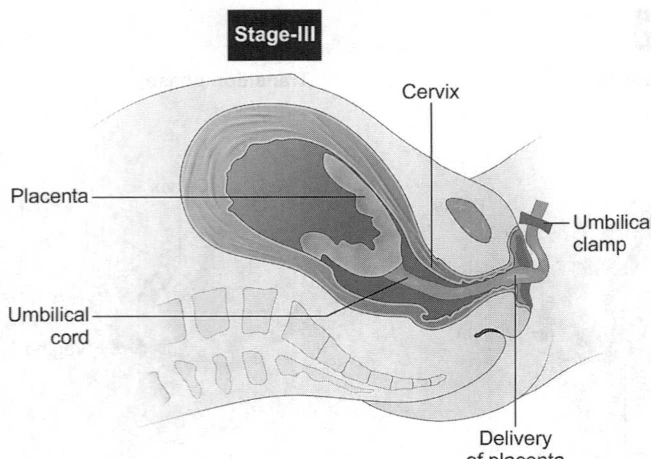

Fig. 21.6: Events in third stage of labor.

After complete separation of the placenta, it is forced down into the flabby lower uterine segment or upper part of the vagina by effective contraction and retraction of the uterus. Thereafter it is expelled out by either voluntary contraction of abdominal muscles (bearing down effect) or manually.

The occlusion of uterine and ovarian vessels is affected by complete retraction as they are literally clamped. It occurs by the mechanism of hemostasis. Apposition of the walls of the uterus following expulsion of the placenta contributes for minimization of loss of blood.

Management

It is done by either employing watchful expectancy or by active management in cases where oxytocin 10 units IV or IM/methergine 0.2 mg IV is administered within 1 minute following delivery of the baby. Placenta is delivered by controlled cord traction soon following delivery of the baby. Uterine massage may be given to make it hard. The placenta and membrane should be examined following their expulsion.

Fourth Stage of Labor

Fourth stage is the stage of recovery which begins immediately after expulsion of the placenta and membranes and remains for one hour. During this period, APGAR score **(Box 21.4)** needs to be recorded first immediately after birth and second at the end of 5th minute of birth.

Box 21.4: APGAR score.

APGAR score is a rapid assessment of the clinical status of a newborn at 1 minute and 5 minutes of age to analyze the need of intervention to establish breathing. It has five components:
1. Color
2. Heart rate
3. Reflexes
4. Muscle tone
5. Respiration

TYPES OF DELIVERY

Vaginal Delivery

Vaginal delivery is commonest type of delivery. It is the safest for infant and mother when fetus is full term with the gestational age is of 37–42 weeks. This follows all the stages of normal labor and delivery of fetus can be done with or without episiotomy. Sometimes instrumental assistance may be required to perform safe delivery (Also *see* Chapter 19: Pregnancy—Clinical). Recently immersion during first stage of labor or water-birth is also becoming popular method of vaginal delivery.

Episiotomy

Between 60 to 90% primigravida women who deliver vaginally, undergo episiotomy. It may prevent perineal tear or pelvic floor injury. It is usually performed after infiltration with local anesthesia. There are three types of incisions of episiotomy **(Fig. 21.7)**.
1. Median
2. Mediolateral
3. J-shaped.

Post episiotomy discomforts and pain at the site become the major concern for the treating physiotherapist.

Instrument-assisted Delivery

It may be necessary to assist the delivery of the baby in the second stage of the labor. Two methods are used to assist—forceps and vacuum extraction.
- **Forceps:** Obstetric forceps have blades with the contour of the baby's head which helps in delivery of the fetus in case of fetal distress. The cervix must be fully dilated

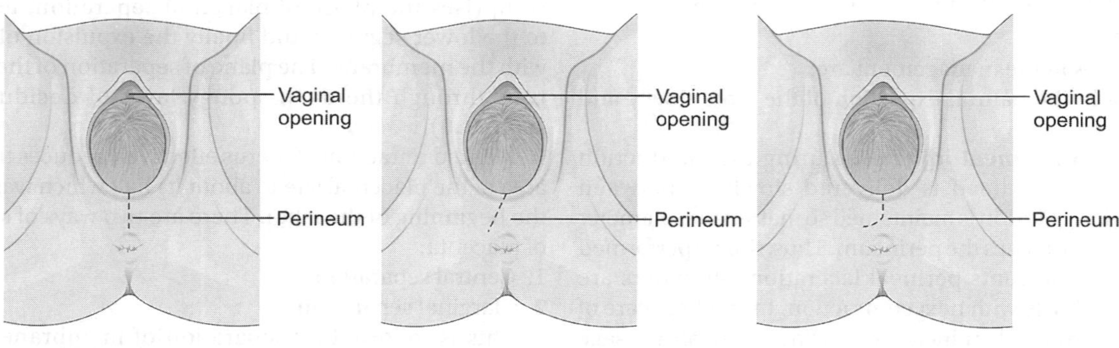

Fig. 21.7: Sites of episiotomy.

with the fetal head partially descended in the birth canal. Delivery is effected by steady traction with each uterine contraction. Complications like bruising of bladder base, perineal trauma, occult anal sphincter tear, etc., can occur **(Fig. 21.8)**.

- **Vacuum extractions:** A metal or silicone rubber cap of the appropriate size is placed over or near the posterior fontanelle, and then suction is applied with traction in each of the uterine contraction till the head passes through the introitus. A red raised circular ring will be seen over the scalp of the fetus post-delivery **(Fig. 21.9)**.

Water-birth

In water-birth, woman remains in the water during the entire labor process including propulsion phase of 2nd stage of labor and baby is delivered vaginally under water. Then the baby is brought to the surface of the water. This may be followed by the delivery of the placenta out of the water. But if the trained staff is not available then immersion in water tub or pool of warm water during first stage of labor can also be practiced. Research shows that there are many potential benefits of waterbirths. It reduces incidence of episiotomy, use of pain-relieving medications, increases incidence of normal vaginal delivery and reduces the length of first stage of labor **(Fig. 21.10)**.

Cesarean Section

Cesarean section (C-section) is a surgical method of delivering a baby in an emergency condition to prevent any complications to the mother and baby or in it can be elective when a mother has medical conditions which may anticipate complications with normal delivery.

It may be carried out under epidural or general anesthesia at any stage of labor. There are two types of incision:

1. Classical vertical paramedian incision
2. Lower segment transverse Pfannenstiel incision

The latter one is performed commonly nowadays due to its cosmetic results and easy healing **(Fig. 21.11)**.

Indications

Indications of emergency C-section

- Antepartum hemorrhage
- Prolapse of umbilical cord
- Failure to progress labor
- Grade II or IV of placenta previa
- Fetal or maternal distress
- Premature rupture of membrane
- Failed surgical induction

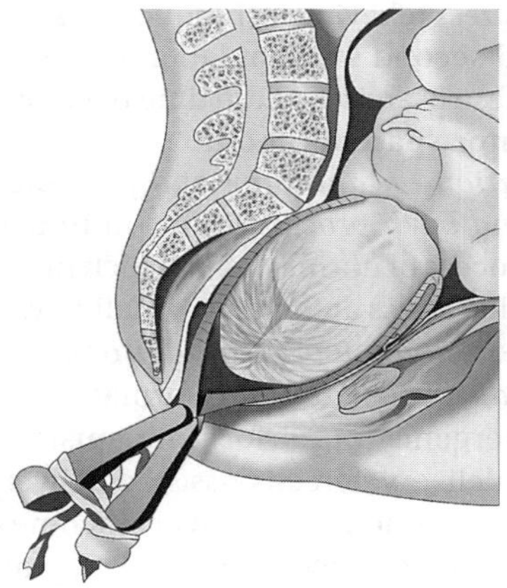

Fig. 21.8: Forceps delivery.

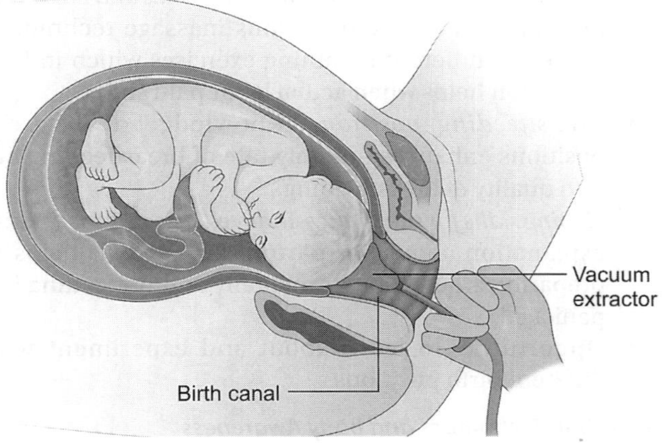

Fig. 21.9: Vacuum extraction delivery.

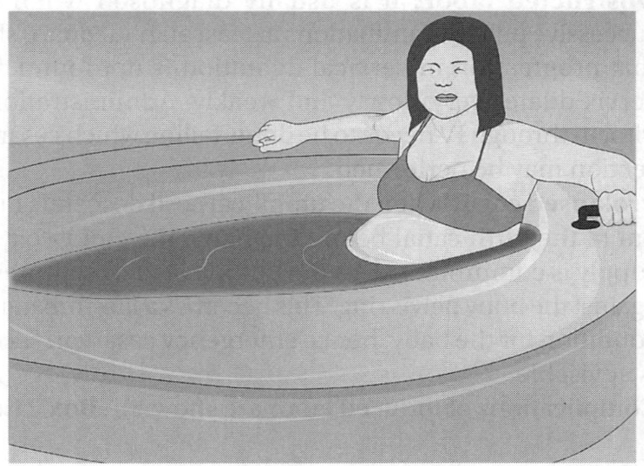

Fig. 21.10: Water-birth.

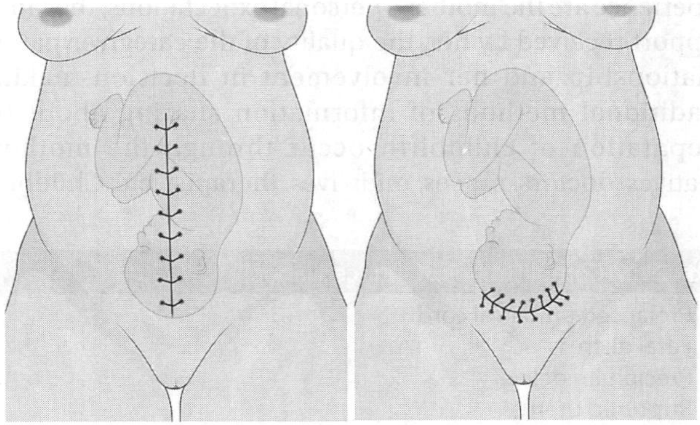

Fig. 21.11: Incisions for cesarean section.

Indications of elective C-section

- Cephalopelvic disproportion (CPD)
- Diabetes or eclampsia
- Previous C-section
- Breech presentation or unstable lie
- Multiple pregnancy like twins or triplets
- Bad obstetrics history
- On maternal request

COMPLICATIONS OF LABOR

Although modern obstetric practice has reduced the risk associated with childbirth, many complications can arise which may influence conduct and outcome of labor. They are:

- **Fetal distress:** This is observed in up to 30% of labors. Causes can be maternal hypotension, dehydration, prolonged uterine activity, premature separation of placenta, cord compression and fetal infection or hemorrhage. Hence intermittent or continuous monitoring of fetal heart rate is very important. Presence of meconium stained (fetal gut contents) liquor is also a sign of distress. In this emergency situation cesarean section is to be performed.
- **Uterine dystocia:** Difficult or abnormal labor can be assessed by considering the strength of the uterine contraction, dilatation of the cervix and descent of the presenting part.
- **Obstructed labor:** It is usually diagnosed when two successive pelvic examinations at least an hour apart, show that progression in cervical dilatation is not found. The cervix dilates very slowly and weakly. Administration of Pitocin through IV needs to be done, failing which cesarean section may be performed.
- **Prolapsed cord:** When the umbilical cord descends down out of the birth canal before the baby, the child's oxygen supply is compromised, as the umbilical cord compresses against the bony pelvis ring. This becomes a life-threatening condition for the baby, hence emergency cesarean section is advisable.

Complications of induced labor are shown in **Box 21.5**.

Box 21.5: Complications of induced labor.

- Prolapsed umbilical cord
- Fetal distress
- Precipitate delivery
- Ruptured uterus
- Infection

ROLE OF PHYSIOTHERAPIST IN LABOR

The important factors in determining her childbirth experience are the mother's personal expectations, the family support received by her, the quality of the caregiver-patient relationship and her involvement in decision-making. Traditional methods of information sharing about the preparation of childbirth occur through the mothers, relatives, doctors, nurses, midwives, therapist, etc. Childbirth educators are professionals who are formally trained and focused on the basic anatomy and physiology of labor and birth and simple but effective strategies including relaxation and breathing to cope with the pain of contractions.

Studies have shown the effectiveness of these methods for relief of pain, along with continuous emotional and physical support during parturition. Research has also proved the effect of movements during labor, physiologic pushing and the upright position for second stage.

Antenatal Preparation

- Antenatal visits educate and prepare the future parents and other members of the family about normal labor and delivery, pain relief, possible complications, and procedures, breastfeeding, newborn care and postpartum care.
- A written plan for birth and for unexpected adverse events should be given to the future parents which includes complications and emergencies that may arise during antenatal period, labor and immediate postnatal period at the antenatal visit at least 1 month prior to the birth.
- Antenatal classes practice relaxation exercises, breathing exercises, stress relieving techniques, positions to be taken in first and second stage of labor, etc., so that they can perform these exercises at the time of labor.
- **Educate future parents about:**
  - *Information on anatomy and physiology of normal labor and birth process:* Helps in understanding the exact process of normal labor which minimizes anxiety and undue stress at the time of delivery.
  - *A brief explanation of medical procedures that may be needed during childbirth:* Information about the need and emergency of performing episiotomy, vacuum suction delivery, forceps-assisted delivery etc., and its use by experts helps in positive outcome of delivery.
  - *A guide to pain relief choices:* Explanation about pharmacological and nonpharmacological interventions of pain relief and how to use them with their effectiveness, advantages and disadvantages.
  - *Chances to learn and try out massage skills and breathing techniques:* Practice of various massage techniques as well as different breathing exercises which induce relaxation helps when actual labor pain starts.
  - *Breastfeeding positions:* Knowledge of different positions enhances not only rate of breastfeeding but also quality of breastfeeding.
  - *Coping skills for pregnancy-induced discomforts:* A brief explanation about postpartum discomforts helps in preparing a new mother mentally and not getting her panicked.
  - Opportunity to learn about and experiment with different birth positions.

Relaxation Techniques and Body Awareness

The ability to diminish tension and restore equilibrium are the most important skills a mother needs to acquire during

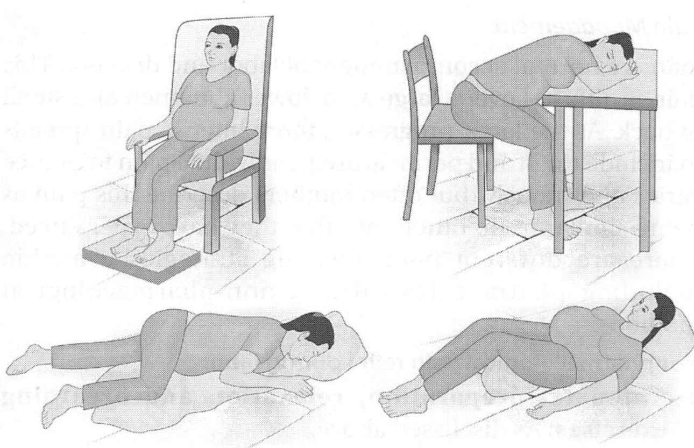

Fig. 21.12: Relaxation positions in first and second stage of labor.

the childbearing period and beyond. This is a very positive and essential approach towards life. It helps the mother in coping with the physical, psychological and emotional disturbances during pregnancy and reduce fatigue and undue stress.

- Various postures in supine, side lying and sitting positions help in inducing relaxations during labor and pushing the baby well providing enough amount of oxygen to the baby **(Fig. 21.12)**.
- Alternate contraction and relaxation of muscle group or individual muscle (Jacobson's relaxation) can help in relaxation of muscle groups. Contraction of agonist and relaxation of antagonist (Mitchell relaxation) results in relaxation of antagonist.
- Guided imagery or visualization techniques are also useful.
- Music therapy helps in relaxation by helping in reliving the sounds, touch, emotions and all sensations pertaining to that of memory. Choose harmonious and rhythmic, pleasant to hear music for inducing relaxation.
- Physical activities like gentle walking release tension and promote relaxation.

Breathing Awareness

Breathing in labor is important to prevent the side effects of hyperventilation which is very much associated with pain and anxiety of labor and to induce relaxation.

Hyperventilation leads to increase in oxygen consumption and is found in women who are very anxious or who experience intense pain. This can cause maternal cerebral and placental vasoconstriction, causing reduction in placental blood flow and fetal oxygen resulting in fetal hypoxia. The physiotherapist must be aware of this situation and relaxation must be practiced to come out of the situation.

Breathing exercises help in providing oxygen to mother, baby and hard-working uterus. They also reduce pain, promote physical and mental relaxation and facilitate distraction from painful contractions.

Lamaze breathing technique is very effective for labor pain management which includes slow breathing for 3–5 counts and exhaling for the same count. Monitor this normal breathing pattern where inhalation is from nose and exhalation by mouth in the form of blowing for one minute. A cleansing breath is done where deep slow breathing is done by nose and exhaling with a deep slow breath out is done by mouth.

Breathing during first stage of labor

It generally begins and ends with slow cleansing breathing as it is comfortable and leads to relaxation. Mother can practice light breathing which begins with one deep cleansing breath followed by quicker and shallower breathing and ends with cleansing breath.

Breathing techniques for second stage of labor

It has been shown that discussing, demonstrating and rehearsing the proper breathing exercises during the antenatal period helps the woman to understand what exactly is required at the time of labor. Maternal expulsive effort is supplementary to the expulsive efforts of the uterus. Coordination of mother's physical efforts with the correct breathing pattern results in proper usage of mother's energy. Completely relaxed body in between pushing efforts and breathing normally in this period minimizes extra efforts during labor. Bearing down efforts can be practiced when the fetal head starts to descend the perineum and mother has an urge to push. Mother must breathe normally and comfortably until the doctors give instructions to push. Then take a deep breath and hold the same or slowly release while bearing down for 5–7 seconds, then release the breath. Take one or two deep breaths, and repeat until rest and end with cleansing breath.

Positions during Labor

In addition to the lithotomy position, many positions are successfully used by midwives and traditional birth attendants worldwide like squatting, standing, kneeling on all fours (quadruped). There are many physiological advantages of upright positions like gravity, reduced risk of aorto-caval compression, better alignment of fetus, etc. Pelvic outlet can be increased during squatting and kneeling positions. Mother should be informed and encouraged to be in a position she finds most comfortable throughout the labor.

During first stage

- Most important and useful position is upright position. Mother should avoid lying flat and encourage walking around.
- As the uterus is anteverted in the first stage of labor, forward lean sitting position is the best position **(Fig. 21.13)**.
- Mother should be informed that bearing down efforts in this stage are useless, they will not only exhaust themselves without any positive outcome but also lead to uterine/genital prolapse, hence she should not be practicing the bearing down in first stage of labor.
- Other positions which can be practiced in this stage are resting over the bean bag, sitting backwards on chair, leaning forward on the wall in standing, rocking in quadruped position, etc. **(Fig. 21.14)**.

During second stage

- Most commonly used recumbent positions are lithotomy and semi-recumbent positions with wedges.

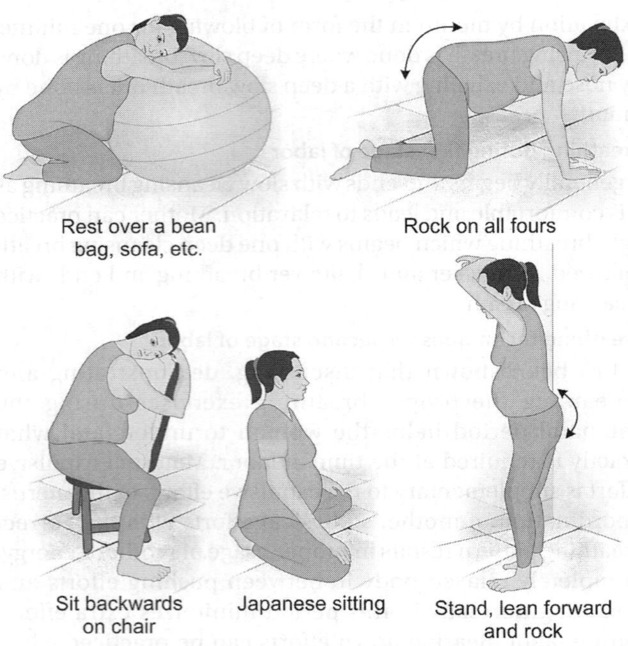

Fig. 21.13: Positions for anteversion of the uterus during first stage of labor.

- Sometimes upright positions include sitting 45 degrees elevated from horizontal, squatting, or kneeling **(Fig. 21.15)**.

Pain Management

Pain is a normal accompaniment of labor and delivery. This pain is diffused over a large area, lower abdomen and small of back. As the labor progresses, more intense pain spreads to include thigh and perineal area. Individual pain tolerance varies enormously, but often mothers describe this pain as being similar to no other pain that they have experienced. There are different pain-relieving strategies available including pharmacological and non-pharmacological methods.

Nonpharmacological pain relief during labor

- **Antenatal preparation, relaxation and breathing exercises:** As discussed above.
- **Music therapy:** It enhances relaxation as it calms the mind and releases the body stress. A soft soothing music in the labor/operative room may lead to relaxation and reduce anxiety and undue stress.
- **Soft tissue techniques:** Soft tissue techniques like massage help in relieving pain by inducing relaxation, inhibition of sensory pain pathways, enhancing blood flow to the part and oxygenation of the tissue. They can be applied for lower back, neck, perineal, abdominal and hand areas. Women should be in comfortable and acceptable position supported by pillows and cushions. Therapist or assisting caregiver can perform the various techniques gently over the painful areas with maximum precautions **(Fig. 21.16)**.
- **Immersion in warm water:** Immersion in warm water during any stage of labor is used for relaxation and pain relief

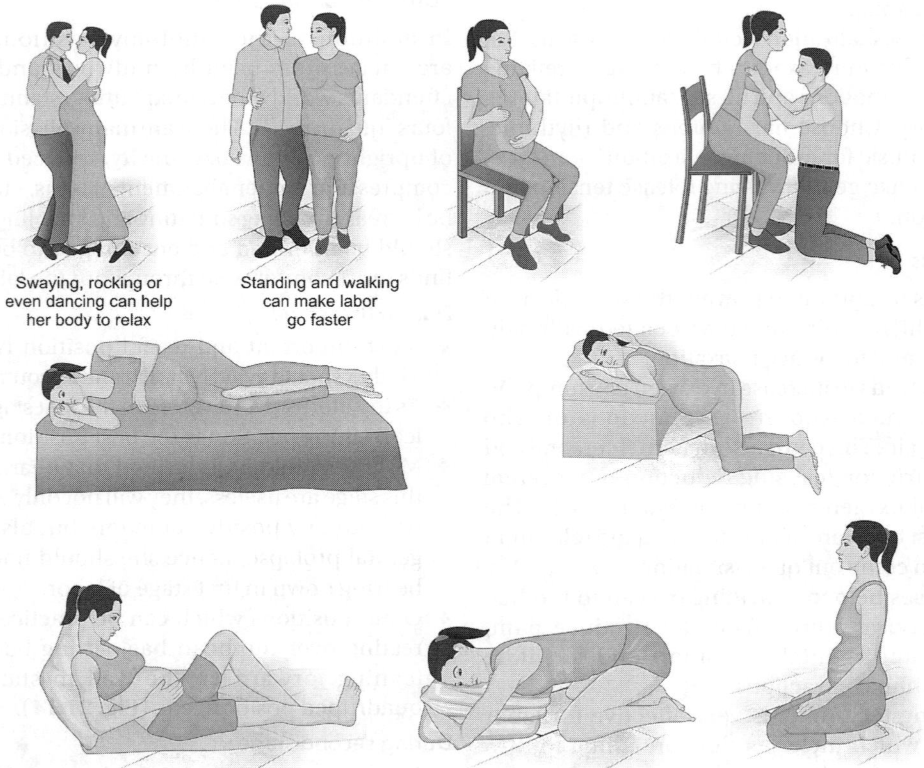

Fig. 21.14: Various positions that can be adopted by the mother during first stage of labor.

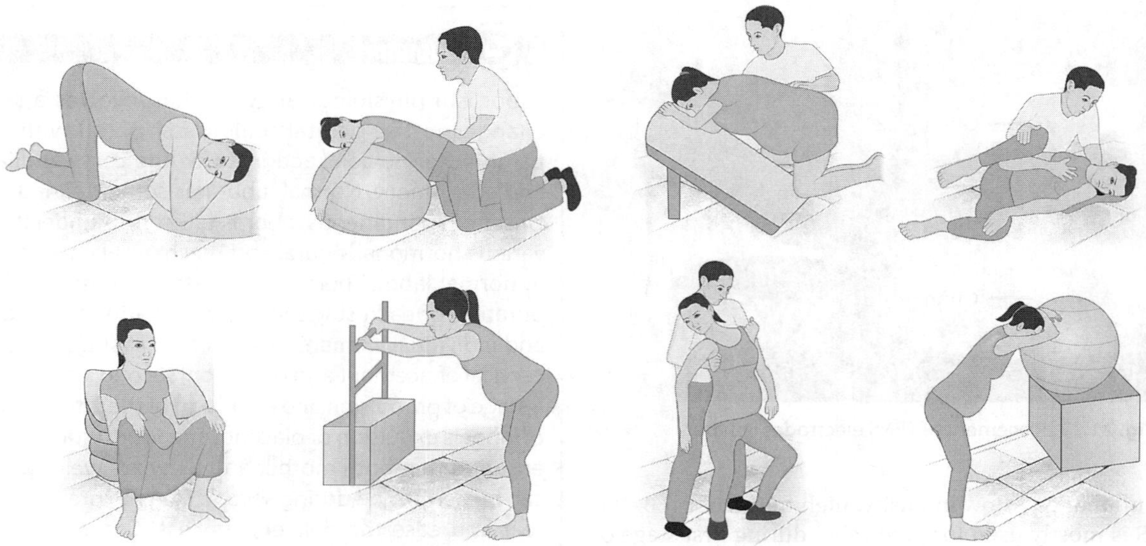

Fig. 21.15: Positions that can be adopted in the second stage of labor.

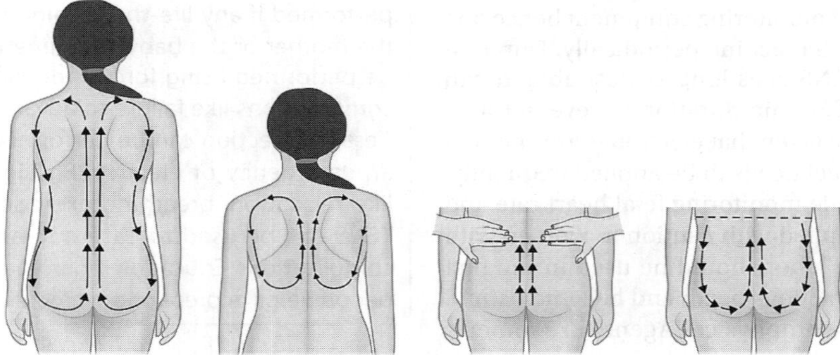

Fig. 21.16: Soft tissue techniques.

where the woman's abdomen is completely submerged in water. This may take place in a receptacle that may be a pool, tub or bath. It is associated with improved uterine perfusion and less painful contractions.

Precautions to be taken are:
- Membrane should be intact
- Body should be immersed in warm water in a position of comfort
- The woman should never be left alone, as labor progresses
- The woman will need to come out of the pool at regular intervals for monitoring.

- **Acupressure:** It is used in labor for relief of pain and other discomforts. With the help of thumb pad, pressure is applied on the desired areas like shoulders, neck, low back, small toes, soles of the feet, etc. This helps in stimulating mechanoreceptors and through gate control theory, pain reduces or it becomes bearable.
- **Hypnosis:** The main effect of hypnotherapy is to induce relaxation and to eliminate or reduce the need of analgesia and shorten labor. Once the mother is trained for autohypnosis during the antenatal period, she can practice the same during labor even without an instructor effectively.
- **Biofeedback:** It is another technique of relaxation that can be used during labor. A woman needs to be educated to become aware about her body, the stressful/contracted conditions of muscles so that she can practice how to relax using biofeedback technique. A biofeedback machine can be used to reduce the stress.
- **Transcutaneous electrical nerve stimulation (TENS):** TENS is a non-invasive, self-controlled form of pain relief without any side effects, uses low voltage electrical impulses which vary in pulse duration, frequency and intensity. TENS works in two ways: It inhibits the transmission of impulses which send pain signals to the brain and releases natural analgesics like endorphins and encephalins.

  Electrodes can be placed on either side of thoracic and sacral spine, or one pair at the T10–L1 spine and other pair on S2–S4 spine. Sometimes other pair of electrodes can be moved to the lower abdomen but less evidences are available **(Fig. 21.17)**.

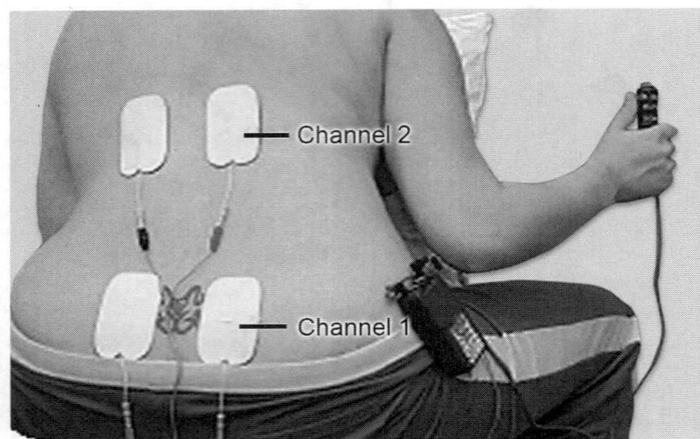

Fig. 21.17: Placement of TENS electrodes in labor.

Conventional type/low intensity, high frequency (80–100 Hz) TENS is mostly used for pain relief during first stage of labor and when contraction occurs, intensity can be raised. A battery-operated equipment can be used which has the control with the woman herself. This stimulation may affect the parameters of the fetal monitoring equipment hence one may need to remove TENS machine periodically. Duration of the treatment with TENS is as long as desirable. It can be used for minimum of 30 min duration to several hours after birth. Care should be taken that electrodes are checked periodically, conducting gel needs to be applied frequently, it should be removed while monitoring fetal heart rate and taking bath. It is to be applied with caution in women with metal implants. TENS in labor should be used in the first stage of labor when contractions begin and become painful (Also *see* Chapter 17: Electrophysical Agents in Women's Health).

Pharmacological Methods to Relief Pain

- **Oral medications:** They are not commonly used by the mother as it may cause adverse effect on the fetus.
- **Inhalation of nitrous oxide:** Inhalation of nitrous oxide with oxygen in 50–50% mixture (called as Entonox) is effective and still in use by some obstetricians. It is self-administered, readily available, does not have any effect on progress of labor and does not affect fetal heart rate. It may cause some adverse effects like light headedness, nausea/vomiting, confusion, disorientation, etc. Hence it should be administered with utmost care.
- **Epidural analgesia:** It is the most effective form of pain relief practice since many years. It should be performed by a medical practitioner, who is trained and skilled in this technique. The consulting professional should also be skilled in performing instrument assisted delivery as many times women will not to be able to put their maximum bearing down effort due to anesthesia effect. Some risks involved with this are:
  - Infections
  - Neural damage
  - Dural puncture

Summary

Labor is a physiological event that involves a series of changes in the genital region associated with regular painful uterine contractions with the cervical dilatation and effacement. Normal labor has some defined criteria. Onset of spontaneous labor is difficult to understand but various hormonal, neural and mechanical changes results in normal labor. There are four stages of normal labor—duration of each stage varies with parity, status of labor and individual women's condition. First stage is a stage of cervical effacement and dilatation, second stage of labor is a stage of propulsion and expulsion of the fetus, third stage of labor is expulsion of placenta and fourth stage of labor is ensuring that both mother and baby are well. Episiotomy can be performed during second stage to prevent perineal tear and ease the delivery process. Complications may develop at any stage during labor and early recognition and appropriate interventions may prevent serious complications. Lower segment caesarian section can be performed if any life-threatening complications arise for the mother or the baby. Instrument-assisted delivery can be performed using forceps or vacuum extraction if any complications like failure to advance in the second stage. Cesarean section can be performed as per indications as an emergency or elective. Physiotherapy interventions like relaxation, breathing exercises, proper positioning, TENS can be used to ease out labor pain and mininize complications. Education regarding labor during antenatal period helps in preparing women for the delivery.

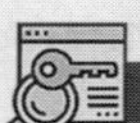

Review Questions

1. Describe various stages of labor.
2. Discuss the various physiotherapy interventions that can be used during labor to reduce pain and minimize complications.
3. What are the various modes of delivery?
4. What causes the initiation of spontaneous labor?
5. Describe the detail the use of TENS during labor.

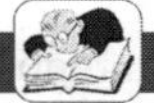

Bibliography

1. American College of Obstetricians and Gynecologists. Operative Vaginal Birth: ACOG Practice Bulletin No. 219. Obstet Gynecol. 2020;135(4):e149-59. doi:10.1097/AOG.0000000000003748.
2. Arya R, Whitworth M, Johnston TA. Mechanism and management of normal labor. Obstet Gynecol Reprod Med. 2007;17(8):232-7.
3. Azizmohammadi S, Azizmohammadi S. Hypnotherapy in management of delivery pain: a review. Eur J Transl Myol. 2019;29(3):8365. doi:10.4081/ejtm.2019.8365.
4. Baker PN. Obstetrics by Ten Teachers, 18th edition. London: Hodder Education; 2006.

5. Barragán Loayza IM, Solà I, Juandó Prats C. Biofeedback for pain management during labor. Cochrane Database Syst Rev. 2011;(6):CD006168. doi:10.1002/14651858.CD006168.pub2.
6. Bergström M, Kieler H, Waldenström U. Effects of natural childbirth preparation versus standard antenatal education on epidural rates, experience of childbirth and parental stress: a randomized controlled multicentre trial. BJOG. 2009;116(9): 1167-76. doi:10.1111/j.1471-0528.2009.02144.x.
7. Bloom SL, Casey BM, Schaffer JI, McIntire DD, Leveno KJ. A randomized trial of coached versus uncoached maternal pushing during the second stage of labor. Am J Obstet Gynecol. 2006;194(1):10–3. doi:10.1016/j.ajog.2005.06.085.
8. Changela PK. Role of Physiotherapist in Obstetric and Gynecological Conditions. New Delhi: Jaypee Brothers Medical Publishers; 2016.
9. Dowswell T, Bedwell C, Lavender T, Neilson JP. Transcutaneous electrical nerve stimulation (TENS) for pain management in labor. Cochrane Database Syst Rev. 2009;(2):CD007214. doi:10.1002/14651858.CD007214.pub2.
10. Friedman EA. Labor: Clinical Evaluation and Management, 2nd edition. New York: Appleton-Century-Crofts; 1978.
11. Gupta JK, Sood A, Hofmeyr GJ, Vogel JP. Position in the second stage of labor for women without epidural anaesthesia. Cochrane Database Syst Rev. 2017;5(5):CD002006. doi:10.1002/14651858. CD002006.pub4.
12. Harrison RF, Shore M, Woods T, Mathews G, Gardiner J, Unwin A. A comparative study of transcutaneous electrical nerve stimulation, Entonox, pethidine, promazine and lumbar epidural for pain relief in labor. Acta Obstet Gynecol Scand. 1987;66(2): 99-104. doi:10.3109/00016348709022011.
13. Hofmeyr G, Nikodem VC, Wolman WL, Chalmers BE, Kramer T. Companionship to modify the clinical birth environment: effects on progress and perception of labor and breastfeeding. Br J Obstet Gynaecol. 1991;98(8):756-64. doi:10.1111/j.1471-0528.1991. tb13475.x.
14. Johnson JH, Figueroa R, Garry D, Elimian A, Maulik D. Immediate maternal and neonatal effects of forceps and vacuum-assisted deliveries. Obstet Gynecol. 2004;103(3):513-8. doi:10.1097/01. AOG.0000114984.83322.1F.
15. Jones L, Othman M, Dowswell T, Alfirevic Z, Gates S, Newburn M, et al. Pain management for women in labor: an overview of systematic reviews. Cochrane Database Syst Rev. 2012;2012(3):CD009234. doi:10.1002/14651858.CD009234. pub2.
16. Konar H. DC Dutta's Textbook of Obstetrics, 9th edition. New Delhi: Jaypee Brothers Medical Publishers; 2018.
17. Lamaze International. Promoting Safe, Healthy Birth Practices. Washington DC: Lamaze International; 2009.
18. Mantle J, Haslam J, Barton S. Physiotherapy in Obstetrics and Gynaecology, 2nd edition. New Delhi: Reed Elsevier India; 2005.
19. Melzack R, Schaffelberg D. Low back pain during labor. Am J Obstet Gynecol. 1987;157(3):636-9. doi:10.1016/S0002-9378(87)80003-4.
20. Nichols F, Humenick S. Childbirth Education: Practice, Research, and Theory, 2nd edition. Philadelphia: WB Saunders; 2000.
21. Nutter E, Meyer S, Shaw-Battista J, Marowitz A. Waterbirth: an integrative analysis of peer-reviewed literature. J Midwifery Womens Health. 2014;59(3):286-319. doi:10.1111/jmwh.12194.
22. Oats J, Abraham S. Llewellyn-Jones Fundamentals of Obstetrics and Gynaecology. 9th edition. St. Louis: Mosby Elsevier; 2010.
23. O'Driscoll K, Meagher D. Active Management of Labor, 2nd edition. London: Saunders; 1986.
24. Pates JA, Satin AJ. Active management of labor. Obstet Gynecol Clin North Am. 2005;32(2):221-30. doi:10.1016/j.ogc.2005.01.001.
25. Sapsford R, Bullock-Saxton J, Markwell S. Women's Health: A Textbook for Physiotherapists. London: WB Saunders; 1998.
26. Simkin P. Reducing pain and enhancing progress in labor: a guide to nonpharmacologic methods for maternity caregivers. Birth. 1995;22(3):161-71. doi:10.1111/j.1523-536X.1995.tb00571.x.
27. Smith CA, Levett KM, Collins CT, Armour M, Dahlen HG, Suganuma M. Relaxation techniques for pain management in labor. Cochrane Database Syst Rev. 2018;3:CD009514. doi:10.1002/14651858.CD009514.pub2.
28. Smith CA, Levett KM, Collins CT, Dahlen HG, Ee CC, Suganuma M. Massage, reflexology and other manual methods for pain management in labor. Cochrane Database Syst Rev. 2018;3:CD009290. doi:10.1002/14651858.CD009290.pub3.
29. Society of Obstetricians and Gynaecologists of Canada. Advances in labor and risk management (ALARM) course manual. 23rd ed. Ottawa: SOGC; 2016-2017.

Multiple Choice Questions (MCQs)

To test your understanding and recall of key concepts.

1. **Which of the following is *not* the most common events that occur in the last weeks of pregnancy:**
   A. Lightening B. Shelfing
   C. Dilatation of the cervix D. Nausea
2. **Which hormone is most closely associated with the onset of labor?**
   A. Progesterone B. Estrogen
   C. Oxytocin D. Relaxin
3. **What is the normal duration of the first stage of labor for a primigravida?**
   A. 3–5 hours B. 6–8 hours
   C. 12–16 hours D. 18–24 hours
4. **Why is the APGAR score recorded at 1 and 5 minutes after birth?**
   A. To monitor maternal health in postpartum period
   B. To evaluate the effectiveness of labor pain management
   C. To assess the newborn's clinical status and need for immediate intervention
   D. To calculate the duration of the labor process
5. **'Lightening' during the prodromal stage of labor signifies__________.**
   A. Full dilatation of the cervix
   B. Fetal head engagement
   C. Imminent delivery
   D. Uterine rupture
6. **Upright positions are encouraged during the first stage of labor to__________.**
   A. Reduce the risk of perineal tears
   B. Enhance uterine perfusion and alignment of the fetus
   C. Minimize uterine contractions
   D. Increase the duration of labor

7. Which of the following statements is the most accurate about the use of TENS for pain relief during labor ?

A. TENS poses significant risks to the fetus but is effective for maternal pain relief
B. TENS provides non-invasive pain relief with minimal side effects for both mother and baby
C. TENS should only be used during the second stage of labor
D. TENS is not recommended due to a lack of evidence supporting its effectiveness

8. A 30-year-old primigravida in active labor complains of lower back pain and exhaustion. She has been using Lamaze breathing techniques but feels they are no longer effective. The obstetrician has requested non-pharmacological support to manage her pain and enhance labor progression. As a physiotherapist, what combination of interventions would you prioritize?

A. Introduce TENS for pain relief, advise on upright positions, and perform soft tissue massage on the lower back
B. Suggest complete bed rest and administer manual relaxation techniques to the patient in supine
C. Focus exclusively on deep breathing exercises and avoid physical interventions
D. Encourage supine positioning and provide passive ROM exercises to the mother

ANSWERS

1. D	2. C	3. C	4. C	5. B
6. B	7. B	8. A		

Chapter **22**

Postnatal Care

Anu Arora

Life is a flame that is always burning itself out; but it catches fire again every time a child is born.
—George Bernard Shaw

LEARNING OBJECTIVES

At the end of the chapter, the reader will be able to:

- Describe the health interventions to be delivered during the postnatal period.
- Describe health behaviors to be practiced during this period to care for mother and child.
- Facilitate devising an exercise and relaxation plan for new mothers assisting their physical and mental recovery.
- Learn to prescribe exercises for restoration of muscle strength and tone, treatment of any musculoskeletal concerns in the postnatal period.
- Learn about proper ergonomics during breastfeeding, baby handling, and household chores.
- Learn about the nutritional requirements of pregnancy.
- Learn about the contraception needs of the new mother.
- Educate regarding the assessment and management of postpartum depression.

CHAPTER OUTLINE

INTRODUCTION

The **postpartum period** is a unique period in the life of a new mother that is characterized by a swift withdrawal of ovarian hormones, which inevitably induces a wide range of adaptive responses. Puerperium is defined as the period of time in postnatal life which comprises of the 6–8 week period from the time of delivery of the placenta up to the resumption of normal ovulatory function.

CONSTITUENTS OF POSTNATAL CARE

Systemic supervision and management of the female in the postpartum period is referred to as the **postnatal care (PNC)**.

Postnatal physiotherapy care entails:

- Careful history taking and examination (general and obstetrical)
- Identifying and managing any concerns encountered by the new mother
- Advice of appropriate exercise intensity, frequency and type to prevent common problems and enhance general functions in postnatal females
- Ergonomic advice regarding baby handling and breast-feeding positions
- Nutrition in lactation
- Structured exercise regime to regain the pre-pregnancy functional capacity
- Making new mothers aware of the normal developmental chronology, and advice on environmental and baby handling techniques to facilitate the physiological process
- Making the new mothers aware of the need for an appropriate contraception
- Emphasizing upon the new mothers, the importance of following the vaccination schedule for the infant.

PHASES OF POSTPARTUM PERIOD

The puerperium may be prolonged because of the effects of lactation on hormonal balance in nursing mothers. Lactation usually inhibits the ovulatory cycles during the puerperium. The mean time to ovulation post-delivery is about 6 months. In non-breastfeeding women, the routine cyclic hormonal milieu is rapidly restored and the mean time to ovulation after delivery is 45 days. This is an important time for the new mother and newborn to recover from the birth process and for their physiological and psychological adjustment to the postnatal period.

The postpartum period is termed in some literature as the **"fourth stage of labor". It can be subdivided into** three distinct but continuous phases **(Fig. 22.1)**.

1. **Acute postpartum period:** Rapidly changing phase with a potential for immediate crises such as postpartum hemorrhage, uterine inversion, amniotic fluid embolism, and eclampsia.
2. **Subacute postpartum period:** This phase is characterized by major changes in the body systems including the hemodynamic, genitourinary health retrieval, metabolism, and emotional well-being.
3. **Delayed postpartum period:** This phase is characterized by extremely gradual changes leading to recovery of muscle tone and connective tissue to the prepregnant physiology.

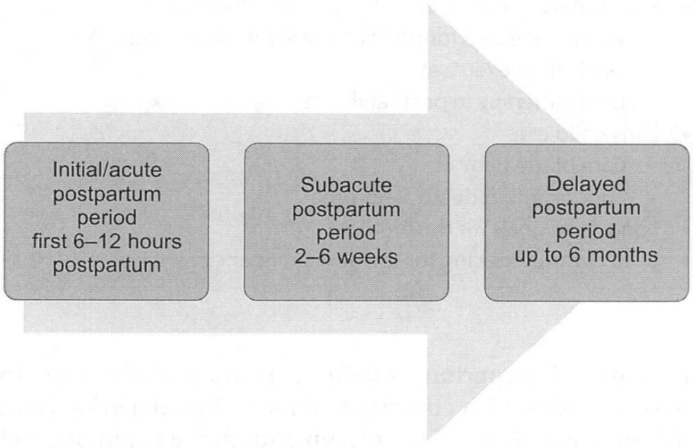

Fig. 22.1: Three phases of postpartum period.

Post-birth

The third stage of labor is characterized by the separation and expulsion of the placenta and membranes. The physiological changes that occur in the third period of labor are designed to facilitate the separation and expulsion of the placenta and fetal membranes, and to ensure control of maternal bleeding. These include:

- The birth of the baby fast tracks the retraction of uterine muscles.
- Strong uterine contractions that squeeze the placenta forcing blood from the intervillous spaces into the spongy layer of the decidua.
- Retraction of the uterine oblique muscle fibers which prevents blood from entering the maternal system
- Seeping of blood between the thin septa of the spongy layer and the placental surface, aiding its separation.
- Formation of a retroplacental clot exerts further pressure.
- The uterine contractions causing the placenta and membranes to descend into the lower uterine segment from where they are eventually expelled.

Factors Affecting Recovery in the Postpartum Period

- Patient's intrinsic collagen support
- The size of the infant
- The route of delivery
- The degree of perineal trauma occurring either naturally (lacerations) or iatrogenically (episiotomy).

EARLY ATTACHMENT AND SKIN-TO-SKIN CARE

Mothers and babies should not be separated from the time of delivery onwards. Early attachment to the breast should be encouraged with skin-to-skin contact. This kind of skin-to-skin contact immediately after birth has multiple benefits for both mother and baby as shown in **Table 22.1**.

Table 22.1: Advantages of skin-to-skin contact of baby and mother immediately after birth.

Advantages for the mother	*Advantages for the baby*
• Stimulates maternal oxytocin production • Facilitates earlier expulsion of the placenta • Reduced bleeding • Increased breastfeeding self-efficacy • Lowered maternal stress levels • Mother–infant bonding	• Decrease in the birth-related stress in the newborn • More optimal thermoregulation • Less crying

Clinical Pointer

Kangaroo mother care: An embrace of life

Kangaroo mother care, a comprehensive newborn care, involving skin-to-skin contact with the mother or other caregiver.

- Reduces mortality in infants with low birth weight by creating an optimal environment for adaptation of newborn infants to extrauterine life.
- Promotes infant survival, neurodevelopment, the quality of mother-infant bonding, and decreases maternal postpartum depressive symptoms.
- Reduces hospital expenditure.

BREASTFEEDING

Breastfeeding is the most significant early life contribution to neonatal, infant and child health growth development. It serves as a nutritional link between the baby and the mother that continues even in postpartum life. This advantage, incurred with breastfeeding starts within an hour or so after birth.

It is recommended that breast milk be the infant's only source of nutrition for the first 6 months of life. It is further recommended that complementary foods be added to the infant's diet only after 6 months of age and that breastfeeding continues up to two years of age and beyond as per choice and prevailing conditions. Breastfeeding is considered as one of the most effective ways to ensure child health and survival. Benefits of breastfeeding are given below and in **Table 22.2**.

- The secretory IgA present in the breast milk are protective against infections of ears, nose, throat and digestive tract, respiratory tract.
- The carnitine level in breast milk helps in the utilization of fatty acids as an energy source and thus reduces the cholesterol levels.
- Lactoferrin in breast milk prevents the growth of iron-dependent bacteria in the GI tract.
- Lysozyme in breastmilk is protective against *Salmonella* and *E. coli*.
- Essential fats in milk are important for cognitive development.
- Breastfeeding is associated with improved cognitive development, and prevention of obesity, hypertension, and insulin-dependent diabetes mellitus, thus lowering the rate of illness and consequently the rate of hospital admission.

Clinical Pointer

Hormonal profile of lactation

Lactation is characterized by:

- Increased levels of prolactin
- Decreasing levels of estrogen
- Elevated release of antinociceptive neuropeptides like oxytocin and vasopressin

In view of the strong evidence of the benefits of breastfeeding for women and babies the World Health Organization (WHO) has recommended that babies should be exclusively breastfed for the first six months "to achieve optimal growth, development, and health".

Ideally breastfeeding should begin as the infant demonstrates spontaneous signs of readiness through salivation, rooting, sucking, etc. In the first couple of hours of life, the baby is alert, active, and ready to feed. Immediately after birth a healthy, term baby, when placed on the mother's stomach, is able to crawl towards the breast. This is called a ***breast crawl***. Breastfeeding should be facilitated as soon as the baby shows signs of readiness for a feed.

Breastmilk contains distinctive bioactive molecules that protect the infant against infection, inflammation and contribute to organ development, immune maturation and healthy microbial colonization. **Figure 22.2** depicts the importance of sucking for generation and release of breastmilk.

For the baby of an unmedicated mother, this will occur within about an hour after delivery. **Colostrum** is the milk produced during the first few days after birth and contains high levels of immunoglobulins, antimicrobial peptides, and growth factors. Colostrum is important for supporting the growth, development, and immunologic defense of neonates.

Table 22.2: Benefits of breastfeeding.

For the mother	*For the baby*
Helps burn calories, and return to pre-pregnancy weight, stimulates involution of uterus	Complete and adequate nutrition for the infant
Delayed return of ovulation and menstruation	Better survival: Less diarrhea as breastmilk stimulates the growth of intestinal flora, no risk of allergy, has laxative action
Decreased risk of ovarian, and breast cancer	Decreased morbidity: Less infections/diseases like pneumonia
Better mother-baby bonding	Better for premature babies, better growth especially in low birth weight (LBW) infants
Easy, safe baby food, makes life easier for the mother	Reduced cardiac risk
Natural, healthiest food for the baby	Easy to digest and has low osmotic load
Readily available at no cost and at body temperature	Promotes bone growth, provides protection to the child against rickets, and helps in neurological development

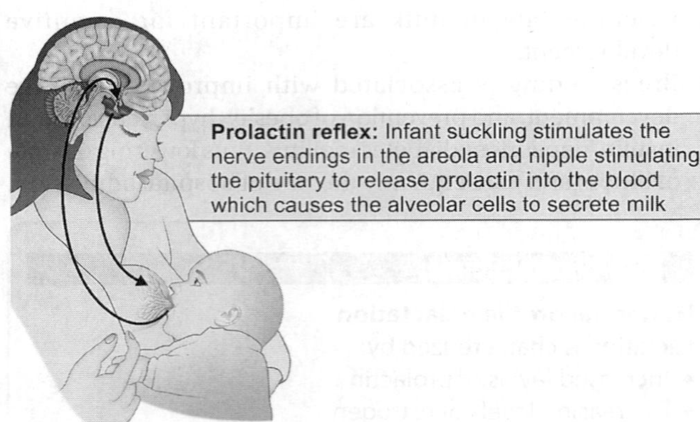

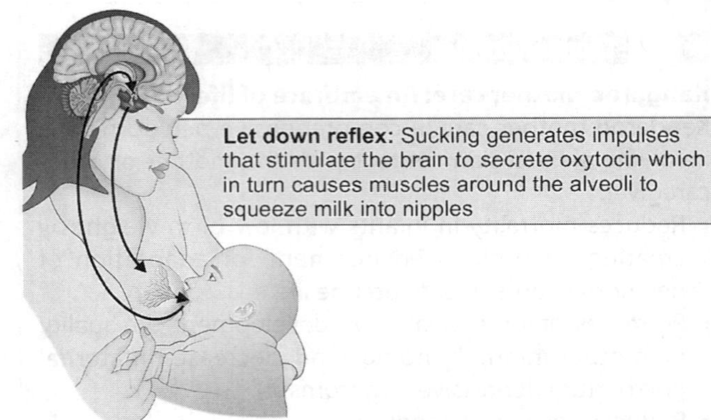

Fig. 22.2: Importance of sucking for generation and release of breastmilk.

Frequency and Duration of Breastfeeding

- Feeding on demand is encouraged. Baby is put to the breast when it is hungry with no restriction of number of feeds and duration.
- Initial feeding should last for 5–10 minutes at each breast to condition the letdown reflex. The suckling time should be gradually increased after that. Complete feeding from one breast before moving to the other is encouraged so the baby gets both the foremilk and hindmilk (richer in fat, possessing more calories and providing better satiety to the infant). The next feed should be started with the other breast first.

Breastfeeding Positions

Optimum positioning of the mother and infant and the attachment of an infant at the breast are the foundation of sustainable and effective breastfeeding. The position of the baby should be close to the mother's body straight to the level of the breast to achieve good attachment. An effective sucking technique is vital to establish breastfeeding, ensure milk transfer, and prevent breastfeeding-related problems.

Baby's position during breastfeeding: The baby's positioning and attachment to the breast during breastfeeding are decisive in the occurrence of different sorts of nipple trauma. The nipple and areola should be guided by the mother to the baby's mouth for proper milk transfer. Chest-to-chest contact between the mother and baby should be maintained for milk transfer; the baby's ear, shoulder, and hip should be in one line.

Evidence in the literature points to a significant association between position and holding variables for causing nipple lesions, wherein **neck flexion, chins held away from the breast, improper suction, and inward lips** are all risk factors for nipple trauma.

Methods for Breastfeeding

Cradle, cross-cradle, side-lying, under-arm posture (football hold), Australian hold, and supine positions (lying face upward) can be used for breastfeeding.

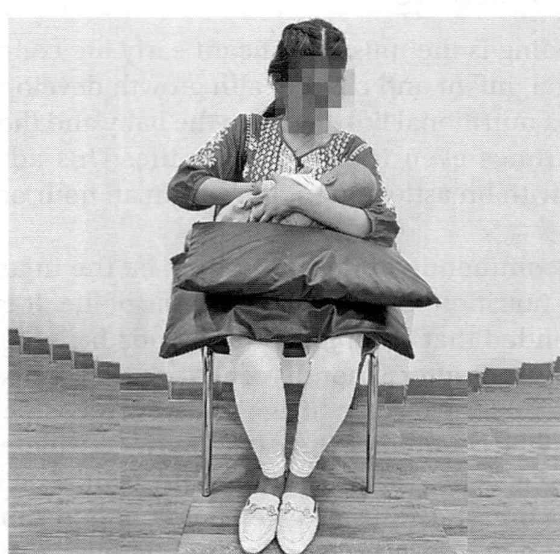

Fig. 22.3: Cradle position.

I. Cradle Position

Position: Baby facing the mother. The baby's head rests in the mother's arm at the elbow. The baby's body rests on the forearm **(Fig. 22.3)**.

 **Clinical Pointer**

Breastfeeding position

Position of the mother: Back supported, knee flexed, pillow under the knee

Position of the baby: Neck supported, latching proper, esophagus as vertical as possible as it not only puts the diaphragm in a position of mechanical advantage but also facilitates the action of gravity to propel the milk from the mouth to the stomach and prevents regurgitation. This is especially important in vulnerable infants

II. Cross-cradle Position

Raising an infant to the same level of the breast with the support of a pillow. The cross-cradle method is one of the most frequently used breastfeeding methods, as the infant is held very intimately to the mother with the head and shoulder

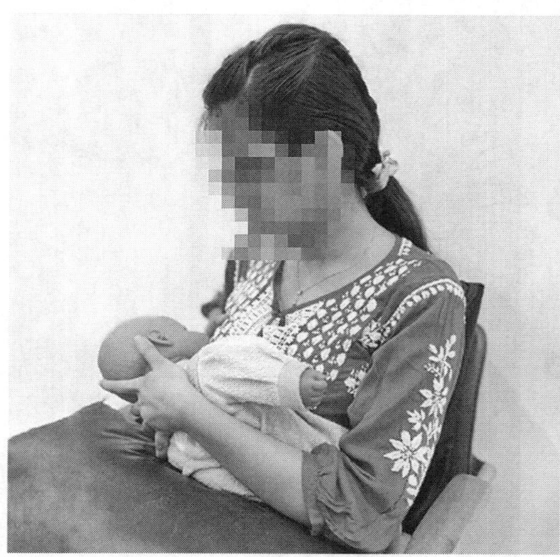

Fig. 22.4: Cross-cradle position.

of the infant supported, and other body parts aligned. The baby's nose pointed to the breast opposite to the nipple is visible to the mother **(Fig. 22.4)**.

Position: The baby is facing the mother. The mother's hand is at the back of the baby's neck. The baby's body rests on the mother's forearm.

III. Football Hold Position

Position: The baby is next to the mother with its legs toward the mother's back. The baby is between the side and the arm with its legs near the mother's elbow. The mother's hand is on the back of the baby's neck **(Fig. 22.5)**.

Clinical Pointer

Feeding premature babies: The most appropriate position is the football position or underarm posture

Benefit: Helps mothers to see their baby's face better therefore ensuring good control of the infant's head

IV. Feeding in Sidelying Position

Position: The infant and mother lie down, stomach-to-stomach, and the mother uses one of her hands to cover the infants head with the other hand covering the baby and drawing close to her body in the laying down method **(Fig. 22.6)**.

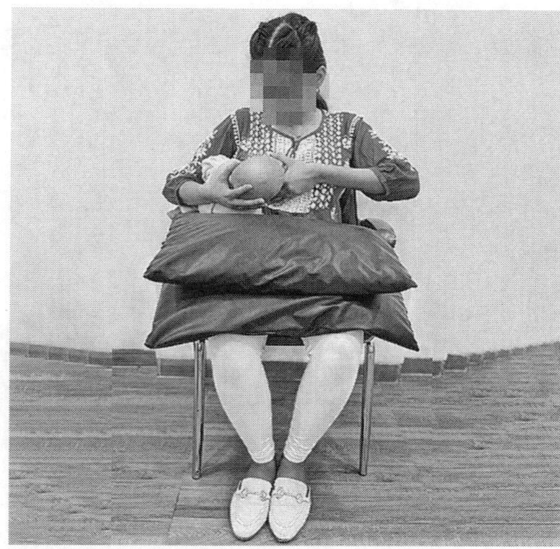

Fig. 22.5: Football hold position.

V. Australian Hold Position

Position: The baby is held vertically and straddles the mother's thigh, facing her. The mother's knee, supports the baby's bottom, while one hand is low on the baby's head to give control as the mother brings the baby to the breast to latch **(Fig. 22.7)**.

Breaking the Wind (Burping)

The air swallowed by the baby during breastfeeding can cause abdominal colic, hiccough, and even regurgitation. To break up this wind, the child should be held upright against the chest and general patting of the child's back is done till it burps the air out.

Assessment of Breastfeeding

Assessment of breastfeeding is shown in **Boxes 22.1** and **22.2**.

Barriers to the Normal Breastfeeding Process

Many factors can act as barriers to the normal breastfeeding process:

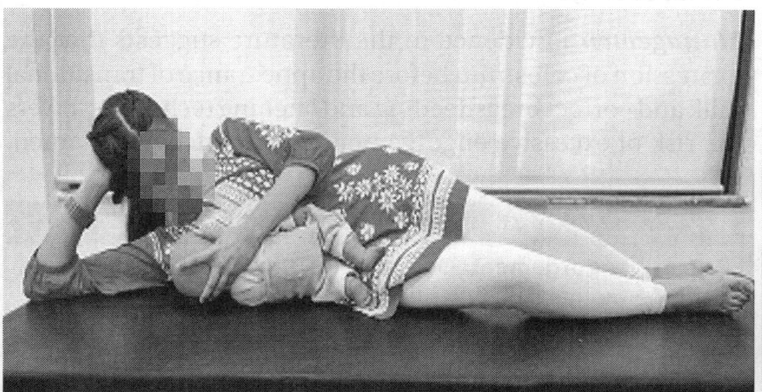

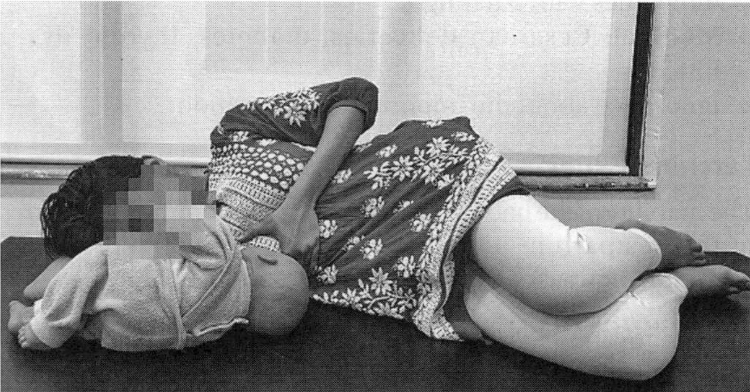

Fig. 22.6: Feeding in sidelying position.

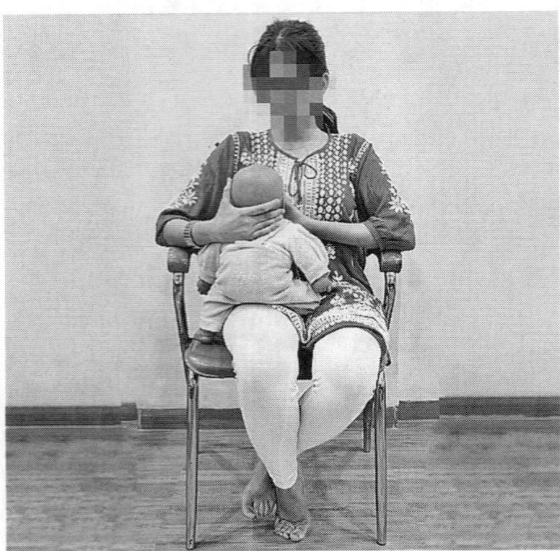

Fig. 22.7: Australian hold position.

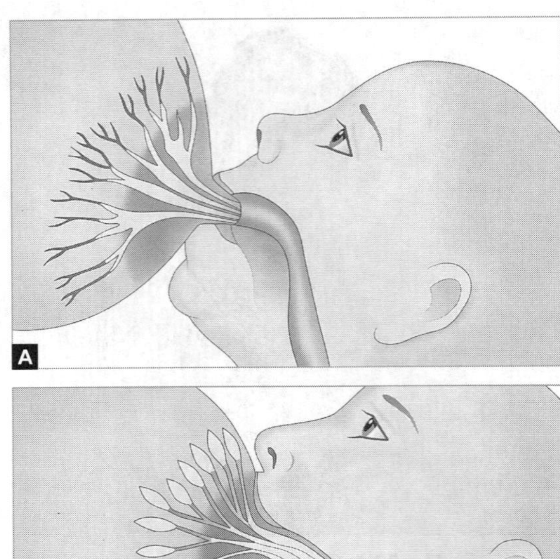

Figs. 22.8 A and B: The technique of breastfeeding: (A) Poor attachment; (B) Good attachment.

Box 22.1: Assessment of breastfeeding.

Screening of lactation assesses behavioral, observational, and psychosocial factors connected to breastfeeding. Five lactation tools that assess maternal behavior/attitude and infant sucking skills in breastfeeding are as follows:
1. BREAST Feed Observation Form
2. Lactation Assessment Tool
3. LATCH Scoring System
4. Mother-Baby Assessment Tool
5. Mother-Infant Breastfeeding Progress Tool

Box 22.2: Assessment on observation.

Observe the baby	Observe the mother
• Position: Anterior surface should face the mother • Observe the ability to latch/suckle • Whether awake/fussy/irritable	• Breast: Shape, size, nipple • Position during feeding • Position of hand on breast • Attitude towards breastfeeding and baby

- **Biological:** Delayed lactation
- **Psychological:** Embarrassment and difficulty in breast-feeding discreetly
- **Mechanical:** Smaller/larger breasts and nipples that create difficulties with latching
- **Medical:** Cesarean deliveries, diabetes, thyroid dys-function
- Ignorance about the importance of lactation.

Latching Issues

The inability of the baby to latch properly is a common concern of the postpartum period contributing to interruption or cessation of breastfeeding **(Figs. 22.8A and B)**.

Assessment: LATCH score is a breastfeeding assessment tool used to assess breastfeeding practices. A low LATCH score at discharge is indicative of the risk of early breastfeeding cessation.

Breast Engorgement

Breast engorgement is the overfilling of breast milk that causes discomfort and pain to the mother. It is thought to be caused by intensified lactogenesis owing to a decline in levels of steroid hormones, in addition to increased prolactin concentrations. This inadequate emptying of breasts can cause concerns like plugged milk ducts, breast infection, and insufficient milk along with discomfort and pain to the mother. It can be of two types as shown in **Box 22.3**.

The condition can be further aggravated by:
- Delay in starting to breastfeed soon after baby's birth.
- Poor attachment, so that milk is not removed effectively.
- Infrequent feeding, not feeding at night or short duration of feeds.

Signs and symptoms: Hard, painful, throbbing, aching and tender breasts.

Management: Evidence in the literature suggests that the expression of colostrum before the appearance of transitional milk and correct breastfeeding and latching technique lowers the risk of excessive engorgement in breastfeeding women.

Box 22.3: Breast engorgement.

Primary engorgement: Occurs in the first few days after birth. Here the mother's body is still trying to adjust to the amount of milk that the baby demands.

Secondary engorgement: Occurs later because of infrequent breastfeeding by the mother, or the baby removes less milk from the breast.

Apart from that, acupuncture, cold cabbage leaves applied to the breasts, cold gel packs, pharmacological treatments, and ultrasound are also effective to vary degrees.

Mastitis

Mastitis is defined as inflammation of the breast with or without infection. It is a common breast condition that is predominantly seen in women during the breastfeeding period. Mastitis with infection may be lactational (puerperal).

Complication: A localized collection of purulent material within the breast is a **breast abscess**. In females of reproductive age, lactational abscesses are predominant.

Treatment: Antibiotics in addition to breast abscess percutaneous drainage and/or surgical incision and drainage could be done.

Clinical Pointer

Inverted/retracted nipple

Nipple that lie flat against the areola or goes inward instead of sticking out.

Management:

Hoffman's technique: Manual exercise regime for drawing out the nipple.

Method: Thumbs are placed on either side of the nipple at its base and firmly pressed into the breast tissue, and separated gently, causing the nipple to point outward.

Suction devices, piercings, and cosmetic surgery can also be used to change the shape of the inverted nipple so that it points outward.

Nutrition in Lactating Mothers

Calori Intake

The energy requirement of a lactating mother refers to the energy intake from food that will balance the energy expenditure needed to maintain body weight, composition, good levels of physical activity, and breast milk production that is consistent with good health for woman and child as well as the ability to perform socially and economically desirable activity.

Breastfeeding mothers require approximately 500 additional kcal/day beyond the requirements for non-pregnant women. During pregnancy, most women store an extra 2 to 5 kg (19,000 to 48,000 kcal) in tissue, mainly as fat, in physiologic preparation for lactation. If women do not consume the extra calories, then body stores are used to maintain lactation. Concern to lose weight rapidly may contradict the mother's nutritional demands, which are increased if she is breastfeeding.

Clinical Pointer

The success of lactation is measured through the amount of weight gain in the infant, i.e., appropriate amount of weight gain implies successful and adequate lactation.

The recommended daily allowance for protein during lactation is an additional 25 g/day. Requirements for many micronutrients also increase compared to pregnancy. Iron supplements should continue in the puerperium and while breastfeeding to restore the iron lost during pregnancy, delivery, and breastfeeding. There are some special dietary recommendations for vegetarians:

- Vitamin D supplements should be consumed by women who do not drink milk or other vitamin D-fortified food.
- Vitamin B_{12} supplements recommended for women who consume ovolactovegetarian and vegan diets.
- 1200–1500 mg/day of calcium to be consumed per day to counter the probable decreased absorption from a plant-based diet.

Clinical Pointer

To ensure the optimum health of the new mother some basic examinations are mandated including the breast examination, determination of the presence of any cervical or perineal tears or infections, and hemoglobin levels assessment.

IMMEDIATE POSTPARTUM CONCERNS

Common immediate postpartum concerns in a new mother are focused on:

- Complete expulsion of the placenta
- Contraction of the uterus
- Absence of bleeding from any site
- Phlebitis

After Pains

Suckling by the baby at the breast stimulates the posterior pituitary to release oxytocin **(Fig. 22.2)**. This initiates bursts of uterine contraction. The sight, sound, or smell of the baby can induce this chain of reaction that causes labor-like pain felt in the lower abdomen or the lumbar region which are called afterpains.

This throbbing, cramping or aching pain is more prevalent in multiparous women than in primipara. The pain could be moderate to severe in intensity as scored on the McGill pain questionnaire.

In addition, retraction of the uterine muscle helps control the postpartum hemorrhage but also gradually reduces the blood supply to the muscle tissue causing degradation of the tissue and pain.

These afterpains can be managed with:

- Heat therapy
- Movement
- Analgesics

Postpartum Hemorrhage

Postpartum hemorrhage (PPH) is defined as a loss of 500 mL of blood or more from the genital tract after the delivery of the baby.

Primary PPH

Causes

- Atonic uterus (due to retained placenta or membranes)
- Genital trauma (spontaneous trauma or trauma due to treatment or interference, e.g., instrument-assisted delivery, e.g., cesarean section, episiotomy)
- Primary hematological disorders (e.g., von Willebrand's or other clotting factor deficiency)
- Disseminated intravascular coagulation (rare)
- Inversion of the uterus (rare)

Secondary PPH

Causes

- Retained fragments of placenta or membranes
- Shedding of dead tissues following obstructed labor
- Breakdown of uterine wound (after cesarean section or ruptured uterus)

Severe blood loss during PPH (>500 mL of blood in one minute) can lead to side effects:

- Exsanguination will occur in 10 minutes
- Effects on vital organs: Kidneys: renal shutdown and cortical necrosis
  - Lungs: Air hunger
  - Brain: Loss of consciousness, nausea, pituitary damage

It is important to recognize primary PPH bleeding from the birth of the baby up to 24 hours after delivery. The uterus which is not well contracted is a warning sign. The uterus feels bulky and the fundus is higher than normal and rising. Recognition of secondary PPH is excessive bleeding from the genital tract after 24 hours and during the first 6 weeks following delivery. The uterus does not involute properly.

Puerperal sepsis marked by offensive lochia, fever, and tachycardia makes secondary PPH graver.

Perineal Pain after Vaginal Delivery

Genital tract trauma leading to pain in the perineum is a common sequel of vaginal delivery that has bearing on the woman's recovery from the process of childbirth.

Perineal Pain

Episiotomy and spontaneous perineal laceration are strongly associated with the presence of perineal pain during the immediate postpartum period. Tight sutures, wound breakdown and infection may also lead to perineal pain.

Lacerations can be classified as shown in **Table 22.3**.

Severe perineal lacerations

Obstetric anal sphincter injuries (OASIS), include third- and fourth-degree lacerations. Internal bleeding may cause hematoma which causes severe pain.

Risk Factors for Postpartum Perineal Pain

- Evidence suggests that perineal and pelvic floor morbidity is greatest among women receiving median episiotomy versus those remaining intact or sustaining spontaneous perineal tears.
- Primiparous and older women are more prone to perineal trauma.
- Fetal weight close to or over four kilograms and occiput posterior position are fetal characteristics that favor perineal trauma.
- Interventions during labor, such as oxytocin induction, increased duration of labor, Kristeller maneuver, use of forceps, and episiotomy, increase the risk of perineal trauma, particularly severe trauma **(Box 22.4)**.

Long-term Consequences of Perineal Trauma

Due to pelvic floor muscle weakening, urinary and fecal incontinence, sexual dysfunction, and perineal pain are seen.

Assessment Scales

Present pain intensity (PPI) and visual analog scale (VAS) components of the short-form McGill Pain Questionnaire can be used to assess pain.

Physiotherapy Management Regime

The following have been found useful along with oral analgesics:

- Ice
- Cold baths
- Warm baths
- Saline baths
- Ultrasound
- Electromagnetic therapy

Box 22.4: Kristeller maneuver.

'Kristeller maneuver' refers to the application of fundal pressure in the form of manual pressure or using an inflatable belt, to the uppermost part of the uterus directed towards the birth canal, in an attempt to assist spontaneous vaginal birth and avoid prolonged second stage or the need for operative birth during the second stage of labor.

Some factors which prompt the obstetrician to go for this controversial maneuver are: Fetal distress, failure to progress, maternal exhaustion or a medical condition where prolonged pushing is dangerous.

Table 22.3: Classification of perineal lacerations.

First degree	*Second degree*	*Third degree*	*Fourth degree*
Involves superficial vaginal mucosa and the perineal skin	Involving the vaginal mucosa and perineal muscles	Involves anal sphincter Has three categories: 1. Only about half of the anal sphincter torn 2. More than half of the anal sphincter torn 3. Torn external and internal anal sphincter	Involves anal sphincter and mucosa

Immediate

- Rest in bed
- Cryotherapy through packs that fit the contour
- Elevation of the part
- Pelvic floor muscle activation (contract-relax)
- Defecation with splinting/assisting pads
- Cushions for sitting (a ring cushion can be used for sitting so that pressure on the perineum is relieved)
- Avoid sitting on a hard surface.

There is some evidence to prove that perineal massage relaxes the perineum, increases perineal blood flow, and stretches the vaginal tissue prior to delivery, resulting in less severe lacerations and reducing the incidence of lacerations requiring sutures.

Postpartum Depression/Peripartum Depression (DSM-V)

The biomedical model dictates that the postpartum period corresponds to the period from the expulsion of the placenta till the return to the pre-gestational physiological functions. However, in the biopsychosocial context, the postpartum period, apart from the biological changes also brings about several psychological and social modifications as a consequence of motherhood making it a principally delicate and variable stage of life in women.

Postpartum depression (PPD) is defined as an episode of major depression that is temporally associated with childbirth. The postpartum period ensues a new routine, new family context, and social role for the female thus provoking physical exhaustion, mood disorders, stress, and depressive symptoms. Hence apart from the intrinsic biological aspects, environmental and personal factors also become important determinants for maintaining or recovering health, functioning, and quality of life in puerperal women.

Postpartum depression comprises a group of depressive-type symptoms that have their onset in the early postpartum weeks or months and can persist for more than a year. The incidence ranges from 3 to 34%.

The postpartum depression presents with extensive and sometimes conflicting symptoms including:

- Exhaustion
- Irritability
- Avid weepiness
- Diminished energy and motivation levels
- Feelings of helplessness and hopelessness
- Anxiety

Vegetative symptoms common in PPD such as:

- Loss of libido
- Appetite
- Sleep disturbance

Psychosomatic symptoms could range from:

- Headache
- Asthma
- Backache
- Vaginal discharge
- Abdominal pain

Cognitive symptoms like:

- Obsessional thinking
- Fear of harming the baby or self
- Overt rejection of the baby

Characteristics

- Sad or depressed mood that persists daily for at least 2 weeks
- Inability to derive pleasure from experiences or lack of interest in things that are normally enjoyable
- Moving or speaking so slowly that others have noticed
- Being so fidgety or restless that one is unable to sit still
- Feeling badly about ones' self- feeling like a failure or have let self or family down, etc.

Assessment/Screening

Self-report assessment tools include:

- The MacArthur initiative on depression and primary care
- Edinburgh postnatal depression scale.

Management

- Antidepressant medication
- **Nonpharmacological interventions:** Psychotherapy (first-line treatment), Repetitive Transcranial Magnetic Stimulation (rTMS) (for further details of management strategies, please refer Chapter 16: Psychosexual Dimensions of Women's Health).

CLINICAL EXAMPLE 1

Ms Asha presents for a follow-up appointment at 9 weeks postpartum.

Chief complaints: Depressed and sad mood most days over the past 5 weeks, and notes that she would prefer to 'just with herself', not talk to anybody that she used to enjoy earlier.

Current status: Breastfeeding.

Loss of appetite, low energy and concentration make it difficult to accomplish tasks at home. She says she is having problem caring for her newborn and is not able to take care of her other responsibilities.

No suicidal or homicidal ideation.

She has not been able to cope with her duties around the home related to childcare and managing their home. Overall she and her husband get along well and she has strong social support. She denies feeling anxious. She denies any substance abuse. She has no significant past medical or family psychiatric history.

Assessment: PPD Scale

Management: Interpersonal Psychotherapy (IPT) and Cognitive Behavioral Therapy (CBT)

Circulatory Issues in Postpartum Period

Varicose Veins

Varicose veins (VV) in lower limbs are a common occurrence in pregnancy (especially primiparous). Pregnancy-induced

VV regain their original shape and competence, particularly after the first pregnancy, in 3 to 6 months.

Causes

Hormonal variations (effect of progesterone on smooth muscle walls of veins) and hemodynamic factors (compression of veins of the lower abdomen) have important implications on dilatation and in determining the decreased venous wall tone during pregnancy.

Signs and symptoms

- Perimalleolar edema on prolonged standing in the evening (measured on an analog scale line ranging from 0–5)
- Presence of small, spider veins clusters
- Leg cramps (considering the percentage of legs with the symptom): Heavier legs, pain on prolonged standing, restless legs, and bruises (measured on visual analog scale line (VASL)

Diagnostic evaluation

- Color duplex and ambulatory venous pressure
- VASL (range 0–10) to evaluate the overall satisfaction

Treatment options

Sclerotherapy, surgery, and/or any medical or conservative treatment (including compression stockings, Buerger's exercises, analgesics, anti-inflammatory agents, and Pycnogenol which is an antioxidative and vasodilator).

Research Pointer

During breastfeeding, mothers are advised not to sit cross-legged, elevate the lower limbs when possible to aid the venous return, and vigorously exercise the calf muscles.

Hemorrhoids

Aggravated by straining which could cause ballooning and prolapse of the veins.

Management

Steroid analgesic creams, cold therapy, oral analgesics, care of pain in the perineum, and defecation training.

Sleep, Fatigue in Postnatal Period

The sleep pattern is greatly disturbed in the postpartum period of new mothers. The erratic sleep patterns of the newborn and having to look after the needs of the infant, contribute to the poor sleep pattern and therefore altered circadian rhythms in new mothers, which could lead to increased maternal morbidity and a high-risk of postpartum depression. Therefore, evaluation for sleep disturbance and depression should be a part of routine postpartum assessments.

Assessment

- Pittsburgh Sleep Quality Index (PSQI)
- Patient-Reported Outcomes Measurement Information System (PROMIS) sleep disturbance instrument.

Physiotherapy Management

As and when required, advice related to optimizing sleep must be a part of postnatal physiotherapy management.

POSTNATAL BACK PAIN

Pregnancy-related low back pain is a common complaint that causes pain between the lower ribs and the gluteal folds/pubic symphysis during the course of pregnancy and could radiate to the posterolateral thigh, to the knee and calf, but never to the foot.

Causes

Pregnancy-related LBP can be due to a combination of mechanical, hormonal, circulatory, and psychosocial factors **(Box 22.5)**.

Box 22.5: Common causes of LBP in postnatal period.

- Decreased postural control and stability
- Labor and delivery induced trauma
- Induced by the physiological and biochemical changes of pregnancy
- Post-delivery uterine contractions (after pains)

Mechanical

During pregnancy, the increased release of the hormone relaxin causes ligamentous laxity that alters the biomechanics of the vertebral column as well as the pelvic girdle, affecting the stability of the spine and leading to back pain. Despite the decrease in relaxin levels post-delivery, it takes some time for the lax structures to revert to their pre-pregnancy status.

Assessment and Management

Table 22.4 describes the assessment and treatment of postnatal back pain.

Epidural Site Pain

Labor epidural analgesia is thought to be associated with an increased incidence of localized pain at the epidural insertion site in the postpartum period. This could be attributed to a small hematoma in the supraspinous ligament following the injection. This pain is transient in nature.

Table 22.4: Assessment and treatment of postnatal back pain.

Assessment	*Treatment*
Subjective examination: Location, type, onset and duration of pain, aggravating and relieving factors, functional movements affected	• Gentle mobilizations • Movement analysis • Low load gradual exercises • Core muscle activation and strengthening • Pelvic floor muscle training • Electrotherapy • Adjunct therapies
Objective examination: Observation for swelling, color, texture, temperature, muscle spasm, palpation, wasting, reproduction of pain with special tests, joint mobility and muscle strength	
Pregnancy-specific self-report questionnaire: Pregnancy Mobility Index (PMI) to assess the ability to do normal household activities	

Management

Goals

- To reduce pain
- To improve mobility

Methods

- Gentle graded mobility exercises
- Hot/ice packs
- Electrotherapy

DIASTASIS RECTI ABDOMINIS

Diastasis rectus abdominis (DRA), divarication of the recti, is abnormal widening of the gap between the two medial sides of the rectus abdominis muscle (increased inter-recti distance) **(Fig. 22.9)**. It is a common health issue affecting both pregnant and postpartum women that involves a stretching of the linea alba with a midline inter-recti separation. The linea alba is also the central insertion point of the rectus abdominis along with the three other crucial abdominal muscles on each side, i.e., the internal obliques, the external obliques, and the transversus abdominis.

The separation of the rectus abdominis is more common in the supraumbilical region and is positively associated with the mother's age as well as the body mass index.

Causes

- Excessive inner-abdominal pressure during pregnancy as the growing uterus stretches the abdominal muscles and connective tissues.
- Relaxin, progesterone and estrogen hormones along with the mechanical stresses by the growing fetus on the abdominal wall as well as a displacement of the abdominal organs lead to elastic changes of the connective tissue, which in turn cause DRA.

Predisposing Factors

- Obesity
- Multiparity
- Fetal macrosomia
- Flaccid abdominal muscles
- Polyhydramnios
- Multiple pregnancies

Implications of DRA

- The growing fetus alters the integrity, mechanical control, and functional strength of the abdominal wall. This reduces further because of the abdominal separation or diastasis recti.
- This alters the trunk mechanics, pelvic stability, and posture, predisposing the lumbar spine and the pelvis to injury, lower back pain, and pelvic instability. The transversus abdominis, pelvic floor, multifidus and diaphragm form the deep core stabilizing muscles akin to a muscular cylinder, work together as a unit to ensure and maintain trunk stability which supports the spine and the pelvis.
- Not only the mechanical functions, but DRA can also adversely affect respiration, parturition, trunk mobility, and support of the abdominal viscera, and pelvic floor functions apart from impairing cosmetics.

Assessment

Details can be referred from Chapter 4: Assessment in Women's Health.

- Clinical assessment of the diastasis recti abdominis muscle using the finger-width method **(Figs. 22.10 and 22.11)**
- Clinical assessment of the diastasis recti abdominis using calipers
- Ultrasound assessment (most reliable and valid method for measurement of the diastasis recti abdominis width).

Management of DRA

- Back care education
- Abdominal exercises with abdominal binders
- External support (e.g., Tubigrip or corset)
- Aerobic exercises
- Activation and strengthening of the core muscles **(Figs. 22.12 to 22.15)**.

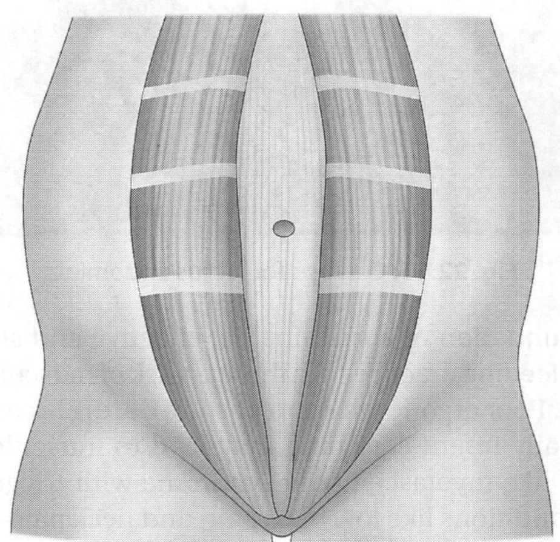

Fig. 22.9: Diastasis recti abdominis.

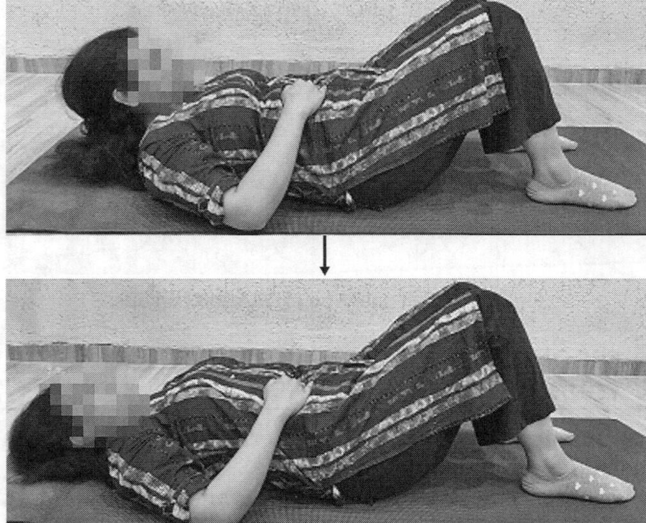

Fig. 22.10: Self-assessment of diastasis recti with finger width.

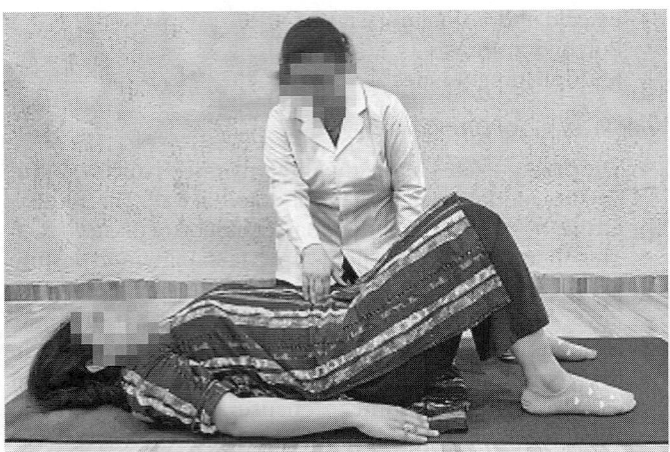

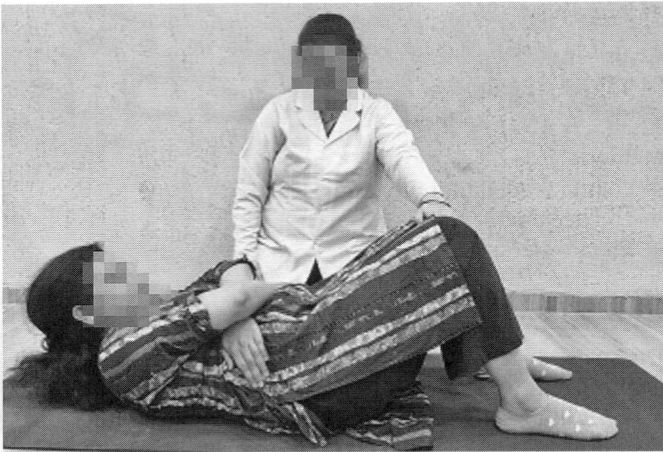

Fig. 22.11: Therapist assessing the diastasis recti with finger width method.

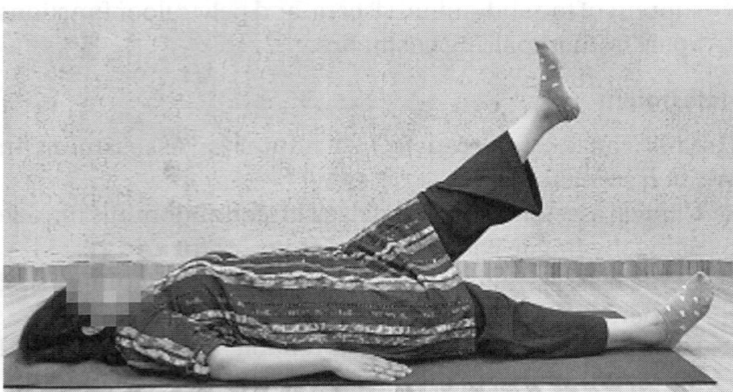

Fig. 22.12: Unilateral SLR.

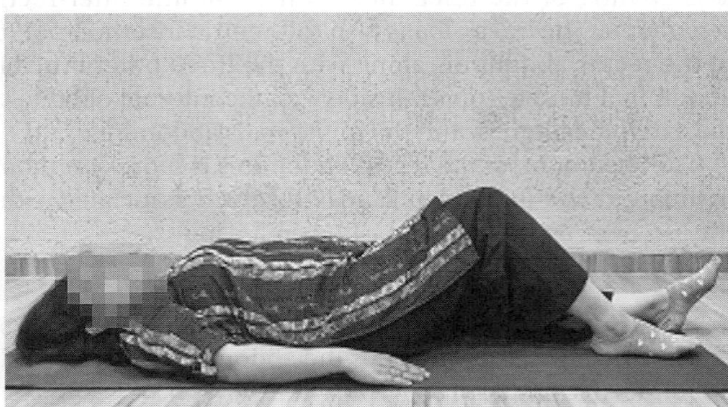

Fig. 22.13: Heel slides.

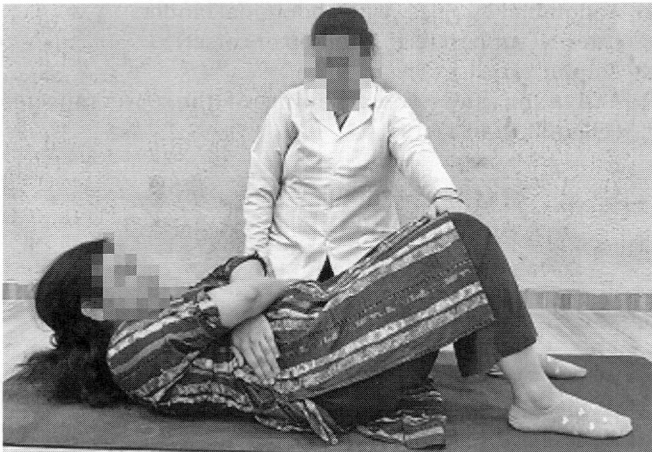

Fig. 22.14: Self-splinting of DRA and curl ups.

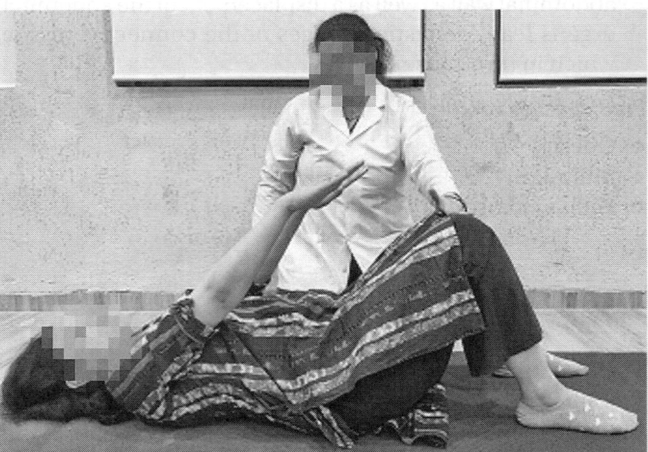

Fig. 22.15: Curl ups for rectus abdominis.

ERGONOMICS FOR THE MOTHER WITH A YOUNG CHILD

Ergonomics is the study of the interrelationships between machines and their human users.

- Adherence to ergonomic principles ensures the comfort, support, and well-being of lactating mothers. Optimal positioning and attachment of an infant at the breast are the foundation of a sustainable, effective and stress-free breastfeeding practice with the least risk of musculoskeletal issues. Poor ergonomics and posture during breastfeeding and daily infant care time may lead to musculoskeletal issues like myofascial pain syndrome with trigger points and conditions like low back pain and neck pain amongst new mothers.

- Physical and mental demands of infant care and self-care on top of the physiological changes of the pregnancy and the postpartum period make the new mothers at risk of musculoskeletal disorders. This could be because of pre-existing risk factors like the following which are further augmented by faulty ergonomics by new mothers during self-care and childcare-related activities:
  - Increased fluid retention in the body
  - Altered posture causing muscle imbalance
  - Hormone-induced laxity of ligaments
  - Irregular sleep patterns
- Some more factors that may contribute to musculoskeletal problems are:
  - Lack of mobility and awkward positions during labor
  - Poor positioning when bathing and feeding the baby
  - Maneuvering the baby in and out of cars, especially when carried in car seats
- The inconvenient position is further exacerbated by the weight of the baby on the mother's lap, and the static breastfeeding position that is held for long, making it a risk factor that synergizes musculoskeletal disorders in lactating mothers.
- Also, increased postpartum breast mass and/or persistent joint laxity further up the risk quotient.

The routine positions of the mother during lactation are uncomfortable, with no back or foot support and unsupported arms. To make it ergonomically viable and safe, the baby should be placed in close apposition to the mother, with its head and body in a straight line **(Figs. 22.16 and 22.17)**.

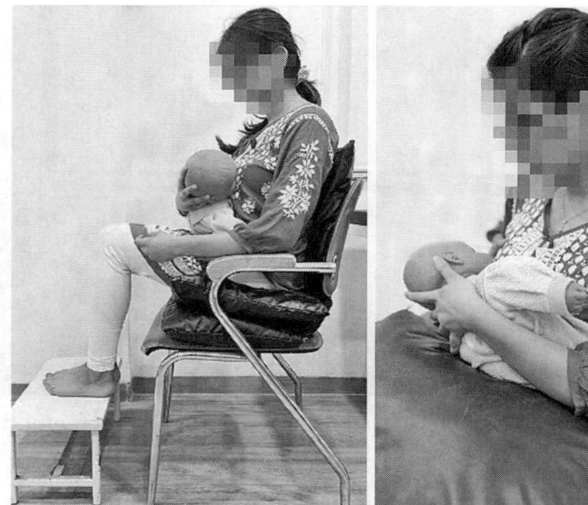

Fig. 22.16: Ergonomically safe positions for breastfeeding.

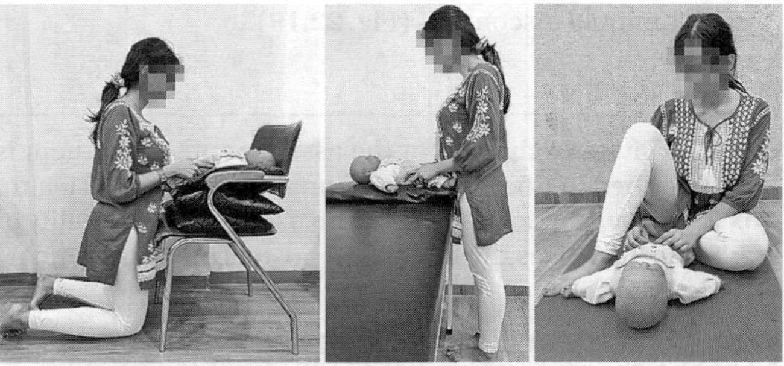

Fig. 22.17: Ergonomically safe and efficient postures for baby care.

Some ergonomic considerations for breastfeeding mothers are:

- Ergonomically designed seating.
- Anthropometric measures must be considered while adopting any chair/furniture.
- Placement of lumbar back support over the lower lumbar spine to support the lumbar lordosis
- Provision of a minimum angle of 105 degrees between the trunk and the thigh to help preserve the lumbar lordotic curve
- Provision of adequate open space for the posteriorly projecting sacrum and buttocks (Seat Pan).
- Provision for unrestricted posterior placement of the shoulders for relaxed sitting by ensuring that the upper limit of the convex primary lower lumbar back support in the chair should be well below the lower angles of the scapulae.
- Flexing the lower limbs at the knee helps reduce tension in the 2-joint muscles thereby reducing the pull on the pelvis.
- Using the hips and knees to bend rather than the spine while picking anything from the ground helps reduce the load on the low back **(Fig. 22.18)**.
- While lifting the baby from a lower surface, bringing the baby as near as possible to the center of mass helps reduce the moment arm of the load and therefore the torque produced.

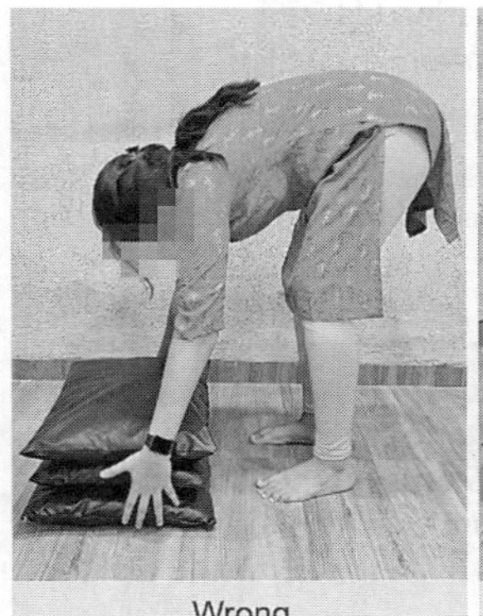

Wrong

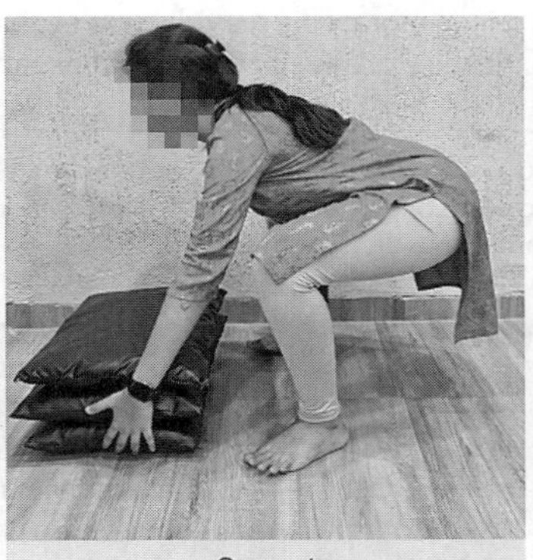

Correct

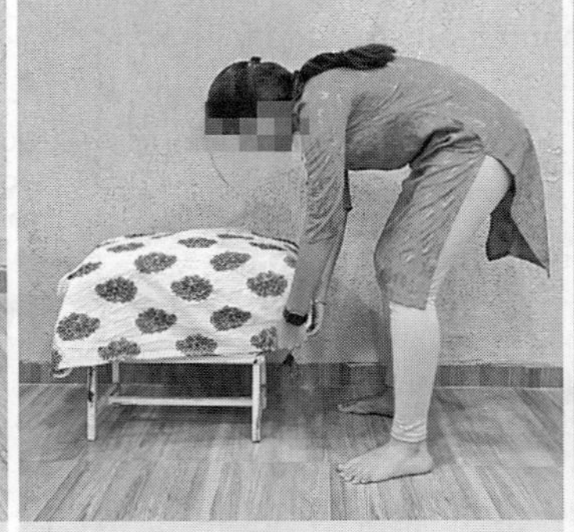

Wrong

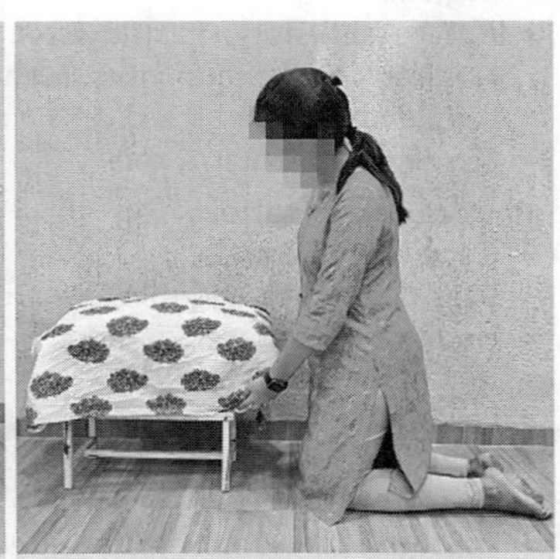

Correct

Fig. 22.18: Incorrect and correct methods of lifting.

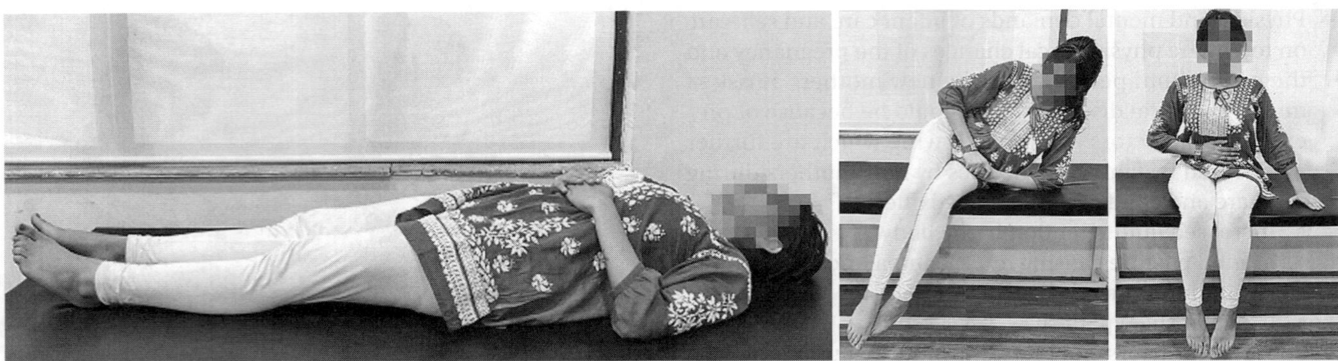

Fig. 22.19: Correct method of supine to sitting transition.

- In postpartum cases after lower segment cesarean section (LSCS), the new mother can utilize log rolling-side turn-sit with elbow support, regime to get up from supine position with minimal discomfort **(Fig. 22.19)**.

ASSESSMENT

Box 22.6 gives a template for the assessment. Assessment is also described in Chapter 4: Assessment in Women's Health. **Box 22.7** gives the scales that can be used to assess quality of life. **Table 22.5** gives the ICF-based postpartum assessment.

Box 22.6: Postnatal assessment template.

History:
- Name, age, date of birth, education
- Occupation, last menstrual period (LMP), expected date of delivery (EDD)
- Obstetrical score
- Delivery details: Type of delivery, date of delivery, time of delivery, blood loss, medications (if given), Episiotomy, Placenta
- Obstetrical history: Past obstetrical history, present obstetrical history
- Past history of illness: Past medical history, past surgical history
- Family history
- Menstrual history
- Marital history
- Contraceptive history
- Personal history: Nutrition—diet, rest and sleep, bowel, bladder, hygiene
- Antenatal history: 1st trimester, 2nd trimester, 3rd trimester, Number of antenatal visits, immunization, iron and folic acid supplementation
- SES, Environmental history

Physical examination:
- General appearance
- Built: Obese/average/thin (endo, ecto and mesomorphic)
- Nutrition: Good/average/poor
- Height, weight, BMI
- Pallor, jaundice, tongue, teeth, gums and tonsils
- Vital signs: Temperature, pulse rate, respiratory rate, blood pressure
- Posture assessment: Rounded shoulders, head-to-foot assessment

Contd...

Contd...

- Obstetrical examination: Breast- ejection of milk? shape, size, color of areola, nipples?, breast engorgement, Colostrum given?; uterus, genitalia.
- Pelvic floor examination: External and Internal examination

In external examination:
- Patient position: Supine position with knees bent, feet apart and pelvic area exposed. Examiner should examine for—red excoriated skin, infection, abnormal lumps, pelvic organ prolapse.
    - Ask patient to cough to check if there is descent.
    - Ask patient to tighten the pelvic muscle and observe the contraction and evaluate the strength of muscle.

PNC assessment:

In internal examination **P** (power), **E** (endurance), **R** (repetition), **F** (fast), **E** (elevation), **C** (co-contraction), **T** (timing), **R** (relax) method of PFM assessment is used.

Modified Oxford Grading Classification:
- Grade 0: No discernible contraction.
- Grade 1: Very weak contraction (flicker)
- Grade 2: Weak contraction (increase in tension without lift or squeeze)
- Grade 3: Moderate contraction with some degree of lift and squeeze
- Grade 4: Good contraction producing elevation with some resistance.
- Grade 5: Strong contraction and strong resistance.

Assessment of Lochia: Odor, color, upper extremity, lower extremity
- Diastasis recti: Above umbilicus, at umbilicus, below umbilicus.
- Linea nigra, stria gravida, scar evaluation (if LSCS)
- Respiratory evaluation: Chest expansion- excursion
- ROM, MMT.

(DOA: date of admission, LSCS: lower segment cesarean section, SES: socioeconomic status, BMI: body mass index, ROM: range of motion, MMT: manual muscle testing)

Box 22.7: Quality of life in postnatal period.
- EPDS: Edinburgh Postnatal Depression Scale.
- IFSAC: The Inventory of Functional Status After Childbirth
- MAPP-QOL: The Maternal Postpartum Quality of Life Tool
- MGI: Mother Generated Index
- SF-36: Short-Form 36

Table 22.5: ICF-based postpartum assessment (ICF-postpartum).

Structures affected	*Functions affected*	*Activity and participation*	*Personal factors*
Cardiovascular systems	Pain	Carrying out daily routine	Age
Respiratory systems	Circulatory function	Walking	Educational background
Urinary systems	Respiratory function	Self-care	Occupational
Pelvic floor	Musculoskeletal-strength, mobility, flexibility	Ensuring one's physical comfort	Socioeconomic status
Reproductive system	Lactation	Doing housework	Marital status
Breast and nipples	Sleep	Assisting dependent	Personal attitudes
Upper extremity	Emotional status	Remunerative employment	Personal habits
Lower extremity	Digestive function	Recreation and leisure	Lifestyle
Muscles of trunk	Bowel and bladder	Socializing	Comorbid factors
	Sexual function		
	Posture and gait		

PHYSIOTHERAPY MANAGEMENT IN POSTPARTUM PERIOD

Postnatal exercises are essential for a variety of reasons.

- In short-term, they help to prevent circulatory problems like deep vein thrombosis and respiratory complications like cough/congestion.
- They help to avoid/decrease perineal discomfort and edema and strengthen the abdominal and perineal muscles.
- They can help to prevent problems in future pregnancies and labor.

The exercises should begin the day after the baby is born and continued until the baby is at least 3 months old.

Box 22.8 describes certain guidelines for exercise in the postpartum period.

Box 22.8: Postpartum exercise guidelines.

- The return to pre-pregnancy exercise intensity should be a gradual but steady process that can be attained through regular exercises.
- The process of reversal to the prepregnant state takes about 6 to 8 weeks, however the physiological and structural effects of relaxin, may persist as long as 12 weeks.
- It is important to correct anemia before engaging in moderately strenuous activities. The lady must stop exercising if vaginal bleeding increases or bright red blood appears.
- Moderate to strenuous activities should be avoided if excessive vaginal bleeding occurs or soreness of an episiotomy persists.
- Exercises that take the hips and pelvis above the chest, such as bridging, knee-chest positions, and inverted postures can put the body at risk for a rare but fatal air embolism through the vagina. Therefore, must be avoided till postpartum bleeding ceases.
- With persistent joint laxity, ballistic movements, end range stretching, and intense weight lifting should be avoided for 3 months.
- It is important to use good supporting brassiere during exercise for better support in nursing mothers. It is advisable for nursing mothers to feed before exercise as it would be more comfortable.
- During puerperium, continue with the care and precautions as during pregnancy to prevent the occurrence of musculoskeletal injury.
- Target heart rates and limits should be carefully established with standard screening and tests if mandated and may be based on the pre-pregnancy fitness level.
- No Pain No Gain is NOT to be followed
- Empty bladder before exercise, avoid GI discomfort by maintaining proper gap between meals and exercise.

WHO Guidelines for Postnatal Care for the Mother

- All women should be given information about the physiological process of recovery after birth.
- Post-delivery, postpartum women should have regular assessments of vaginal bleeding, uterine contraction, fundal height, temperature, and heart rate (pulse) routinely during the first 24 hours starting from the first hour after birth.
- Post 24 hours, inquiries should continue to be made about general well-being and assessments made regarding the following:
  - Micturition and urinary incontinence
  - Bowel function
  - Healing of any perineal wound
  - Headache
  - Fatigue
  - Back pain
  - Perineal pain and perineal hygiene
  - Breast pain
  - Uterine tenderness and lochia
  - Their emotional well-being
  - Family and social support they have
  - Their usual coping strategies
- Breastfeeding progress should be assessed at each postnatal contact.
- Counseling on nutrition, hygiene, birth spacing and family planning.
- **Red flag signs and symptoms:** The following signs and symptoms should be looked out for and in the event of their

occurrence, exercise should be stopped and gynecologist should be contacted immediately.

- ***PPH:*** Sudden and profuse blood loss or persistent increased bloodloss, faintness, dizziness, palpitations/tachycardia.
- ***Preeclampsia/eclampsia:*** Headaches accompanied by one or more of the symptoms of visual disturbances, nausea, vomiting, epigastric or hypochondrial pain, feeling faint, and convulsions (in the first few days after birth).
- ***Infection:*** Fever, shivering, abdominal pain, and/or offensive vaginal discharge
- ***Thromboembolism:*** Unilateral calf pain, redness or swelling of calves, shortness of breath or chest pain.

Clinical Pointer

According to the United States Department of Health and Human Services (USDHHS), "Healthy postpartum women who were not highly active or engaging in vigorous-intensity physical activity should obtain at least 150 minutes of moderate-intensity aerobic activity spread throughout the week".

Advices

- If a patient is in sound health, she is allowed to do her usual duties.
- Postpartum exercises may be continued for another 4–6 weeks.
- Vaccination: Measles mumps rubella (MMR), Hepatitis B.
- To evaluate the progress of the baby periodically and continue breastfeeding for 6 months.

Patient Education

- The patient and family are explained about changes that occur in pregnancy with the help of charts, posters and videos and are assumed that all these changes are normal and will eventually return to pre-pregnancy state.
- Patient is educated about various exercise and its importance and benefits.
- Patient should be made aware of postnatal care.
- Explain to the patient that the maintenance of proper hygiene will prevent infection.
- Genital area to be kept clean and dry.
- Bathing should be regular
- Importance of family planning and its guidelines are explained.
- Sanitary napkins should be changed at regular intervals. Use of cloth to be avoided.
- Breast should be cleaned before and after feeding the baby with the help of cotton cloth.
- Importance of breastfeeding: Exclusive breastfeeding for 6 months should be followed strictly.

Postnatal Physiotherapy

- **Exercises to prevent circulatory complications:** Ankle toe movements, active walking where possible.
- **Exercises to prevent pulmonary complications** and maintain pulmonary health and hygiene: Deep breathing, diaphragmatic breathing
- **Fatigue management:** Pranayama, Jacobson's technique
- **Postural correction:** Stretching and Strengthening Exercises: stretching followed by strengthening exercises for pectorals and upper scapular muscles, chin tucks, shoulder retraction, and shoulder shrugs to improve rounded shoulders.
- **Treatment for swelling:** Healthy diet, rest, and staying hydrated keep swelling down.
  - Avoid standing for a long time and cross-leg sitting which reduces circulation.
  - Massage over the dependent area affected by edema.
  - Elevation and ankle toe movements, hip knee movements.
- **Hydrotherapy** as an adjunct therapy can be used to reduce pain, reduce muscle spasms and promote relaxation in women who do not have any contraindications like infection or non-healing wounds.
- **Diaphragmatic breathing:** To promote efficient respiration, breath control and postural control, promote relaxation, enhance cardiovascular capacity, and improve core muscle stability.
- **Recruit and strengthen the core stability muscles**: To improve function and decrease the risk of low back ache **(Figs. 22.20 to 22.26)**.

Bridge exercise, a closed-chain weight-bearing exercise, is used to strengthen the trunk stability muscles, such as the internal oblique and lumbar multifidus **(Fig. 22.20)**.

Variations: To improve the effects of bridge exercises following variations can be used:

- Modified bridge exercises with single-leg support
- Modified bridge exercises with the feet on an unstable surface

In all four positions, weight of the viscera stretches and inhibits the rectus abdominis, so that the drawing-in maneuver recruits the transversus abdominis **(Fig. 22.22)**.

The Bird Dog exercise is a simple core exercise that strengthens the core, hips, and back muscles **(Fig. 22.25)**. It also:

- Improves the stability
- Encourages a neutral spine
- Relieves low back pain
- Promotes proper posture
- Improves mobility

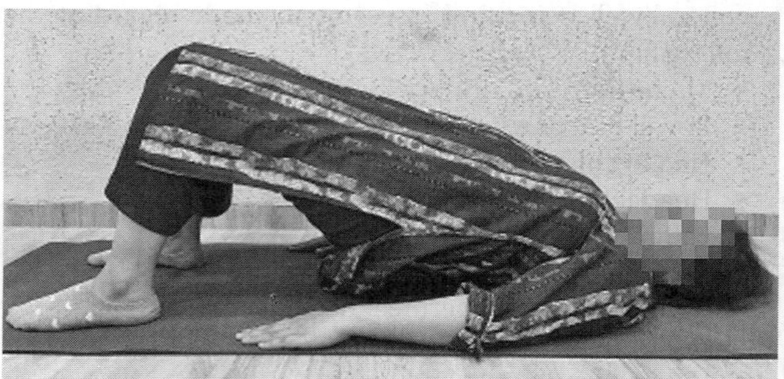

Fig. 22.20: Bridge exercise.

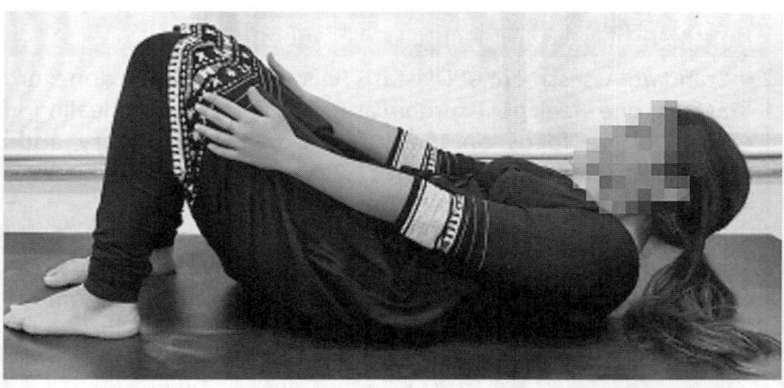
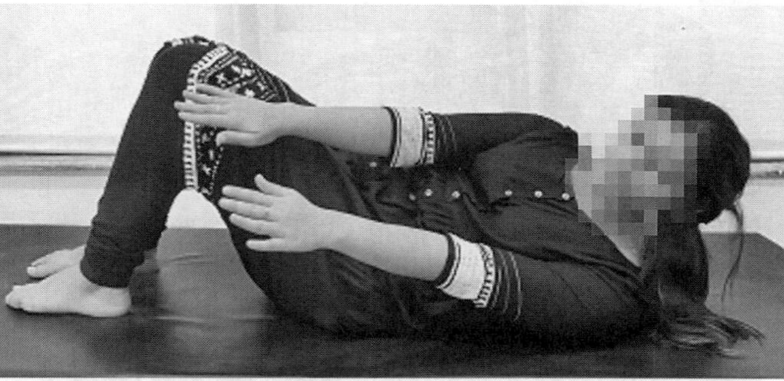

Fig. 22.21: Abdominal curl ups: Straight curl ups and diagonal curl ups.

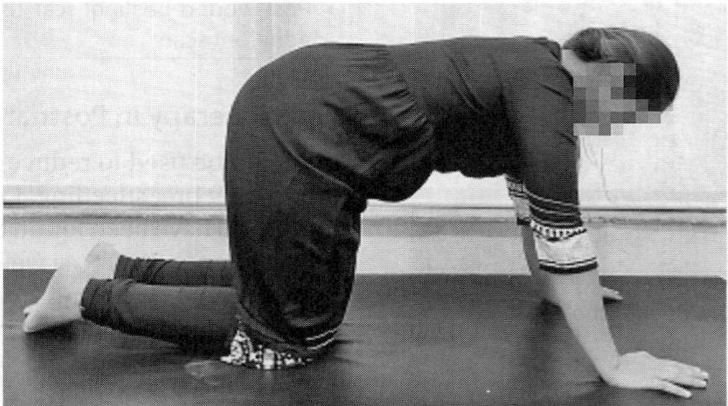

Fig. 22.22: Drawing in maneuver in quadruped position.

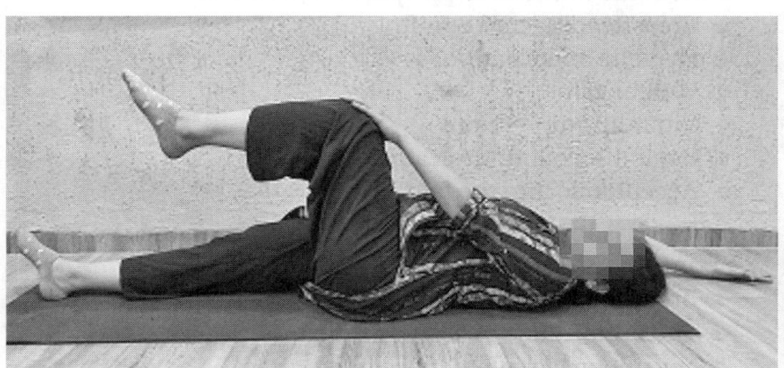
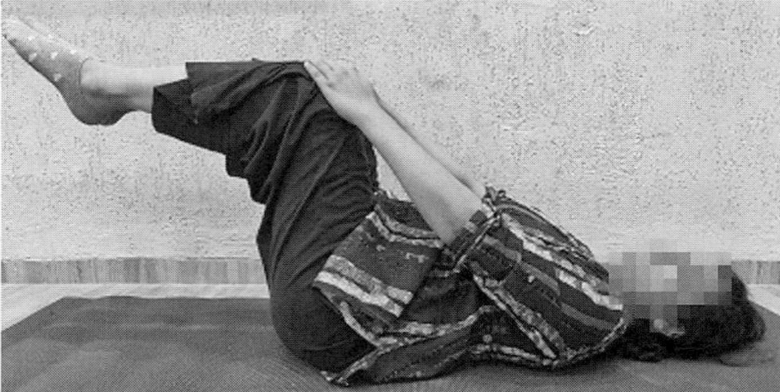

Fig. 22.23: Recruiting the core.

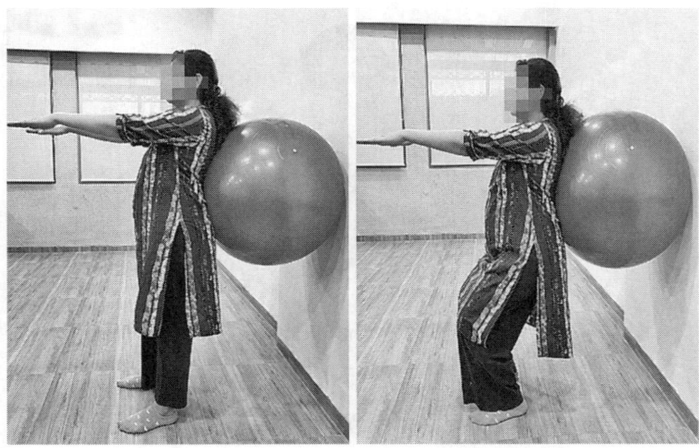

Fig. 22.24: Wall exercises with vestibular ball.

Pelvic Floor Exercises

The pelvic floor muscles may become weakened by pregnancy, vaginal delivery and surgery. This weakness might translate into pelvic floor dysfunctions like urinary incontinence, pelvic organ prolapses, etc. PFM should be assessed using standard assessment protocols as mentioned in Chapter 4: Assessment in Women's Health.

This weakness can be managed using exercises, electrotherapy as well as biofeedback.

Kegel exercises are the most popular and efficient exercises for PFM. For effective strengthening of these deeply situated muscles, it is important to:

- To identify the appropriate muscles
- To contract the muscles in a correct manner
- To repeat the process for the required number of sets

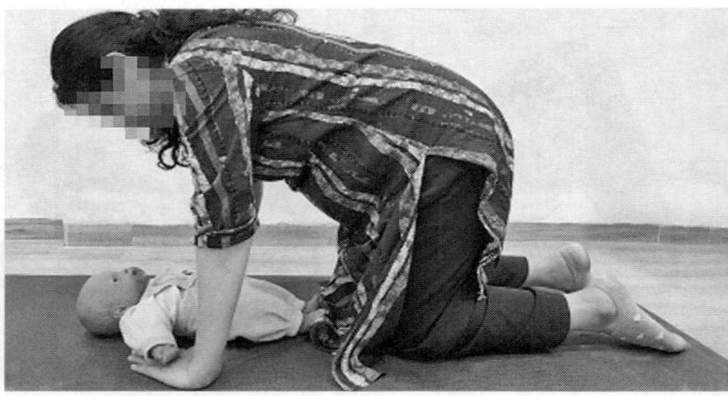

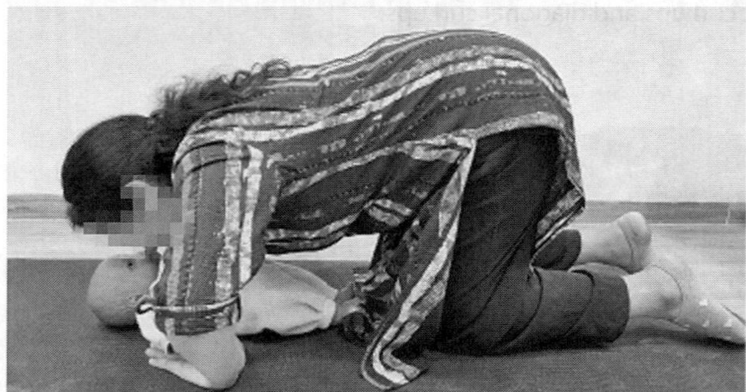

Fig. 22.25: Modified push ups with the baby.

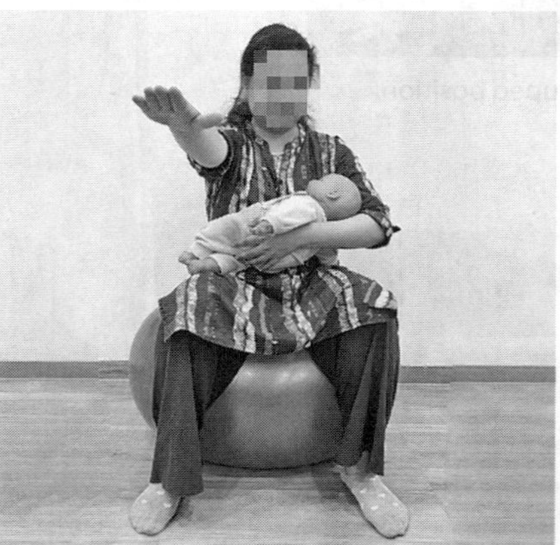

Fig. 22.26: Balance exercise with the baby.

- ❖ Avoid tricky movements like contraction of hip adductor, abdomen, and gluteal muscles, instead of the pelvic floor muscles
- ❖ Target fast contractions wherein, the patient tightens and relaxes the pelvic muscles quickly. This helps train the pelvic floor muscles to adapt to the increased intra-abdominal pressure during coughing and laughing.
- ❖ Target slow contractions wherein, the patient holds the contracted muscles for a longer period and then relaxes. These contractions help to strengthen the muscle.
- ❖ To enhance the treatment effect Kegel's can be used along with biofeedback and electrotherapy. Assisted pelvic floor muscle training with special devices like the Perineometer, Kegelmaster, vaginal cones, etc., can be used for resistance training of the PFM. Also, *see* Chapter 15: Managing the Pelvic Floor.

Box 22.9: Special considerations following surgical delivery: LSCS.

- Standard Assessment of Diastasis Recti should NOT be done for at least one week post-surgery as it may delay wound healing
- Appropriate focus on the prevention of pulmonary and circulatory complications **(Fig. 22.27)**
- TENS and cryotherapy can be used for pain relief
- Log rolling and wound splinting must be taught for pain-free bed mobility
- Electrotherapy modalities like LASER, ultrasound, and infrared can be used for wound healing
- Isometrics for abdominal muscles and pelvic floor can be initiated early on to promote wound healing and pain relief
- Use of pillows and lying positions to facilitate early breastfeeding initiation
- Post-wound healing, scar tissue mobilization can be done for adherent scars

Electrotherapy in Postnatal Care

TENS can be used to reduce postpartum uterine contraction pain during breastfeeding. LASER, ultraviolet radiations, and ultrasound have been found to be effective for surgical wound management of LSCS as well as the perineal lesions. Special considerations following surgical delivery are shown in **Box 22.9.** Sitz bath is also helpful in relieving pain from episiotomy.

EARLY CHILD CARE

Some of the vital concerns for the totally dependent newborn in the immediate postpartum period are:

- ❖ Breastfeeding and bonding
- ❖ Hygiene and cleanliness
- ❖ Weight gain
- ❖ Vitamin supplements
- ❖ Beginning of immunization
- ❖ Acceptance into the family

So, it is important to counsel the mother and the family about

- ❖ Breastfeeding and infant care
- ❖ The importance of immunization
- ❖ Nutritional supplementation required
- ❖ Safety
- ❖ Sleeping arrangement for the baby

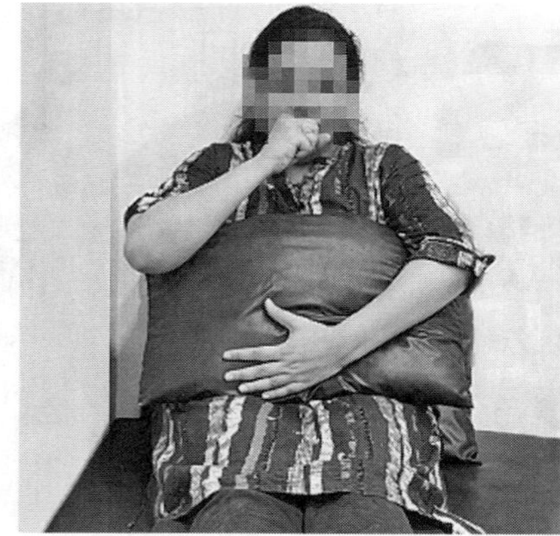

Fig. 22.27: Cough with wound splinting in LSCS patients.

Box 22.10: Newborn assessment.

- Name, mother's name, sex
- Date of delivery, time, type of delivery
- APGAR score, weight of baby
- Length of baby, head circumference, chest circumference, abdominal circumference
- Reflexes

Care of the Baby

The normal newborn baby should be assessed within a few hours of delivery **(Box 22.10)**.

General appearance: In a normal full-term baby

- Weight: Approximately 3.5 kg
- Height: 50 cm in length when extended and head circumference is 34–35 cm
- Attitude: Flexion
- Cry: Lusty
- Skin: Covered in vernix caseosa, a white sticky substance
- Lanugo (fine hairs) cover the skin
- Color: Pink all over
- Movement: The baby should move their limbs equally on both sides.

Apgar score has been used to record the observations on the vitality of the newborn infant for both therapeutic and prognostic purposes Chapter 21: Labor and Childbirth.

Tight swaddling should be discouraged for several reasons:

- Blocking the movement of the diaphragm decreases the ventilation of the lungs.
- It reduces blood circulation in different parts of the body;
- No air space between body and swaddling sheets prevents the baby keeping warm.
- Restricted free movement of the limbs prevents the development of neuromuscular coordination.
- Tight swaddling along with head swaddling can impede breastfeeding as the baby's head movement and mouth opening for correct attachment to the breast are hindered.
- Swaddling makes baby sleepier and less responsive to frequent breastfeeding, which interrupts breastfeeding and lactation establishment.

Sudden Infant Death Syndrome

Sudden infant death syndrome (SIDS) is used to refer to the death of a seemingly healthy infant younger than 1 year of age whose death is unexpected by history and remains unexplained after a thorough case investigation. Though a conclusive mandate is missing evidence has pointed to the fact that the prone sleep position more than triples the risk of SIDS as it is associated with impaired arousal from sleep, reduced vasomotor tone, and diminished laryngeal chemoreflexes and baroreceptor reflexes. Therefore, prone sleep position should be avoided especially in vulnerable infants.

Several genetic, environmental and personal habits of the mother including alcoholism/drug consumption have been implicated in literature as stressors that may cause asphyxia of a vulnerable infant who has immature defense mechanisms that are not fully integrated.

LONG-TERM GOALS FOR THE MOTHER

- To maintain physical fitness and improve cardiovascular endurance by aerobic conditioning program.
- Aerobic activities can include walking, spot marching, stepping, stair climbing, and cycling.
- **Further strengthening:** Core strengthening, progression of TA activation, pelvic tilts and rolling, back strengthening, crunches.
- Ergonomic advices:
    - Using a broom with large and long handle sweeping to avoid squatting or forward bending during the activities
    - Sitting: Thighs fully supported, trunk fully supported, slight even distribution of weight.

BIRTH CONTROL: SPACING FOR THE NEXT PREGNANCY

The carry forward effect of high levels of estradiol (E2) and progesterone during pregnancy initially accounts for the hypothalamic-pituitary suppression during the postpartum period leading to amenorrhea. The hypothalamic hypogonadism of lactation or lactational amenorrhea can persist for more than 12 months depending on the frequency and intensity of suckling. For the postpartum mother, this endogenous contraception allows women to cope with the physiologic demands of the postpartum period. However, for contraception purpose, this method is shown to be effective only when all three specific criteria are met with:

1. Exclusive breastfeeding occurs without routine supplements or delays in feedings
2. The infant is younger than 6 months
3. Menstruation has not recommenced.

For effective birth control, any of the following methods can be adopted as per the advice of the gynecologist:

- Barrier methods
- Long-acting reversible contraceptive methods [e.g., intrauterine devices (IUDs), the implant]
- Hormonal methods (e.g., pills, patches, rings)

Summary

Surviving pregnancy and childbirth can never be the marker of successful maternal health care. It is critical to expand efforts to reduce maternal injury and disability to promote health and well-being. Every pregnancy and subsequent birth is unique. Addressing the specific concerns of puerperal females would ensure optimum recovery to pre-pregnancy functional capacities but also reduce the risk of postpartum issues.

The physiotherapist should seek to prevent deep vein thrombosis, improve the respiratory, cardiac, gastrointestinal, locomotor, postural, and urinary functions (among others), and cesarean the bond between mother and newborn. They should also assist with relieving pain associated with perineal trauma and cesarean sections paving the path for a healing process that uses effective nonpharmacological resources to improve the postnatal well-being of the mother and the infant.

CLINICAL EXAMPLE

A 28-year-old primiparous woman gave birth to a baby boy through a full-term normal delivery with left mediolateral episiotomy two days back. The baby weighed 2.7 kg and cried immediately after birth. Currently, the mother has a complaint of pain at the suture site and difficulty in sitting. Otherwise, the mother and baby are in good health. Discuss her postnatal physiotherapy management program.

Management Goals

- Patient education and ergonomic advice
- Prevent pulmonary/circulatory complications
- Pain management and wound management: Electrotherapy, exercise therapy and sitz bath
- Assistive device: Ring-shaped cushion for sitting
- Encourage general mobility
- Assess and manage diastasis recti
- Assess/teach breastfeeding positions
- Initiate core and pelvic floor muscle activation and training
- Advice on baby handling
- Advice on nutrition and contraception

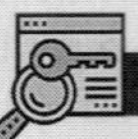

Review Questions

1. Enlist the objectives of postnatal care.
2. Enumerate the various phases of postpartum period.
3. What are the factors affecting recovery in the postpartum period?
4. Discuss the benefits of Kangaroo Mother Care.
5. Discuss the benefits of breastfeeding for the mother and the baby.
6. Describe the commonly used breastfeeding positions.
7. What is the role of prolactin and the let down reflex in lactation?
8. Write in brief about assessment of breastfeeding.
9. Mention some special pointers for nutrition in lactating mothers.
10. Discuss the immediate postpartum concerns.
11. Discuss some ergonomic advices for breastfeeding mothers.
12. Develop an exercise protocol for a female in immediate postpartum period.
13. Give salient points of early child care.

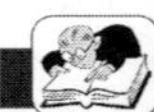

Bibliography

1. ACOG Committee Opinion No. 736. Optimizing postpartum care. Obstet Gynecol. 2018;131(5):e140-50. doi:10.1097/AOG.0000000000002633.
2. Cunningham FG, Leveno KJ, Bloom SL, Dashe JS, Hoffman BL, Casey BM, et al. Williams Obstetrics, 25th edition. New York: McGraw-Hill Education; 2018.
3. Dutta DC. DC Dutta's Textbook of Obstetrics, 9th edition. New Delhi: Jaypee Brothers Medical Publishers; 2018.
4. Mantle J, Haslam J, Barton S. Physiotherapy in Obstetrics and Gynaecology, 2nd edition. Edinburgh: Elsevier; 2004.
5. Oats J, Abraham S. Llewellyn-Jones Fundamentals of Obstetrics and Gynaecology, 9th edition. St. Louis: Mosby Elsevier; 2010.
6. Royal College of Obstetricians and Gynaecologists. Postpartum haemorrhage, prevention and management (Green-top Guideline No. 52). London: RCOG; 2016.
7. Sapsford R, Bullock-Saxton J, Markwell S. Women's Health: A Textbook for Physiotherapists. London: WB Saunders; 1998.
8. Smith CA, Levett KM, Collins CT, Armour M, Dahlen HG, Suganuma M. Relaxation techniques for postnatal recovery: a Cochrane review. Cochrane Database Syst Rev. 2018;(3):CD009514. doi:10.1002/14651858.CD009514.pub2.
9. World Health Organization. WHO recommendations on postnatal care of the mother and newborn. Geneva: WHO; 2014. Available from: https://www.who.int/publications/i/item/9789241506649

Multiple Choice Questions (MCQs)

To test your understanding and recall of key concepts.

1. What is the term for the postpartum uterine contractions stimulated by breastfeeding?

A. After pains
B. Lochia pains
C. Perineal pains
D. Uterine spasms

2. Why is early skin-to-skin contact encouraged immediately after delivery?

A. To prevent infections in the infant
B. To promote thermoregulation and maternal bonding
C. To accelerate maternal recovery
D. To increase milk production

3. The following factors affect recovery of the mother in the postpartum period, *except*:

A. Patient's intrinsic collagen support
B. Size of the infant
C. Route of delivery
D. Duration of labor

4. Diastasis recti in postnatal period signifies ______________.

A. Improved trunk stability and posture
B. Impaired core stability and predisposes to lower back pain
C. Indicates pelvic floor dysfunction
D. Indicates immediate need for surgical intervention

5. A mother reports significant perineal pain one day postpartum following a mediolateral episiotomy. What is the best initial physiotherapy intervention?

A. Start analgesics immediately
B. Provide cryotherapy and suggest resting on a ring cushion
C. Apply heat therapy to the perineal area
D. Begin resistance exercises for the pelvic floor muscles

6. A month postpartum lactating mother experiences breast engorgement and pain. What physiotherapy management should be implemented?

A. Hot packs, massage and temporarily restrict breastfeeding
B. Cold compresses, massage, proper latching and continue breastfeeding
C. Phonophoresis to reduce pain and swelling and restrict breastfeeding
D. Complete cessation of breastfeeding

7. What is the physiological role of prolactin in postnatal lactation?

A. Stimulates uterine contractions to aid recovery
B. Increases milk production and suppresses ovulation
C. Enhances thermoregulation in the newborn
D. Prevents postpartum depression

8. A 32-year-old mother, 3 weeks postpartum, reports lower back pain and difficulty lifting her baby. Assessment reveals diastasis recti and poor core stability. She is eager to resume her pre-pregnancy exercise routine but is unsure where to start. What is the most appropriate physiotherapy intervention?

A. Advise her to start high-intensity core exercises immediately to close the diastasis
B. Begin with pelvic tilts, gentle transverse abdominis activation, and education on proper lifting techniques
C. Recommend complete rest and avoid any physical activity for another 3 weeks
D. Focus solely on aerobic exercises to improve overall fitness

ANSWERS

1. A	2. B	3. D	4. B	5. B
6. B	7. B	8. B		

Chapter 23

Cesarean Section

Gopi Contractor

LEARNING OBJECTIVES

At the end of the chapter, the reader will be able to:
- Describe the prevalence, classification, indications and contraindications of cesarean section (CS).
- Discuss different surgical methods, outcomes of surgery and postoperative complications of cesarean section.
- Gain knowledge of guidelines for prevention of CS during different stages of labor.
- Understand the morbidity and mortality after cesarean section.
- Discuss psychological aspects of cesarean section and understand management strategies for the same.
- Describe physiotherapy assessment and management of patient having cesarean section in brief.

CHAPTER OUTLINE

INTRODUCTION

A cesarean section (CS) is defined as a surgical procedure in which incisions are made through the woman's lower abdomen and uterus to deliver one or more babies. It is the commonest surgical procedure performed in obstetric practice.

Based on the type of incision, there are two types of CS – classical CS and lower uterine segment CS (LSCS). Classical CS involves a large longitudinal incision in the upper uterine segment and allows a comparatively larger space for the baby to be delivered. LSCS involves a transverse incision in the lower uterine segment, just above the edge of the bladder. It causes lesser blood loss and is easier to repair. Classical CS is more prone to complications and hence, is used rarely nowadays.

Common obstetric complications faced by most of the women are obstructed labor and postpartum hemorrhage.

INCIDENCE OF CESAREAN SECTION

Despite the rise in the frequency of cesarean delivery in many countries, cesarean section rates in rural areas of many African and Asian countries remain lower than the 10–15% ideal rates proposed by the World Health Organization (WHO) as a target to optimize maternal perinatal health.

Rise in Cesarean delivery has happened from 5% in 1970 to 31.9% in 2016. For some women, it is the only or safest way to deliver a baby. In 1985, WHO had stated that the rate of CS should not exceed 10% to 15% in any country. The rising frequency of CS in 2015 led the WHO to hold a consensus conference. The conference concluded that there is maternal and neonatal benefit with CS rates up to 19%.

On the basis of data available, WHO concluded the following:

- CS should be provided to women in need, rather than the goal to achieve a specific rate.

- CS can save maternal and infant lives, but only when it is performed for those in whom indicated medically.
- The effects of CS rates on other outcomes, such as morbidity of mother and child, outcomes of pediatric population, and social and psychological well-being are still unclear.
- At population level, higher rates (more than 10%) are not associated with less maternal and newborn mortality rates.
- Permanent complications, disability or death can occur particularly where less advanced facilities regarding surgery, postsurgical care or surgical complications are available.
- CS should ideally only be undertaken when it is medically necessary.
- Further research is needed to understand the health effects of cesarean section on immediate and future outcomes.

CLASSIFICATION

WHO conducted a systematic review of systems in 2011 to classify CS. According to its conclusion, the Robson classification **(Table 23.1)** is the most appropriate system to fulfill current needs. WHO recommended building upon this to develop an internationally applicable CS classification system.

Table 23.1: Robson's classification of CS.

Groups	*Clinical characteristics*
1.	Nulliparous, singleton, cephalic, ≥37 weeks, spontaneous labor
2.	Nulliparous, singleton, cephalic, ≥37 weeks, induced labor or cesarean section before labor
3.	Multiparous without previous cesarean section, singleton, cephalic, ≥37 weeks, spontaneous labor
4.	Multiparous without previous cesarean section, singleton, cephalic, ≥37 weeks, induced labor or cesarean section before labor
5.	Multiparous with prior cesarean section, singleton, cephalic, ≥37 weeks
6.	All nulliparous breeches
7.	All multiparous breeches (including previous cesarean section)
8.	All multiple pregnancies (including previous cesarean section)
9.	All pregnancies with transverse or oblique lie (including those with previous cesarean section)
10.	Singleton, cephalic, ≤36 weeks (including previous cesarean section)

This classification system categorizes all women into 10 groups. The categories are based on five basic obstetric characteristics that are routinely collected in all maternities like:

- Parity (nulliparous, multiparous with and without previous cesarean section)
- Onset of labor (spontaneous, induced or pre-labor cesarean section)
- Gestational age (preterm or term)
- Fetal presentation (cephalic, breech or transverse)
- Number of fetuses (single or multiple)

A new classification relating the degree of urgency to the presence or absence of maternal or fetal compromise was developed later. This modified version **(Table 23.2)** uses a color scale for the classification and was proposed by Lucas et al. It reinforces the need to recognize that a 'continuum of urgency' applies to cesarean section, rather than discrete categories.

INDICATIONS

Main indications for cesarean delivery (more than 75%) are:

- Dystocia, including prolonged or obstructed labor, lasting more than 12–24 hours or with clinical signs of difficulty
- Previous cesarean delivery
- Fetal distress
- Breech presentation

Other ***less common indications*** are:

- Placental abruption
- Multiple pregnancy
- Fetal causes
  - Certain congenital malformations or skeletal disorders
  - Infection
  - Prolonged acidemia
- Maternal causes
  - Infections like human immunodeficiency virus (HIV) or herpes simplex virus (HSV)
  - Obstructive lesions in the lower genital tract, including malignancies, obstructive vaginal septa, etc.
  - Associated medical comorbidities like aortic stenosis or obesity

Most of the indications are relative indications, there are very few absolute indications. CS may not be best for every woman; the outcome may differ from one to another.

Emergent CS is planned when there is:

- Umbilical cord prolapse
- Abruptio placentae
- Partial or total placenta previa (stage III or IV)

Table 23.2: Lucas classification of urgency of cesarean section.

A classification that relates the degree of urgency to the presence or absence of maternal or fetal compromise		
Urgency	***Definition***	***Category***
Maternal or fetal compromise	Immediate threat to life of the female or fetus	1
	No immediate threat to life of the female or fetus	2
No maternal or fetal compromise	Requires early delivery	3
	At a time to suit the female and maternity services	4

- Prerupture syndrome
- Uterine rupture
- Eclamptic seizure
- Acute fetal distress
- Fetopelvic disproportion
- Chorioamnionitis
- Fetal presentation abnormalities
- Fetal heart rate (FHR) abnormalities
- Severe preeclampsia
- Dynamic dystocia

CONTRAINDICATIONS

Absolute contraindications are rare, and relative contraindications depend on clinical context. CS is contraindicated when the expected maternal mortality risk would be greater after the procedure than after any alternative mode of delivery. Relative contraindications of cesarean section are:

- Ethically, a cesarean is contraindicated if the pregnant patient refuses
- Existence of genital tract infection—actual or potential
- A pregnant patient with severe coagulopathy, which makes surgery extremely dangerous
- A patient with an extensive history of abdominal surgery and scarring, e.g., burns
- The convulsive stage of eclampsia
- Intrauterine fetal death
- Gross congenital malformation
- Extreme prematurity
- Lack of a valid indication for the operation

OPERATIVE PROCEDURES

Operative procedures for cesarean section include:

Classic Pfannenstiel-Kerr technique, Joel-Cohen method and Misgav Ladach technique.

- The Pfannenstiel-Kerr technique consists of the Pfannenstiel incision **(Fig. 23.1)** which is a transverse skin incision, two fingers above the symphysis pubis, which is extended towards the anterior superior iliac spine (ASIS), and ends 2–3 cm medial to ASIS on both sides.
- In the Joel-Cohen technique, skin incision is placed 3 cm above the original Pfannenstiel incision **(Fig. 23.1)**. The subcutaneous tissue is incised, manually the lateral tissue is separated then, bluntly the peritoneum is opened with fingers, the uterine cavity is incised, and the incision is extended bluntly laterally by two fingers. After delivery of the baby, the placenta is delivered spontaneously.

 **Clinical Pointer**

The **Joel-Cohen** technique is better than the Pfannenstiel-Kerr technique because it is faster to perform, less postoperative pain, causes less blood loss, shorter hospital stay, less postoperative infection, is more economic, saves more staff time, and utilises less anesthesia. So it has better feasibility.

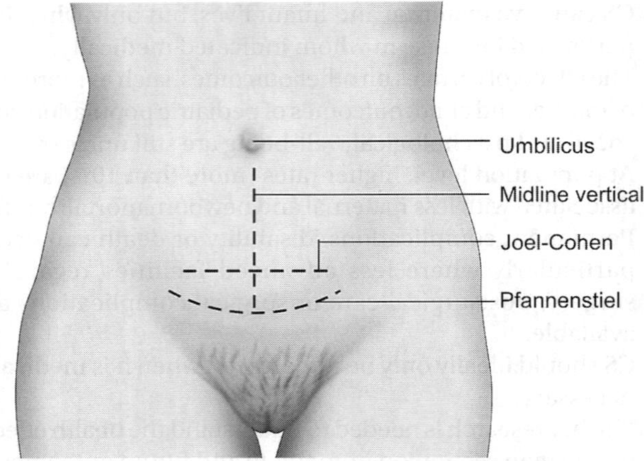

Fig. 23.1: Pfannenstiel incision, Joel-Cohen and midline vertical incision.

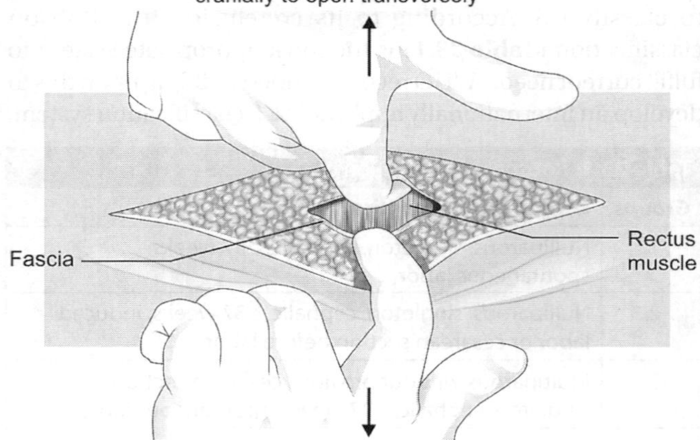

Fig. 23.2: Misgav Ladach technique of cesarean delivery.

- In Misgav Ladach technique **(Fig. 23.2)** a transverse skin incision, 5 cm above the symphysis pubic is made and blunt dissection of all abdominal walls after sharp superficial incision of the facia and uterus is done. Then placenta is removed manually after delivery of the baby. The fascia is closed continuously, the subcutaneous layer is not sutured, and then with the mattress suture, the skin is closed.

 **Clinical Pointer**

Misgav Ladach technique has several advantages over other techniques because of digital manual manipulation instead of invasion using sharp instruments.

- There is least possible trauma to the tissues, faster recovery, less blood loss, less anesthetic time, and less suturing.
- A reduced level of antibiotics and faster return of normal bowel function, shorter maternal hospital stay and less postoperative adhesion formation as well as lower incidence of fever, and urinary tract infection have been suggested.

The Misgav Ladach technique of cesarean delivery may be the least traumatic and most uncomplicated medical intervention in the history of medicine.

OUTCOME OF PROCEDURES

Cesarean section usually requires slightly longer operative time, though recovery outcomes are generally good. Due to intra-abdominal adhesions, very rarely, the patient may experience pelvic pain, which seems to be more intense in those who have multiple procedures.

Possible adverse maternal outcomes of CS include:
- Postpartum fever
- Surgical site infection
- Puerperal sepsis
- Maternal mortality

Possible adverse neonatal outcomes of CS:
- Neonatal sepsis
- Early neonatal death
- Stillbirth
- Perinatal asphyxia
- Low APGAR score
- Prematurity

Complications of Cesarean Section

- **Hemorrhage:** Hemorrhage is the most frequent complication during or after operation. This may be due to hypervolemia that develops from first to third trimester of pregnancy. 1000 mL of bleeding is generally accepted for the cesarean section, and in case of larger amounts, it is termed as obstetric hemorrhage.
- **Urological injuries:** Injuries to the urinary bladder can occur if the bladder is not emptied completely before the surgery, if there are adhesions over the bladder secondary to a previous CS or if CS is done at a later stage in labor. Bladder injuries are the commonest injuries to occur amongst urological injuries. Occasionally, the ureter can be obstructed or partially or completely sectioned by a ligature or due to angulation.
- **Intestinal lesions:** Intestinal lesions are very rare in CS, and if they occur, it may be due to an urgent abdominal approach with intestinal adhesions to the anterior wall.
- **Anesthetic complications:**
  - *Hypotension* caused by sympathetic nerve block aggravated by aorto-cava compression, is the most frequent anesthetic complication.
  - *Headache* may develop by puncture of the arachnoid hard membranes that cause an escape of cerebrospinal fluid with loss of cushioning effect.
  - *Chemical pneumonitis* can occur by aspiration of gastric contents; it has a bad prognosis.
  - There is a chance of *fetal injuries* due to scalpel.
- **Infection:** The infection of the surgical site called surgical wound infection is caused by contamination. Most frequently involved pathogen is the coagulase-negative *Staphylococcus*. There are various risk factors such as poor tissue management, prolonged surgical time, contaminated instruments, nutritional status and previous anemia or caused by surgery.
- **Thromboembolism:** At the site of thrombus formation, symptoms are usually minimal or absent until detached and manifest as a pulmonary or pelvic embolism. In the cases of pulmonary thromboembolism, the picture manifests suddenly with general malaise, tachypnea, dyspnea, severe chest pain and hemoptysis, and in severe cases, it progresses to the state of shock with a high percentage of mortality.
- **Late postsurgical complications:** Late postsurgical complications include the formation of adhesions, endometriosis of the abdominal wall in the surgical scar, and the high possibility of low placental insertion, placental accreta or uterine rupture in later pregnancies.

Morbidity and Mortality after Cesarean Section

Maternal mortality has been defined by WHO as the death of a woman during pregnancy or within 42 days of the termination of pregnancy irrespective of the duration and site of the pregnancy for any cause related to or aggravated by the pregnancy or its management, but not from accidental or incidental causes. Estimates suggest mortality rates after CS to be between 5.81 and 6.1 per 100,000 procedures. Almost 73% of the maternal mortalities are due to direct causes and rest 27% from indirect causes. **Table 23.3** presents the direct and indirect causes of maternal mortality.

WHO has defined maternal morbidity as any health condition related to or aggravated by pregnancy and delivery which causes a negative effect on woman's well-being. These morbidities can lead to short-term and long-term effects on mother and baby. Morbidity after CS births is four times than for vaginal delivery.

Intraoperative or postoperative complications have been reported during hospital stay in 27% women who had CS. Reports suggest severe complications in 10% women and life-threatening complications in only 0.76%.

Short-term morbidities after CS are:
- Hemorrhage
- Blood transfusion
- Peripartum hysterectomy
- Thromboembolic events
- Amniotic fluid embolism
- Wound hematoma
- Postpartum urinary retention
- Anesthetic complications

Long-term morbidities after CS are:
- Adherent placenta/placenta accreta
- Placenta previa
- Placental abruption

Table 23.3: Direct and indirect causes of maternal mortality.

Direct causes	*Indirect causes*
• Hypertensive disorders • Unsafe abortions • Hemorrhage • Sepsis • Embolism	• Cardiovascular disorders • Cerebrovascular accidents • Pulmonary system disorders • Gastrointestinal system disorders • Other indirect causes

- ❖ Uterine rupture
- ❖ Hysterectomy
- ❖ Stillbirth
- ❖ Preterm birth

Neonatal morbidities after CS among others are:

- ❖ Cerebral palsy
- ❖ Stillbirth
- ❖ Delayed maternal adaptation
- ❖ Respiratory morbidity
- ❖ Affected immune system

Clinical Pointer

The risk of morbidity and mortality was high in women after emergency CS and in women with history of previous CS. Neonatal and perinatal mortality and morbidity also increase in CS delivered babies.

Psychological Aspects of Cesarean Section

Current literature focuses on four main psychological outcomes of CS:

1. Maternal depression
2. Satisfaction with the birth
3. The mother-infant relationship
4. Breastfeeding

It can be inferred from recent evidences that mothers having CS are mentally affected.

Research Pointer

A meta-analysis of 43 studies investigating the psychosocial outcomes of cesarean section concluded that women are significantly less satisfied with their birth experience after a cesarean birth than after a vaginal delivery. Almost 10 to 20% of women suffer from postnatal depression which is a very common and debilitating problem in the first year after delivery.

Other maternal psychological outcomes include:

- ❖ Post-traumatic stress disorders
- ❖ Puerperal psychosis
- ❖ Lower self-esteem

Clinical Pointer

Negative psychological outcome is not present in all women who have a cesarean section. At one end of the spectrum, there are women who are extremely happy about having a cesarean birth and whose psychological profile, postcesarean is entirely positive. On the other end of the spectrum, there are women who feel devastated by their cesarean birth experience and have long-term negative psychological outcomes.

Box 23.1 presents the factors that appear to modify the psychological impact of CS.

Box 23.1: Factors which appear to modify the psychological impact of cesarean section: A summary of the research evidence.

Obstetric factors

- Emergency cesarean section
- General anesthesia

Psychological vulnerability

- Psychiatric history

Quality of care received

- Perceived low quality/amount of support received from maternity caregivers
- Perceived lack of involvement in decision to have cesarean
- Perception that the cesarean may have been unnecessary/ avoidable

Management Strategies

As a part of prevention and management strategies, caregivers should be aware of the possible psychological responses to cesarean section so that they may recognize psychological difficulties that may arise in the cesarean mothers they care for.

- ❖ Mother should be informed earlier about the possible outcome of the procedure and according to her own need she should also be involved in each and every decision related to operative procedure.
- ❖ If the procedure is done under general anesthesia, there are a number of steps that can be taken to minimize women's sense of having 'missing pieces' in her experience, of feeling unsure that the baby is genuinely hers, and of feeling that she does not have an image of her baby's birth. These include:
    - ◆ Allowing partners to attend general anesthetic cesareans if they wish
    - ◆ Enabling the partner or midwife to take photographs or a video of the birth
    - ◆ Minimizing all unnecessary separations between mother and child
    - ◆ Arranging for someone present at the cesarean to talk through the birth with the mother soon after delivery.
- ❖ The caregiver should identify the developing negative psychological impact and as a preventive measure postnatal psychological counseling should be done. Also *see* Chapter 16: Psychosexual Dimensions of Women's Health.

PHYSIOTHERAPY ASSESSMENT

Assessment of a woman following CS remains similar to assessment of a woman following vaginal delivery in most aspects. Assessment following vaginal delivery can be found in Chapter 4: Assessment in Women's Health. The differentiating features have been described in **Box 23.2**.

Range of Motion Examination

- ❖ Within the permissible movement
- ❖ Ballistic movement should be avoided
- ❖ End range pressure should be avoided

Box 23.2: Assessment of a woman following CS.

Subjective assessment	Objective assessment
• Demographic details • Chief complaint • Obstetric history • Immunization history • Perinatal history (any complications during the operation) • Postnatal history includes type of cesarean section, duration of cesarean section, site of incision, place of delivery, details about anesthesia • History of incontinence • Pain examination • Past history • Medical history • Drug history • Personal history • Family history • Socioeconomical history • Environmental history • Psychological history • Neonatal history	• Body build • Edema • Trophic changes • Wound/Scar – at lower abdominal region • Posture • Gait ***On palpation*** • Spasm • Wound/scar—healed/non-healed, adherent/non-adherent • Temperature – local/general • Tenderness • Swelling ***On examination*** • Vital signs • Range of motion examination • Manual muscle testing • Gait examination • Diastasis recti assessment • Sacroiliac dysfunction assessment • Pelvic floor muscles strength assessment • Exercise tolerance test (using 6 minutes or 3 minutes walk test) • Functional assessment

- Hypermobility is already present because of laxity of the ligament
- If edema is present, ranges must be restricted for that joint.

Manual Muscle Testing

Extra caution is needed while assessing:
- Abdominals (if permitted by gynecologist usually after 1 month or after soft tissue healing)
- Gluteal muscles
- Perineal muscles

Gait Examination

Observational gait analysis should be done to identify the deviations due to surgical procedure.

Diastasis Recti Assessment

(Also *see* Chapter 22: Postnatal Care).
- Can be conducted usually after 1st week
- Following points should be considered:
  - Maximum diastasis area
  - Length and width of diastasis
  - Degree and bulging of abdomen during recti activation

Functional Assessment

- **Maternal Postpartum Quality of Life (MAPP-QOL) Questionnaire:** It is a self-administered, paper-and-pencil instrument that measures maternal quality of life during the early postpartum period. Here the questions are related to the satisfaction and importance with the areas of life.
- **Mother Generated Index (MGI):** The mother-generated index (MGI) is one of the few existing specific questionnaires for assessing the postnatal quality of life (QoL).
- **Edinburgh Postnatal Depression Scale (EPDS):** The Edinburgh Postnatal Depression Scale (EPDS) is a set of 10 screening questions that can indicate whether a woman is having depression and anxiety during pregnancy and in the year following the birth of the baby.
- **Postpartum Specific Anxiety Scale (PSAS):** The PSAS measures the anxiety in four different areas like: Competence and attachment anxieties; Infant safety and welfare anxieties; Practical baby care anxieties; Psychosocial adjustment to motherhood.

PHYSIOTHERAPY MANAGEMENT

Structural and Functional Impairments

- Risk of pulmonary, vascular and gastrointestinal complications
- Postsurgical pain and discomfort
- Adhesion formation at incisional site
- Faulty/improper posture
- Pelvic floor dysfunction which may lead to urinary incontinence, uterine prolapse, etc.
- Weakness of abdominals
- Diastasis recti development

Aims and Planning

- To maintain and improve pulmonary function and decrease the risk of pneumonia
- To promote postoperative wound healing
- To reduce incisional pain with coughing, movement and while breastfeeding
- To reduce perineal pain (during immediate postnatal period)
- To prevent postsurgical vascular complications
- To correct posture
- To prevent pelvic floor muscle dysfunction
- To treat musculoskeletal problems
- To restore abdominal muscle strength
- Diastasis recti correction
- To improve mental health
- To explain postnatal ergonomics

Management Strategies

To Maintain and Improve Pulmonary Functions and Decrease the Risk of Pneumonia

- Diaphragmatic breathing exercise can be explained by asking the mother to perform slow deep inspiration, asking her to expand the diaphragmatic region, followed by slow expiration **(Fig. 23.3)**.
- Chest expansion exercises can be explained by asking the mother to perform deep inspiration followed by a three-

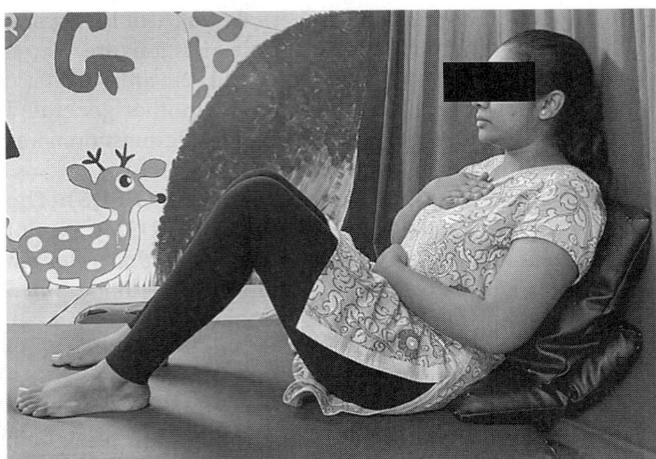

Fig. 23.3: Diaphragmatic breathing exercise.

second pause at maximal inspiratory volume attained, and then slow expiration.

- Mother can be advised to be physically active and mobile as early as possible to avoid pulmonary complications and reduce the risk of infections like pneumonia.
- If mobility outside the bed is difficult, generalized bed mobility with lower limb active movements will enhance respiratory function and also prevent circulatory complications like deep vein thrombosis, varicose veins, oedema, superficial vein thrombosis, etc.

To Promote Postoperative Wound Healing

- Low-level laser therapy (LLLT) promotes angiogenesis, increases amount of collagen production, promotes muscle regeneration thus it promotes metabolic processes and helps in wound healing postsurgery. The dosage can be 4.8 J/cm^2.
- Ultrasound (low intensity pulsed ultrasound: Dosage-0.5 W/cm^2, pulsed mode-20% duty cycle; 1 MHz; 1-2 min/cm^2) facilitates healing of incision in 3–4 weeks. Mechanical vibration produced during ultrasound therapy facilitates healing at cellular level, stimulates protein synthesis and increases cell proliferation.

To Reduce Incisional Pain while Coughing, General Mobility and Breastfeeding

- Support should be given with the pillow to the incision while coughing or breastfeeding. Along with that education regarding incisional care should be given.
- Transcutaneous electrical nerve stimulation (TENS) can be used with four rubber electrodes in a crook lying position. Conventional TENS (high frequency, low intensity pulses, 12–30 mA, 100–150 Hz) significantly decreases post-operative pain intensity.
- High-intensity laser therapy (HILT) can be used with pulsed emission (1,064 nm), very high peak powers (3 kW), high levels of energy density (from 810–1,780 mJ/cm), very short pulse duration of (120–150 µs), a duty cycle of approximately 0.1%, and frequency (10–40 Hz).

To Reduce Perineal Pain (During Immediate Postnatal Period)

- For the relief of perineal pain, repeated contraction and relaxation of the pelvic floor musculature can be performed. The resulting pumping action assists in venous and lymphatic drainage and removal of traumatic exudate, thus reducing stiffness and restoring function.

Clinical Pointer

Perineal pain tends to be maximal with the first contraction of pelvic floor muscles and decreases with repetition as edema disperses.

- Effects can be enhanced by asking the mother to perform pelvic floor muscle exercises in other possible positions like stride crook lying, prone lying, stride standing, or stride sitting **(Fig. 23.4)**.
- Mother should be educated for comfortable positions for feeding, relaxation and sleep, using pillows and

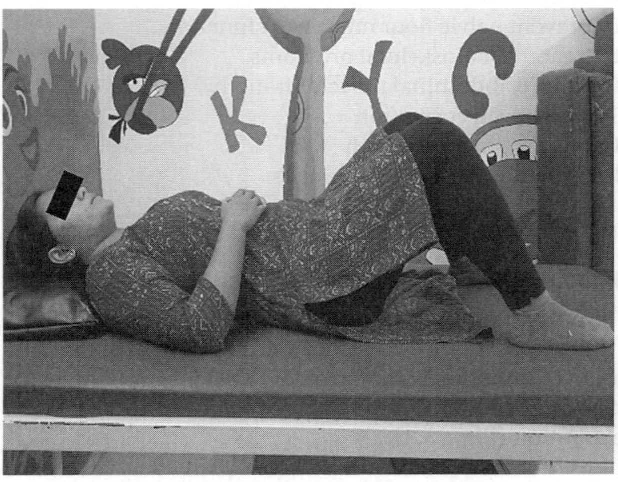

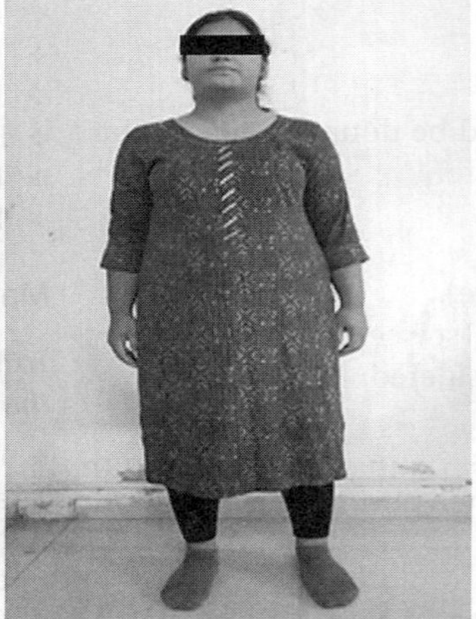

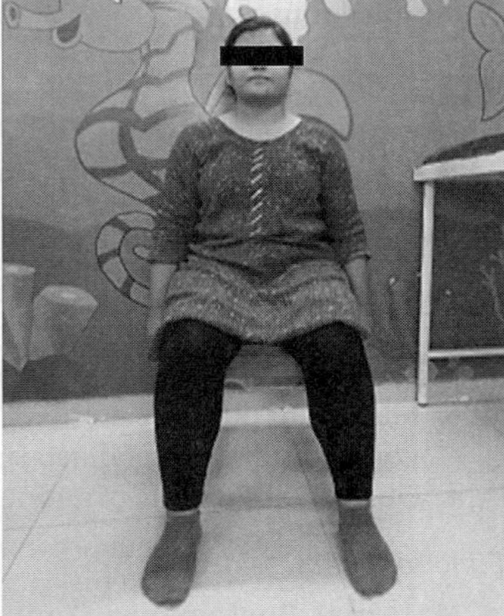

Fig. 23.4: Pelvic floor muscle exercises in stride crook lying, stride standing and stride sitting.

pressure-relieving cushions. Pain relief can occur rapidly if positioning is appropriate.

- Crushed ice, wrapped in damp disposable gauze or a disposable wash cloth and applied to the affected area for 5–10 minutes can be used.
- Ultrasound has shown to increase tissue temperature, which in turn leads to increased blood flow and increased repair.
- Pulsed short-wave diathermy or pulsed electromagnetic energy (PEME) can be given in the early postnatal period for bruising, large hemorrhoids, extensive suturing, post-cesarean birth hematomas, and inflamed or infected wounds.

To Prevent Postsurgical Vascular Complication

Early postsurgical vascular complications are edema, varicose vein, hemorrhoids and superficial and deep vein thrombosis.

- Ankle dorsiflexion and plantar flexion movements vigorously throughout the day can be effective.
- Frequent position modification by keeping the lower extremities elevated **(Fig. 23.5)** and avoiding cross leg sitting can be beneficial.

To Correct Posture

Excessively increased lumbar lordosis or sway back posture with protracted shoulders are the commonest postural deviations to address. Regaining good posture is important —standing, sitting, lying or being active with ideal posture is an important aspect.

- The mother should be asked to try to stand tall, avoid slumping of the shoulders and gently draw in the lower tummy for postural support.
- Visual biofeedback can be effective by standing in front of mirror and faults in the posture can be corrected.
- Stretching of shortened muscles like back extensors, scapular protractors and internal rotators of the shoulder should be emphasized to maintain neutral position of spine and scapula.
- Strengthening of weak muscles like abdominals, shoulder external rotators, lower neck and upper thoracic extensors and upper neck flexors should be done.

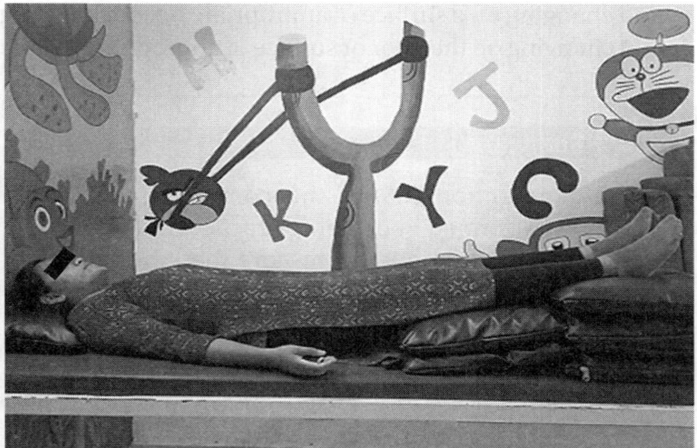

Fig. 23.5: Positioning to prevent postsurgical vascular complications.

- Recruitment of core muscles can be emphasized to develop the spinal stability and maintain the posture in a correct alignment throughout.

To Prevent Pelvic Floor Muscle Dysfunction

Pelvic floor muscle dysfunction can be prevented by activating the pelvic floor muscles.

- The first step is to find a comfortable position - side lying or supine lying; and progressing to sitting and standing. In the beginning the mother should be asked to try to relax all muscles, and focus on a steady breathing pattern.
- To activate the anterior pelvic floor muscles, the subject is asked to replicate the action of stopping the flow of urine midstream.
- To activate the posterior pelvic floor muscles, replicate the action of stopping passing gas.
- To activate both the anterior and posterior pelvic floor muscles, combine the two above actions.
- Elevator/graded isometric exercises—ask the mother to visualize that she is traveling in an elevator. So as elevator travels from one floor to another, she has to increase the amount of contraction. She has to contract little more every time.
- Progression can be done by moving from stable to dynamic surface like mat or balance board and same exercise can be performed.

Also *see* Chapter15: Managing the Pelvic Floor.

To Treat Musculoskeletal Problems

Low back pain, pain in epidural site, coccydynia and thoracic pain are most common musculoskeletal problems.

- Low back pain can be because of improper posture and weak abdominal muscles. Lumbosacral corset can be effective. Ergonomic principles can be explained during all functional activities. Specific mobilization techniques for sacroiliac, lumbar and lumbosacral region may be appropriate.
- Pain at epidural site can be because of tiny hematoma in the dura and epidural space. Heat in the form of hot pack application can be soothing.
- Thoracic pain can be relieved by postural correction especially during functional activities.
- Coccydynia can be due to damaged ligament or displacement of coccyx during pregnancy. Active physiotherapeutic measures, such as ultrasound, ice or hot packs and TENS, can give relief. In sitting, a cushion or pillow, arranged in such a way as to take away the pressure on the ischial tuberosities and thighs, may assist comfort. Prone lying will be the most comfortable position, and frequent gluteal contractions can be advised to reduce initial pain.

To Restore Abdominal Muscle Strength

Abdominals are divided into superficial including rectus abdominis and obliques and deep muscles including transversus obliquus.

- Superficial abdominals can be strengthened by performing trunk curls **(Fig. 23.6)** and pelvic lifts **(Fig. 23.7)**.
- For deep abdominals activation, the abdominal hollowing exercise ('core exercise') can be performed.

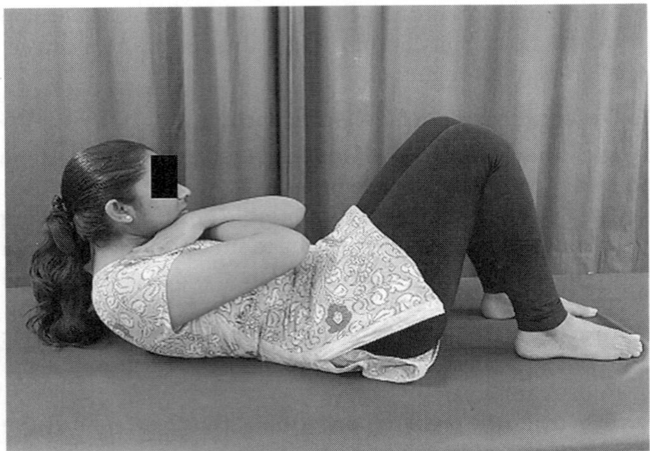

Fig. 23.6: Trunk curls.

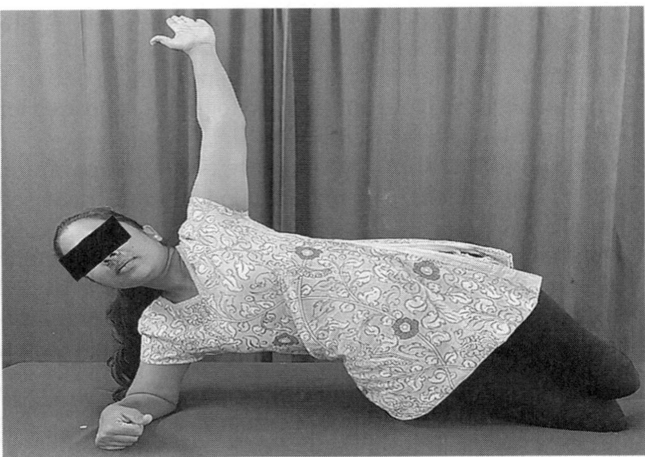

Fig. 23.7: Pelvic lifts.

- Start with lying on back or side with knees bent, or sitting with back well supported.
- Place one or both hands on the abdomen, below the level of umbilicus ('tummy button'). Breathe in through nose, and as you breathe out, draw in your lower abdomen, pulling it gently away from your hands towards your back and then relax.
- Progress to perform the same exercise in standing.
- Further progression is made by adding a holding period of 3 seconds which can be gradually increased to 10 seconds for a maximum repetition of 10 times performed at least thrice daily or as often as the subject can.
- Hollowing should be performed throughout the day to recruit the deep muscles - before and during any physical activity requiring effort, e.g., when lifting.

Diastasis Recti Correction

Also *see* Chapter 22: Postnatal Care

- Start with isometric abdominal exercises in all functional activities which should be repeated hourly.
- Once the condition progresses, exercise can be loaded with increase number of repetitions with limb loading.
- If the diastasis is larger, all such exercises can be performed with abdominal binder. As the symptom resolves, one can reduce the use of abdominal binder.

To Improve Mental Health

- General body exercise has antidepressant effects in clinical depression including major depression. It may have both preventive and treatment applications in postpartum depression. It also promotes general wellbeing.
- Cognitive behavioral therapy is one of the best ways to treat major depression.
- Yoga and meditation can be an effective means to improve mental health of a mother.
- Partner and parental support can be the best way to treat psychiatric issues.
- Music therapy by listening to soft music can be effective.

To Explain Postnatal Ergonomics

- **While sitting in chair:** Back should be supported, the sitting surface should not extend as far as the popliteal fossa to avoid impingement; feet should be flat on the floor; weight should be equally distributed over both buttocks; sitting surface should be soft enough to allow for pressure distribution; trunk should be supported with maintained natural spinal curves.
- **While standing:** Feet slightly apart, weight evenly distributed over both feet, shoulders relaxed, arms held loosely at the side, head in line with trunk.
- **While in lying position:** Body should be fully supported with pillows—head, knees, low back, etc., legs should not be crossed.
- **While feeding baby:** Ergonomic principles must be followed to avoid musculoskeletal discomfort, or maybe even pain. Back flexion should be avoided while feeding a baby. Different feeding positioned **(Fig. 23.8)** should be taught by keeping baby in such a way that strain is avoided in any area of the mother's body.
- Nappy changing is another activity that can result in pain if done with bad posture. Positions that increase risk to the mother should be avoided. Suggested positioning for nappy changing could be: sitting and changing on the lap, and changing on a surface of appropriate height, kneeling and changing on the floor or surface of appropriate height.

Summary

A cesarean section (CS) is the commonest surgical procedure performed in obstetric practice. Over the past three decades it is important to note that, the cesarean section rate has increased significantly worldwide. Main indications for cesarean delivery (more than 75%) are Dystocia, previous cesarean delivery, fetal distress and breech presentation. Other indications, such as placental abruption, multiple pregnancy, fetal and maternal disease, placenta previa are less common. CS is contraindicated

Contd...

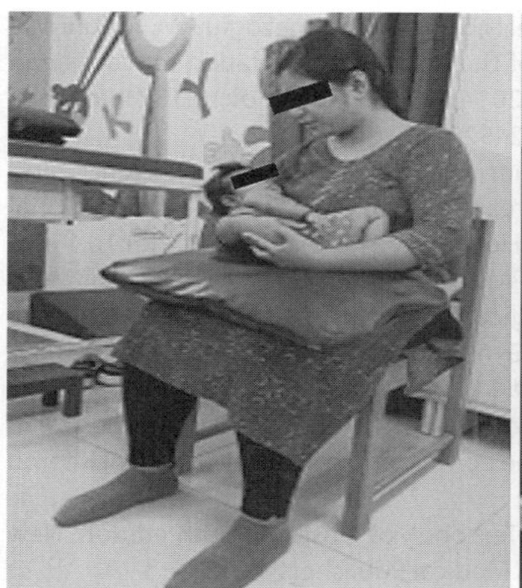
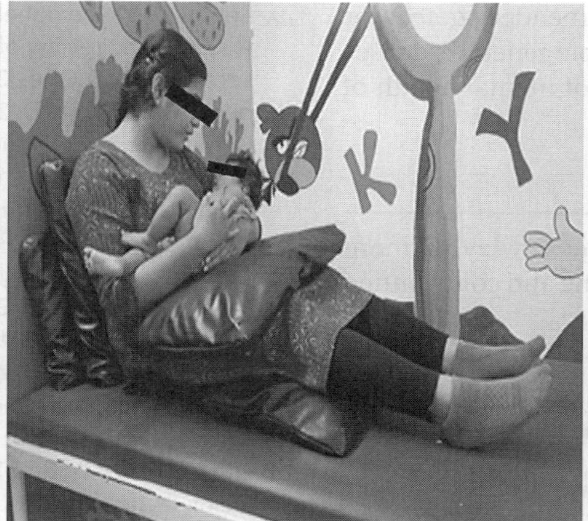
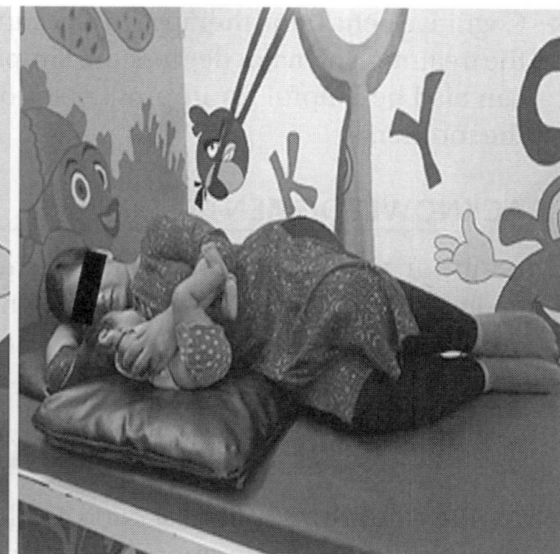

Fig. 23.8: Different feeding positions.

Contd...

when the expected maternal mortality risk would be greater after the procedure than after any alternative mode of delivery. Various techniques are performed for operative delivery of a baby such as, Classic Pfannenstiel-Kerr technique, Joel-Cohen method and Misgav Ladach technique. Hemorrhage, urological injuries, intestinal lesions, anesthetic complications, infection, thromboembolism and late postsurgical complications like formation of adhesions, endometriosis of the abdominal wall in the surgical scar, and the high possibility of low placental insertion, placental accreta or uterine rupture are the commonest complications after CS. The American College of Obstetricians and Gynecologists (ACOG) and the Society for Maternal-Fetal Medicine (SMFM) released joint guidelines for the safe prevention of primary cesarean delivery. Current literature focuses on four main psychological outcomes of cesarean section: maternal depression, satisfaction with the birth, the mother-infant relationship, and breastfeeding. While looking at various recent evidences we can infer the finding against mental health of mothers having CS. Various physiotherapeutic techniques are available to treat the outcome of CS in a best possible way.

CLINICAL EXAMPLES

Example 1

A 35-year-old female presented with a history of G2P2A0L2. When she was 32 weeks pregnant, she was diagnosed with pregnancy-induced hypertension (PIH). The gynecologist advised her to go for lower section cesarean section (LSCS). 1.5 months after LSCS procedure, she complained of severe low back pain which increased with prolonged sitting without support and prolonged standing. Stress urinary incontinence was also one of her complaints which increased with strenuous activities.

Suggested Physiotherapy Management

- Thorough examination should be performed to find out the cause for LBP. Expected cause can be due to poor posture, affected spinal stability (due to generalised laxity of ligaments during pregnancy) or poor ergonomics.
- Core stability exercises with postural correction can be recommended to reduce LBP.
- Proper ergonomic education can be provided for proper sitting, lying, kneeling, feeding and nappy changing positioning.
- Appropriate work—rest intervals should be explained with proper ergonomics.
- For stress urinary incontinence, pelvic floor muscle strengthening exercises should be explained during all functional activities.

Example 2

A 27-year-old female developed placental abruption at 34 weeks of her gestational age. So the obstetrician advised her for emergency cesarean section at the time of diagnosis. Right now, she is postoperative day 22. She is having incisional site pain throughout the day. Since last few days she is not feeling well. She is experiencing frequent episodes of mood swings. She is also complaining of the neck and back pain. As she is a classical dancer, she is more concerned about her posture and fitness.

Suggested Physiotherapy Management

- For incisional site pain, TENS or High Intensity LASER Therapy can become an effective intervention.
- Pillow can be provided for support while coughing or sneezing. Education regarding incisional care should be provided.
- Pulsed Ultrasound therapy can be given to promote wound healing.
- According to the described symptoms, it seems that the mother is having postnatal depression. So appropriate psychological counseling can be done.

- Cognitive behavioral therapy is a recommended strategy for the treatment of major depression. Simple general exercises can also be helpful for improvement of mental health of the mother.

ACKNOWLEDGMENTS

The author would like to thank Harsha Yewley, Himani Kapadiya and Yachana Vasave for reviewing and contributing photos to the chapter.

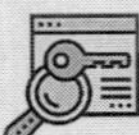

Review Questions

1. Write a note on cesarean section. Explain in detail about physiotherapy assessment and management for the same.
2. Explain in detail about classification of cesarean section.
3. What are the indications and contraindications of cesarean section?
4. Explain in brief about cesarean section. Explain surgical procedure for the same.
5. What is included in postoperative care following a cesarean section?
6. Write a note on complications of cesarean section.
7. What are the possible morbidity and mortality issues associated with CS?
8. Explain different factors affecting psychological aspects of CS. Explain physiotherapy management for the same.
9. Explain in detail about postoperative physiotherapy management after cesarean section.

Bibliography

1. ACOG Practice Bulletin No. 205: Vaginal birth after caesarean delivery. Obstet Gynecol. 2019;133(2):e110-27. doi:10.1097/AOG.0000000000003078. PMID: 30681539.
2. Ali SM, Hassan SA, Ghani RM. Effect of early post-caesarean section exercises on early resumption of women's functional activities. Egypt Nurs J. 2020;17(2):135-40.
3. American College of Obstetricians and Gynecologists; Society for Maternal-Fetal Medicine. Safe prevention of the primary caesarean delivery. Obstet Care Consensus No. 1. Am J Obstet Gynecol. 2014;210(3):179-93. doi:10.1016/j.ajog.2014.01.026.
4. Androutsopoulos G, Shendy M, editors. Caesarean Section. Norderstedt: BoD–Books on Demand; 2018.
5. Assefa EM, Janbo A, Ghiwot Y. Comparative analysis of caesarean section using the Robson's Ten-Group Classification System in private and public hospitals, Addis Ababa, Ethiopia. Obstet Gynecol Int J. 2021;4(2):81-91.
6. Aubrey-Bassler K, Newbery S, Kelly L, Weaver B, Wilson S. Maternal outcomes of caesarean sections: do generalists' patients have different outcomes than specialists' patients? Can Fam Physician. 2007;53(12):2132-8. PMID: 18077746.
7. Aujang ER. Complications of caesarean operation. In: Androutsopoulos G, Shendy M, editors. Caesarean Section. London: IntechOpen; 2018. p. 89-104.
8. Baker PN, Kenny L, editors. Obstetrics by Ten Teachers, 19th edition. London: CRC Press; 2011.
9. Betran AP, Vindevoghel N, Souza JP, Gülmezoglu AM, Torloni MR. A systematic review of the Robson classification for caesarean section. PLoS One. 2014;9(6):e97769. doi:10.1371/journal.pone.0097769. PMID: 24926787.
10. Betran AP, Ye J, Moller AB, Souza JP, Zhang J. Trends and projections of caesarean section rates: global and regional estimates. BMJ Glob Health. 2021;6(6):e005671. doi:10.1136/bmjgh-2021-005671. PMID: 34130991.
11. Clement S. Psychological aspects of caesarean section. Best Pract Res Clin Obstet Gynaecol. 2001;15(1):109-26. doi:10.1053/beog.2000.0150. PMID: 11359324.
12. Dempsey A, Diamond KA, Bonney EA, Myers JE. Caesarean section: techniques and complications. Obstet Gynaecol Reprod Med. 2017;27(2):37-43.
13. Dutta DC. DC Dutta's Textbook of Obstetrics, 9th edition. New Delhi: Jaypee Brothers Medical Publishers; 2018.
14. Ebneshahidi A, Mohseni M. The effect of patient-selected music on early postoperative pain, anxiety, and hemodynamic profile in caesarean section surgery. J Altern Complement Med. 2008;14(7):827-31. doi:10.1089/acm.2007.0755. PMID: 18803489.
15. Fitelson E, Kim S, Baker AS, Leight K. Treatment of postpartum depression: clinical, psychological and pharmacological options. Int J Womens Health. 2011;3:1-14. doi:10.2147/IJWH.S6938. PMID: 21339932; PMCID: PMC3036554.
16. Gürşen C, Inanir A, Kucuksen S, Kucuk A, Erdem SS, Altan L. The effect of exercise on functional activity level, fatigue, and quality of life in pregnancy: a randomized controlled trial. J Matern Fetal Neonatal Med. 2016;29(5):779-83. doi:10.3109/14767058.2015.1012063. PMID: 25719775.
17. Keag OE, Norman JE, Stock SJ. Long-term risks and benefits associated with caesarean delivery for mother, baby, and subsequent pregnancies: systematic review and meta-analysis. PLoS Med. 2018;15(1):e1002494. doi:10.1371/journal.pmed.1002494. PMID: 29360829.
18. Lavender T, Hofmeyr GJ, Neilson JP, Kingdon C, Gyte GM. Caesarean section for non-medical reasons at term. Cochrane Database Syst Rev. 2012;(3):CD004660. doi:10.1002/14651858.CD004660.pub3. PMID: 22419295.
19. Mantle J, Haslam J, Barton S, (editors). Physiotherapy in Obstetrics and Gynaecology, 2nd edition. Edinburgh: Butterworth-Heinemann; 2004.
20. Mohamed O, El-Sayed W, Abd El-Monem AM. Effect of pelvic floor exercises on post-caesarean section women. J Nurs Health Sci. 2020;9(3):1-7.
21. Molina G, Weiser TG, Lipsitz SR, Esquivel MM, Uribe-Leitz T, Azad T, et al. Relationship between caesarean delivery rate and maternal and neonatal mortality. JAMA. 2015;314(21):2263-70. doi:10.1001/jama.2015.15553. PMID: 26624825.
22. Norman E, Sherburn M, Osborne RH, Galea MP. An exercise and education program improves well-being of new mothers: a randomized controlled trial. Phys Ther. 2010;90(3):348-55. doi:10.2522/ptj.20090139. PMID: 20093325.
23. Royal College of Obstetricians and Gynaecologists. Caesarean section. Green-top Guideline No. 45. London: RCOG; 2015.
24. Sandall J, Tribe RM, Avery L, Mola G, Visser GH, Homer CS, et al. Short-term and long-term effects of caesarean section on the health of women and children. Lancet. 2018;392(10155):1349-57. doi:10.1016/S0140-6736(18)31930-5. PMID: 30322585.
25. Sapsford R, Bullock-Saxton J, Markwell S, (editors). Women's Health: A Textbook for Physiotherapists. London: WB Saunders; 1998.

26. Thabet AA, Mahran HG, Ebid AA, Alshehri MA. Effect of pulsed high-intensity laser therapy on delayed caesarean section healing in diabetic women. J Phys Ther Sci. 2018;30(4):570-5. doi:10.1589/jpts.30.570. PMID: 29765119; PMCID: PMC5944453.
27. Torloni MR, Betran AP, Souza JP, Widmer M, Allen T, Gulmezoglu M, et al. Classifications for caesarean section: a systematic review. PLoS One. 2011;6(1):e14566. doi:10.1371/journal.pone.0014566. PMID: 21283801; PMCID: PMC3029286.
28. Weerasinghe DS, Fernando S, Samarasinghe G. Physiotherapy management following caesarean section: a randomized controlled trial. Sri Lanka J Obstet Gynaecol. 2022;44(1):19-27.
29. Williams JW, Cunningham FG, Leveno KJ, Bloom SL, Spong CY, Dashe JS, et al. Williams Obstetrics, 25th edition. New York: McGraw-Hill; 2018.
30. World Health Organization. WHO recommendations: non-clinical interventions to reduce unnecessary caesarean sections. Geneva: WHO; 2018. Available from: https://www.who.int/publications/i/item/9789241550338

Multiple Choice Questions (MCQs)

To test your understanding and recall of key concepts.

1. **What is the most common indication for a cesarean section?**
   A. Placenta previa
   B. Breech presentation
   C. Fetal distress
   D. Labor dystocia
2. **Which surgical technique for cesarean section is considered the least traumatic and most efficient?**
   A. Pfannenstiel-Kerr technique
   B. Misgav Ladach technique
   C. Joel-Cohen method
   D. Classical cesarean section
3. **Misgav Ladach technique is preferred over other cesarean methods because__________.**
   A. It ensures minimal blood loss, quicker recovery, and reduced postoperative adhesions
   B. It is faster to perform but involves more postoperative complications
   C. It focuses on incision precision and longer hospital stays
   D. It eliminates the need for abdominal fascia closure
4. **The primary goal of postoperative physiotherapy after a cesarean section is_______________.**
   A. Prevent pulmonary complications and enhance abdominal muscle recovery
   B. Focus exclusively on pelvic floor exercises
   C. Delay mobility to ensure complete healing of the incision
   D. Avoid all physical activity for 6 weeks to prevent complications
5. **A postpartum female complains of incisional pain while coughing and breastfeeding. The most appropriate intervention in this case is__________.**
   A. Complete bed rest for next 2 weeks
   B. Wound splinting during coughing and breastfeeding along with TENS therapy
   C. Initiate curl-up exercises for abdominal strengthening
   D. Suggest pain medications and put breastfeeding on hold
6. **Delayed mobility of a cesarean section patient can lead to increase in the risk of________.**
   A. Pulmonary and vascular complications
   B. Delayed scar healing and better muscle recovery
   C. Scar tissue adhesions
   D. Diastasis recti of the rectus abdominis muscle
7. **A 29-year-old woman, two weeks post-cesarean section, reports persistent lower abdominal pain, difficulty moving from bed to standing, and poor posture while breastfeeding. On examination, there is mild tenderness at the incision site, a palpable gap suggesting diastasis recti, and generalized weakness of the core muscles. As a physiotherapist, what should be the prioritized plan of care?**
   A. Begin advanced core strengthening exercises like planks and crunches to close the diastasis
   B. Focus on isometric exercises for the transverse abdominis, posture correction while breastfeeding, and gradual functional mobility training
   C. Advise complete bed rest to avoid further strain on the abdominal muscles
   D. Use ultrasound therapy to reduce tenderness at the incision site before initiating any exercises

ANSWERS

1. D	2. B	3. A	4. A	5. B
6. A	7. B			

Chapter 24

Neonatal and Early Pediatric Problems

✍ *Archana Shah, Priyasingh Rangey*

LEARNING OBJECTIVES

At the end of the chapter, the reader will be able to:

- Learn neonatal and infant care.
- Gain knowledge about the WHO recommendations for neonatal care.
- Discuss common conditions occurring before and after birth.
- Know role of physiotherapy in neonatology, infanthood and early pediatrics.

CHAPTER OUTLINE

- Introduction
  - Problems developing before birth
  - Problems occurring after birth
- Care of the newborn after delivery
  - Essential care
  - Neonatal resuscitation
  - Prevention of neonatal infections
- Common conditions seen during infancy and early pediatric period
  - Hypoxic-ischemic encephalopathy
  - Neonatal seizures
  - Neonatal sepsis
  - Neonatal meningitis
  - Neonatal respiratory distress syndrome
  - Neonatal jaundice
  - Congenital syphilis
  - Other neonatal and early pediatric disorders
- Physiotherapy in pediatric patients
  - Scope of pediatric physiotherapy
  - Goals of treatment
  - Benefits of pediatrics physiotherapy
  - Physiotherapy in various neonatal conditions

INTRODUCTION

Neonatal Intensive Care Unit (NICU) is a specially equipped nursery where critically ill and unstable neonates (babies up to 28 days of life) receive diagnostic, therapeutic and life support care for a wide range of illnesses and conditions **(Fig. 24.1)**.

According to the World Health Organization (WHO), there were 2.4 million newborn deaths in 2019 globally. Most of childhood deaths occur in period from birth to the first 28 days. This occurs due to lack of quality care during antenatal period, at birth, immediately after birth or in the first 28 days of birth. Neonatal deaths can be reduced by 16% if quality care is provided by a midwife led team. India ranked first among all countries in the number of neonatal deaths in 2019. This shows that there is a great extent of scope of improvement in the maternal and neonatal care we provide in our country. **Box 24.1** shows strategies recommended by the WHO for newborn care.

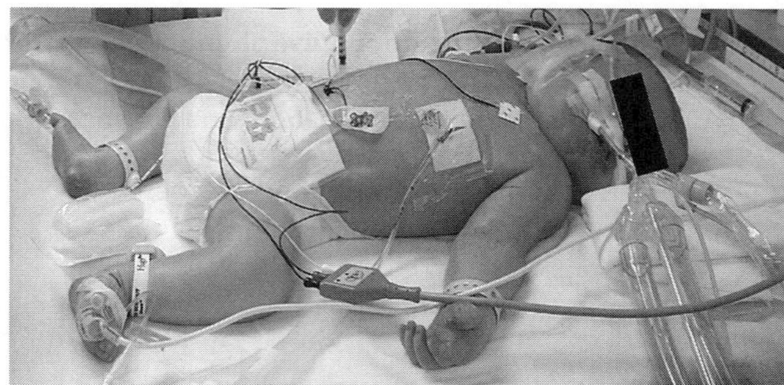

Fig. 24.1: A baby in the NICU.

Box 24.1: WHO recommendations for newborn care.

- All newborns should be provided thermal protection (e.g., kangaroo mother care), early and exclusive breastfeeding by the mother, hygienic care of the umbilical cord and skin, detailed assessment for need of additional care or serious health concerns and preventive treatment in form of vaccination, immunization and supplementation.
- Prompt medical care should be sought by the family if the baby shows any signs of danger, e.g., feeding problems, reduced activity, fever, convulsions or fits, difficulty in breathing or jaundice in the first 24 hours of birth.
- Every low-birthweight neonate should be shifted to a hospital or care facility and extra care should be taken.
- Mothers having human immunodeficiency virus (HIV) infection and their newborns should be administered preventive antiretroviral treatment (ART) to prevent opportunistic infections, HIV testing should be done for exposed neonates and infants and mothers should be counseled regarding feeding.

Newborns can be classified depending on the gestational age (time from last date of menstruation of the mother to the date of delivery):

- **Preterm:** Delivered before 37 weeks of gestation
- **Full-term:** Delivered between 37–41 weeks of gestation
- **Late-term:** Delivered between 41–42 weeks of gestation
- **Post-term:** Delivered at or after 42 weeks of gestation.

Babies who have critical illnesses are kept in NICU for management including those who have:

- Prematurity
- Low birth weight
- Perinatal problems
- Congenital abnormality
- Respiratory disorders
- Neuromuscular disorders
- Undergone surgical procedures
- Some risk

NICU care often requires multidisciplinary team work which includes among others:

- Neonatologists
- Orthopedic surgeons
- Pediatric surgeons
- Physiotherapists
- Nursing team
- Lactation supporting experts

Neonatal and early pediatric problems can arise from causes that are antenatal or postnatal.

Problems Developing Before Birth

Problems may develop before the birth of the child due to maternal problems since before pregnancy or maternal problems developing during pregnancy or conditions related to the fetus. Good quality and appropriate antenatal care can help in early diagnosis and management of these problems. Maternal health problems that can affect the fetus include:

- Anorexia
- Bulimia
- Malnutrition
- Asthma
- Cancer (cancer treatment drugs may affect the fetus)
- Diabetes (may lead to birth defects, hypoglycemia of the fetus, etc.)
- Epilepsy or other seizure disorders (seizures themselves may harm the fetus and anticonvulsant drugs too may produce harmful side effects)
- Hypertension, cardiac and kidney disorders
- Systemic lupus erythematosus (may cause increased risk of prematurity and miscarriage)
- Preeclampsia
- Thyroid disorders

Maternal drug use can also affect the fetus. Medicinal drugs like insulin, opioids, antidepressants and anticonvulsants can affect the fetus. Active or passive smoking or alcohol or abusive drug consumption can lead to birth defects, prematurity, miscarriage and stillbirth.

Clinical Pointer

It is essential for the mother to avoid harmful substances, take prenatal vitamins, get prenatal care and maintain healthy weight and diet.

Problems Occurring After Birth

Problems in the newborn occurring immediately or in a few days after birth include:

- Apnea
- Bronchopulmonary dysplasia
- Hypo- or hyperthyroidism
- Neonatal jaundice
- Meconium aspiration syndrome
- Pneumothorax
- Respiratory distress syndrome
- Anemia
- Polycythemia
- Necrotizing enterocolitis

In the early developing years, the child may develop asthma, interstitial lung disease, heart disorders, brain injuries, musculoskeletal disorders, etc.

CARE OF THE NEWBORN AFTER DELIVERY

Essential Care

Essential care should be provided to all newborns. It includes:

- Drying of the infant with a clean towel
- Observation of the infant for any abnormalities, especially breathing
- Resuscitation, if required
- Maintenance of skin-to-skin contact between mother and infant
- Covering the infant to prevent heat loss
- Clamping and cutting of the umbilical cord at least 1 min after delivery
- Initiation of breastfeeding in the first hour of birth
- Measures to prevent infection.

Box 24.2: WHO's four essential elements of newborn care.

1. Immediate and thorough drying of the infant
2. Skin-to-skin contact between mother and infant
3. Delayed cord clamping (severing umbilical cord at least 1 minute after delivery or once the cord stops pulsating)
4. Early initiation of breastfeeding

Table 24.1: Common causes and results of birth asphyxia.

Causes	• Oligohydramnios • Preeclampsia or eclampsia • Prolonged and arrested labor • Premature birth • Premature rupture of the membranes • Umbilical cord problems • Placental abruption • Placenta previa • Ruptured uterus • Fetal stroke • Uterine hyperstimulation • Postmaturity syndrome • Anesthetic complications • Delayed emergency cesarean section
Results	• Acidosis • Ischemia • Hypoxia • Hypercarbia • Hypotension • Developmental delays • Cerebral palsy • Seizure disorders • Motor disorders • Behavioral and emotional disorders • Speech delays • Learning disabilities • Hearing impairments, visual and feeding impairments

Skin-to-skin contact and breastfeeding keep the infant warm and prevent hypogylcemia. **Box 24.2** shows the four essential elements of newborn care given by the WHO.

Neonatal Resuscitation

According to WHO statistics, 4 million neonatal deaths occur every year due to birth asphyxia. The incidence rates are low in developed countries but quite high in developing and under-developed countries. American College of Obstetricians and Gynecologists (ACOG) and American Academy of Pediatrics (AAP) label a neonate as asphyxiated if following signs are present:

- Arterial pH of umbilical cord <7
- APGAR score of 0–3 lasting more than 5 minutes
- Neurological manifestations like hypotonia, coma or seizures
- Multisystem organ dysfunction.

Table 24.1 enlists the common causes and results of birth asphyxia.

Approximately 1% of newborn infants require resuscitation measures. Neonatal resuscitation aims to prevent and minimize morbidity and mortality associated with hypoxic-ischemic tissue injury and to re-establish cardiac output and spontaneous respiration. **Box 24.3** lists infant characteristics that can help rule out need for neonatal resuscitation.

Box 24.3: Infant characteristics that can rule out need for neonatal resuscitation.

All four below-mentioned criteria should be fulfilled to rule out neonatal resuscitation:
1. Infant born after full term
2. Amniotic fluid clear of meconium and signs of infection
3. Breathing or crying infant
4. Infant having good muscle tone

If any of the characteristics listed in **Box 24.3** are not present, there may be a need to take the following steps in sequential manner.

Each step should be completed for 30 seconds, the infant should be re-evaluated (check for respiration, heart rate and color), if the infant does not improve, a move should be made to the next step.

- Step 1: Initial stabilization by:
  - Providing warmth by putting the infant under radiant heat source
  - Positioning the head of the infant in a 'sniffing' position to open the airways
  - Clearing airway using a bulb syringe or suction catheter
  - Drying the infant
  - Stimulating breathing
  - Re-positioning
- Step 2: Ventilation
- Step 3: Chest compressions
- Step 4: Administration of epinephrine and/or volume expansion

Post-resuscitation Care

Even after the vital signs have returned to normal, there is risk for infants who have received neonatal resuscitation to deteriorate. Hence, once adequate respiration and circulation has been established, the infant should be shifted to an environment where continuous monitoring can be done and anticipatory care can be provided, possibly a NICU **(Fig. 24.2)**.

Prevention of Neonatal Infections

Table 24.2 shows the strategies to prevent neonatal infections.

Prophylactic antibiotics (intravenous or intramuscular gentamicin and ampicillin for at least 2 days, followed by re-assessment, and continuation of treatment only if signs of sepsis are present) can be administered for infants at risk of developing infections.

COMMON CONDITIONS SEEN DURING INFANCY AND EARLY PEDIATRIC PERIOD

Hypoxic-Ischemic Encephalopathy

Hypoxic-ischemic encephalopathy (HIE) is a common complication seen among full-term births. A hypoxic-ischemic event occurring during the prenatal, intrapartum or postnatal period results in inadequate blood flow to the

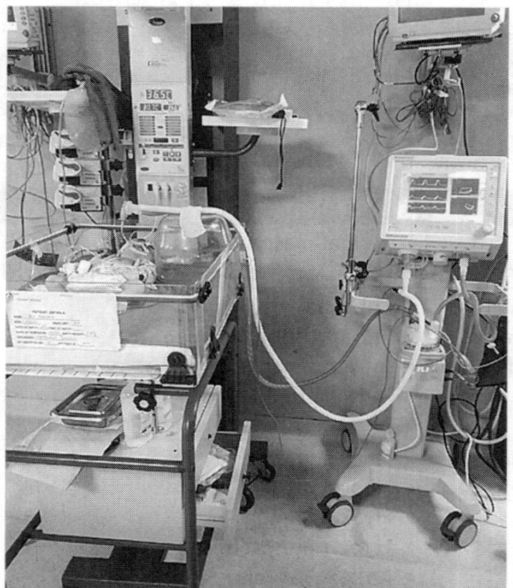

Fig. 24.2: Neonate on artificial ventilation and under monitoring in an NICU.

Table 24.2: Strategies to prevent neonatal infections.	
Early infections	• Avoid unnecessary separation of mother and infant • Washing hands before delivery and handling the infant • Ensure good hygienic condition during delivery • Appropriate care of the umbilical cord and eyes
Late infections	• Exclusive breastfeeding • Washing hands or using alcohol rubs before and after handling the infant • Maintaining body temperature of infant using Kangaroo mother care, incubator **(Fig. 24.3)** or water humidification • Maintaining sterility during all procedures and injection administration • Removal of intravenous drips when no longer required

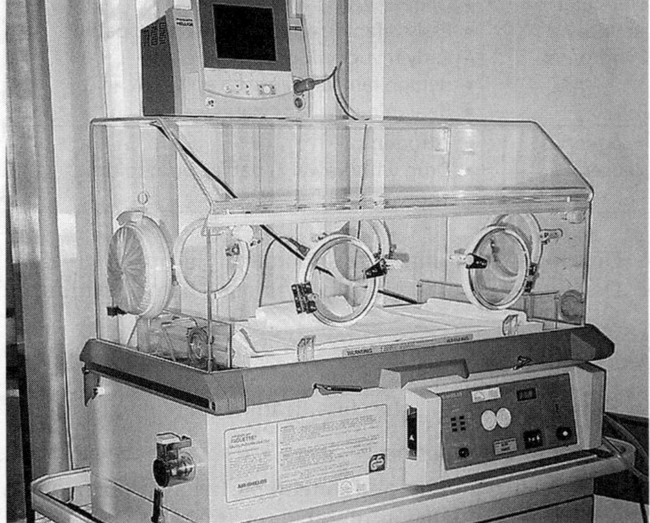

Fig. 24.3: Incubator.

infant brain resulting in a brain injury, known as HIE. It results in death or severe disability in the form of cerebral palsy, mental retardation and epilepsy.

Pathophysiology

The exact cause is not known but the causes listed in **Table 24.3** have been stipulated.

The pathologic events of HIE occur in two stages—primary energy failure and secondary energy failure as shown in **Figures 24.4 and 24.5** respectively.

Table 24.3: Probable causes of HIE.	
Antenatal causes	• Maternal hypotension • Maternal diabetes with vascular disorder • Preeclampsia • Maternal respiratory disorders like asthma and penumonia • Severe maternal anemia • Fetal lung malformations • Placenta previa
Intra-partum causes	• Placental abruption • Uterine rupture • Cord prolapse • Breech presentation • Tight nuchal cord • Prolonged labor
Postnatal causes	• Meconium aspiration • Severe hyaline membrane disease of the neonate • Congenital heart anomalies • Prematurity • Serious neonatal infections

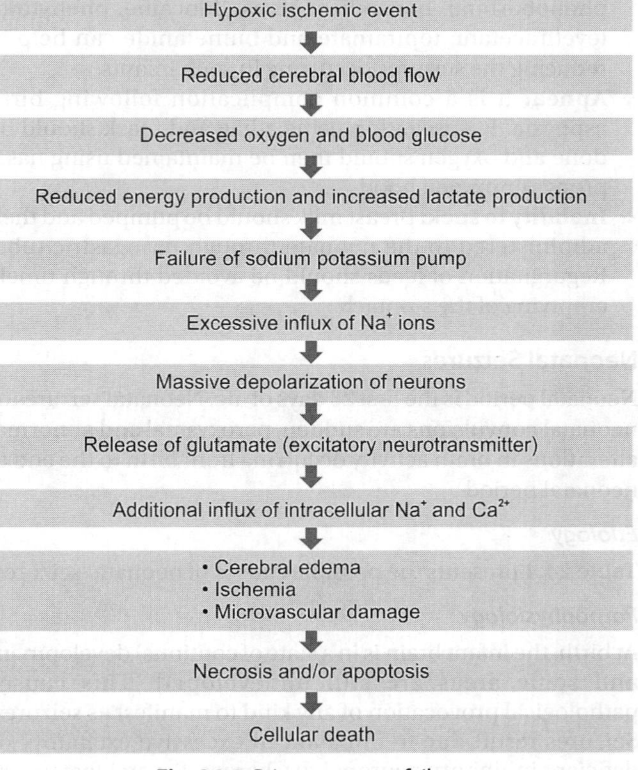

Fig. 24.4: Primary energy failure.

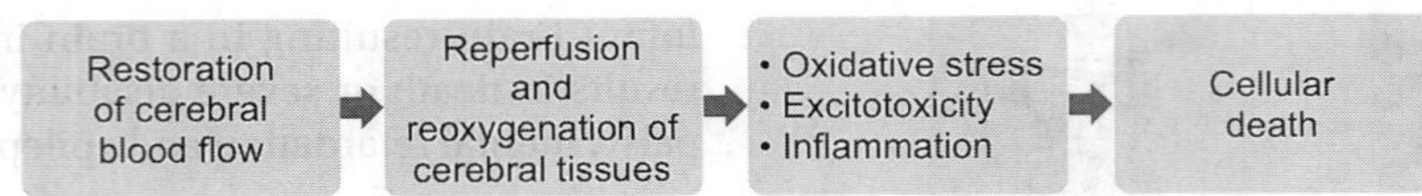

Fig. 24.5: Secondary energy failure.

Clinical Manifestations

- Low APGAR score
- Metabolic acidosis in cord blood
- Neonate may develop signs of apnea and seizures with abnormal electroencephalographic findings
- Convulsions
- Poor motor tone
- Inability to suck or breast feed

Management

Moderate hypothermia: It decreases free radicals and glutamate, reduces oxygen demand and apoptosis, thereby reducing neuronal loss. As per the latest guidelines from the American Academy of Pediatrics (AAP) and the Cochrane Collaboration, the standard of care for neonates with moderate-to-severe hypoxic-ischemic encephalopathy (HIE) is therapeutic hypothermia with a target core body temperature range of 33°C to 34°C maintained for a duration of 72 hours followed by gradual rewarming.

Recent advances have suggested the use of erythropoietin (EPO), stem cell therapy and xenon gas for the management, but these are still in the early stages of research.

Supportive management includes:

- **Seizures:** Infants with moderate or severe HIE are at risk of developing seizures. Administration of drugs like phenobarbital, benzodiazepines, lidocaine, phenytoin, levetiracetam, topiramate and bumetanide can help in reducing the seizures occurring in such infants.
- **Apnea:** It is a common complication following birth asphyxia. Resuscitation using a bag and mask should be done and oxygen should then be maintained using nasal prongs or oxygen hood.
- **Inability to suck:** Breast milk should be pumped and then administered to the neonate through nasogastric tube. Regurgitation of feeds should be avoided through timely emptying of the stomach.

Neonatal Seizures

Neonatal period is the first 28 days of life. Neonatal seizures or neonatal convulsions are sudden, paroxysmal and abnormal alterations in brain activity occurring from birth to the end of neonatal period.

Etiology

Table 24.4 presents the possible causes of neonatal seizures.

Table 24.4: Etiology of neonatal seizures.

Hypoxic conditions	• Perinatal asphyxia • Hypoxic ischemic encephalopathy (HIE)
Intracranial hemorrhage (ICH) and infarction	• Subdural • Subarachnoid • Intraparenchymal • Intraventricular • Cerebral artery and vein infarction
Metabolic disturbances	• Hypoglycemia • Hyponatremia • Hypocalcemia • Hypomagnesemia • Hypernatremia • Infants of toxemic and hypoglycemic mothers • Pancreatic disease
Infection	• Intrauterine infection • Viral encephalitis • Bacterial meningitis • Brain abscess • Postnatal infections like herpes simplex virus, beta-hemolytic streptococci, *Mycoplasma*, *Escherichia coli* infection
Thromboembolic	• Sinus venous thrombosis • Arterial ischemic stroke
Inborn errors of metabolism	• Pyroxidine deficiency • Peroxisomal disorders • Urea cycle defects • Molybdenum cofactor deficiency • Amino acid deficiencies • Organic acidemias
Congenital brain malformations	• Lissencephaly • Schizencephaly • Hydranencephaly • Holoprosencephaly
Neonatal epilepsy syndromes	• Genetic epilepsy syndromes • Early infantile epileptic encephalopathy • Early myoclonic encephalopathy • Benign familial neonatal epilepsy • Benign neonatal seizures
Exogenous causes	• Iatrogenic • Drug withdrawal in babies born to drug abusive mothers

Pathophysiology

At birth, the infant brain is in a state of continual development and some areas are still undeveloped. This causes pathological provocation of any kind to manifest as seizures. Seizures result due to imbalanced excessive excitatory or deficient inhibitory neuronal discharges. Several factors are responsible for this imbalance:

- Developmental state of the neonatal neuron
- Development of excitatory synapses before inhibitory synapses
- Early maturation of voltage-gated ion channels specific to depolarization.

Table 24.5 presents the classification of neonatal seizures.

Diagnosis and Evaluation

- Abnormal, repetitive and stereotypic behaviors of neonate should be evaluated as possible seizures.
- Thorough history focussing on prenatal and family history should be taken.

Table 24.5: Classification of neonatal seizures.

Classification	*Characteristics*
Subtle seizures	• Most common type of neonatal seizures • Named 'subtle' since the clinical manifestations are frequently overlooked • Imitate normal actions and behaviors
Tonic seizures	• May be focal, multifocal or generalized • May be symmetrical or asymmetrical • Sustained contraction of facial, axial, limb and other muscles is present • Imitates decerebrate or decorticate posturing
Myoclonic seizures	• Rapid, single or repetitive arrhythmic jerks • May affect focal areas like a finger, or a limb or the entire body • More frequently seen in preterm infants • May suggest poor prognosis as they are associated with severe brain damage • May mimic Moro reflex or startling responses
Clonic seizures	• Rhythmic jerks localized to some part of the face or limbs, axial muscles and diaphragm • May occasionally be hemiconvulsive or multifocal

- Thorough physical examination of the neonate, especially ocular movements, muscle tone and reflexes should be done.
- Pathological tests should include:
  - Blood glucose levels to rule out hypoglycemia
  - Electrolyte panel to rule out hypo- or hypernatremia, hypocalcemia and hypomagnesemia
  - Complete blood count, blood cultures, C-reactive protein and cerebrospinal fluid (CSF) levels to rule out sepsis, meningitis and encephalitis
  - Meconium analysis to determine presence of illicit substances like abusive drugs or alcohol
  - Blood gas analysis followed by additional laboratory tests to rule out inborn errors of metabolism
  - Specific blood testing for genetic or epilepsy syndrome
- Radiographic and advanced investigations include:
  - Computed tomography (CT), ultrasonography and magnetic resonance imaging (MRI) of the brain to rule out stroke, structural defects of the brain and hemorrhage or infarction of the brain
  - Polygraphic studies with simultaneous video electroencephalography (EEG) recording to confirm presence of seizures and determine area of brain affected.

Management

- Managing a patent airway, hemodynamic stability and intravenous access comprise first-line of management.
- For clinically evident and prolonged seizures, administration of phenobarbital or fosphenytoin should be done. Other agents like levetiracetam and lidocaine can be used in selected settings. If there is any delay in administering these agents, short-acting benzodiazepines like midazolam can be administered.
- Targeted therapy for the identified underlying pathology responsible for the seizures should be undertaken.
  - Management of HIE as mentioned earlier in the chapter
  - Antibiotics based on the blood culture reports for sepsis or meningitis or encephalitis
  - Administration of dextrose for hypoglycemic neonates
  - Correction of electrolyte imbalance for respective pathologies
  - Referral to neurosurgeon and subsequent interventions if intracranial hemorrhage is diagnosed
  - Stopping feeding, correction of metabolic derangements, and empiric therapy with vitamin and cofactor replacement in case of inborn errors of metabolism.

Neonatal Sepsis

Neonatal sepsis refers to a systemic infection that has spread to the bloodstream of a neonate. It can be:

- Early onset sepsis (EOS)—sepsis occurring in neonates at or before 72 hours
- Late onset sepsis (LOS)—sepsis occurring after 72 hours.

Clinical Features

- Irritability, lethargy and feeding problems
- Temperature instability
- Apnea
- Respiratory distress
- Bulging fontanelles
- Jaundice
- Seizures
- Skin lesions may occur with staphylococcal, Candida and Listeria infections.

Sepsis Screening

This includes:

- Complete blood count (CBC)
- C-reactive protein (CRP)
- Micro erythrocyte sedimentation rate (ESR)
- Procalcitonin
- CSF
- Urine
- Blood culture—which is the gold standard

Diagnosis

- Blood cultures
- CSF culture and analysis—may reveal elevated white cell count and protein level positive culture, reduced glucose concentration and positive polymerase chain reaction
- Elevated C-reactive protein levels
- Complete blood count—neutropenia and elevated immature to total neutrophil (I/T) ratio
- Elevated procalcitonin levels

Management

Initially, empiric treatment with antibiotics should be started as soon as sepsis is suspected. For EOS, the general treatment should include intravenous administration of ampicillin and aminoglycosides to cover majority of the bacteria. For LOS, nosocomial coverage should be given for *Staphylococcus aureus*, coagulase negative *Staphylococcus* and *Pseudomonas* species. A combination of vancomycin and aminoglycoside is also recommended. For central nervous system (CNS) infections, a third generation cephalosporin should be considered since aminoglycosides have poor CNS penetration.

Neonatal Meningitis

Neonatal meningitis is the inflammation of meninges in a neonate. It is one of the most disabling conditions with a morbidity rate of 20–60%.

Risk Factors

Risk factors for neonatal meningitis include:
- Preterm infants
- Male gender
- Infants in daycare
- Babies of mothers with a history of sexually transmitted infection, particularly genital herpes
- Babies of mothers with positive group B *Streptococcus infection*
- Consumption of certain foods by the mother which may pass down *Listeria* infection.

Pathophysiology

The child may be exposed to the pathogen during the birth process. Contact of the neonate's skin to the birth canal during delivery or transmission to ruptured amniotic membranes through the vagina may introduce the pathogens to the neonate's body. Poor hand hygiene, endotracheal tubes, catheters, feeding tubes and ventilators may also transmit infection between infected and uninfected infants.

Since the blood-brain barrier is still undeveloped when a child is born, it becomes easier for the pathogen to cross it and reach the brain tissue. Also, the cerebral vessels are fragile and this creates more devastating effects. An immature immune system in the neonate adds to this complex and makes the effects even worse.

Diagnosis

- Fever, irritability, fussiness, lethargy, respiratory distress, vomiting, or poor feeding in a neonate should raise an alarm and a septic work up should be done.
- Bulging fontanelle **(Fig. 24.6)** and seizures are seen commonly in such neonates.

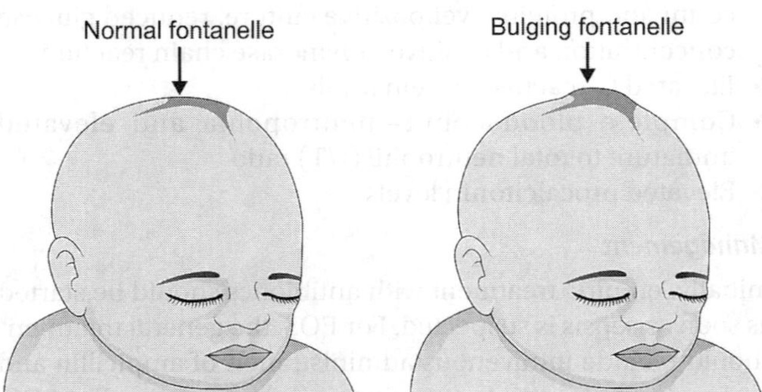

Fig. 24.6: Bulging fontanelle.

- Diagnostic work up includes complete blood count, blood culture, urine culture, lumbar puncture and chest radiograph.
- CSF analysis is the gold standard for testing bacterial meningitis. WBC count in CSF ranges from 200–100,000/mL in bacterial meningitis and 25–1,000/mL for viral meningitis.

Management

- Aggressive treatment should be begun as soon as possible and the child should be hospitalized. Cultures should be followed until negative for 72 hours.
- Broad spectrum antibiotics should be started as soon as possible. Treatment for bacterial meningitis should include ampicillin and gentamicin or cefotaxime. Treatment for HSV related meningitis should include acyclovir.
- If signs of hypoxemia are present, oxygen therapy should be started.
- For seizures, phenobarbital can be administered.
- If hypoglycemia is present, IV glucose should be started.

Neonatal Respiratory Distress Syndrome

Neonatal respiratory distress syndrome (RDS) is respiratory distress occurring in a newborn immediately after birth. It more commonly occurs in preterm infants due to surfactant deficiency. This surfactant deficiency occurs due to either inadequate production of surfactant or inactivation of surfactant on immature lungs.

RDS is a self-limiting condition as birth triggers increased surfactant production. However, the neonate needs to be supported till then as morbidity and mortality associated with neonatal RDS are quite high. Incidence of RDS and gestational age of infant are inversely proportional to each other, with smaller and more premature infants showing more severe disease. The incidence of RDS can be reduced by administration of dexamethasone (2 doses of 12 mg 24 hours apart) to the mother at risk of preterm delivery, e.g., premature rupture of membranes or premature uterine contractions.

Risk Factors

Increased risk of developing RDS is seen in neonates with:
- Prematurity and low birth weight
- Twin (especially monozygotic twins) or multiple births
- White race
- Male gender
- Siblings with history of neonatal RDS
- Cesarean section delivery especially delivery in absence of labor
- Diabetic mother
- Infection
- Hypothermia

Pathophysiology

Figure 24.7 describes the pathophysiology behind neonatal RDS.

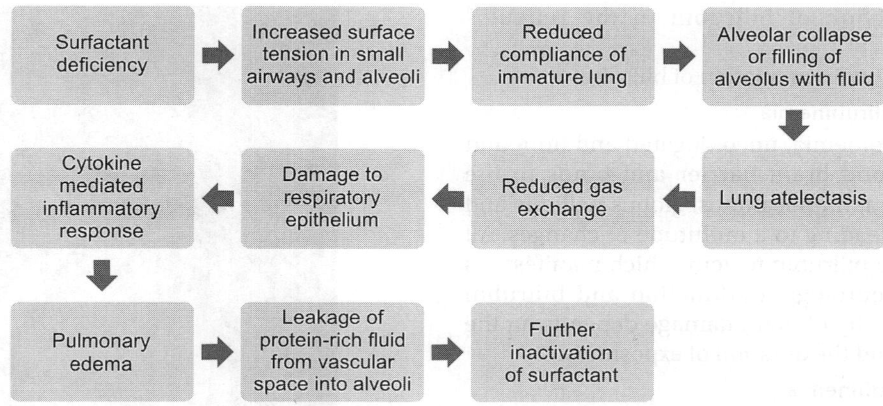

Fig. 24.7: Pathophysiology of neonatal RDS.

Clinical Features

- Occasionally premature birth
- Signs of respiratory distress immediately after birth or few minutes after birth
- Decreased breath sounds
- Diminished peripheral pulses rarely
- Signs and symptoms of increased work of breathing (expiratory grunting, tachypnea, excessive use of respiratory muscles, nasal flaring, cyanosis, poor peripheral perfusion and retractions)
- Reduced air entry on auscultation
- Decreased urine output and peripheral edema may develop in some children.

Diagnosis

- Chest radiograph shows ground-glass reticulogranular appearance with air bronchograms and low lung volumes which are suggestive of homogenous lung disease with diffuse atelectasis
- Arterial blood gas analysis shows hypoxemia
- Echocardiogram is helpful in ruling out any congenital heart diseases.

Management

Goals of management include:

- Antenatal corticosteroids for prevention of neonatal RDS in at risk patients
- Respiratory support
- Surfactant therapy
- General care of the newborn.

Management strategies include:

- Monitoring ventilation and oxygenation using arterial blood gas analyses and noninvasive pulse oximetry
- Assisted ventilation using continuous positive airway pressure, nasal intermittent positive pressure ventilation (NIPPV), high flow nasal cannula or mechanical ventilation
- Intratracheal surfactant replacement therapy through an endotracheal tube (commonly used exogenous surfactants are Beractant, Poractant alfa and Calfactant)
- Supportive care like caffeine therapy, fluid and electrolyte management.

Neonatal Jaundice

The term 'jaundice' has been derived from a French word 'jaune' meaning yellow. Neonatal jaundice or hyperbilirubinemia results due to elevated total serum bilirubin (TSB) levels. Clinical manifestations include yellowish discoloration of skin, sclera and mucous membranes. Jaundice can be normal or abnormal **(Box 24.4).**

Abnormal jaundice may occur due to:

- Hypothyroidism
- Congenital syphilis or other intrauterine infection
- Liver disease
- Hemolytic disease
- Bacterial infection

Pathophysiology

Newborn infants have higher levels of TSB due to:

- Higher levels of hemoglobin at birth
- Shorter red blood cell lifespan
- Limited ability of the newborn liver to conjugate unconjugated bilirubin.

Causes of Pathological Jaundice in Newborns

- Impaired hepatic uptake
- Insufficient conjugation of bilirubin

Box 24.4: Normal and abnormal jaundice.

- *Normal or physiological jaundice:* Almost all babies (85% term neonates and almost all preterm neonates) appear yellow for a few days after birth, but recover without any intervention. A rise of bilirubin levels to 12 mg/dL in newborn is considered physiologic.
- *Abnormal or non-physiological or pathological jaundice:* Yellowish discoloration of skin and sclera
  - Appearing on the first day of life
  - Associated with fever
  - Lasts for >14 days in term infants and >21 days in preterm infants.

  It may result in kernicterus, acute bilirubin encephalopathy or even jaundice-related death. A total bilirubin of >95th percentile on the hour-specific Bhutani normogram or >0.2 mg/dL/hour rate rise in total serum bilirubin or transcutaneous bilirubin is considered hyperbilirubinemia.

- Increased production of bilirubin in the reticulo-endothelial system
- Increased enterohepatic circulation of bilirubin

Unconjugated hyperbilirubinemia

In severe hyperbilirubinemia, unconjugated and unbound bilirubin crosses blood brain barrier and binds to the brainstem, cerebellum, hippocampus, globus pallidus and subthalamic nuclei, leading to a multitude of changes. All these changes lead to bilirubin toxicity which manifests as bilirubin-induced neurologic dysfunction and bilirubin encephalopathy. Severity of brain damage depends on the amount of bilirubin and the duration of exposure.

Conjugated hyperbilirubinemia

It occurs due to abnormal uptake, metabolism, transport and/or excretion of bilirubin and bile salts. This results in elevated levels of bile acid in the liver which promotes proliferation of bile ducts and fibrosis and causes inflammation and apoptosis of hepatocytes, which ultimately results in hepatocellular injury and cirrhosis of liver.

Diagnosis

- Detailed history taking including birth and family history
- Examination should be done in daylight, but may be unreliable if child has dark skin or has received phototherapy
- Evaluate for pallor, petechiae, extensive bruising, subgaleal bleed, cephalhematoma, hepatosplenomegaly, signs of dehydration and weight loss
- Signs and symptoms of bilirubin encephalopathy include:
  - Poor feeding
  - Seizures
  - Altered sleep
  - Lethargy
  - Abnormal tone
- Bilirubin levels should be examined using a transcutaneous measurement device or taking blood samples for TSB.
- Other tests include complete blood count, neonatal and maternal blood type, Coombs test, reticulocyte count, serum albumin and blood smear.
- Bilirubin/albumin ratio should be assessed.
- In infants with bilirubin encephalopathy, T1 weighted MRI shows hyperintensity during acute stages, whereas T2 weighted images show hyperintensity as the disease evolves.
- For conjugated hyperbilirubinemia, serum aminotransferases, alkaline phosphatase, gamma-glutamyl transferase levels and prothrombin time/INR should be checked in addition to the above mentioned tests.
- In conjugated hyperbilirubinemia, hepatic ultrasonography may show triangular cord sign, gallstones, choledochal cysts, inspissated bile and sludging in the biliary tree.

Management

- Phototherapy **(Fig. 24.8)** using visible light in the blue-green range (460–490 nm) is the first-line treatment for unconjugated hyperbilirubinemia. It induces bilirubin photoisomerization and converts bilirubin to lumirubin which helps in excretion of bilirubin. Eyes of the infant should be covered during phototherapy as it can cause retinal injury.

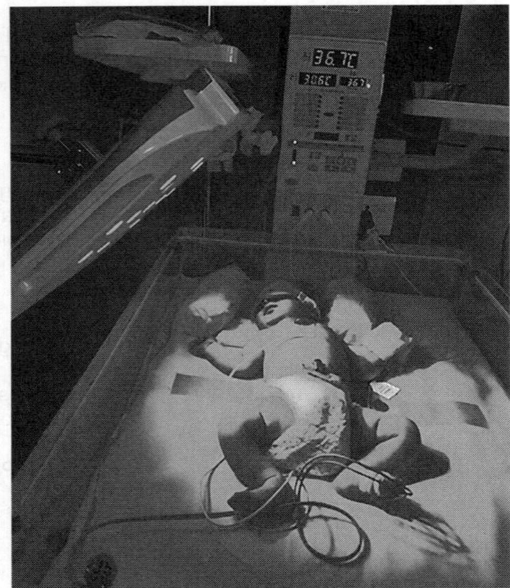

Fig. 24.8: Neonate receiving phototherapy in NICU.

- The second-line treatment is exchange transfusion, which is used when phototherapy fails. It involves double volume blood transfusion to remove bilirubin from the bloodstream. It can effectively and immediately remove about 60% TSB.
- Intravenous Ig infusion is also recommended in select cases by the American Academy of Pediatrics.
- Management of conjugated hyperbilirubinemia should focus on the specific etiology.

Congenital Syphilis

The transmission of *Treponema pallidum* from the mother to the fetus results in congenital syphilis. It may lead to premature birth or stillbirth in some instances. In few others, the child may be asymptomatic or may present with clinical signs and symptoms.

Pathophysiology

T. pallidum is directly released into the bloodstream of the fetus, causing spirochetemia. It then spreads to all the different organs like bones, kidneys, liver, spleen and heart. The spread causes inflammation in all these organs leading to a multitude of clinical manifestations.

Diagnosis

- Most infants are asymptomatic at birth, but clinical manifestations may develop at around 3 months of age. These include hepatomegaly, rhinitis, jaundice, rash and generalized lymphadenopathy.
- If congenital syphilis is not diagnosed early and inflammation persists, it may result in scarring and gumma formation. Late congenital syphilis may manifest as:
  - Saber shins (anterior bowing of shins)
  - Facial changes—saddle nose, frontal bossing and prominent maxilla

- Perioral fissuring or scarring along with skin and mucous membrane gummas
- Hutchinson teeth—hypoplastic notched permanent teeth, usually the upper central incisors
- Sensorineural hearing loss and visual abnormalities
- Intellectual disability
- Cranial nerve palsies
- Eye involvement may lead to secondary glaucoma, interstitial keratitis and corneal scarring

❖ Histological examination of placenta and cord for presence of spirochetes.

❖ If nasal discharge is present then it should be examined using darkfield microscopy.

❖ Radiographs of long bones may show osseous destruction, localized demineralization, pathological fractures and metaphyseal serration; chest radiograph shows diffuse opacification of bilateral lung fields.

❖ Non-treponemal and treponemal specific tests like venereal disease research laboratory (VDRL), rapid plasma reagin (RPR), fluorescent treponemal antibody absorption (FTA-ABS) and/or micro-hemagglutination test can be done.

❖ CSF examination may show elevated CSF protein, pleocytosis and reactive CSF VDRL.

Clinical Pointer

Hutchinson teeth, sensorineural hearing loss and interstitial keratitis form the Hutchinson triad which is specific for congenital syphilis.

Management

❖ Congenital syphilis can be prevented by treating the pregnant mother with penicillin.

❖ For infants with confirmed syphilis, intravenous aqueous crystalline Penicillin G or intramuscular procaine Penicillin G.

Other Neonatal and Early Pediatric Disorders

Table 24.6 presents some of the other common neonatal and early pediatric disorders.

Table 24.6: Other common neonatal and early pediatric disorders.

Condition	*Description*	*Clinical manifestations*	*Diagnosis*	*Management*
Cleft lip and palate	Improper formation of the mouth during gestation	Opening in the roof of mouth and lips	It is visible deformity	Surgical closure can be done of the palate at 1 year of age and of the lips at 6 months of age
Bowel obstruction	Can be due to bowel atresia, hypertrophic pyloric stenosis, meconium plug syndrome, malrotation with volvulus, Hirschsprung disease or imperforate anus	Vomiting and abdominal distension	Bile-stained vomit Ultrasonography and radiography of the abdomen confirm the obstruction	• Stop oral feeding; start nasogastric feeding • IV fluids can be started • Combination of ampicillin, gentamicin and metronidazole can be used • Surgery may be required
Abdominal wall defects	Incomplete development of abdominal wall	Open defect on the abdominal wall is visualized with exposed bowel (gastroschisis) or thin layer covering abdomen (omphalocele)	Prenatal ultrasonography and fetal MRI can help in prenatal diagnosis	• Fetal surgeries can be tried, though success has not yet been established • Postnatal surgery to repair the defect can be done
Myelomeningocele	Incomplete closure of the spinal neural tube	Neural tissue or meninges are exposed with a fluid filled sac protruding out of the affected vertebral level	Amniocentesis in the first trimester showing elevated levels of alpha-fetoprotein and ultrasonography in the second trimester help in prenatal diagnosis	• Prenatal surgical repair has proven quite successful • Postnatal surgical correction is relatively complication free
Cerebral palsy	Group of disorders affecting a person's ability to move, sense, maintain balance or posture	• May affect several systems of the body like sensory system, musculoskeletal system, neurological system, etc. Clinical manifestations may depend on the system affected • Growth and development may be retarded	Developmental monitoring and screening needs to be done; ultrasound, MRI, CT scan and EEG help in diagnosis	Management is a blend of medications, physical therapy, occupational therapy, speech therapy and surgical techniques

Contd...

Contd...

Condition	Description	Clinical manifestations	Diagnosis	Management
Congenital dislocation of hip or developmental dysplasia of hip (CDH or DDH)	Complete or partial displacement of head of femur from acetabulum due to incomplete development of the roof of socket	Shortening of limb, restricted abduction when hip is flexed and asymmetrical skin crease on the back of hip	Positive Ortolani, Barlow and Galeazzi test	Maintenance of hip in flexion and abduction using abduction brace or cast for milder cases; surgical correction may be required for more severe cases
Congenital talipes equinovarus (CTEV) or clubfoot	Genetic disorder where the foot remains inclined inwards	Supination, varus and adduction of foot	Ultrasound can help in prenatal diagnosis; radiography can be done postnatally	Simple stretching for mild deformity; serial manipulations and splinting for moderate deformity and surgical repair for severe deformities
Pneumonia	Acute respiratory infection affecting the lungs; caused usually by *Streptococcus pneumoniae, Hemophilus influenzae* type B or respiratory syncytial virus	Cough with/without difficulty in breathing and fever, rapid breathing with chest wall retraction during inhalation	Chest radiograph and blood tests help in diagnosis	Immunization can be done to prevent pneumonia; oral antibiotics form the first line of treatment
Tuberculosis	Chronic respiratory illness caused due to *Mycobacterium tuberculosis*; sometimes may spread to other organ systems as well	• Fever, cough lasting longer than 3 weeks, chills, weight loss, poor growth, easy fatigue • Other symptoms may depend on the system involved	Chest radiography, sputum examination, tuberculin skin test, CT scan and MRI	Prevention involves immunization using bacillus Calmette–Guérin (BCG) vaccine; first line drugs are isoniazid, rifampicin, pyrazinamide and ethambutol
Asthma	Chronic inflammatory disease of the airways, characterized by recurrent episodes of airflow obstruction occurring due to bronchospasm, edema, and increased mucus production	Cough, wheezing, shortness of breath and chest tightness; episodic symptoms triggered by exposure to allergens, upper respiratory tract infections or irritants like tobacco smoke; may worsen at night	Spirometry with assessment of bronchodilator response, exercise testing, methacholine challenge and allergy testing	Avoiding exposure to irritants; short-acting beta-2 agonist for asthmatic episode; low, medium or high dose inhaled corticosteroid (depending on age in progression) or montelukast for persistent asthma
Interstitial lung disease	Group of rare lung disease affecting airways, alveoli and/or interstitial tissue of lungs	Tachypnea, chest wall retraction during inhalation, difficulty in breathing, chronic cough (occasionally hemoptysis), wheezing, clubbing, poor growth, hypoxemia	Chest radiography and CT scan, lung function tests, lung biopsy	Supplemental oxygen, airway clearance techniques, anti-inflammatory drugs (preferably steroids) like oral prednisolone, intravenous methylprednisolone and hydroxychloroquine
Cystic fibrosis	Chronic respiratory condition affecting lungs, sinuses and pancreas; caused by genetic mutation in a gene on chromosome 7	Newborns may present with meconium ileus, early respiratory infections and neonatal jaundice; infants and children may present with poor weight gain, failure to thrive, anemia, recurrent sinopulmonary infections and distal intestinal obstructive syndrome with/without pancreatic insufficiency	Sweat chloride test, test for immunoreactive trypsinogen, chest radiography and pulmonary function testing	• Poor prognosis • Respiratory infections should be treated using antibiotics, supplemental oxygen may need to be administered, anti-inflammatory agents to relieve airway obstruction and chronic supportive therapy including pancreatic enzymes, mucolytics, fat soluble vitamins and bronchodilators

PHYSIOTHERAPY IN PEDIATRIC PATIENTS

Physiotherapists who work in the field of pediatrics provide support and treatment services to pediatric population. Children are different from adults. A good understanding of child development and how it relates to body systems is required.

Goals of Treatment

The main goal is to achieve maximal daily living activity independence in accordance with the child's educational, social and cultural needs. Goals focus on components of the international classification of functioning, disability and health (ICF).

This is done through addressing pain management, improving strength and endurance as well as providing the learning opportunities needed for skill acquisition.

The physiotherapists work as a team member along with family and other health professionals like pediatrician, neurologist, orthopedic/surgeons, nurse, occupational therapist, pharmacist, nutritionist, teacher, etc.

Benefits of Pediatric Physiotherapy

- Improves gross motor skills, posture, integral reflexes, muscle balance and strength, balance and coordination, range of motion, muscle tone, gait and learning difficulties.
- Addresses respiratory difficulties.

Physiotherapy in Various Neonatal Conditions

The role of physiotherapy in NICU has historically mainly been associated with the care of neonatal lungs. But now we have its active involvement in many neurological and neuromuscular conditions as well as in babies with birth injuries.

- Chest physiotherapy is useful for maintenance of a clear airway and to re-expand collapsed segments of the lungs, maintain adequate levels of oxygenation, facilitate early weaning of support and reduce the probabilities of re-intubation. Chest physiotherapy commonly includes techniques like percussion, vibrations, positioning for postural drainage and airway suctioning.
- Neuromuscular physiotherapy includes positioning, skin to skin holding (kangaroo care), therapeutic holding, orofacial stimulation, taping, range of motion exercise, soft tissue mobilization for surgical scar release, hydrotherapy and parent education for feeding, dressing, positioning of infants for sleep, interaction/play. These developmental strategies are beneficial for promotion of posture and movement appropriate to gestational age and medical stability, to modulate sensory stimulation in the baby's NICU environment, to promote behavioral organization and physiological stability, to foster infant-parent attachment and provide direct intervention for neonatal feeding dysfunction and oromotor deficits.
- Preterm babies—immature musculoskeletal systems and exposure to prolonged atypical positioning in NICU may be associated with torticollis, positional plagiocephaly, reduced movement quality and lower extremity malalignment—supportive positioning may enhance the development of normal skeletal alignment and provide opportunities for normal movement patterns. Passive range of motion is given to infants with congenital restriction of joint mobility which increases bone mineral density and weight gain in premature babies.

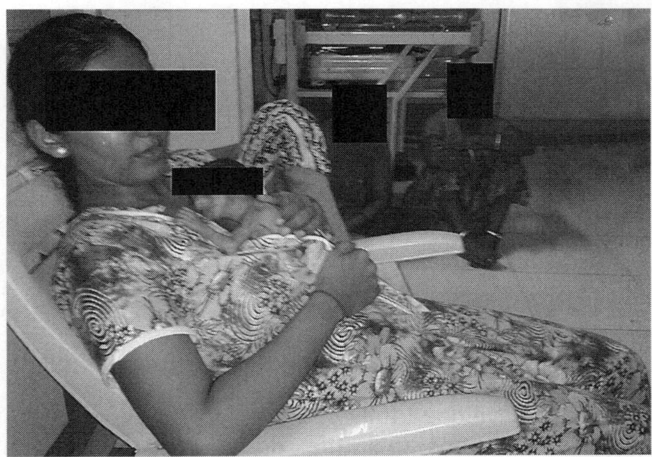

Fig. 24.9: Skin-to-skin contact by mother.

- Therapeutic handling improves development. Orofacial stimulation hastens feeding progression and decreases the transition time to oral feeding. Kangaroo care or skin to skin holding **(Fig. 24.9)** showed improvement in physiological stability, promoted temperature regulations, improved feeding, oxygen saturations and respiratory stability and fostered infant parent bonding. Multimodal sensory stimulation helps shorten length of hospital stay. Tactile stimulation also improves short-term growth. Neonatal massage has shown to produce favorable effects in reducing stress levels and improving infant parent bonding.

Pain

- In NICU, neonates experience long-term sequel of pain borne during invasive medical procedures. Hydrotherapy helps in pain reduction and improvement in sleep cycle of hospitalized babies.
- Musculoskeletal malformations are quite commonly seen in newborn babies (~13 to 20/1,000 live births). The position of a baby whilst in uterus as well as during delivery or the position they adopt as newborns can all contribute to the development of musculoskeletal problems.
- Other factors like genetic, congenital or chromosomal abnormalities are also implicated.
- Low birth weight, non-vaginal delivery, maternal age >30 years and multiparity are factors significantly associated with increased incidence of congenital malformations. If unchecked, these problems can lead to pain or limited mobility.
- Foot abnormality are most commonly seen followed by hand and spinal abnormality. Flat head syndrome or plagiocephaly, congenital talipes equinovarus (CTEV)

or clubfoot and torticollis or wryneck are the frequent conditions requiring physiotherapy.

- Traumatic conditions like fractures of clavicle, humerus and femur bones are commonly reported. A flail upper extremity secondary to brachial plexus injury during child birth or lower limb weakness secondary to myelodysplasia are also commonly seen. Parental education is needed for continuation of the physiotherapy care after discharge.

Summary

Neonatal and early pediatric period is a time period when the children are most vulnerable as their immune systems have not developed fully yet. They are susceptible to various infections and other diseases due to these reasons. Preterm neonates and infants are especially prone to such diseases as they do not have full developed organs. Such children should be cared for in special environments like the neonatal or pediatric intensive care unit. Early diagnosis and management are imperative for a better prognosis and lower morbidity and mortality. Management should include medical and surgical management, physiotherapy, general nursing care and family support. Various modalities such as massage, heat therapy, exercises, electrotherapy, patient education and advice for treating injuries, ailments or deformities form the physiotherapy management.

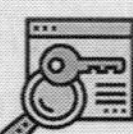

Review Questions

1. Why preterm neonates and infants are especially vulnerable to infections?
2. Enlist the problems occurring immediately after birth and later on.
3. Describe essential neonatal care.
4. How to prevent infections in neonates?
5. Write short notes on:
   a. Hypoxic ischemic encephalopathy
   b. Neonatal sepsis
   c. Congenital syphilis
   d. Neonatal respiratory distress syndrome

Bibliography

1. Allen KA, Brandon DH. Hypoxic ischemic encephalopathy: Pathophysiology and experimental treatments. Newborn Infant Nurs Rev. 2011;11(3):125-33. doi: 10.1053/j.nainr. 2011.07.004. PMID: 21927583; PMCID: PMC3171747.
2. Ansong-Assoku B, Shah SD, Adnan M, et al. Neonatal Jaundice. In: StatPearls [Internet]. Treasure Island (FL): StatPearls Publishing; 2022. [Updated 2022 Jun 4]. Available from: https:// www.ncbi.nlm.nih.gov/books/NBK532930/.
3. Bryce E, Mullany LC, Khatry SK, et al. Coverage of the WHO's four essential elements of newborn care and their association with neonatal survival in southern Nepal. BMC Pregnancy Childbirth. 2020;20:540. https://doi.org/10.1186/s12884-020-03239-6.
4. Bundy LM, Noor A. Neonatal Meningitis. In: StatPearls [Internet]. Treasure Island (FL): StatPearls Publishing; 2022. [Updated 2022 Jun 21]. Available from: https://www.ncbi.nlm.nih. gov/books/NBK532264/
5. Camacho-Gonzalez A, Spearman PW, Stoll BJ. Neonatal infectious diseases: evaluation of neonatal sepsis. Pediatr Clin North Am. 2013;60(2):367-89. doi: 10.1016/j.pcl.2012.12.003. Epub 2013 Jan 17. PMID: 23481106; PMCID: PMC4405627.
6. Chadha IA. Neonatal resuscitation: Current issues. Indian J Anaesth. 2010;54(5):428-38. doi: 10.4103/0019-5049.71042. PMID: 21189881; PMCID: PMC2991653.
7. Clement A, Nathan N, Epaud R, et al. Interstitial lung diseases in children. Orphanet J Rare Dis. 2010;5:22. https://doi.org/10.1186/1750-1172-5-22.
8. Eichenwald EC, Hansen AR, Martin CR, Start AR. Cloherty and Stark's manual of neonatal care, 8th edition. Wolters Kluwer Pvt Ltd. India. 2021.
9. Fitzgerald MP, Kessler SK, Abend NS. Early discontinuation of antiseizure medications in neonates with hypoxic-ischemic encephalopathy. Epilepsia. 2017;58(6):1047-53. doi: 10.1111/epi.13745. Epub 2017 Apr 12. PMID: 28401998; PMCID: PMC5462843.
10. https://www.physio-pedia.com/Neonatal_Intensive_Care_Unit_(NICU).
11. https://www.who.int/news-room/fact-sheets/detail/newborns-reducing-mortality.
12. Hussain SA, Vaidya R. Congenital Syphilis. In: StatPearls [Internet]. Treasure Island (FL): StatPearls Publishing; 2022. [Updated 2022 Jan 19]. Available from: https://www.ncbi.nlm.nih. gov/books/NBK537087/.
13. Khalessi N, Afsharkhas L. Neonatal meningitis: risk factors, causes, and neurologic complications. Iran J Child Neurol. 2014;8(4):46-50. PMID: 25657770; PMCID: PMC4307368.
14. Kliegman RM, St. Geme J. Nelson Textbook of Pediatrics, 21st edition. Elsevier Publications; 2020.
15. Krawiec C, Muzio MR. Neonatal Seizure. In: StatPearls [Internet]. Treasure Island (FL): StatPearls Publishing; 2022. [Updated 2022 Apr 30]. Available from: https://www.ncbi.nlm.nih. gov/books/NBK554535/.
16. Lizzo JM, Cortes S. Pediatric Asthma. In: StatPearls [Internet]. Treasure Island (FL): StatPearls Publishing; 2022. [Updated 2022 May 8]. Available from: https://www.ncbi.nlm.nih.gov/books/NBK551631/.
17. Marais BJ, Schaaf HS. Tuberculosis in children. Cold Spring HarbPerspect Med. 2014;4(9):a017855. doi: 10.1101/cshperspect.a017855. PMID: 25037105; PMCID: PMC4143109.
18. Musculoskeletal implications of preterm infant positioning in NICU. J Perinat Neonat Nurs. 2002;16(1):58-70.
19. Panayiotopoulos CP. The Epilepsies: Seizures, Syndromes and Management. Oxfordshire (UK): Bladon Medical Publishing; 2005. Chapter 5, Neonatal Seizures and Neonatal Syndromes. Available from: https://www.ncbi.nlm.nih.gov/books/NBK2599/
20. Pocket Book of Hospital Care for Children: Guidelines for the Management of Common Childhood Illnesses, 2nd edition. Geneva: World Health Organization; 2013. 9, Common surgical problems. Available from: https://www.ncbi.nlm.nih.gov/books/NBK154433/.
21. Practice patterns of physiotherapists in neonatal care units: a national survey. Indian J Crit Care Med. 2013;17(6).
22. Singh M, Alsaleem M, Gray CP. Neonatal Sepsis. In: StatPearls [Internet]. Treasure Island (FL): StatPearls Publishing; 2022. [Updated 2022 May 17]. Available from: https://www.ncbi.nlm.nih. gov/books/NBK531478/.

23. Western pediatrics physiotherapy—musculoskeletal problems in babies.
24. Workineh Y, Semachew A, Ayalew E, Animaw W, Tirfie M, Birhanu M. Prevalence of perinatal asphyxia in East and Central Africa: systematic review and meta-analysis. Heliyon. 2020;6(4):e03793. doi: 10.1016/j.heliyon.2020.e03793. PMID: 32368646; PMCID: PMC7184262.
25. Yadav S, Lee B, Kamity R. Neonatal Respiratory Distress Syndrome. In: StatPearls [Internet]. Treasure Island (FL): StatPearls Publishing; 2022. [Updated 2021 Jul 31]. Available from: https:// www.ncbi.nlm.nih.gov/books/NBK560779/.
26. Yozawitz E, Stacey A, Pressler RM. Pharmacotherapy for seizures in neonates with hypoxic ischemic encephalopathy. Paediatr Drugs. 2017;19(6):553-67. doi: 10.1007/s40272-017-0250-4. PMID: 28770451.
27. Yu E, Sharma S. Cystic Fibrosis. In: StatPearls [Internet]. Treasure Island (FL): StatPearls Publishing; 2022. [Updated 2021 Aug 11]. Available from: https://www.ncbi.nlm.nih.gov/books/NBK493206/.

Multiple Choice Questions (MCQs)

To test your understanding and recall of key concepts.

1. **Which neonatal condition is characterized by inadequate surfactant production?**
   A. Neonatal jaundice
   B. Respiratory distress syndrome
   C. Neonatal meningitis
   D. Neonatal seizures
2. **Delayed cord clamping in neonates leads to________.**
   A. Reduced risk of infection
   B. Increased blood volume and iron stores in the neonate
   C. Prevention of respiratory distress syndrome
   D. Reduced likelihood of neonatal jaundice
3. **Kangaroo mother care in neonatal care____________.**
   A. Reduces neonatal hypothermia
   B. Prevents neonatal seizures
   C. Improves muscle tone in neonates
   D. Reduces bilirubin levels in neonatal jaundice
4. **A neonate born at 34 weeks of gestation shows signs of respiratory distress. What is the most appropriate initial management ?**
   A. Administer surfactant therapy and provide oxygen
   B. Begin immediate intravenous antibiotics
   C. Initiate phototherapy to prevent jaundice
   D. Perform exchange transfusion
5. **Which factor is least likely to contribute to neonatal sepsis?**
   A. Premature rupture of membranes
   B. Low birth weight
   C. Normal APGAR score at one minute
   D. Maternal urinary tract infection
6. **Following can be the potential consequence of untreated neonatal jaundice:**
   A. Kernicterus leading to neurological damage
   B. Severe dehydration causing hypovolemic shock
   C. Increased surfactant production causing lung collapse
   D. Hypercarbia leading to respiratory failure
7. **What is the primary benefit of hypothermia therapy in neonates with hypoxic-ischemic encephalopathy?**
   A. Increases free radicals in the brain
   B. Reduces neuronal loss and apoptosis
   C. Enhances oxygen demand in brain tissue
   D. Prevents electrolyte imbalance
8. **What is the best course of action in a neonate with meconium aspiration syndrome who is showing severe respiratory distress?**
   A. Immediate suctioning followed by ventilatory support
   B. Administer intravenous fluids to maintain hydration
   C. Begin empirical antibiotic therapy
   D. Perform a chest X-ray and wait for diagnostic results
9. **A neonate born at 35 weeks of gestation has respiratory distress and a chest radiograph showing 'ground-glass' appearance. Despite surfactant therapy and oxygen supplementation, the condition persists. Which intervention should be considered next?**
   A. Exchange transfusion
   B. High-frequency oscillatory ventilation (HFOV)
   C. Bronchodilator therapy
   D. Empirical corticosteroid administration
10. **A neonate is diagnosed with hypoxic-ischemic encephalopathy (HIE). Which combination of therapies should be included to maximize neuroprotection?**
   A. Moderate hypothermia and phenobarbital for seizures
   B. Hyperthermia and intravenous antibiotics
   C. High-dose corticosteroids and oral glucose
   D. Early feeding and diuretics for cerebral edema
11. **What is the main mechanism by which phototherapy in neonatal jaundice reduces bilirubin levels?**
   A. Enhances hepatic conjugation of bilirubin
   B. Facilitates renal excretion of unconjugated bilirubin
   C. Converts bilirubin into water-soluble photoisomers
   D. Stimulates bone marrow to reduce hemolysis

ANSWERS

1. B	2. B	3. A	4. A	5. C
6. A	7. B	8. A	9. B	10. A
11. C				

Chapter **25**

Early Intervention

Amruta Nerurkar

LEARNING OBJECTIVES

At the end of the chapter, the reader will be able to:

- Describe in brief the events in the embryological development of the nervous system and the neurodevelopmental pathologies resulting from possible insults.
- Explain and apply the knowledge related to the gross motor, fine motor, oromotor, social cognitive domains of normal development.
- Recall and apply the knowledge of biological and environmental risks encountered by a preterm infant and the related special needs.
- Recall and practice the neuroprotective and therapeutic strategies for an infant born preterm.
- Understand the process of endogenous and experience dependent neuroplasticity in an infant.
- Enlist the screening tools and neurodevelopmental outcomes applicable to early intervention.
- Have a basic understanding of the application of neurodevelopmental therapy and sensory integration therapy in caregiving of infants faced with neuromotor and sensory challenges.
- Get introduced to play theories related to the continued, holistic development from infanthood to childhood.

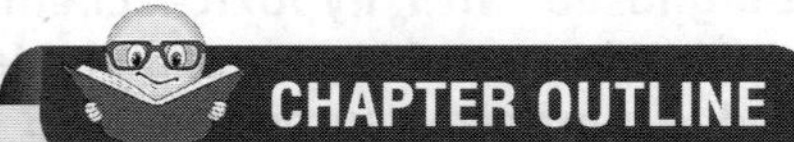

CHAPTER OUTLINE

- Introduction
- Phases of intrauterine development
- Needs of an infant born preterm
  - Factors that make the brain of a preterm infant vulnerable to insult
  - Neuroprotective core measures
- Neonatal hydrotherapy
- Oromotor therapy in NICU
- Assessment in early intervention
- Normal development
  - 0–4 months
  - 5–8 months
  - 9–12 months
- Play theories associated with development
- Application of schools of neurophysiotherapy like Neurodevelopmental therapy and sensory Integration in early intervention of infants at risk

INTRODUCTION

Nurturance is the constant work of nature in every form which supports the ability of the being to survive, to sustain its survival and to gain all the necessary skills needed to bring manifestation to its unique traits in a productive way.

For a child to be able to respond to its own innate drives, to be able to choose the appropriate strategy to fulfill the drive in the wake of the challenges posed by life at every stage in a healthy manner, it is essential for the child to have some basic ingredients or building blocks in place. Though the needs of every human child are unique due to the unique genetic predisposition, epigenetic influence and effects of learning, a few common ingredients or domains of development have been identified as the basic foundation which facilitates the child's ability to respond to these needs. This chapter will attempt to elucidate all those phases of neurological development in the intrauterine life and development across the 1st year of life which are commonly experienced across all human infants globally.

PHASES OF INTRAUTERINE DEVELOPMENT

The most important events in the embryological development of the nervous system along the three trimesters are:

- Organogenesis
- Neuronogenesis from the stem cells
- Migration
- Proliferation
- Differentiation
- Myelination

The developmental abnormalities of the human brain depend on the stage at which an insult has taken place. The insult to the developing brain can be caused by a trauma, nutritional deficiency, hormonal imbalance in the mother, infection, maternal drug abuse with studies indicating the relative impact of each. However, these factors have a different impact depending on the stage of embryological development.

In the **1st trimester**, as the neural tube is getting formed, a nutritional deficiency (Folate/Vitamin B9) can result in malformation of the neural tube leading to neural tube defects like spinal dysraphisms, or structural malformations of the brain.

The **2nd trimester** of pregnancy is marked by formation of the neuronal cells from the germinal matrix that migrate to their specific destinations and proliferate. Thus, the process of neuronal proliferation, migration and cortical organization may get impacted due to an insult in the 2nd trimester.

In the **3rd trimester** of pregnancy, infants are particularly vulnerable to white matter injury between 24 and 36 weeks of gestation, whereas gray matter injuries more commonly occur in the late trimester, after 36 weeks of gestation.

The age of the infant at the time of the brain insult influences an infant's ability to receive afferent sensory information.

Thus, if there is a periventricular insult causing damage to the internal capsule in the early part of the 3rd trimester, the thalamocortical pathways can get formed bypassing the area of periventricular lesion and can reach the primary somatosensory cortex. But if the insult happens after the pathways are laid, in the later part of the 3rd trimester, the formed pathways through the internal capsule will be damaged and will have trouble making connections with the somatosensory cortex.

This information is important for a caregiver and the therapist because it suggests the possibility of infants having suffered from any hypoxic insult or a major stressor during the late prenatal, perinatal or postnatal period, having impairments with the somatosensory system. The therapist or the caregiver in such situations may have to engage the infant through visual or verbal cues to facilitate the learning of the basic structure of a movement.

NEEDS OF AN INFANT BORN PRETERM

According to the data by World Health Organization, preterm is defined as babies born alive before 37 weeks of pregnancy are completed. There are subcategories based on gestational age: extremely preterm (less than 28 weeks), very preterm (28 to 32 weeks), moderate to late preterm (32 to 37 weeks).

In a baby born preterm, the various systems of the body like the neurological and cardiopulmonary systems are still in the process of maturation and are not yet completely prepared to function in the extrauterine environment.

The various sensory systems have a schedule of maturation along the period of gestation and slowly become equipped to cope up with the stressors that the extrauterine environment can offer. Similarly, the physiological organization dependent on fetal circulation needs to transition to one where the lungs become the primary organs of gas exchange and this transition is dependent on the anatomical development of lungs.

The immaturity of various anatomical structures makes the preterm infant biologically vulnerable to factors like infections, invasive procedures, and environmental changes. Moreover, the physiological instability of the preterm infant mandates stay in the NICU away from the mother for a greater duration making them exposed to unnatural environmental stressors and depriving the baby of the essential nurturing stimuli coming from the mother.

When the baby is born at term and the umbilical cord is clamped, the ability to cry depends on maturity of the brainstem centers that sense the change in blood gases and the presence of surfactant that enables the lungs to expand.

The preterm infant is susceptible to **cardiopulmonary dysfunction** because of the following reasons:

- Capillary bed not well developed till 26 weeks
- Increased pulmonary resistance
- Sustained right to left shunt
- Type 2 alveolar cells and surfactant production not matured till 35 weeks of gestation
- Decreased lung compliance
- Elastic properties of lung not developed
- Chances of airway collapse
- Lung space decreased by relative size of heart
- Type I fibers in diaphragm not developed
- Diaphragm can fatigue faster
- Lack of fatty tissue, high surface area/body weight ratio
- Hypothermia and increased oxygen consumption
- Reflexes depressed—cough, gag reflex depressed, chances of aspiration, infection high.

There are biological, established and environmental risk factors explained in literature which are guidelines for referral of a preterm infant for therapy **(Table 25.1)**.

Besides these, **environmental risk factors** have been enlisted that disturb the process of neuroplasticity and can create maladaptive behavioral responses in the child. This topic demands special attention.

Neuroplasticity refers to the ability of the brain to make short- or long-term modifications to the strength and number of its synaptic neuronal connections in response to

Table 25.1: Risk factors for referral of preterm infant for therapy.

Biological risks	*Established risk factors*
Factors that increase the vulnerability of the preterm infant to additional stressors and predispose the infant to neurodevelopmental abnormalities	The confirmed abnormalities detected at birth which are certain to alter the course of development
• Birth weight of 1,500 g or less ➢ Gestational age of 32 weeks or less ➢ Small for gestational age ➢ Prenatal exposure to drugs, alcohol ➢ Ventilator requirements for 36 hours or more • Intracranial hemorrhage grade 3 • Periventricular leukomalacia • Muscle tone abnormalities (hypotonia, hypertonia, asymmetry of movement) • Recurrent seizures • Feeding dysfunctions • Symptomatic TORCH infection • Meningitis • Asphyxia with APGAR <4 at 5 minutes • Multiple births	• Hydrocephalus • Microcephaly • Chromosomal abnormality • Musculoskeletal abnormality (CDH, arthrogryposis, torticollis) • Brachial plexus injury • Myelodysplasia • Congenital myopathies • Metabolism errors • HIV • Down syndrome

(TORCH: toxoplasmosis, Others (syphilis, hepatitis B), rubella, cytomegalovirus, herpes simplex; CDH: congenital dysplasia of hip; HIV: human immunodeficiency virus)

incoming stimuli associated with activity and experience. Neuroplasticity is a lifelong property of the human brain, although it is most prominent from birth until late childhood.

The development of neural networks depends on both molecular cues that guide synapse development and activity-dependent mechanisms that use patterned activation to adjust the strength and number of synaptic connections.

The events of development of the central nervous system in the 1st and 2nd trimesters are endogenously stimulated and the synaptic connections are then built based on experience. The more a certain neural network is stimulated, the more will there be internalization of the behavioral response or expectation and the neuronal connections which are not stimulated will be lost over the time.

Neuroplasticity happens at various levels including:

- Physiological (i.e., the release of more neurotransmitters to compensate for cell death)
- Anatomic (i.e., the extension of existing axons into space vacated by deleted axons)
- Metabolic (i.e., the brain's ability to grow capillaries in an area to suit a new function such as occurs with learning).

There are two aspects of synaptogenesis in response to stimulation explained by Dr Rita H Pickler in '*a model of neurodevelopmental risk and protection for preterm infants*'.

- The first is referred to as '*experience expectant mechanism*'. This means that the stimulation experienced by the brain creates a largely scattered excitability across brain areas that make the system expect certain experiences or forming a structural substrate of expectations. These synapses which are functionally excitable get strengthened if they receive repeated stimulation.
- The other aspect is '*experience dependent mechanism*' which refers to the formation of synapses in response to repeated stimulation in a more specific way leading to specific learning.

Factors that make the Brain of a Preterm Infant Vulnerable to Insult

They are as follows:

- Some of the factors implicated in poor neurobehavioral or cognitive outcomes in preterm infants include:
  Hypoxic/ischemic insults, maternal infection with overproduction of cytokines, and other proinflammatory agents, excessive glutamate release initiating the excitotoxic cascade, oxidative stress, growth factor deficiency, specific maternal drugs, maternal stress.
- Prenatal and perinatal events and conditions—prolonged time between membrane rupture and delivery and multiple placental lesions. The presence of proinflammatory cytokines decrease the threshold of the nervous tissue to hypoxia making the neonatal brain more susceptible to damage due to hypoxia if the inflammatory cytokines are already high.
- Other associations include:
  - Pharmacologic treatment during pregnancy with steroids and other medications
  - Primiparity
  - Maternal diseases such as pregnancy-induced hypertension, diabetes mellitus, or chorioamnionitis.
- Genetic factors like the alteration in apolipoprotein E (ApoE), a lipid transport protein that also plays a role in repair after cell injury, have been linked to injuries to the developing brain. The alteration in this factor may impede post injury repair and the primary synaptogenetic process.
- Neonatal jaundice is known to exist due to increased circulation of free unconjugated bilirubin due to greater turnover of RBCs, inadequate serum bilirubin available for binding, immaturity of the transporter pump, and inadequate or absent intestinal flora. The immature, developing neuronal pathways are more susceptible to damage due to deposition of bilirubin which when

deposited in areas of the brain like the basal ganglia can lead to a condition like kernicterus. These events are more pronounced in a preterm infant.

- Environmental factors in the NICU:
  - There may be a stress response generated due to this constant overstimulation and an inability to counter the same with movements, because of the inadequate muscle activity and the fact that the baby may be restricted to the surface due to the tubes in the NICU. Stress is known to be accompanied by the release of cortisol which is known to suppress the expression of neurotrophic proteins.

Neuroprotective Core Measures

Keeping in mind the challenges mentioned above, there are **neuroprotective measures** recommended by The Joint Commission (TJC) of the US Centers for Medicare and Medicaid Services. Using the TJC model of disease-specific core measures that are related to specific medical conditions, Coughlin et al proposed five developmental care core measures that are focused on care actions, which are disease-independent yet essential to promote healthy growth and development of the preterm infant and family.

To provide more practical guidance for NICU staff in delivering developmental care to preterm infants in the NICU, the five neonatal core measures first introduced by Coughlin et al. have been recategorized and expanded into seven distinct family-centered developmental core measures of neuroprotective neonatal care by Altimier et al. This expansion enables additional focus on developmentally appropriate positioning and handling, optimizing nutrition and feeding, and protecting skin, all areas that are fundamental to providing developmental neonatal care. The **seven neuroprotective core measures** for family-centered developmental care described in the Neonatal Integrative Developmental Care Model **(Fig. 25.1)** include the following:

- Healing environment
- Partnering with families
- Position and handling
- Safeguarding sleep
- Minimizing stress and pain
- Protecting skin
- Optimizing nutrition

NICU Brain Sensitive Care Committee Swedish Medical Center have thus recommended 7 core areas for implementation of neuroprotective strategies for a preterm infant.

Core Measure 1: Safeguarding Sleep

The goal here is to assess infant sleep-wake state before caregiving, and to safeguard prolonged periods of uninterrupted sleep whenever possible.

A fetus at 32 weeks of gestation is known to spend 90–95% of its time asleep and this duration decreases to 85–90% by term.

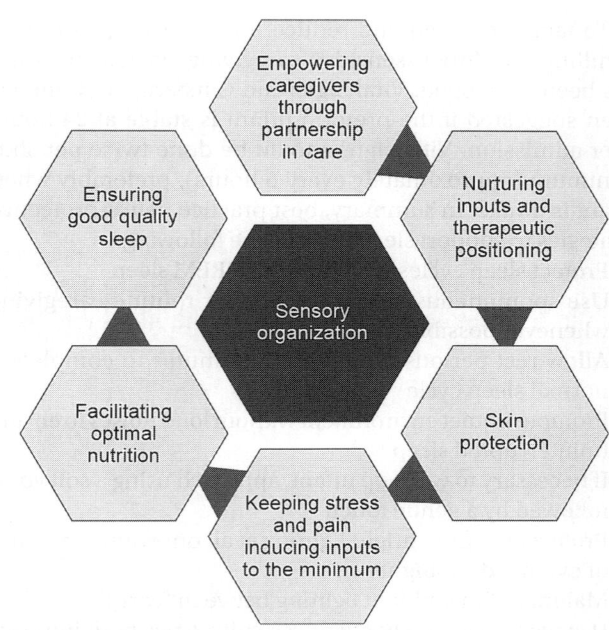

Fig. 25.1: The main tenets of care given in the neonatal care unit.

Sleep patterns begin to form in the last months of pregnancy, with predominantly active (rapid eye movement or "REM") sleep initially, followed by longer periods of quiet (non-REM) sleep. Preterm infants have shorter sleep cycles of 30–40 minutes with 80% of sleep being active/REM sleep. As a preterm infant matures (by approximately 36 weeks) sleep cycles average between 50–60 minutes with time divided more evenly between active and quiet sleep. Term infants begin and end their sleep cycle in active sleep and have longer periods of awake, alert time.

Both REM (rapid eye movement) sleep and Non-REM sleep are important in the life of a preterm infant. Sleep plays a critical role in early neurosensory development, impacts memory and subsequent learning, and preserves brain plasticity. Sleep deprivation reduces both brain size and plasticity, and is associated with enduring consequences for learning, behavior, and function. Neurosensory development depends upon appropriate stimuli from both internal and external sources. Endogenous stimulation occurs only during REM sleep, something that a fetus at 32 weeks would be engaged in for the vast majority of the time. Once these sensory systems are formed using endogenous input from the baby's own central nervous system (CNS), they are ready for exogenous stimuli from the external world. Fetal development of the sensory system occurs in a specific sequence: Tactile (touch), Vestibular (proprioception), Olfactory (smell), Gustatory (taste), Auditory (hearing) and then Visual (sight).

Disrupting this predetermined sequence of sensory development can interfere with later function. Since the visual system matures towards the end of the normal gestation, preterm infants are not ready for light or any kind of visual experience prior to 36–40 weeks gestation. Protecting sleep cycles, especially REM sleep, is absolutely essential for optimal neurosensory and visual development.

To facilitate sleep and reduce unnecessary procedural handling, the "brain-sensitive caregiving" vital signs order has been developed. Vital Signs and Clustering of Care has been suggested if the preterm infant is stable at 24 hours after admission. Vital signs should be done twice per shift minimum (approximately every 6 hours), preferably when infant is awake. In summary, best practice neuro-protective strategies to support sleep include the following:

- Protect sleep cycles, and especially REM sleep
- Use spontaneous awake periods for routine caregiving whenever possible
- Allow rest periods of at least 60 minutes to complete a normal sleep cycle
- Promote a quiet environment without loud noises to ensure uninterrupted sleep
- If necessary to wake up infant, approach using a soft voice followed by a gentle touch
- Protect eyes from bright lighting at all times and avoid use of overhead spotlights
- Maintain dim ambient lighting between "cares"
- Use narcotics and sedatives carefully, since both interfere with REM and non-REM sleep
- Facilitate prolonged skin-to-skin to promote normal sleep pattern.

Core Measure 2: Part 2A—Positioning for Success

Here, the goal is to eliminate or reduce positional deformities by maintaining infants in a midline, flexed, contained, and comfortable position.

When born prematurely or critically ill, gravity forces weak infants into an uncomfortable flat and extended resting posture, with the extremities abducted and externally rotated. The baby's head falls asymmetrically to one side, usually the right side and causes uneven flattening of the skull. Over time, neuronal connections are reinforced that support these abnormal postures as a baseline. Developmental delays and permanent disabilities may ensue. In utero, the fetus kicks and moves freely against boundaries that provide constant somaesthetic (touch), kinesthetic (movement), and proprioceptive (position) feedback.

What can we do in the NICU?

- Aim for containment, rather than restraint
- Flexible enough to allow spontaneous movement, firm enough to limit excessive activity
- When possible, hands should be able to move towards face/mouth for self-comfort.

Positioning to support optimal alignment and containment should be provided for all infants.

A **"positioning checklist"** has been suggested which can be used, before leaving the bedside:

- Shoulders softly rounded forward?
- Hands towards midline, able to touch face/mouth if possible for self-comforting?
- Hips aligned and pelvis tucked?
- Knees, ankles, feet aligned and softly flexed?
- Neck neutral or slightly flexed, no hyperextension?
- Head midline, or turned slightly right or left? Avoid turning more than 45° to either side.

When the infant is positioned in prone:

- Select appropriate size for the positioner. If infant is between sizes, use smaller size to prevent abduction of legs and shoulders, and to allow shoulders and hips to flex around the positioner.
- Bottom of prone positioner should end around the umbilicus.
- Avoid turning head to a full 90° angle by allowing it to rest slightly off edge of positioner.

Reposition if infant appears restless, uncomfortable, and/or during "hands on care". Teach parents how to position properly and solicit their input on baby's comfort and preferences.

Supportive containment with positioning aids can be used to approximate the defined boundaries the fetus experiences in utero. These aids are selected based upon individual infant needs, e.g., the Freddy Frogs, Dandle Roos, Roo-Wrap are some of the aids mentioned in literature that help attain the position that simulates the intrauterine position while allowing the infant to kick and perform active movements.

Part 2B: Handling with Care

Here the goal is to maintain autonomic stability throughout positioning changes and caregiving activities, as well as during periods of rest and sleep.

Moving infants quickly may be efficient for caregivers, but is very stressful for infants and often leads to autonomic instability (i.e., apnea/bradycardia/desaturation "events"). Rapid and unsupported movement (such as the "premie flip") triggers sensory distress and excessive motor activity, as infants attempt to stabilize themselves to a fixed surface during the vestibular disturbance. Infants may remain disorganized, nauseated, and dizzy for up to 30 minutes following a "premie flip", and more "events" are likely to occur later in a delayed response to handling.

What can we do in the NICU?

Minimize stress and support autonomic stability during rest and caregiving interventions by utilizing careful handling and containment techniques. Consider using a second person to assist with position changes for intubated infants. Whenever possible, avoid disturbing infants during sleep and try to use spontaneous awake periods for caregiving. If it is necessary to awaken the infant, start with a soft voice, followed by a gentle touch. "Containment", also known as a "facilitated tuck" or "hand hugs", refers to the parent's or caregiver's hands being used to maintain an infant in a flexed midline position. This technique provides support for the infant and the opportunity to control their own body. Infants who are not adequately "contained" demonstrate more physiologic instability, agitation, and stress cues. Containment is indicated for all handling, caregiving and procedures. When an additional caregiver is unavailable to assist, Dandewraps/Roos or blanket swaddles can beused.

Clinical Pointer

Intracranial pressure (ICP) is lowest when the head is in midline and elevated as compared to the body. Caution should be taken when changing diapers to prevent sudden fluctuations in ICP when the feet are raised above the head. This is important during the first several days of life for prevention of Intraventricular hemorrhage but should also be avoided throughout hospitalization to minimize gastrointestinal (GI) reflux.

- Avoid raising feet above head whenever possible
- Slide new diaper under infant and lift slightly at hips to remove old diaper
- To clean diaper area, lift knees to the chest while supporting the back and buttocks
- Consider placing the infant on one side to clean buttocks and diaper area.

Miscellaneous strategies to prevent increased ICP include:

- Suction (endotracheal tube or ETT, deep nasal/oral) only when clinically indicated
- Minimize pain and stress
- Flush and draw from umbilical lines very slowly (1 mL over 30–45 seconds)

Part 3: Protecting Skin

Here the goal is to protect newborn skin integrity and to provide opportunities for nurturing input through this vital sensory organ.

The skin is the largest organ of the body, and makes up about 13% of weight in a preterm, versus 6–10% of adult's weight. Skin integrity is essential to survival and any break provides a portal of entry for infection. The skin is one of five sensory organs designed to help protect the body by relaying information about the environment via sensory neurons to the brain. Touch is the first of the senses to develop early in fetal life, with sensory neurons found around the mouth and face by week 7, and covering the entire body by week 20. The fetus (and preterm infant) has more sensory nerve endings than the adult, which are closer to the surface of the skin. The infant's hands, feet, and mouth are especially sensitive to touch due to the density of sensory nerve fibers that send constant messages to the cerebral cortex.

The skin is comprised of several distinct layers:

- The epidermis (outer layer) acts as a protective barrier against the environment and assists with temperature management. Term infants have 10–20 protective epidermal layers whereas preterms <30 weeks GA may only have 2–3 layers and those <25 weeks have negligible epidermal barriers. Thus, they are vulnerable to absorption of toxins, and prone to insensible heat and transepidermal water loss (TEWL).
- The dermis (middle layer) is made up of collagen fibers that provide strength and elasticity, and contains both blood vessels and nerves. Thin fibrils connect the dermis and epidermis. Because preterm infants have fewer fibrils connecting the skin layers, they are susceptible to "epidermal stripping" with tape removal. Epidermal stripping occurs when the bond between tape and skin is stronger than the bond between epidermal and dermal layers and the epidermal layer is accidentally removed with the tape.
- The bottom layer of skin is fatty connective tissue that accumulates during the third trimester and provides shock absorption and insulation. Most preterm infants have minimal "padding" to maintain heat or protect from the discomfort of hard surfaces.

What can we do in the NICU?

To provide nurturing touch:

- Role model use of gentle but firm touch, which is tolerated better than stroking.
- Skin to skin care (Kangaroo Care) provides an excellent means of offering safe, nurturing touch to minimize/avoid injury and noxious inputs.
- Provide humidity for the first two weeks of life to reduce Transepidermal water loss for extremely low birth weight (ELBW) infants.
- Reduce unnecessary exposure to topical products, and rinse off with water if possible.
- Assess intravenous (IV) line hourly for evidence of phlebitis and/or infiltration.
- Change diapers every 2–4 hours during spontaneous awake periods to avoid diaper rash.
- Handle preterms gently and provide soft bedding to compensate for lack of "padding", but remind parents that soft bedding and "nests" are safe only in hospital setting.
- Apply and remove adhesives cautiously, as these are the primary source of skin breakdown in the NICU protective skin strategies. To achieve this:
  - Avoid skin breakdown from common sources such as adhesive removal, thermal injury, abrasion/friction, diaper dermatitis, continuous positive airway pressure devices, pressure ulcers, and/or infection
  - Consider applying Tegaderm to clean, dry skin at risk for abrasion/friction, moisten adhesive-skin interface with either water, saline, or Vaseline and use silicone-based, alcohol-free, adhesive removers when available, as they are the safest adhesive removers currently available for the neonatal population
  - Minimize the use of tape, adhesive products, and bonding agents
  - Whenever possible, leave adhesives in place until adhesive bond starts to lessen
  - To remove tape, hold surrounding skin in place and slowly pull tape at a very low angle, parallel to the skin surface rather than straight up at a 90° angle.

Core Measure 4A: Minimizing Stress

Here the goal is to reduce stress whenever possible, and to promote both self-regulation and neurodevelopmental organization. Neonatal stress is greatly exacerbated by maternal separation, exposure to repetitive and uncomfortable caregiving interventions, painful procedures, and unfiltered noise and lighting. Short-term, stress may increase energy expenditure and cortisol levels, and cause cardiorespiratory instability. Long-term, there is evidence that repeated stress during this vulnerable period of brain development may result in permanent structural and functional changes. Minimizing stress may support the preterm's capacity for neuroplasticity and decrease the likelihood of encoding abnormal stress responses.

Strategies known to reduce infant stress and improve outcomes include:

- Skin to skin care (refer to section 7-A for Kangaroo care)
- "Cue based caregiving"
- Safeguarding sleep.

Much infant stress can be reduced by thoughtful use of **parental nurturing touch**, either with skin-to-skin care or containment ("hand hugs"). Parents should provide nurturing touch whenever possible, especially following caregiving or procedures until the infant has returned to baseline and/or fallen asleep as it is known to activate the parasympathetic nervous system ("rest and digest response"). Procedural touch activates the sympathetic nervous system ("fight or flight response"), which increases stress and disrupts sleep.

"Cue based caregiving" is based upon the concepts of neurobehavioral organization, which refers to a smooth balance between an infant's physiologic and behavioral systems. Individualized caregiving is dictated by different cues that tell caregivers to either continue with handling, or to pause temporarily to provide for recovery.

- **Stress cues** are physiologic signals that the infant is overwhelmed, and needs gentle containment and a break to avoid energy loss and decompensation.
- **Stability cues** indicate that it is safe to interact or proceed with caregiving.
- **Self-help cues** should be supported, since they indicate that an infant is trying to "organize" himself within the NICU environment.

It is necessary to help parents identify and respond to cues.

Protect sleep by clustering of care whenever possible, but be aware that the infant may not tolerate all of the caregiving measures that have been bundled into a single session. Clustering of care is intended to provide longer rest periods but may actually result in more physiologic alterations (changes in blood pressure, cardiorespiratory stability, altered cortisol levels, and heightened pain responses) than single care-taking events. Clustered care appears to be especially stressful for preterms < 28 weeks gestational age (GA), so individualized cue-based caregiving is essential to avoid overwhelming an infant.

Part 4B: Minimizing Pain

Here the goal is to minimize the intensity, duration and physiologic cost of the pain experience, and to maximize the infant's ability to cope with and recover from painful experiences.

Afferent nerve pathways are fully intact by 24–26 weeks GA. Efferent nerve pathways that send protective impulses back to motor neurons, and trigger reflexive withdrawal from pain also regulate neuromodulators (such as serotonin) that control pain signals by reducing or blocking the continued transmission of painful stimuli. Efferent pathways are largely undeveloped until 36–40 weeks GA, and continue to mature postnatally. Hence, infants may not withdraw in response to pain and are often unable to inhibit persistent pain signals, leading to some acute physiologic changes, including elevated heart rate, respiratory rate, blood pressure and intracranial pressure.

The following comfort measures are known to minimize pain and stress, while maximizing an infant's regulatory and coping abilities:

- After pain exposure, sensitivity is accentuated by increased excitability of nociceptive neurons in the spinal cord, causing routine handling and caregiving to be perceived as painful due to heightened activity in nociceptive pathways. The infant should be allowed to fully recover from painful stimulus before resuming caregiving.
- Containment should be provided with hands (facilitated tuck or "hand hugs"), Dandleroos/wraps or standard swaddling. Maintaining flexion and allow hand to mouth can be used for self-comforting.
- Skin-to-skin contact significantly diminishes pain responses during and after blood collection through heel for preterm and term infants.
- Non-nutritive sucking (NNS) during painful procedures is thought to activate nonopioid pathways, creating temporary pain relief. A systematic review found that breastfeeding and breast milk reduced pain responses and can be used to minimize procedural pain.
- Sucrose, if applied to the tip of tongue 2 minutes before the procedure, is effective in reducing pain responses, especially when combined with sucking (i.e., dipped pacifier) and other comfort measures. The two-minute interval is thought to coincide with the endogenous opioid release triggered by the sweet taste.

Core Measure 5: Optimizing Nutrition

Here the goal is to provide the best nutritional support available, and to support a positive infant-driven breast- or bottle-feeding experience.

Breast milk is the most tolerated substrate for preterm infants and it allows enteral feedings to be reached earlier, reducing the need for parenteral feeding. Studies have reported decreased risk of necrotizing enterocolitis, retinopathy of prematurity and sepsis as well as improved neurodevelopmental outcomes, higher intelligence quotient (IQ) and larger brain volumes in preterm infants who are fed breast milk. Care must be taken to provide a safe, functional, nurturing, and developmentally appropriate feeding experience. The use of an infant driven feeding approach and appropriate feeding techniques is vital to provide for a successful experience and to avoid oral aversion.

What can we do in the NICU?

- Minimize negative perioral experiences such as suctioning, vigorous oral care, and saline for oral care
- Use colostrum for gentle oral care
- Promote non-nutritive sucking (NNS) at mother's pumped breast during gavage feeds
- Provide the taste and smell of breast milk during gavage feedings (binky dips)
- Focus on quality of feeding rather than quantity of feeding.
- Glucose should be infused within 30–60 minutes after birth

Oromotor stimulation and hydrotherapy with swaddling before feeding has been shown to improve the oromotor activity during feeding. These are explained separately in another section.

Positioning of the infant in sidelying while feeding allows the tongue to move in the gravity eliminated plane thus enabling feeding with ease.

Core Measure 6: Parent Partnerships

Here the goal is to support parents in their role as the most important caregivers for their infant, and to promote secure attachment.

What can we do in the NICU?

- Discuss infant's clinical condition and needs in a culturally appropriate, clear manner
- Use active, empathetic listening with parents as they express their concerns and fears
- Acknowledge and identify the stage of grief and loss of the parents and provide support accordingly
- Assist parents in accessing resources such as support groups, counseling whenever needed
- Create a welcoming environment where parents know that they are valued
- Allow parents to join in infant's care to the extent they choose, whenever they desire
- Encourage containment ("hand hugs") both during and after caregiving
- If able to do so without awakening, allow parents to provide containment during sleep
- Parents may hold "between" cares as tolerated, but stress the critical need for infant to sleep as much as possible
- Encourage parents to read to infant when awake to support language development
- Promote skin-to-skin as soon as possible, as often as possible, for as long as possible
- Empower parents to recognize and respond to infant cues appropriately
- Explain that when dealing with infants, "the infant leads and the adult follows"
- Help parents become competent in infant care, building confidence towards discharge.

Part 7: Healing Environment

Here the goal is to provide an environment that promotes healing by minimizing the impact of NICU environment on the infant's developing central nervous system **(Table 25.2)**.

Table 25.2: Strategies to provide an environment that promotes healing.

Core measure	*Environment*	*Goal and strategies*
7A	Temperature	Our goal is to provide a neutral thermal environment in which the infant is able to maintain a normal core temperature with minimum oxygen consumption and calorie expenditure. • Infants who are admitted to pre-warmed warmers for initial stabilization should be transferred to incubators with quiet motors as soon as possible • Humidity should be used for ELBW infants • Medically stable infants may be weaned from incubators to open cribs around 1,500–1,600 grams. • Kangaroo care is now widely practiced with the goal of reducing stress in the infant and achieving thermosynchrony. Thermosynchrony refers to the mother's ability to increase the temperature of her chest as much as 2°C to warm a cool infant and decrease by 1°C to cool an overheated infant.
7B	Touch	Touch is the first of the senses to develop early in fetal life. Preterms are exposed to a significant amount of painful "procedural touch" as part of medical therapy. It is vital to offset these negative experiences with positive tactile encounters such as nurturing touch, reassuring the preterm infant that all touch is not noxious. In the NICU: • Because preterm infants are not able to modulate sensory input well, light touch or gentle stroking can seem over-stimulating and irritating • Demonstrate gentle but firm "static containment" ("quiet hands" or "hand hugs") • Encourage frequent and extended periods of skin-to-skin care (Kangaroo Care) • When parents are uninvolved or unable to visit frequently, encourage consistent use of cuddlers or available staff to provide swaddle holding
7C	Vestibular-proprioceptive	The vestibular and proprioceptive systems develop after the sense of touch. The secure boundaries of the uterine wall promote generalized flexion and gentle containment, supporting the development of proprioception. Maternal movement and fetal activity within warm amniotic fluid offer vestibular and tactile stimulation. • Provide containment during caregiving, change infant's position slowly and without sudden movements • Utilize supportive positioning devices such as the DandleRoos/Wraps • Facilitate skin to skin opportunities

Contd...

Contd...

Core measure	*Environment*	*Goal and strategies*
7D	Taste and smell	The **gustatory (taste) system** is intact by 24 weeks GA and even young preterm infants are capable of responding to bitter, sweet, or salty flavors. Maternal diet and flavors are identified in amniotic fluid, and flavonoids in amniotic fluid are identical to those in maternal breast milk. Providing the scent and taste of mother's milk has been shown to promote infant cueing, sucking, and arousal in anticipation of eventual oral feedings. "Pacifier dips" with mother's milk increase nonnutritive sucking, intake, and growth. The **olfactory system** is functional by 28 weeks GA, with olfactory input communicated directly from the nose to the cerebral cortex. The emotional context of different smells is significant because odors are processed by the limbic system, the same area of the brain that manages emotion and memories. Maternal odor is also known to influence neonatal behavior by facilitating state regulation, the ability to transition gradually through the different levels of consciousness, from quiet sleep to full cry. • Maintain a scent-free unit for staff, and encourage parents to limit use of fragrances • Avoid the odor of smoke on caregiver clothing and bodies • Provide mother's scent when possible, with breast pad or soft cloth • Offer "Pacifier dips" with mother's milk • Use colostrum for oral care
7E	Auditory	Auditory development is a slow process that begins early in gestation, with crucial stages of maturation occurring during the final weeks of pregnancy and well beyond. The neural connections between the cochlea and auditory cortex are fully intact by 30 weeks GA. At this point a complex "mapping" of hair cells (sensory receptors) begins to occur within the cochlea creating "tonotropic columns", which will continue to develop over the first 6 months of life. Low-frequency tonotropic regions of the cochlea are able to mature before high-frequency regions. As the walls of the uterine lining begin to thin towards the end of pregnancy, more high frequency sounds make their way through to the fetus. After term delivery and until about 6 months of age, the auditory system requires thoughtful external input (speech, music, and meaningful sound) in order to complete the essential "tuning" and mapping of the cochlear hair cells into functional tonotropic columns. Preterm delivery impacts the development of the auditory system by eliminating the natural sound barrier provided by the womb. Short-term impact on vital signs such as heart rate (HR), blood pressure (BP) and oxygen saturations. Long-term impact on the quality and quantity of sleep. The following interventions are useful to decrease noise, encourage uninterrupted sleep, and facilitate normal auditory development: • Speak as quietly as possible within patient bays, avoid loud laughter or conversations • Avoid talking over incubator or allowing medical rounds too close to bedside • Empty sloshing water in ventilator tubing • Quiet alarms as quickly as possible, and remember to reset them • Use blankets or covers over incubator to attempt to muffle noise • Avoid placing items on incubator, do so gently if necessary • Close incubator portholes, drawers and refrigerator gently • If able, use pagers/cell phones on vibrate mode rather than audible alarm mode • Transfer infants from warmers to incubators with quiet motors as soon as possible • Infants should remain in incubators only as long as needed to maintain heat balance • Use padding on trash can lids and cupboard doors • Use earmuffs for infants • Safeguard both REM and non-REM sleep, but especially REM sleep • Provide day-night cycles when auditory stimulation is decreased
7F	Vision	The structural elements of the eye form early in fetal life, but the majority of essential neural mechanisms and connections develop during the final 12 weeks of pregnancy. The endogenous stimulation needed to trigger neural migration and formation of directional columns for vision occurs only during REM sleep, which occupies much of fetal life. Adequate sleep is essential for healthy retinal development and intact pathways to the visual cortex. The visual experience for term infants should include light directed onto objects rather than the infant's face, novelty, and motion. Since color perception begins to develop slightly later, exposure to color is not necessary in the infant's visual field until after 2–3 months. The focal distance for term infants is 10–12 inches and gradually increases with time and the ability to focus. There is mixed data about the use of day/night cycled lighting The following interventions are thought to promote good visual function: • Protect sleep, especially REM sleep • Use adjustable lighting at each bedside, strive towards a day/night cycle for the NICU

Contd...

Contd...

Core measure	*Environment*	*Goal and strategies*
		• Use minimal amount of light needed to accurately assess and manage infant • Consider the use of penlights and flashlights whenever possible • Protect eyes from direct light during assessments, rest periods, and after pupil dilation for Retinopathy of Prematurity (ROP) exams • Use heavy incubator covers to limit excessive light exposure during sleep, underside of these covers should be solid and dark colored to minimize unnecessary visual stimulation • Mobiles and high contrast patterned toys are suitable for use under supervision only with term infants, and for periods of 5–10 minutes at a time • Limit visual stimuli early on, with focus on parent's faces

Box 25.1: Hydrotherapy.

- A standard plastic bassinet serves as the hydrotherapy tub, and the water temperature is prepared at 37.8 to 38.3°C (100 to 101°F).
- An overhead radiant heater is used to decrease temperature loss and enhance thermoregulation in the undressed infant.
- Medical clearance is acquired along with the maximum acceptable limits for blood pressure, heart rate, color changes. The baseline heart rate and blood pressure values are recorded and pre-treatment posture and behavioral states are observed.
- The undressed infant is swaddled and moved into a semiflexed, supine position. After being lifted into the water, the swaddled infant is given a short period of quiet holding in the water without body movement or auditory stimulation to allow behavioral adaptation to the fluid environment. A second caregiver (e.g., nurse or parent) stabilizes the infant's head and shoulder girdle region while the neonatal therapist provides support at the pelvis.
- Within the loosened boundaries of the swaddling blanket, the movement techniques involve midline positioning of the head and slow, graded movement incorporating slight flexion and rotation of the trunk, followed (if tolerated) by progression distally to the pelvic girdle region and finally to the shoulder girdle region.
- After guided trunk extension flexion with partially dissociated movement at the shoulder or pelvic girdle, most infants will demonstrate active extremity movement in the water and the swaddling blanket is adjusted (or removed) to allow more movement or more stability depending on the response of the infant. The improved range and smoothness of spontaneous extremity movement is facilitated by the buoyancy and surface tension of the water.
- If the movement therapy becomes stressful, with agitation or crying by the infant, body movement is stopped immediately, and the infant is either consoled or removed from the water and held with warmed towels.
- Possible risks involve hypothermia, increase in heart rate and blood pressure and intolerance. Hence, careful monitoring of temperature, blood pressure, oxygen saturation, behavioral state, skin color, heart rate and respiratory rate is extremely essential.

NEONATAL HYDROTHERAPY

Indications for referral of medically stable infants to the hydrotherapy component of the neonatal therapy program include: Behavioral state abnormalities leading to feeding dysfunction and barriers in social interaction, limited range of motion due to connective tissue factors, muscle tone abnormalities, affecting posture, movement, feeding and medically stable infant, i.e., when intravenous lines are discontinued, temperature, heart rate instabilities and apnea are resolved **(Box 25.1)**.

Box 25.2 describes the benefits of a 10 minutes hydrotherapy session.

OROMOTOR THERAPY IN NICU

Table 25.3 shows the factors that feeding difficulties in preterm neonates may be related to.

Three instruments for assessing oral-motor and feeding behaviors in the nursery are:

1. The neonatal oral-motor assessment scale (NOMAS)
2. The nursing child assessment of feeding scale (NCAFS)
3. The early feeding skills (EFS) assessment for preterm infants.

Box 25.2: Benefits of a 10-minute hydrotherapy session.

- Improved postural tone with semiflexed posture is obtained with higher behavioral tolerance by the infant. These maintained for 2 to 3 hours when aquatic intervention is followed by flexed, midline body positioning in the side-lying or prone on a water mattress or supported against rolls.
- Mild flexion contractures of knees and elbows and dynamic hip adduction contractures can be safely and quickly reduced by gentle muscle elongation techniques in warm water.
- Enhancement of visual and auditory orientation responses (e.g., visual fixing and tracking, auditory alerting, and localization to human voices), prolonged high-quality alertness, and longer periods of social interaction with caregivers.
- Improved sleep quality and behavioral organization.
- Feeding performance may improve when hydrotherapy is scheduled 30 minutes before feeding due to better alertness and posture, reflected in decreased duration of feeding, consumption of more percentage of the required feeds and weight gain.

General strategies during feeding may include:

- Specific arousal or calming procedures before feeding.
- Positioning: Semiflexed, upright positioning with light support under the chin. Feeding infants in the side-lying

Table 25.3: Factors that may be related to feeding difficulties in preterm neonates.

Neurological immaturity	Decreased tongue mobility	Tactile hypersensitivity in the mouth
Depressed oral reflexes	Presence of tongue thrusting	Inefficient and uncoordinated respiratory patterns
Prolonged use of an endotracheal tube for mechanical ventilation and subsequent oral tactile hypersensitivity	Decreased lip seal on nipple	Insufficient proximal stability from hypotonic neck and trunk musculature
Insufficient postural tone	Nasal regurgitation	Hypertonic posturing of the neck and trunk in extension

position may improve tongue position, particularly if marked tongue retraction is present.

- Techniques such as tactile facilitation of the facial muscles,
- Use of a pacifier during gavage feedings,
- Light manual support to the jaw or lip and thickening of formula are recommended.
- Scheduling of feeding based on the infant's readiness (behavioral cues of hunger and alertness) is usually implemented by neonatal nurses and shown to be effective in helping infants advance the frequency of oral (rather than gavage) feedings. The timing of movement therapy or neonatal hydrotherapy 30 minutes before feeding may improve performance by preparing postural tone, facilitating oral musculature, and enhancing alertness.

Clinical Pointer

For some infants, oral intake by bottle may be improved by individualizing nipple selection according to contour, length, hole size, texture, and compression resistance.

Expected outcomes of oral-motor intervention supported by clinical research include:

Increased number of nutritive sucks after perioral stimulation, increased volume of fluid ingested during nipple feedings, decreased number of gavage feedings and earlier bottle feeding, accelerated weight gain and earlier hospital discharge.

Monitoring the infant's physiological tolerance, breathing pattern, and work of breathing is critical during oral motor examination, intervention, and feeding trials. Regurgitation with aspiration of milk or formula into the lungs may occur during feeding trials, with complications of pneumonia, cardiopulmonary arrest, and associated asphyxia. Because of these risks, feeding trials should not be attempted by neonatal therapists untrained in managing the respiratory and general physiological monitoring components of neonatal feeding.

ASSESSMENT IN EARLY INTERVENTION

Assessments in the infant at every stage are carried out with a certain purpose. It can be to determine whether the infant is adequate for gestational age, to determine and track the neurodevelopmental outcomes in an infant across the first two years of life (sometimes in response to specific care-giving strategies), to determine or predict a risk for neurodevelopmental abnormalities and for referral for therapy, for assessment of processing of various sensory systems, etc.

Many of the measures fall short on predictive validity as the status of the infant may change based on various other systemic health conditions and also based on the quality of care giving. As the infant reaches 6 months of age, the ability of a scale to determine prognosis becomes more possible.

Following is a list of the various assessments, each one of which is carried out with a specific purpose.

- **Pain assessment**: The following tools have been identified as part of the Neonatal Individualized Developmental Care and Assessment Program (NIDCAP) as signs of excessive stimulation and stress in the preterm infant.
  - The Premature Infant Pain Profile (PIPP)
  - The face, legs, activity, cry, and consolability behavioral tool (FLACC)
  - The neonatal pain, agitation, and sedation scale (N-PASS).
- **To determine the gestational age** as per physical and neurological signs:
  - A method for clinical assessment of gestational age in the newborn infant was developed by **Dubowitz** and colleagues from data derived from a total of 167 preterm and term infants (28 to 42 weeks' gestation) tested within 5 days of birth. The tool focuses on criteria for calculation of gestational age from a composite of 10 neurological and 11 external (physical) characteristics. This test rates criteria on a 4-point scale; it is commonly administered by nurses or physicians in the newborn nursery.
  - **Newborn maturity rating—Ballard score:** Ballard and colleagues designed a simplified modification of the Dubowitz gestational age tool. It has been widely adopted because of the time efficiency (3 to 4 minutes versus 10 to 15 minutes) and the elimination of active tone items, which are difficult to evaluate reliably in physiologically unstable newborns. The Ballard instrument involves only six physical and six neurological criteria, with a 0 to 5 scale and a maturity rating. It is designed to be used for neonates (20 to 44 weeks gestation) from birth through 3 days of age and has demonstrated concurrent validity with the Dubowitz gestational age calculation tool.
- **The neurological examination of the full-term infant was designed by Prechtl** to identify abnormal neurological signs in the newborn period. Significant findings from the examination are summarized in the following categories:
  - Quality of posture, spontaneous movement, and muscle tone (consistency and resistance to passive movement)

- Presence of involuntary or pathological movements (clonus, tremor, athetoid postures or movements)
- Behavioral state changes and quality of cry
- Threshold or intensity of responses to stimulation.

(Because of the transient pattern of neurological signs and rapid changes in the developing nervous system, Prechtl advised repeated examinations to monitor neurological status.)

- **Prechtl's general movement (GM) assessment:** During the neonatal period through 1 to 2 months after term (40 weeks of gestation), clinical signs suggestive of neuromotor abnormality including stiff, jerky movements or a paucity of movement may be observed.
- **Neonatal Behavioral Assessment Scale (NBAS):** To document individual behavioral and motor differences in infants at term gestation to 2 months of age. Four dimensions of new bornbehavior are analyzed in NBAS:
  - Interactive ability
  - Motor behavior
  - Behavioral state organization
  - Physiological organization.
- **The neurological assessment of the preterm and full-term newborn infant** is a streamlined neurological and neurobehavioral assessment to provide both a systematic and quick newborn examination applicable to infants born preterm or at term gestation and a longer infant examination for children up to 24 months of age. The test can be performed with relatively less training. The test includes the six behavioral state categories of NBAS and seven orientation and behavior items scored on a 5-point grading scale and sequenced according to the intensity of response.
- **Assessment of preterm infants' behavior (APIB):** Als et al. designed the APIB to structure a comprehensive observation of a preterm infant's autonomic, adaptive, and interactive responses to graded handling and environmental stimuli. It involves six maneuvers with increasingly challenging and complex interactions with a highly structured format.
- **Individualized Developmental Care Assessment Program (NIDCAP):** Als and colleagues developed NIDCAP to document the effects of caregiving environment on neurobehavioral stability of neonates. This naturalistic observation protocol includes continuous observation and documentation at 2-minute intervals of an infant's behavioral state and autonomic, motor, and attention signals, with simultaneous recording of vital signs and oxygen saturation.
- **Test of infant motor performance:** Developed by Campbell and colleagues, the 42-item Test of Infant Motor Performance (TIMP) is focused on evaluating postural control, spontaneous movement, and head control **for neonates at 32 weeks of gestation to 16 weeks postterm,** assessed through observation of infant movement and through responses to various body positions and to visual or auditory stimuli.
- **Infant Neurological International Battery (INFANIB):** The Infant neurological international battery (INFANIB) is an observational scale used to assess the neuromotor status of neonates and infants aged 1 to 18 months. It consists of 5 factors: Spasticity, vestibular functions, head and trunk, French angles and legs.
  It can be used for referral for early intervention and for monitoring.
- **Alberta infant motor scale (AIMS):** The AIMS was designed to evaluate gross motor function in infants from birth to independent walking, or birth through 18 months. The stated purposes of the AIMS are:
  - To identify infants who are delayed or deviant in motor development
  - To evaluate motor maturation over time.

  The AIMS is described as an "observational assessment" that requires minimal handling of the infant by the examiner. The test includes 58 items, organized by the infant's position, designed to evaluate three aspects of motor performance: weight bearing, posture, and antigravity movements.
- **The movement assessment of children:** The Movement Assessment of Children (MAC) assesses functional gross motor and fine motor skills of children from age 2 to 24 months. The motor assessment is composed of three sections including head control, upper extremities and hands, and pelvis and lower extremities. In addition, there are four assessment sections (general observations, special senses, primitive reactions, and muscle tone) that contribute to the interpretation of MAC findings for any one child.
- **Bayley scales of infant and toddler development (BSID):** The 4th edition of the BSID (BSID-III), published in 2019, is the most recent update.

  BSID 4 has the following number of items:
  - Cognitive scale: 81 items
  - Language scale: 42 items in the receptive and 37 items in the expressive domain
  - Motor scale: 46 items in the fine motor and 58 items in the gross motor domain
  - Social-emotional scale is unmodified from Bayley III

  The adaptive behavior scale utilizes the Vineland behavior assessment system.

  BSID helps in the following ways:
  - Early identification of intellectual delay. Re-assessments can help to monitor progress over time.
  - To individualize the management and to accommodate a child's developmental and learning needs.
  - To assess individual domains of development: For example, cognitive delay.
  - To help researchers as a research tool.

  BSID III and BSID-4 are used for the age group starting from 16 days to 42 months.
- **Tests for assessing sensory processing:**
  - **Infant toddler sensory profile** is used with infants and toddlers from birth to 36 months of age and enables professionals to gather information about the child's sensory processing abilities, and evaluate how those patterns either support or interfere with functional

performance, as reported by the caregiver. The primary features of this model include the consideration of a person's neurological threshold (i.e., reactivity/ responsivity), self-regulation strategies (behavioral response), and the interaction among thresholds and responding strategies thus illustrating the four basic patterns of sensory responsiveness including low registration (high neurological threshold and passive self-regulation strategy), sensation seeking (high neurological threshold and an active self-regulation strategy), sensory sensitivity (low neurological threshold and passive self-regulation strategy), and sensation avoiding (low neurological threshold and active self-regulation strategy). Items are grouped into six sensory sections: general processing, auditory processing, visual processing, tactile processing, vestibular processing, and oral sensory processing.

- **The test of sensory function in infants** primarily measures sensory defensive behaviors (e.g., avoidance behaviors and sensitivity to stimuli) between the ages of 4 months and 18 months. The test focuses on evaluation of tactile deep pressure, visual tactile integration, vestibular functions, and ocular motor control.
- **The sensory rating scale** is a parent report measure that is used to identify and quantify sensory responsiveness in children 0 to 3 years of age. The items included in the Sensory Rating Scale are: touch, movement and gravity, hearing, vision, taste and smell, and temperament and sensitivity.

- **Tests for congenital dislocation of hip:** Barlow and Ortolani Tests: Barlow test is done by gently adducting the hip while palpating for the head of femur falling out the back of the acetabulum and that no posterior directed force be applied. Ortolani test involves stabilizing the pelvis by holding the contralateral hip and using hand to gently abduct the hip being tested while exerting upward force through the greater trochanter on the lateral side. The perception of a palpable click indicates a positive Ortolani sign and represents reduction ofdislocated hip.
- **Tests for congenital talipes equinovarus:** There are several clubfoot classification systems like Ponseti and Smoley, Manes et al., Harrold and Walker, Catterall, Dimelgo clubfoot. Golden and Fitch. The most frequently used are the ones by Dimelgo et al., and the Pirani Score.

Based on the assessments done over time, the prediction of the neurodevelopmental status is attempted and referral for therapy is done when indicated.

Parent education is extremely important and special efforts should be taken to empower parents as primary caregivers in order to bridge the gap created by the separation between the parents and the infant due to the NICU stay.

NORMAL DEVELOPMENT

As the system is subjected to experiences, there is more precise selection of postural and peripheral movement patterns that turn out to be safe, efficacious and energy efficient and hence get strengthened.

The entire description of Normal development through each domain is beyond the scope of the chapter. Hence, the text pertaining to normal development has been restricted to explanation of the biomechanical sequence of certain events and the relationship between different domains of development. Readers are requested to refer to Normal Development of Functional Motor Skills, First Year of Life by Alexander et al. and Illingworth, The Normal Child.

0–4 Months

At birth, the normally developing full term neonate is found have an attitude of physiological flexion **(Box 25.3 and Fig. 25.2)**. This position is formed as the size and weight of the baby increase in the uterus and the uterine contours hold themselves around the body of the baby in a circle of containment. It is a position where the head and the limbs are closely in contact with each other and the baby receives a warm hug from all sides. The movements performed in the uterus supported by the amniotic fluid and then by the uterine walls are responsible for the gradual development of the active tone and the position creates shortening of certain muscle groups that elongate over the course of extrauterine development.

There are certain biomechanical events that unfold as the baby learns to raise the head up **(Figs. 25.3A and B)** against gravity:

- Elongation of the short muscles is needed for the alignment to be achieved and then for the activation of muscles. Unless the muscles have a minimum essential length, they cannot activate.
- In supine, the baby performs random movements of the upper limbs in the gravity eliminated plane largely, which help open out the anterior chest wall.

Box 25.3: Physiological flexion of the body of a newborn infant is characterized by the features like.

- C shape of the spine
- Elevated scapulae
- Internal rotation and adduction at the glenohumeral joints
- Elbow flexion
- Pronation
- Fisted hands
- Hips and knees in flexion
- Dorsiflexion

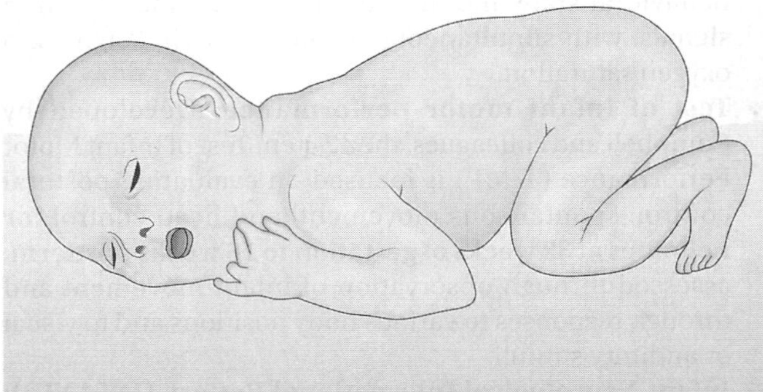

Fig. 25.2: Full-term neonate assuming a flexion attitude in prone.

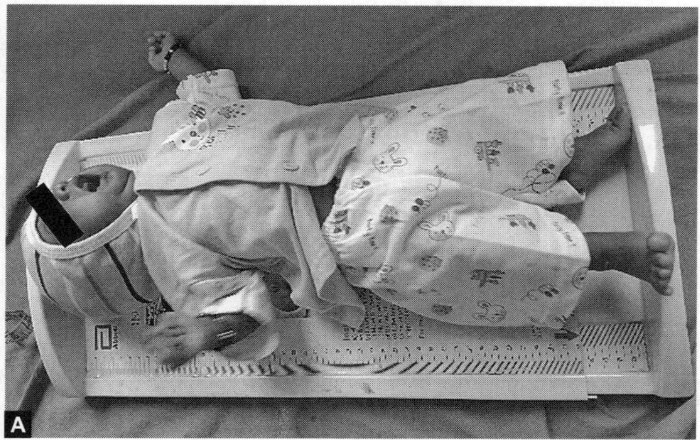

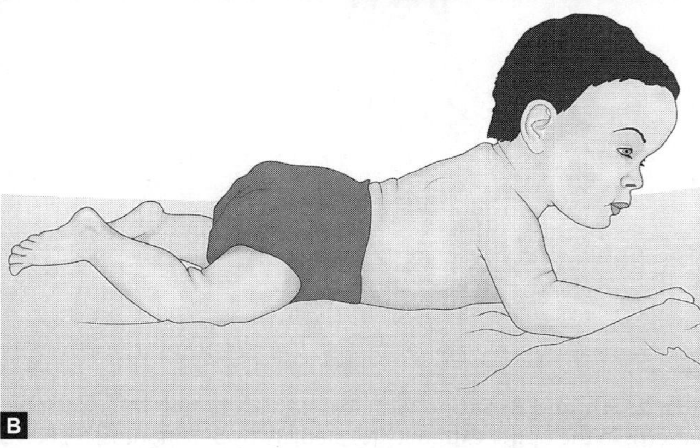

Figs. 25.3A and B: (A) Neonate in supine with horizontal arm movements facilitating anterior chest wall mobility; (B) Three-month-old infant extending upper body on forearms.

- These movements help elongate the pectorals thus allowing the descent of the ribcage which is in an elevated position in a newborn infant.
- In prone, the child pushes on the forearms (in response to visual vertical).
- This is an important phase where the ribcage that is slowly increasing in its mobility enjoys more freedom and as a consequence there is release or elongation of the muscles that take origin from the ribcage. These mainly include the serratus anterior which is a scapular stabilizer. Once this is elongated, it starts working as a couple along with the middle lower trapezius to bring the scapulae down from the elevated position as observed in physiological flexion to the more appropriate anatomical position.
- As the scapulae descend, the posterior cervical muscles (capital and cervical extensors) get elongated. With elongation, comes the ability to get activated. This facilitates the upward movement of the head against gravity from prone.

In the fine motor domain:

- The child progresses from stereotypical synergies to better voluntary dissociation between the shoulder and hand.
- An anticipatory grasp is an important event because it gives evidence of the child being able to form a motor plan in response to the visual image of the specific object being approached and this develops by 3–4 months.

Fine Motor and Gross Motor Connection

- As the child comes up on forearms, it shifts from side to side.
- While the coming up on forearms from the initial physiological flexion position involves movement of forearms from pronation to supination, the weight shifts in the frontal plane in prone involve shifting between pronation and supination. This increases the mobility within the forearm.
- This also helps hand opening and formation of palmar arches. As the weight shifts laterally the weight comes on the ulnar border of the hand and an arch is functionally created. The intrinsics of hand develop in this process of weight shifts.

Visual Contribution to Reach and Grasp

- The gaze of a newborn infant is first on the periphery of objects and later settles in the center by 1–2 months.
- Gaze fixation and optic righting reaction develop along the 1st and 2nd months.
- As head gets stabilized by 3 months with better coactivation of the cervical muscles, gaze stabilization improves.
- Smooth pursuits also improve by 3–4 months and can get controlled gradually.
- As gaze stabilization and convergent gaze improve, the infant is able to localize the object in terms of distance and also able to judge the 3-dimensional form of the object. This facilitates creation of anticipatory grasp and the selection and execution of motor plan for reach become better refined.

Relationship between Ribcage Mechanics, Gross Motor Function and the Oromotor System

As described earlier, the ribcage dynamics play an extremely important role in allowing the scapulae to be mobile and this in turn allows elongation of the cervical muscles and the resultant head holding. The oromotor system is also largely dependent on the ribcage, its position and mobility. As the ribcage descends, with more spinal extension developing in supine and in prone, the diaphragm develops a better-defined dome shape and the intercostals become prepared to support the ribcage. The infrahyoids are the muscles that take their origin from the sternum and along with suprahyoids control the alignment of the hyoid bone. Abnormal ribcage mechanics including an inability of the ribcage to descend can cause the hyoid bone to be unstable which in turn will fail to provide anchorage to the muscles connecting the hyoid bone with the jaw (mylohyoid, geniohyoid), with the tongue (hyoglossus), with the skull (stylohyoid) and the scapula (omohyoid).

If we try to integrate these links, one can surmise the possible contribution of altered mechanics of ribcage towards the disarticulation and feeding problems in children with neuromotor disorders. Some texts on normal development and on cerebral palsy give elaborate description of the way a child with quadriplegic cerebral palsy uses their tongue in peculiar fashion to pull the head into extension and also to keep the hyoid bone from impinging on the surrounding structures. One can also see the possibility that the children with altered ribcage mechanics may be dependent on their accessory muscles for movement of the ribcage and may use the reverse insertion pattern by pushing the neck into extension.

Cognition-Communication-Motivation-Learning

- Learns to expect a response and expresses surprise, joy, relief through a social smile.
- One sees the emergence of the cause effect associations reflected in repetition of effort, shaking of rattles, movements performed to see water splashed by 4 months.
- There is eye contact and mimicking of expressions.
- Development of the cognitive domains like attention (focus, disengagement and enhancement), perceptual abilities (body image and schema development, visual form and spatial perception), learning and memory formation ability are dependent on the optimal arousability nurtured during the early postnatal period.

5–8 Months

In this phase the infant is able to push on hands in prone to ascend upwards. This phase is mainly characterized by the shift of body weight towards the lower lumbar spine in prone and the sensory motor maturation of the lower body segments. There is elongation of the hamstrings, iliopsoas, rectus abdominus muscles and better activation of glutei. This phase also helps in reduction of the anteversion of the femoral head thus increasing the distance between the fulcrum of the hip joint and the lateral trochanter, creating a mechanical advantage for the hip abductors, essential for weight acceptance in the future.

While every new position is attained by the child, there is movement first in the sagittal plane, followed by lateral weight shifts in the frontal plane and finally movements in the transverse plane involving rotations and diagonal weight shifts **(Figs. 25.4A and B)**.

In the oromotor domain: The infant achieves the important feeding function of munching which requires selective lateral jaw movements and lateral and later diagonal movements of the tongue within the mouth. Thus, there is development of selective control of the jaw and the tongue with better stability versus mobility balance. In the speech domain this reflects as emergence of babbling or pronunciation of consonants using lip closure and tongue movements.

9–12 Months

The dynamic sitting balance develops during this phase. The child unknowingly engages the feet in its associated reactions while engaging in play in sitting and this prepares the feet for weight bearing in terms of the intrinsic activity and proprioceptive awareness.

The rotations or transverse plane weight shifts that develop during this period make the child explore the space behind. This in itself is an important event as this makes the child aware of there being a world other than the one that is immediately visible. This becomes a stepping stone to the further development of imagery skills, anticipation and a sense of continuity between the experienced and the imagined.

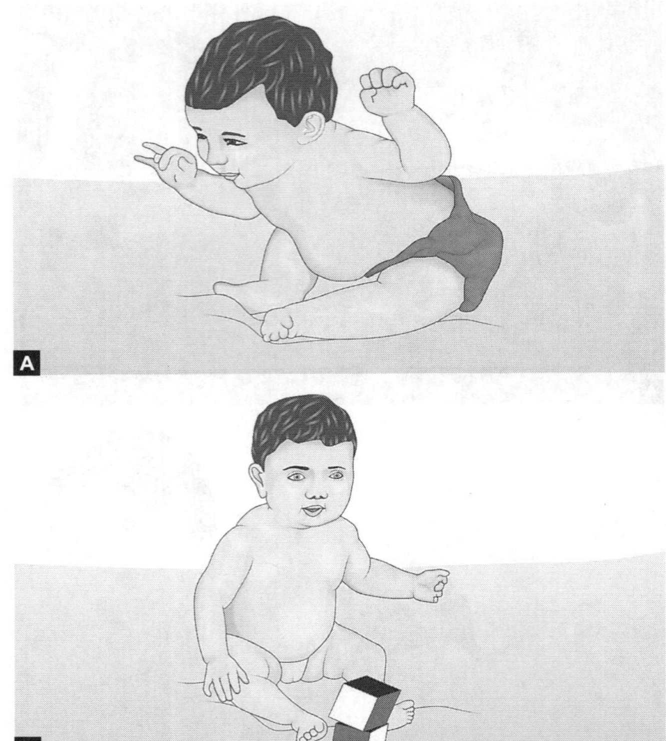

Figs. 25.4A and B: Sitting with less pelvic control: (A) associated patterns in the upper extremity for stability by 5–6 months; (B) Pelvis becomes more stable through co-activation by 7–8 months.

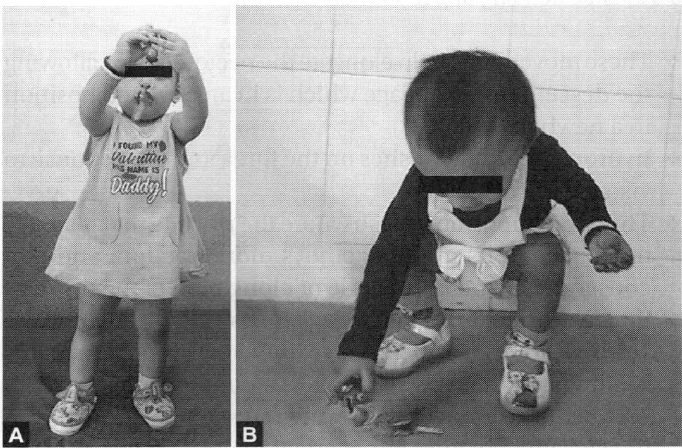

Figs. 25.5A and B: Playing with both hands.

Pulling to stand progresses to pushing to stand. There is greater duration of standing and gradual weight acceptance on feet. The infant starts cruising with lateral weight shifts by 11 months. Playing with options while performing supported standing, the child learns to step, turn and gradually starts walking **(Figs. 25.5 and 25.6)**.

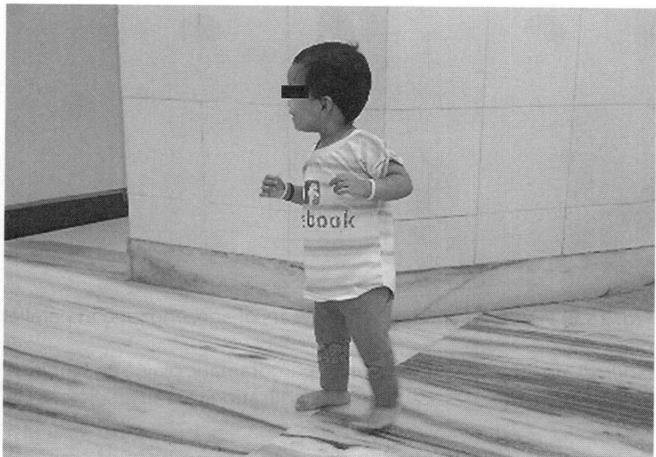

Fig. 25.6: Standing.

As the upper limbs get less involved in postural stability, they can be used for exploration of objects in different ways. Pincer grasp and its variations develop by around 9 months of age **(Figs. 25.7A and B)**.

Early walking involves taking steps with minimal support (wide base of support, high guard posture, medial weight bearing, spine held in a rigid posture).

Independent walking evolves from the high guard posture with anterior tilt of pelvis, excessive lordosis, wide base of support to a more neutral spine and pelvis, dissociation between pelvis and femur in the transverse plane and use of hands for holding objects while walking.

- Child starts speaking meaningful monosyllables and then bisyllables to express needs by 12–14 months which evolve in quality and grow in number.
- Child develops object permanence by 9–10 months
- Develops stranger anxiety around the same time as now has the concept of safe and unsafe (based on memories)

The development of Play across toddlerhood and childhood has been briefly explained in a later section of the chapter.

PLAY THEORIES ASSOCIATED WITH DEVELOPMENT

Though play is perceived as an activity that comes into being through a medium and has a certain form, play is essentially an experience and there are some features that may be identified as the lowest common denominators across all types of play.

- Play involves being engaged with the moment with a sense of complete immersion. It brings a sense of curiosity, happiness and a feeling of being connected with abundance and hence the person voluntarily seeks the play experience.
- Play involves imagination and a feeling of assuming an alternate reality to be the truth, and being able to suspend every other assumed reality.
- It is now understood that the playfulness and an ability to play starts very early in infanthood and according to some theorists in the intrauterine life itself.

The ability to be playful demands that the individual engages in a process of discovering a potential connection across elements, gets curious about the experience and builds on it. A play situation if created with sensitive understanding of the needs of the child with the kind of material which creates balance between stimulating the imagery and modulating the sensory inputs can be therapeutic and can help achieve the very states of arousal and attention upon which further play can be built.

Anita Bundy in her text on playfulness, explained the features of play to be Intrinsic Motivation, Internal Control, Freedom to suspend reality and Framing. From her literature one can understand that as a care giver or a therapist, it is essential to provide material or opportunities to the child to explore the play possibilities. It may be necessary for the adult to initiate play for the child, but thereafter the child needs to take over and discover the narrative that is unique to the child and to the moment. Too much emphasis on a predetermined process may defeat the very purpose of play which is discovery, fun and happiness.

To evaluate a child's playfulness, Anita Bundy developed the Test of Playfulness (ToP). The ToP is an observational

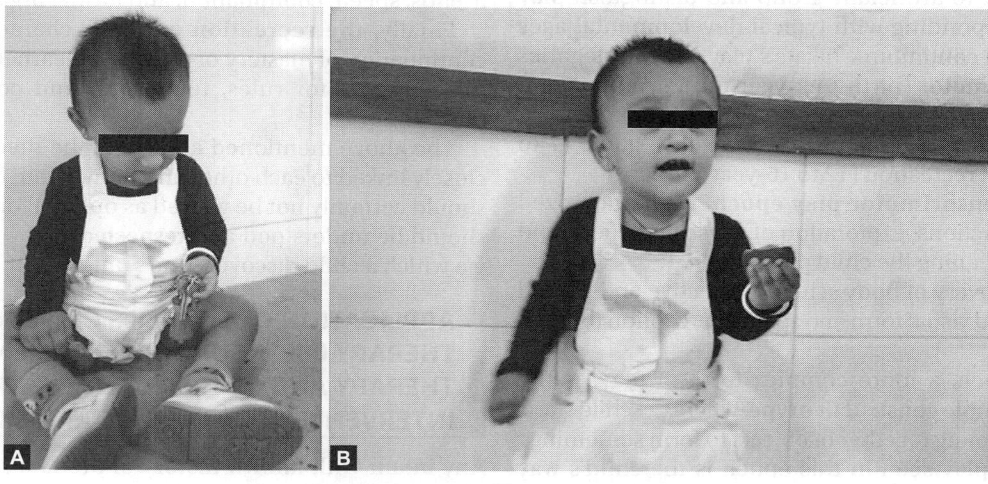

Figs. 25.7A and B: Fine motor activities.

assessment tool for children 6-months to 18-year-old, which consists of 29 items, and is used to assess intrinsic motivation, internal control, freedom to suspend reality, and the transaction being framed.

Neurodramatic play: Sue Jennings in her book ' Healthy Attachments and Neurodramatic Play' explains the essential playfulness that exists or should exist between the mother and her child that is still in the uterus and through the first 6 months of life. Neurodramatic play is the use of sensory play, rhythmic play and dramatic play between the baby and the primary care giver, mostly the mother. Sensory play creates a sense of containment boundaries through which the baby gradually develops a sense of body schema awareness and an ability to initiate movements within a space which is felt as safe. There is self-efficacy developed as a result of this experience. This is referred to as the 'Theatre of Containment'.

Rhythm is a way of life and the baby while in the uterus experiences it in the form of mother's heart beats as well as the rocking that it receives due to the heartbeats and also while the mother walks. Rhythm can be used as a circle of predictability which holds the emotional and physical experience together within its constant structure.

Dramatic play is an emotional give and take between the mother and the infant in which the mother takes cues from the infant or talks to the infant assuming that the infant understands. The infant is engaged in this sequence and responds through vocalizations, facial expressions, body movements. The infant anticipates, waits for the response, looks for feedback and feels surprise, curiosity etc. Thus, the infant gets its experience of an emotional journey within a safe space that is referred to as the 'theatre of resilience'.

An extension of the Neurodramatic play into the next phase is called the Embodiment-Projection-Role (EPR) play which is active till 7 years of life according to this theory.

The EPR can be experienced in numerous ways and uniquely by every child. The ways to nurture EPR are slightly beyond the scope of this chapter and students can refer to the text 'Healthy Attachments and Neurodramatic Play' by Sue Jennings for better understanding of this topic.

Another author **Takata developed a series of play epochs** as a way to artificially group and distinguish play activities, corresponding with typical developmental ages and existing on a continuum. Takata's play epoch categories include: sensorimotor (birth to 2-year-old), symbolic and simple constructive (2 to 4-year-old), dramatic, complex constructive, and pre-game (4 to 7-year-old), game (7 to 12-year-old), and recreation (12 to 16-year-old).

Within the **sensorimotor play epoch**, is characterized by repetition of actions, exploration of cause and effect, and solitary play - meaning the child plays alone.

There is discovery of body schema, selective and graded motor control and visual form and spatial perception through this kind of play.

The next epoch, a more complex form of play, is **the symbolic and simple constructive type**, where the child starts imagining the coming together of objects to form something.

The pretend play seen in this epoch is the child's way of chasing a short narrative or dramatic experience with someone by briefly enacting an adult or an animal or using an object to indicate something else.

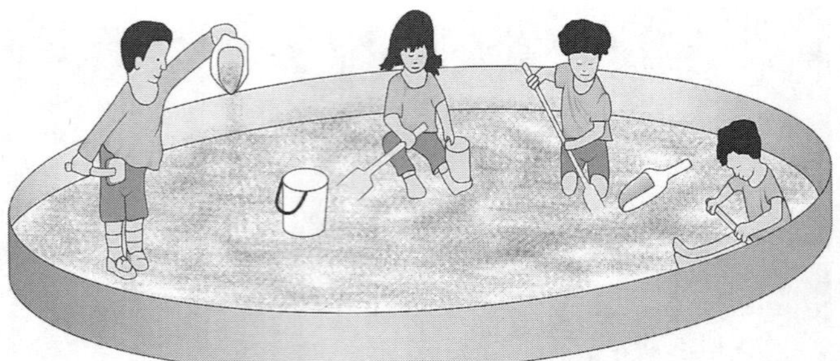

Fig. 25.8: Picture of children, 2 to 4 years of age, engaged in parallel play.
(*Source:* 'Healthy attachments and neurodramatic play', Sue Jennings, Philadelphia, USA, Jessica Kingsley publication; 2014).

The children are not yet in position to imagine a group to be one's extended identity. This experience however in an inchoate stage can be nurtured through echo play with an adult. Here the child either repeats the same activity as the adult or may continue a trail taking cues from the adult.

Children engaged in parallel play are shown in **Figure 25.8**.

Following this play epoch, children enter into **the dramatic, complex constructive (Fig. 25.9) and pre-game epoch, which involves role-playing and reality-based imaginative play**. Other characteristics of this epoch include locomotion, action and novelty, as children participate in associative play, which adds a component of social engagement. In this epoch, the child is able to be part of a group and in every action is knowingly or unknowingly contributing to the group performance. This type of play is cooperative play. This involves tolerance, imagery, understanding the basic rule of things coming together to form an organized whole. This is also reflected in Complex constructional play where the constructions are guided by some theme. The motor coordination and imagery skills improve through this epoch from 4 to 7 years of age.

Proceeding from this epoch is **the game epoch**, in which children are interested in games with rules, cooperating with friends, speed, coordination, and formal organizations.

Finally**, the recreation epoch** is characterized by the continuation of mastery of previously learned skills through play, respect for rules, teamwork, and competitiveness (Takata, 1974).

The above mentioned are few of the theories which are closely linked to each other and derive from each other. Play should certainly not be viewed as optional or peripheral but should be understood and respected as the very substance via which a child discovers one's unique self.

APPLICATION OF SCHOOLS OF NEUROPHYSIO THERAPY LIKE NEURODEVELOPMENTAL THERAPY AND SENSORY INTEGRATION IN EARLY INTERVENTION OF INFANTS AT RISK

Any infant with known history of prenatal, perinatal and/ or postnatal risk factors including prematurity needs to be

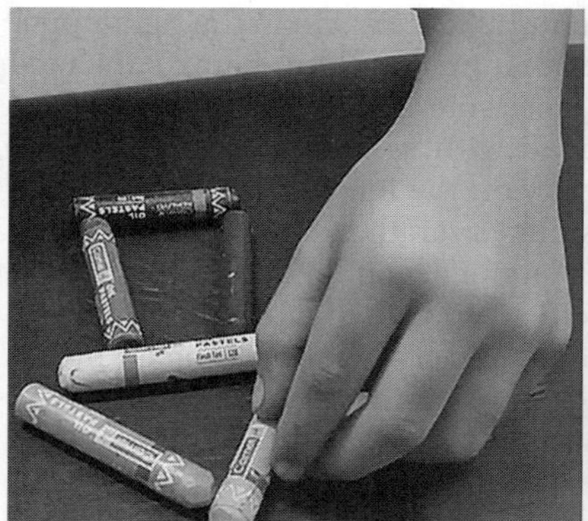
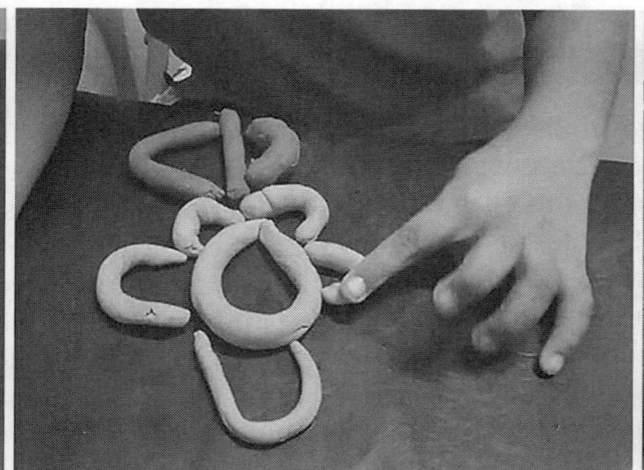
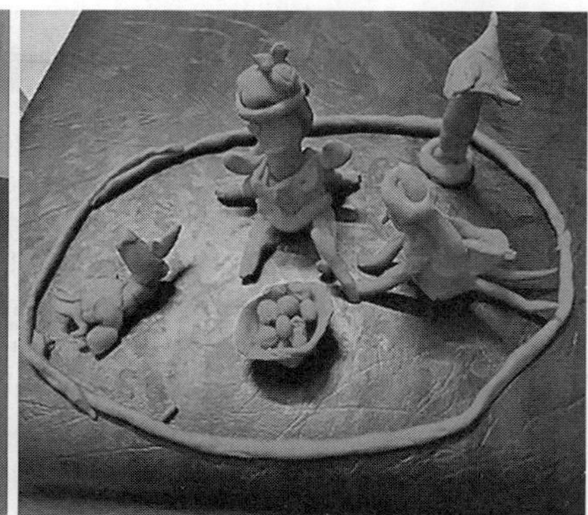

Fig. 25.9: A stage between simple to complex constructional play.

closely monitored throughout the infanthood as well as through early childhood for the motor function, sensory-behavioral profile and cognitive function. Infants are accordingly referred for the appropriate therapy discipline like Physiotherapy, Occupational therapy, Speech therapy or for remedial and special education support.

Neurodevelopmental therapy (NDT) is a holistic and interdisciplinary clinical practice model informed by current and evolving research that emphasizes individualized therapeutic handling based on movement analysis for habilitation and rehabilitation of individuals with neurological pathophysiology. Though NDT is commonly viewed as a Neurotherapeutic skill aimed at facilitation of neuro-motor function, which it is, it is a holistic discipline that derives from the International Classification of Function for its Assessment and employs a rigorous process of identifying the specific impairments that impede the attainment of a certain functional ability that is most relevant to the participation need of the individual. This helps the therapist prioritize relevant integrities and impairments as a basis for establishing achievable outcomes with clients and caregivers. In early intervention using NDT, the therapist will thoroughly observe the posture, responsiveness and self-initiated movements of the infant. She will identify the abnormal movements and will try to determine the reasons for the same, e.g., the internal or external triggers that activate the dystonic posture or the sensory inputs that cause the infant to go into an opisthotonic posture and also the cues that help modulate tone and allow the infant to feel integrated and initiate a purposeful movement. There is an identification of multisystem and single system impairments wherein the observable impairments in muscle tone, postural alignment, weight shifts, base of support are first determined and then each impairment is analyzed for the contribution coming from the neuromotor, musculoskeletal, sensory, gastrointestinal, respiratory systems, etc.

Thereafter, goals are identified for the infant using the SMART criteria (specific, measurable, attainable, relevant and time bound). The goal is then task analyzed and there is again a reverse engineering process deployed, wherein the impairments that create barriers in attainment of the goal get enlisted based on the task analysis. Treatment is then designed and implemented for attainment of goals by using preparatory strategies like rib cage mobilization, elongation, preparation of the weight bearing surfaces, etc., then by using Simulating activities where the goal as a whole or in parts is simulated in the exercise or in the play activity and finally by practice of the actual functional goal keeping in mind the principles of motor learning. There is also the very essential carryover of therapy which is implemented as a home program by the primary caregiver and by the family at large.

Sensory issues in infants, especially in preterm infants and also the full-term infants who have suffered an insult to the developing brain exists due to either the inadequate maturation of the sensory systems or inappropriate connections that are formed due to the infant having been exposed to certain stimuli. These may present as Sensory Modulation disorders (low registration, overresponsive or seeking) and/or may manifest as planning disorders (dyspraxias like somatodyspraxia or bilateral integration and sequencing problems) or processing problems associated with specific sensory systems like visual perception, auditory perception etc., or a combination of the above. **Sensory integration** as a therapy discipline incorporates a thorough assessment of all the sensory systems and their interaction in the context of age-appropriate activities. Assessment measures like the Sensory Profiles and the Sensory Integration and Praxis Test are used to qualitatively describe as well as Quantify the impairment. Based on these and a few other assessments (some of them carried out informally while the therapy takes shape), therapy is gradually built up. Many activities and equipment are chosen based on the systems that need modulation and those that need enhanced input to create a sensory ambience in which the specific skill is trained in the child. Sensory integration therapy starts as early as in the NICU and continues till infanthood and childhood. Essential part of the therapy is parent and teacher education as they need to carry over the training atmosphere into spaces and across spaces which the child inhabits through most of the day.

The application of NDT and SI in early intervention is described in the clinical example.

Summary

Early intervention in an infant involves understanding of the natural process of maturation of each system including the central nervous system and its constant reorganization in response to environmental inputs. In order to formulate the strategies of early intervention, it is necessary to identify all the factors biological and environmental that facilitate or impede the organized development of the infant as a platform for acquisition of skills in various domains as a toddler and then as a child. As a therapist, it is important to educate the caregivers about all those neuroprotective and nurturing inputs that can be created within the immediate environment and to keep monitoring the development using standardized measures which are valid predictors of neurodevelopmental outcomes. In case of a delay in acquisition of skills or detection of abnormal neurobehavioral profile, it is necessary to form a thorough functional physical therapy diagnosis and to uphold an interdisciplinary approach to ensure that the appropriate remedies are made available to the infant at the right age. A disciplined attitude and diligent execution of strategies can help minimize the impact of the biological and environmental risk factors and maximize the opportunities for skill development.

CLINICAL EXAMPLE

Presently 18 months of age, Baby R was born full term through vaginal delivery. The **significant aspects of his history** were: prolonged second stage of labor and perinatal asphyxia with Intermittent Positive Pressure Ventilation for 5 minutes, ventilation started on Day 1 and extubation on the day 16 of life followed by Continuous Positive Pressure ventilation and exogenous oxygen, APGAR score was 1 at 1 minute, 5 at 5 minutes and 7 at 10 minutes, weight of 2,900 grams at birth, convulsions within the first 6 hours of birth. He was diagnosed with Sarnat grading of Hypoxic Ischemic Encephalopathy as Grade II towards III. EEG indicated severe diffuse Encephalopathy and USG skull revealed Periventricular Leukomalacia Grade 4. He was discharged on the 22nd day of life with anticonvulsants and vitamins and other nutritional supplements.

The **parents were educated** by the NICU personnel and the physiotherapist about the positioning of Baby R for facilitation of midline activity and hand to mouth activity in flexion of the trunk in a car seat or in side-lying and also for feeding of Baby R in a reclined position with a bowl and spoon, monitoring of skin color, respiratory pattern, sleep cycle, any signs of convulsions, the visual inputs and auditory inputs to be provided in the midline and at the eye level or slightly below that for facilitation of convergent gaze and flexion and to avoid the asymmetrical extensor posturing that the baby had demonstrated in the NICU.

From 3 months onwards, there was hypertonia observed in an asymmetrical pattern with extension in the left upper and lower extremities and flexion in the right upper and lower extremities that increased on being subjected to tactile inputs on face, sole of the feet and posterior aspect of trunk or head with associated asymmetry in the trunk with convexity on the left and concavity to the right side with occasional overall extension of the trunk and neck. There was a lateral deviation of eyes to the right upwards and no specific response to auditory inputs, no visual regard to objects in peri-personal space and no indication of recognition of mother. The INFANIB score of the baby at 3 months was 48 indicating abnormality in neurodevelopment.

In physiotherapy, the therapy **goals focuszed on** improving symmetrical coactivation of postural muscles from prone and subsequently in sitting, improving visual regard for objects with an ability to use eyes for exploration and an ability to unilaterally and bilaterally reach and explore objects in supported sitting in the peripersonal space with simultaneous activations in the postural muscles for stability.

While applying the principles of NDT and SI, preparatory strategy was gentle **rib cage mobilization** to facilitated elongation and alignment of the ribcage for better alignment of the primary muscles of inspiration and of the core muscles that take origin from the rib cage. Baby R was treated on an inclined surface on the right side with graded inputs into the right hip to **facilitate active elongation** and turning towards the right side. He was facilitated to bear weight on the right forearm making use of the movable surface of the vestibular ball in small amplitudes to increase proprioceptive awareness and the resultant pushing on the right side. Baby R was subjected to **visual inputs** with enhanced contrast placed in the central eye field for convergent gaze in a reclined position on the arc of a ball with support at the rib cage. He was also subjected to **auditory inputs** to which he responded by raising the upper extremity towards flexion with an open hand and occasional grasp without an obvious visual fixation. To improve function in the **oromotor domain**, the baby was given oral support below the lower lip and under the chin in a 2-finger support fashion to grade the opening and closure of jaw, to facilitate lip closure and to stimulate the tongue movement for facilitation of oral phase of feeding. This was coupled with graded offering of paste like food in small quantities.

By 9 months, Baby R was able to push on forearms in prone and on hands with facilitation at forearms. He still had asymmetry in the trunk and would pull his pelvis up on the right side. The feet were prepared for weight acceptance. After this he was slowly transitioned to sitting on a stool with feet supported under the knees, with the right forearm supported. This could be progressed to taking weight on the right hand as he elongated the trunk actively to the right and could extend the right elbow. Over the months, the visual regard for objects has improved and there is intermittent movement of eyes within head to track the object in space. Baby R has started reaching to objects more consistently and shifts them into positions purposefully in order to engage in sensory cause effect play. There is constant but moderate cueing in the form of a diagonal input needed from the left ribcage or upper extremity towards the right hip to inhibit the tendency to pull and rotate to the right with an attempt to reach with the left hand.

At 18 months, he can be facilitated to perform transition from sit to stand and vice versa with an anterior support where he responds with a controlled descent and an antero-inferior weight shift in ascent. He has started smiling occasionally and is able to vocalize more often to indicate discomfort and hunger. Baby R needs consistent therapy and the parents continue to follow the advice regarding positioning, oral support and stimulation and graded sensory inputs in the different domain at home.

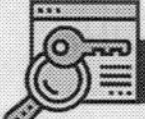

Review Questions

1. Explain the stages of embryological development of central nervous system.
2. Explain the abnormalities that can result from insults to central nervous system in different trimesters of gestation.
3. Explain the possible reasons for cardiopulmonary complications in a preterm infant.
4. Explain the core neuroprotective measures to be employed in the neonatal intensive care unit.
5. Explain the assessments measures applicable for screening of neurodevelopmental abnormalities in an infant.
6. Explain the development of gross motor function in the first 4 months of life of a normally developing infant.
7. Explain the relationship between the various domains of development in the first 4 months of life.
8. Explain the development of dynamic sitting balance in a normally developing infant.
9. Explain in brief the various play theories.
10. An infant born at 28 weeks of gestation is in the NICU currently at day 14 of life. On examination, he is found to show signs of hyperresponsiveness. Explain the assessment and the neuroprotective and nurturing strategies applicable for this infant.

Bibliography

1. Alexander R, Boehme R, Cupps B. Normal Development of Functional Motor Skills—The First Year of Life. University of Virginia, USA: Psychological Corporation; 1993.
2. Altimier L, Phillips R. The Neonatal Integrative Developmental Care Model: Seven Neuroprotective Core Measures for Family-centered Developmental Care. Newborn and Infant Nursing Reviews.
3. Balasundaram P, Avulakuntal. Bayley Scales of Infant and Toddler Development. StatsPearls Publishing, Treasure Island; 2021.
4. Bierman J, Hazzard C, Girolami G, Shiratori T. A guide to NDT Clinical practice: 8 Key Nutrients to support developmental treatment: Chapter 15-'Neuroplasticity and Recovery). New York: Thieme Publishers; 2016.
5. Bundy AC. Play Theory and Sensory Integration. In: Fisher AG, Murray EA, Bundy AC (Eds). Sensory Integration: Theory and Practice. Philadelphia: FA Davies; 1991;48-68.
6. Burton G, Roller M. Neurodevelopmental outcome of high-risk newborns discharged from special care baby units in a rural district in India. J Public Health Res. 2012;4(1):318.
7. Canavese F, Dimeglio A. Clinical examination and classification systems of congenital clubfoot: a narrative review. Ann Transl Med. 2021;9(3):1097.
8. Chambers S, et al. Highly efficient neural conversion of human ES and iPS cells by dual inhibition of SMAD signalling. J Nat Biotech. 2009. 10.1038/nbt.1529.
9. Coonc L, Nurkse S. Using Play to Facilitate Motor Skill Development of Children with Cerebral Palsy in Mexico. Masters Thesis, University of Puget Sound; 2014.
10. Copp A, Greene N. Neural tube defects: Prevention by folic acid and other vitamins. Indian J Pediatr. 2000;67:915-21.
11. Das DS, Bhattacharya DM, Sanyal DD, Basu DS, et al. Growth and neurodevelopment outcome of NICU graduates till 1 year at a tertiary care centre in eastern India and identification of the clinical and electrophysiological predictors of adverse developmental outcome. Pediatric Review. Int J Paediatr Res. 2017;4(2):155-56.
12. Dunn W. Infant/Toddler Sensory Profile. User's Manual. San Antonio, TX: The Psychological Corporation;2002.
13. Eeles A, Spittle A, Anderson P, et al. Assessments of Sensory Processing in Infants: A Systematic Review. Developmental Medicine and Child Neurology Reviews; 2012.
14. Elshazzly M, Lopez MJ, Reddy V, et al. Embryology, Central Nervous System. Treasure Island (FL): StatPearls Publishing; 2022.
15. Glennon TJ. Test of Sensory Functioning In Infants. In: Volkmar FR. (Ed). Encyclopedia of Autism Spectrum Disorders. Springer, New York; 2013.
16. Illingworth R. The Normal Child, 10th edition, Elsevier; 1997.
17. Jennings S. Healthy Attachments and Neurodramatic Play. Philadelphia, USA: Jessica Kingsley Publishers; 2011.
18. Kenner C. McGrath Developmental Care of Newborns and Infants, 3rd edition. National Association of Neonatal Nurses. USA: Walter Kluwers Publication; 2010.
19. Lazaro R, Umphred D. Neonates and Parents: Neurological Rehabilitation (Chapter-Neurodevelopmental Perspectives in the Neonatal Intensive Care Unit and Follow-Up, 6th edition. Missouri, USA, Mosby, Inc., an affiliate of Elsevier Inc. 2013: 283-84.
20. Lee EJ, Lee SY. Environmental impact of the NICU on developmental outcomes. J Pediatr Nurs. 2018;3(5): 279-89.
21. Millichap JG. Neural tube defects. Spina Bifida, Pediatric Neurology Briefs. 1987;1(3):59-60.
22. Novak I, Morgan C, Adde L, et al. Early, accurate diagnosis and early intervention in cerebral palsy. JAMA Pediatr. 2017;171(9):897-907.
23. Pickler R, McGrath J, Reyna B, et al. A model of neurodevelopmental risk and protection for preterm infants. J Perinat Neonatal Nurs. 2010;24(4):356-65.
24. Provost B, Oetter P. The sensory rating scale for infants and young children: Development and reliability. Physical Occupational Therapy in Pediatrics. 1993;13:15-35.

Multiple Choice Questions (MCQs)

To test your understanding and recall of key concepts.

1. **What is the definition of preterm as per the World Health Organization?**
   A. Babies born alive before 28 weeks of pregnancy
   B. Babies born alive between 32 and 37 weeks of pregnancy
   C. Babies born alive before 37 weeks of pregnancy
   D. Babies born alive after 37 weeks of pregnancy
2. **Which sensory system matures last during fetal development?**
   A. Tactile
   B. Auditory
   C. Vestibular
   D. Visual
3. **What role does neuroplasticity play in early childhood development?**
   A. It fixes neuronal connections permanently
   B. It involves long-term changes in synaptic strength in response to stimuli
   C. It reduces the brain's ability to adapt to external stimuli over time
   D. It has no role in sensory development
4. **How does neonatal hydrotherapy benefit preterm infants?**
   A. It promotes musculoskeletal rigidity
   B. It enhances sleep quality and behavioral organization
   C. It disrupts sensory processing for adaptation
   D. It replaces feeding interventions in NICU
5. **The neuroprotective strategy critical to promote healthy sleep cycles in preterm infants is __________.**
   A. Frequent use of bright light therapy
   B. Ensuring loud noise during wake periods
   C. Using spontaneous awake periods for caregiving
   D. Increasing handling frequency regardless of sleep state
6. **If a preterm infant shows feeding difficulties due to hypertonic posturing of the neck, it is most suitable to __________.**
   A. Feed the infant in a fully reclined supine position
   B. Implement oromotor therapy with positioning support
   C. Use gavage feeding indefinitely without oral intervention
   D. Administer sedatives before feeding sessions
7. **The critical vulnerabilities of the preterm brain to hypoxic insults can be attributed to __________.**
   A. Overproduction of cytokines, oxidative stress, and maternal infection
   B. High oxygen saturation, excessive surfactant, and low bilirubin
   C. Advanced pulmonary maturity, reduced neuroplasticity, and hypotonia
   D. Fully developed sensory networks, lack of synaptic pruning, and stable autonomic systems
8. **Delay in ribcage descent could affect an infant's oromotor and feeding capabilities because __________.**
   A. It enhances feeding reflexes and improves nutrient intake
   B. It stabilizes the hyoid bone, enabling better tongue movement
   C. It leads to instability in the hyoid bone, affecting anchorage of feeding muscles
   D. It has no significant impact on feeding mechanics
9. **A 28-week preterm infant shows delayed motor responses and inadequate weight gain despite NICU interventions. Which combined strategies would be most effective?**
   A. Kangaroo care and minimal visual stimulation while continuing gavage feeding
   B. Increased parental involvement, hydrotherapy, and oromotor stimulation 30 minutes before feeding
   C. Early introduction of solid foods and eliminate sleep protection protocols
   D. Replace all neurodevelopmental interventions with pharmacological therapy
10. **A preterm infant diagnosed with periventricular leukomalacia (PVL) shows difficulty integrating sensory stimuli. Which of the following therapeutic approach should be prioritized in this case?**
    A. Intensive visual stimulation and reduced auditory input
    B. Neurodevelopmental therapy with sensory integration focusing on tactile and proprioceptive systems
    C. Strictly environmental sensory deprivation to avoid overloading neural pathways
    D. Advanced cognitive tasks to compensate for sensory deficits

ANSWERS

1. C	2. D	3. B	4. B	5. C
6. B	7. A	8. C	9. B	10. B

Section 5

Cancer in Women

Section Outline

Chapter **26**

Breast Diseases

Shefali Desai, Anshumi Desai

"Seeds of faith are always within us;
Sometimes it takes a crisis....
To nourish and encourage their growth"

—Susan Taylor

LEARNING OBJECTIVES

At the end of the chapter, the reader will be able to:

- Discuss the occurrence, incidence, patterns and trends of breast cancer.
- Understand the modalities and methods to detect breast cancer at an early stage.
- Describe the management and treatment of breast cancer including comprehensive care and team or a multidisciplinary approach.
- Understand the prevention and management of complications.
- Learn about the role of physiotherapy in management of the disease and complications of the disease.

CHAPTER OUTLINE

- Introduction
- Anatomy and physiology of the breast
  - Blood supply and lymph nodes
- Benign breast disease
- Breast cancer
  - Epidemiology of breast cancer
  - Risk factors for occurrence
  - Types or classification of breast cancer
  - Signs and symptoms
  - Diagnosis—triple assessment
  - Staging breast cancer
  - Treatment
- Breast cancer and pregnancy
- Role of a physiotherapist in breast cancer management

INTRODUCTION

The breast is an important organ in women. Breast is a physiologically dynamic structure in which cyclic variations are superimposed on changes of development and involution throughout a woman's life. There are certain conditions which are just physiological changes and not a disease.

Breast diseases can be classified into benign and malignant (cancer). All breast conditions are not cancers. 70–80% of the breast diseases are benign, only 20–30% are malignant.

Cancer is an incessant or uncontrolled growth of abnormal cells, which invades the normal tissue. Cancer develops when normal control mechanisms stop working, resulting in tumors, damage to the immune system and other impairments that can increase the morbidity and mortality.

The incidence of cancers in women is less than in men **(Fig. 26.1)**. The most commonly occurring cancers in woman are:

- Breast
- Gynecological cancers
- Colorectal
- Lungs
- Skin
- Thyroid
- Lymphomas

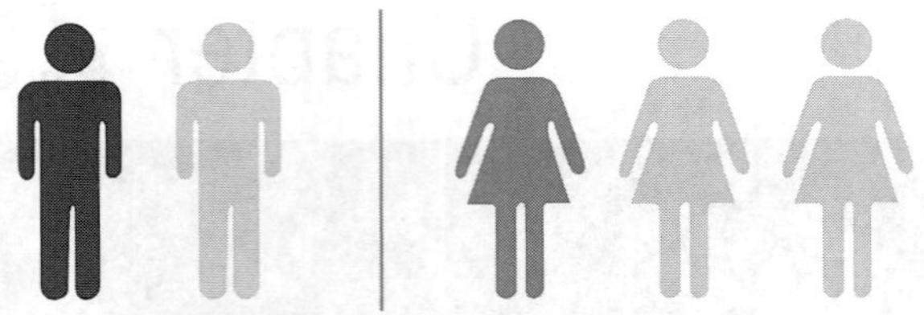

Fig. 26.1: Incidence of cancer.

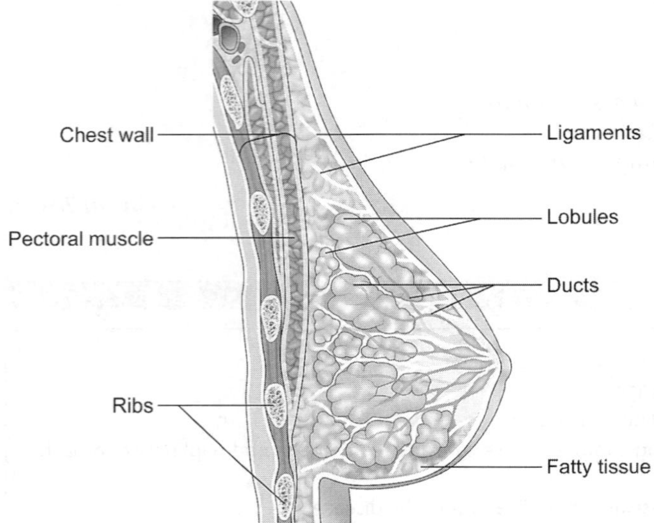

Fig. 26.2: Anatomy of the breast.

Breast cancer has been threatening women, not only of the older age group but younger too! The pattern of occurrence and management of breast cancer has undergone a major paradigm shift. Newer modalities for diagnosis and treatment have emerged in the past few years, which has revolutionized the management of breast cancer. All breast cancers are not the same and today the treatment is TAILORED—it is modified and moulded according to the type of cancer and the needs of the patient. There is no treatment that "Fits for all".

ANATOMY AND PHYSIOLOGY OF THE BREAST

The breast is an organ whose structure reflects its special function: the production of milk for lactation. The breast has 15–20 segments, each of which has lobules, which in turn drain into the ducts, which end up into the nipple **(Figs. 3.8 and 26.2)**. Most cancers of the breast arise from the cells which form the terminal ductal lobule (TDLU). Anatomically, the adult breast lies over the pectoralis muscle, vertically from 2nd to the 6th ribs and horizontally from the edge of the sternum out to the midaxillary line. A tail of breast tissue, called the "axillary tail of Spence", extends into the axillary area. This is important because breast cancer can develop in this axillary tail. The breast tissue is encircled by a fascia. The deep layer of this fascia lies snugly over the pectoralis major muscle, and the superficial layer is just under the skin. The skin covering the breast is same as the skin elsewhere on the body and with similar sweat glands, hair follicles, and other features.

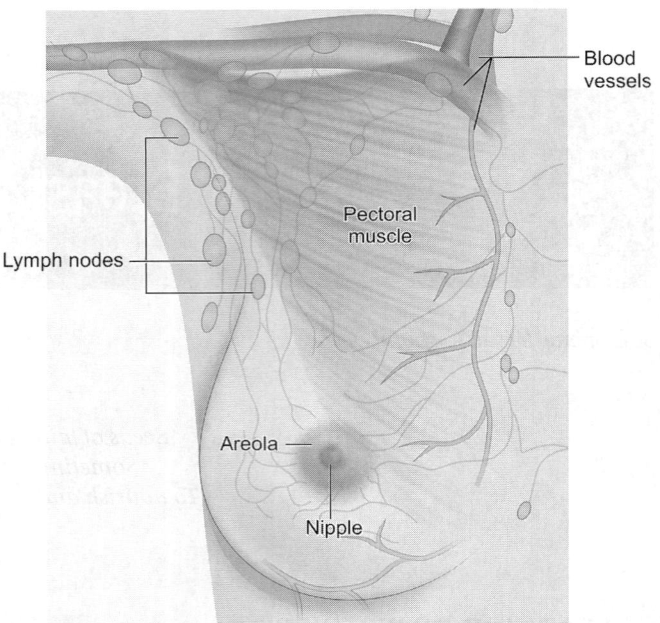

Fig. 26.3: Blood supply and lymphatics.

Blood Supply and Lymph Nodes

The blood supply from the breast comes primarily from the internal mammary artery. The lymphatic vessels of the breast drain into axillary lymph nodes and the internal mammary nodes. It is through these lymphatic vessels that breast cancers metastasize or spread to lymph nodes. The axillary nodes are a group of lymph nodes. Clinically they are divided into Level I, II, III according to their location lateral, behind or medial to the pectoralis minor muscle. The axillary lymph nodes lie in the axilla around the axillary vein and its tributaries and the nerves emerging from the brachial plexus supplying the chest wall and the upper limb **(Fig. 26.3)**.

BENIGN BREAST DISEASE

Benign breast disease (BBD) encompasses a huge gamut of conditions and lesions **(Fig. 26.4 and Table 26.1)**.

Fibrocystic Changes

These are exaggerated physiological changes in which cysts, adenosis and fibrosis are found. It is a variant of the cyclical changes of the breast tissue. It is best treated conservatively with medications, vitamin supplements and with reassurance.

Fibroadenoma

It is the commonest benign tumor in breast occurring commonly in younger women.

- When small, only reassurance is required.
- It has very rare chances of turning into a malignancy hence, conservative approaches are preferred,

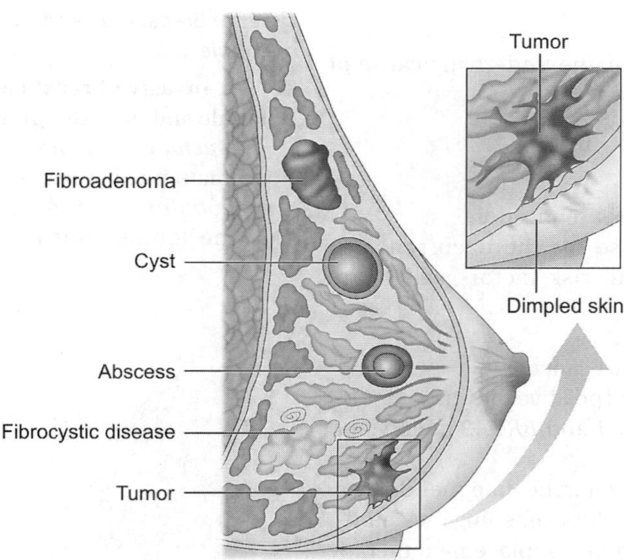

Fig. 26.4: Breast diseases *(For color version, see Plate 7)*.

Table 26.1: Types of benign breast diseases (BBD).

Common BBD	Fibrocystic changes	Fibroadenoma	Cyst	Phyllodes tumor	Mastitis	Abscess
Less common BBD	Hamartoma	Radial scars	Sclerosing adenosis	Fat necrosis	Lipoma	Antibioma galactocele

- Surgery is required if the tumor is larger.
  - Minimally invasive surgery: Vacuum assisted extraction by vacuum assisted breast biopsy (VABB) system can be done in lesions up to 2.5–2.8 cm.
  - If larger removal by surgery with a cosmetic incision is done.

Cyst

Cysts are fluid-filled tumors. They are classified as:
- Simple
- Complicated
- Complex

Cysts could be single or multiple. They are treated conservatively or by aspiration if large and symptomatic. If complex and with a solid component, the cyst should be biopsied to rule out malignancy. Cysts need to be operated if they recur after repeated aspirations (up to 2–3 times) or they appear to be complex on imaging or biopsy.

Phyllodes Tumor

It is a tumor of the breast, which is not so common, with a high potential of recurrence and can be benign, borderline or malignant.

Mastitis

Inflammation of the breast can be:
- Acute
- Chronic granulomatous mastitis
- Tuberculosis

Granulomatous mastitis is a terrifying condition for some as it is difficult to treat.

Abscess

Most commonly occurring during lactation due to incorrect feeding habits and incomplete evacuation of the milk. Prevention is the best treatment, but if it occurs, aspiration is the choice of treatment. Surgery is sometimes required.

Others Benign Tumors of Breast

These include, among others:
- Hamartoma
- Radial scars
- Sclerosing adenosis
- Fat necrosis
- Lipoma
- Antibioma
- Galactocele

BREAST CANCER

Epidemiology of Breast Cancer

Breast cancer is the second most common cancer in the world and the commonest cancer amongst women.

Breast cancer has been ranked number one cancer among Indian females with age adjusted rate as high as 25.8 per 100,000 women and mortality 12.7 per 100,000 women. Data reports from various latest national cancer registries were compared for incidence, mortality rates. Mortality-to-incidence ratio was found to be as high as 66 in rural registries whereas as low as 8 in urban registries.

Risk Factors for Occurrence

Most breast cancers are sporadic, the underlying cause of which is a combination of:
- Internal or hormonal exposures
- Lifestyle factors
- Environmental factors
- Normal physiology, such as DNA replication

Since there is no exact cause for the occurrence of breast cancer, there are certain risk factors which are attributed for:
- Age more than 50 years
- Previous history of having breast cancer
- Family history of breast cancer (positive only in 5–10%)
- Genetic predisposition—*BRCA1* and *BRCA2* mainly and other genes
- Hormonal influence—early menarche, late menopause, bearing a child at a late age, not breastfeeding the child
- High estrogen containing hormonal replacement therapy and contraceptive pills
- Dense breasts
- Lifestyle—food, alcohol, radiation exposure at young age.

Types or Classification of Breast Cancer

Breast cancer is not one disease. There are different types and subtypes **(Table 26.2 and Figs. 26.5A and B)**.

Types of Breast Cancer According to Site of Origin, i.e., Duct or Lobule

- **Non-invasive breast cancers:** Restricted to the duct or lobule and not extending beyond it:
  - *Ductal carcinoma in situ (DCIS):* **(Fig. 26.6)**. It is an anatomical precursor of cancer.
  - *Lobular carcinoma in situ (LCIS):* It arises from the lobules but does not invade the surrounding

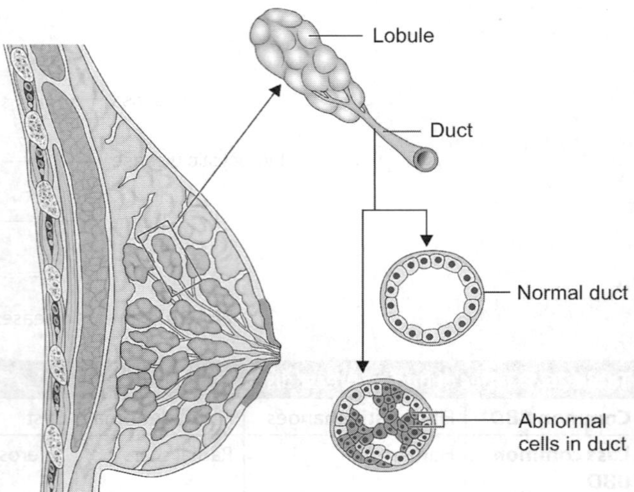

Fig. 26.6: Ductal carcinoma in situ.

Table 26.2: Types of breast cancer.

Site of origin	Ducts	Noninvasive ductal carcinoma in situ (DCIS)	Invasive ductal carcinoma (IDC)
	Lobules	Noninvasive lobular carcinoma in situ (LCIS)	Invasive lobular carcinoma (ILC)
Extent	Early breast cancer (EBC)	Locally advanced breast cancer (LABC)	Metastatic breast cancer (MBC)
Gene expression	Hormone positive breast cancer	HER2Neu positive breast cancer	Triple negative breast cancer (TNBC)

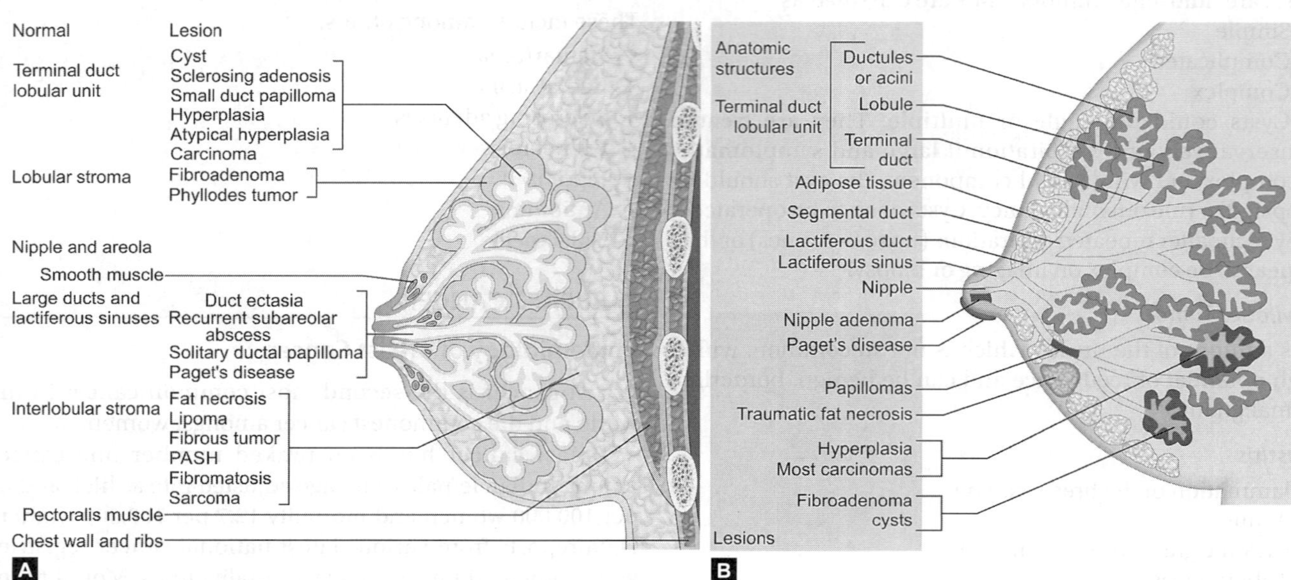

Figs. 26.5A and B: Lesions that are commonly seen according to the breast structure *(For color version, see Plate 7)*.
(PASH: pseudoangiomatous stromal hyperplasia)

breast tissue. It is no longer considered cancer, but precancerous. It is a physiological precursor of cancer.

- **Invasive breast cancers (70–80% of all breast cancers):** Cancer has invaded or spread into surrounding breast tissue.
  - *Not otherwise specified (NOS):* It is the most common type of invasive breast cancer.
  - *Invasive ductal carcinoma (IDC):* It is the commonest type of breast cancer. The cancer spreads beyond the duct lining into the surrounding breast tissue **(Fig. 26.7)**.
  - *Invasive lobular carcinoma (ILC):* ILC is the second commonest breast cancer. The presentation is not a typical lump but more diffuse lesion is found and it could be bilateral.

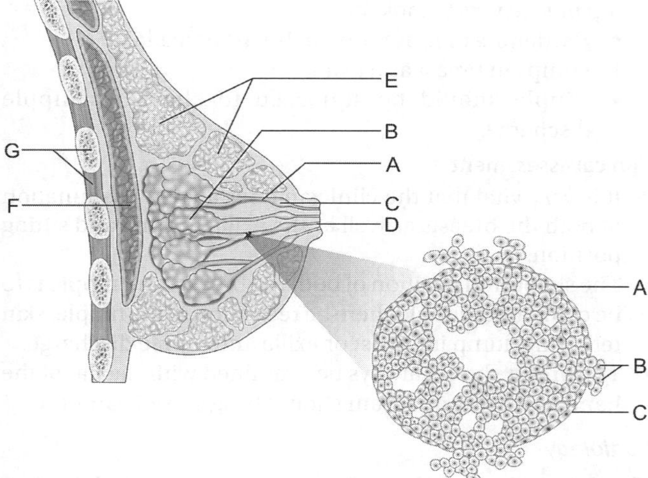

Fig. 26.7: Normal breast with invasive ductal carcinoma (IDC) in an enlarged cross-section of the duct breast profile: (A) Ducts; (B) Lobules; (C) Dilated section of duct to hold milk; (D) Nipple; (E) Fat; (F) Pectoralis major muscle; (G) Chest wall/rib cage) [In enlarged image: (A) Normal duct cell; (B) Ductal cancer cells breaking through the basement membrane; (C) Basement membrane].

Types of Breast Cancers According to the Extent

- **Early breast cancer (EBC):** Cancer which is confined to breast tissue or to axillary lymph nodes (Stage 1 and 2)
- **Locally advanced breast cancer (LABC):** Cancer which has spread to the skin of the breast or chest wall or the tumor is very large (Stage 3)
- **Metastatic breast cancer (MBC):** Cancer which has spread to distant sites (Stage 4).

Subtypes of Breast Cancer

The subtypes of breast cancer are based on the genes a cancer expresses. Breast cancer cells may have receptors (proteins) that hormones—estrogen and progesterone, or a protein called HER2 can attach to and encourage the cells to grow.

- **Hormone receptor positive breast cancer (80%):** About 80% of all breast cancers are "ER-positive." That means the cancer cells grow in response to the hormone estrogen. About 65% of these are also "PR-positive." They grow in response to progesterone. Tumors that are ER/PR-positive are much more likely to respond to hormone therapy than tumors that are ER/PR-negative. Hormone positive cancers have better prognosis.
- **HER2-positive breast cancer (15–20%):** Targeted therapy is used to treat these cancers. HER2-neu positive cancers are aggressively growing cancers.
- **Triple negative breast cancer (15–20%):** Cancer that does not have any receptors for either hormones or HER2 is called triple negative breast cancer (TNBC). It has the worst prognosis amongst all breast cancers.

Signs and Symptoms

Figure 26.8 shows the common signs and symptoms of breast cancer.

Lump in Breast and/or Axilla-painless usually

- Lump which is painless is likely to be malignant.
- Lump could be in the breast or axilla or both.

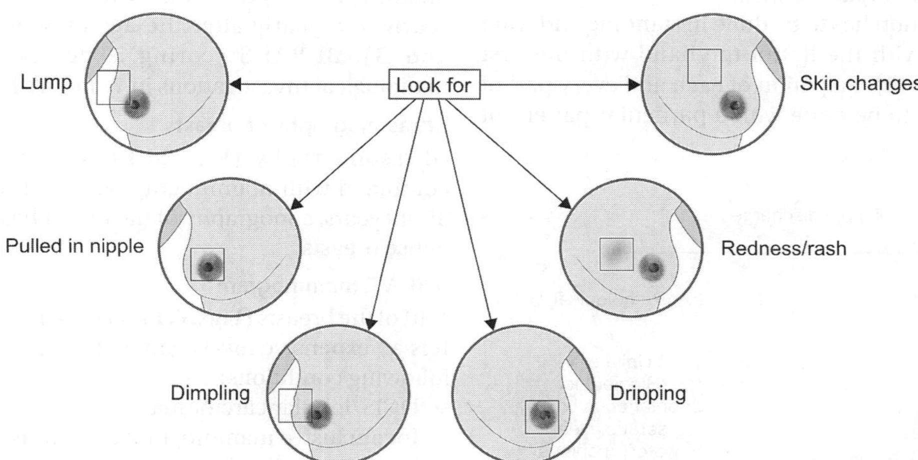

Fig. 26.8: Signs and symptoms of breast cancer.

Nipple Discharge

- Discharge could be clear, greenish, yellowish, brownish or bloody. Multiple duct discharge on expressing manually is more likely to be physiological and is not to be treated aggressively **(Fig. 26.9)**.
- Unilateral, single duct, copious spontaneous discharge is a pathological nipple discharge—**PND**. If bloody, it is likely to harbor papilloma or papillary carcinoma, and requires investigations and proper treatment. Mammary ductoscopy (endoscopic examination of breast ducts) can be done and removal of the discharging duct can be done under endoscopic guidance to avoid major surgery, especially in benign disease.

Other Signs of Breast Cancer

- Redness
- Itching
- Ulceration
- Nipple retraction
- Skin tethering—orange peel or peau de' orange appearance.

Diagnosis—Triple Assessment

Figure 26.10 shows the triple assessment approach for diagnosis of breast cancer.

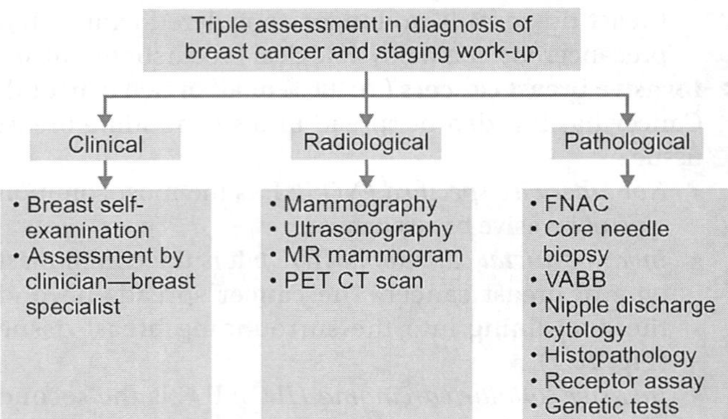

Fig. 26.10: Triple assessment approach for diagnosis of breast cancer.

Clinical

Breast self-examination (BSE)

BSE is a very important part for diagnosis of breast tumors—benign or malignant. All girls/women should begin BSE starting at the age of 20 years every month.

Breast self-examination is divided into:

1. **Inspection:** One should stand in front of the mirror with hands by the side and then, lifting up the arms **(Fig. 26.11)**. Look for:
   - Bilateral symmetry
   - Position of nipple
   - Retraction of nipple
   - Skin of the breast—discoloration, redness, ulceration, tethering
   - Visible lumps in breast or axilla
2. **Palpation:** Palpation has to be done in standing and lying down position, with the flat of the hand with the first 3 fingers **(Fig. 26.12)**. Palpation of each and every part of the breast needs to be done with a particular pattern of one's own choice, it could be circular or from bottom to top or vice versa. Look for:
   - Hardening or induration in breast or axilla
   - Lumps in breast and axilla
   - Nipple should be squeezed to check for nipple discharge.

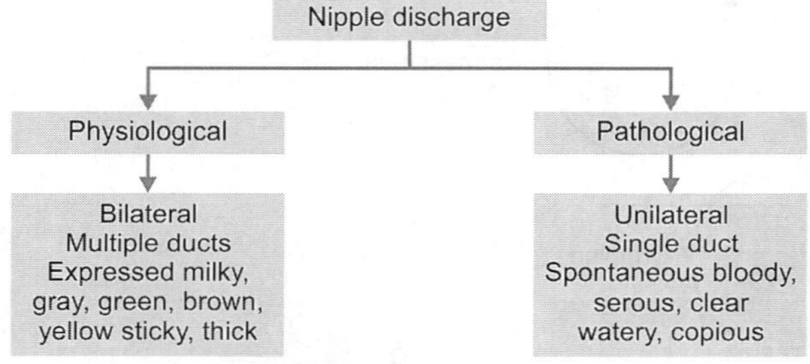

Fig. 26.9: Nipple discharge.

Clinical assessment

- It is very vital that the clinician does a good examination of both the breasts as well as the axilla in lying and sitting position.
- The shape and position of both the breasts and nipple is to be compared, should there be retraction of the nipple, skin tethering, lump in breast or axilla and nipple discharge.
- The breast should always be examined with the flat of the hand and every quadrant should be assessed carefully.

Radiology

The following radiological investigations are advised as indicated. (*Refer* Chapter 6: Radiological Investigations in Women's Health for further details).

Mammography

Mammography is the gold standard for the diagnosis for breast cancer. Digital mammography gives a better result than the regular Mammography picture. Hence, a screening mammogram is advised after the age of 40 years every two yearly and yearly after the age of 50 years **(Figs. 26.13A and B)**. BI-RADS scoring is described in Chapter 6: Radiological Investigations in Women's Health.

Ultrasonography of breasts

Ultrasonography **(Fig. 26.14)** of the breasts is always combined with mammography. In girls and women under 35–40 years, sonography of the breast has to be done, due to dense breasts.

MRI–MR mammogram

MRI of the breasts **(Figs. 6.1 and 6.2)** has specific indications. It is an expensive investigation, hence has to be done in the following conditions:

- DCIS/lobular carcinoma
- Inconclusive mammogram and ultrasonogram
- Genetic/family history with suspicious lesions
- Bilateral disease

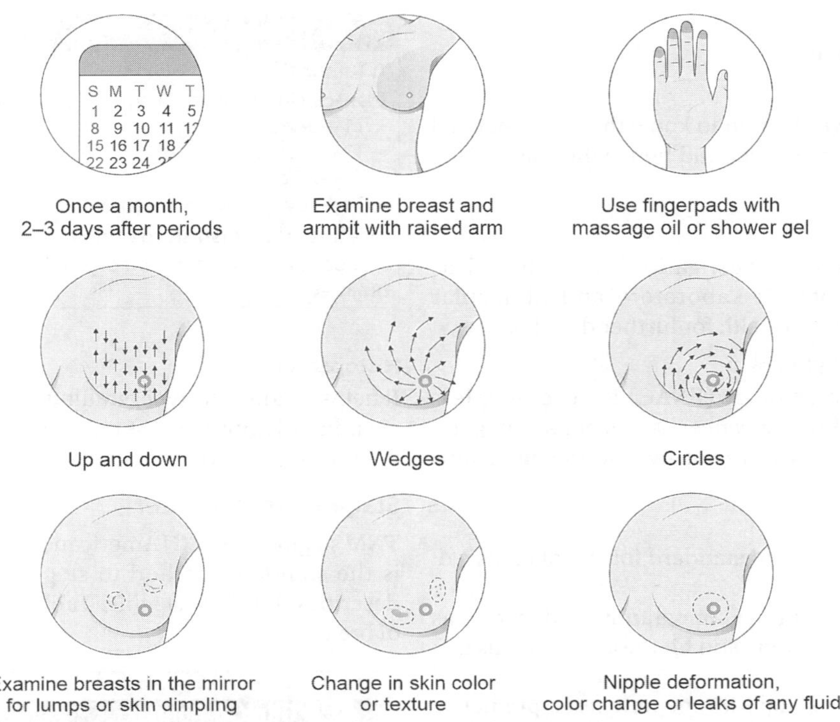

Fig. 26.11: Breast self-examination (inspection).

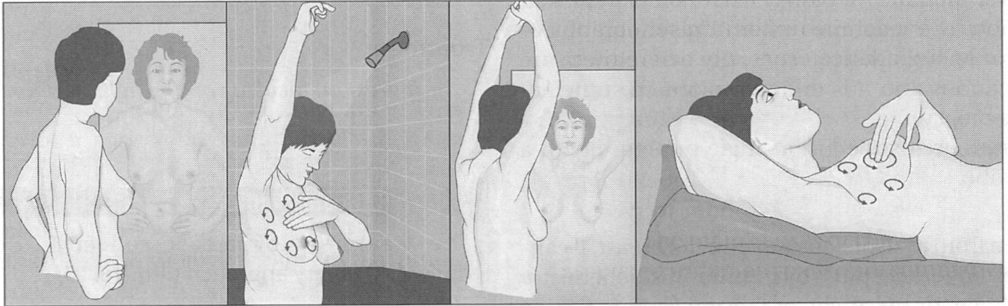

Fig. 26.12: Breast self-examination (palpation).

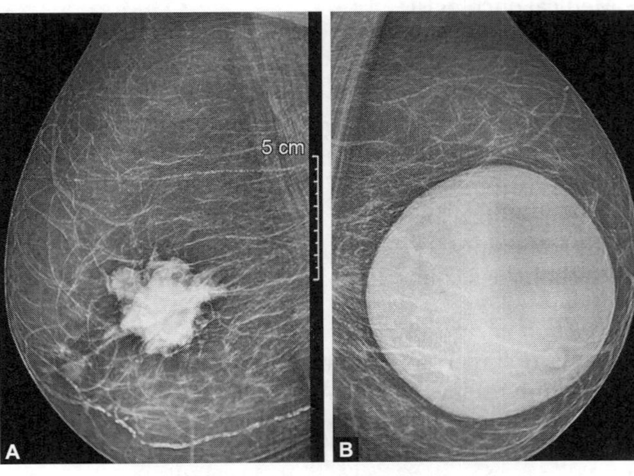

Figs. 26.13A and B: Mammography showing: (A) Cancer; (B) Benign tumor.

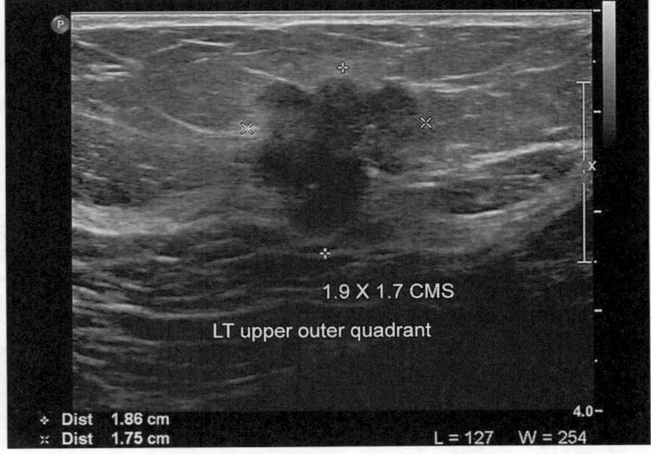

Fig. 26.14: Ultrasound of the breast.

- Microcalcifications
- Breast implants in situ

PET CT Scan

PET scan is a single investigation to know the local, regional and distant spread of the cancer and hence the stage of the disease.

Pathology

The following pathology investigations are advised as indicated (*Refer* Chapter 5: Laboratory and Molecular Investigations in Women's Health for further details).

Fine Needle Aspiration Cytology

Fine needle aspiration cytology (FNAC) is becoming less popular in detection of breast cancer as it is not a very good tool for tissue diagnosis and does not give the receptor status as do other tests.

Core needle biopsy

Core needle biopsy is the gold standard for the diagnosis of breast cancer.

- A better way is to do it under sonography guidance so as not to miss the small lesions and hit the correct focus in a larger lesion.
- Other prognostic tests like Ki67, genetic tests, predictive tests can be done from the core needle biopsy tissue.

Vacuum assisted breast biopsy system (VABB)

- This is a newer modality of biopsy where biopsy is taken from the lesion by a machine under ultrasonography or stereotactic or MRI guidance especially where there are microcalcifications and it is difficult to obtain sufficient tissue in core biopsy.
- Multiple tissues are excised in a single puncture with a large bore probe.

Receptors assay

The biopsy taken from a suspicious lump in the breast, if cancerous is also tested for receptors by immunohistochemistry (IHC). The positivity or negativity of these receptors decide the treatment of breast cancers by systemic therapy and it also has a role in the newer staging of the disease as well as prognosis.

Genetic testing

- 5–10% of breast cancers are hereditary.
- The genes responsible for this are mainly *BRCA1* and *BRCA2*.
- Genetic testing has revolutionized the management of breast cancer with newer tests and molecules coming up for management.
- *BRCA1* positive tumors are usually triple negative and more aggressive.

Tests for prognostic and predictive value

There are certain tests which have a prognostic and predictive value. These are:

- Ki67
- Oncotype Dx
- MammaPrint
- CANASSIST (Indian test)

Box 26.1: TNM staging.

T: Tumor size

T is—carcinoma in situ, Paget's disease of the nipple

- T1—0–2 cm
- T2—2–5 cm
- T3—>5 cm
- T4—any size but involvement of skin or/and chest wall

M—distant metastasis to other organs

Tumor has spread to distant organs like ovaries, lungs, liver, bones, brain, etc.

Histopathology

It helps to know the type, grading, extent of tumor, margins of clearance, lymph node status, thereby helping the staging of the tumor and further management after surgery.

Staging Breast Cancer

TNM staging by AJCC (American Joint Committee on Cancer) is the standard method to stage breast cancer. **Box 26.1** describes the TNM staging. **Table 26.3** describes the stages of breast cancer.

Clinical Pointer

The stage grouping depends not only on TNM but the tumor grade, receptor assay and genetic tests.

Treatment

It is about focusing on the fight and not on fright.

—Robin Roberts

Clinical Pointer

The treatment of breast cancer is done using a multidisciplinary approach **(Fig. 26.15)**.

A multidisciplinary team approach includes:

- Breast surgeon
- Medical oncologist
- Radiation oncologist
- Pathologist
- Radiologist
- Plastic/reconstructive surgeon

There is also a role of the following in the management of breast cancer:

- Genetic counselors
- Physiotherapists
- Psychological counselors

Surgery and its Complications

The types of surgery for primary tumor done in breast cancer are described below.

Breast conservation surgery (BCS)

The tumor with surrounding margins (lumpectomy) is removed and the breast is preserved. With younger women

Table 26.3: Stages of breast cancer.

Stage	*Substages*	*Characteristics*
Stage 0	—	Carcinoma in situ
Stage I (small lump in breast with no/minimal nodes)	Ia	Lump less than 2 cm with no nodes involved (T1N0M0)
	Ib	No lump or less than 2 cm, (T0 or T1,N1M0) Axillary lymph nodes 0.2–2 mm deposits
Stage II	IIa	No primary tumor but 1–3 axillary nodes (T0N1M0) Tumor <2 cm and 1–3 nodes (T1N1M0) Tumor 2–5 cm and no lymph nodes (T2N0M0)
	IIb	T 2–5 cm and 1–3 nodes (T2N1M0) T >5 cm and no nodes (T3N0M0)
Stage III	IIIa	Any T and 4–9 nodes/internal mammary nodes (T0,T1,T2,T3, N2, M0)
	IIIb	Inflammatory breast cancer or tumor chest wall or skin ulceration Nodes 0–9 (T4,N0,N1,N2,M0)
	IIIc	Any T with >/= 10 nodes, internal mammary or infraclavicular nodes (Any T, N3, M0)
Stage IV	—	Any T but spread to other organs, chest wall (Any T, Any N, M1)

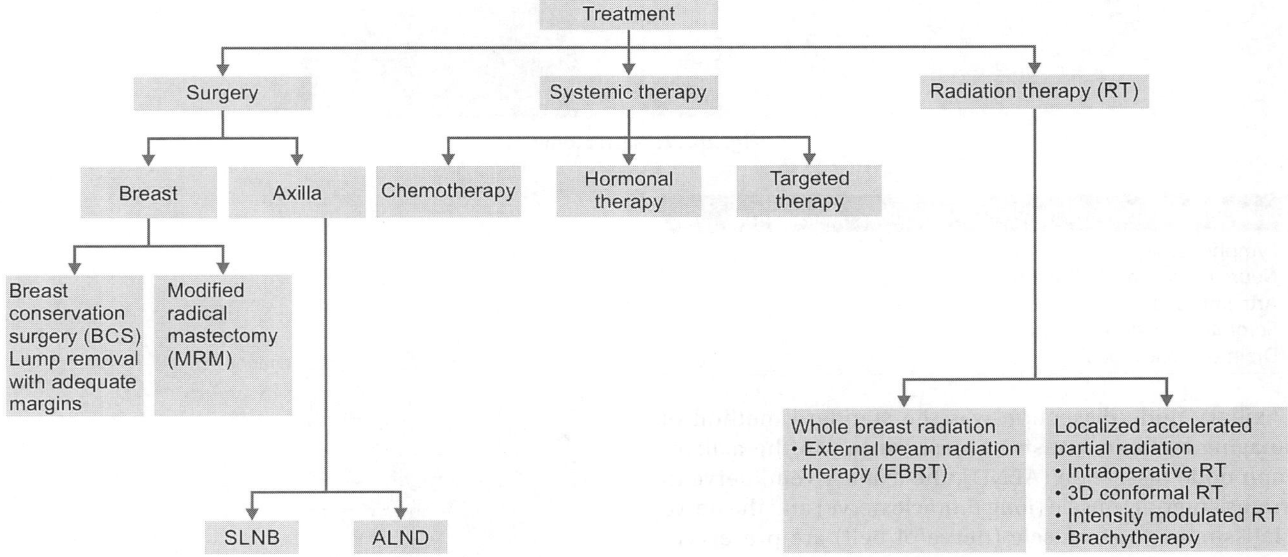

Fig. 26.15: Team approach in management of breast cancer.
(SLNB: sentinel lymph node biopsy; ALND: axillary lymph node dissection)

having breast cancer and detection done at an early stage, BCS is being advocated more and more.

- Oncoplasty for reconstruction of the anatomy and contour of the breast after lumpectomy is usually done, which gives a huge psychological benefit to the patients **(Figs. 26.16A to C)**.
- Radiation therapy is given to the rest of the preserved breast tissue.

Modified radical mastectomy (MRM)

It is removal of the breast with the axillary nodes. This is done in larger tumors, multifocal, multicentric disease and patients who are not willing for radiation therapy or want their breast to be removed **(Fig. 26.17)**.

Radical mastectomy, when originally performed, involved removal of both the Pectoral muscles but it caused a lot of debility and morbidity. Hence, the procedure was modified to remove the facia covering the pectorals but preserve the Pectorals, and yet have oncological clearance.

Axillary lymph node surgery

They are of two types:

1. SLNB: Sentinel lymph node biopsy
2. ALND: Axillary lymph node dissection

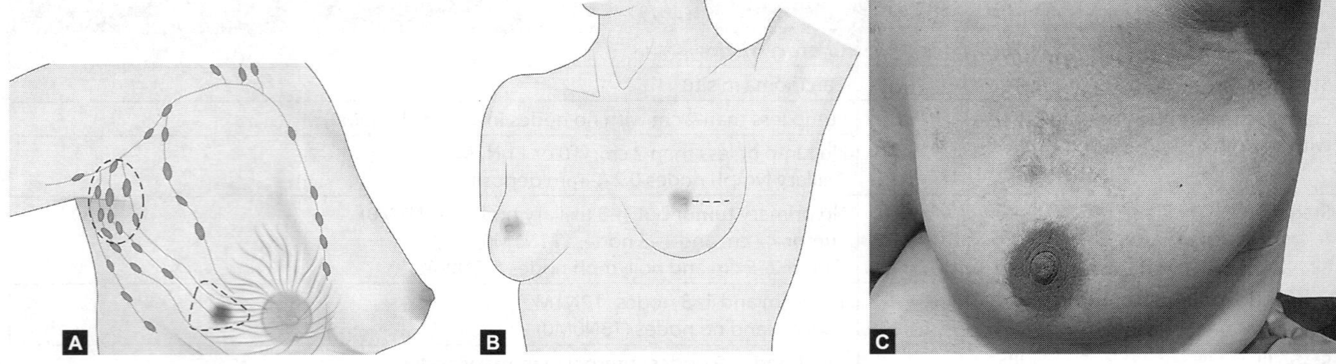

Figs. 26.16A to C: Breast conservation surgery.

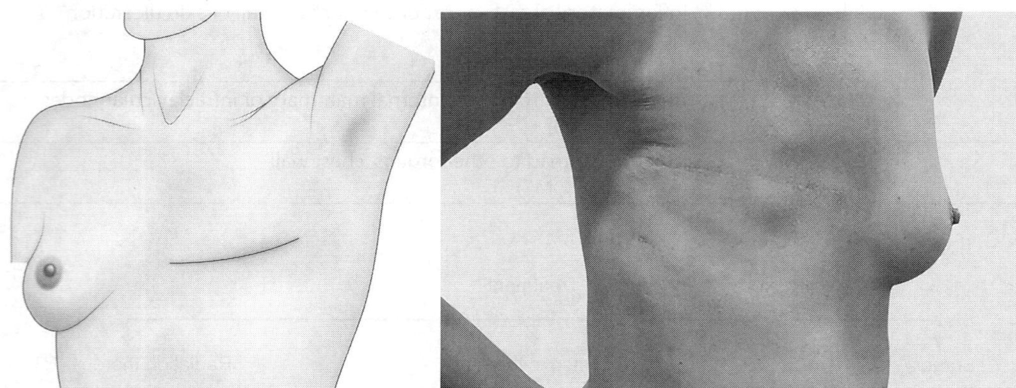

Fig. 26.17: Mastectomy.

Box 26.2: Side effects of removal of all axillary lymph nodes.

- Lymphedema
- Neurological pain in the arm
- Arm immobility
- Seroma formation
- Drain complications

Axillary node dissection was the standard method of managing axilla in invasive breast cancer. In the axillary lymph node dissection (ALND), the axillary vein, nerve to serratus anterior muscle (long thoracic nerve) and the nerve to latissimus dorsi muscle (nerve of bell) are preserved. The intercostal nerves can be sacrificed in order to have a complete axillary clearance according to the oncological principles. But there are a lot of side effects of removal of all axillary nodes as enlisted in **Box 26.2**.

In order to prevent these now sentinel lymph node biopsy (SLNB) **(Fig. 26.18)**, is done to sample at least 3 nodes which are stained by the blue dye or picked up on radionuclide gamma probe. If these nodes are not involved then the axillary dissection can be spared and the patient can be spared of the complications.

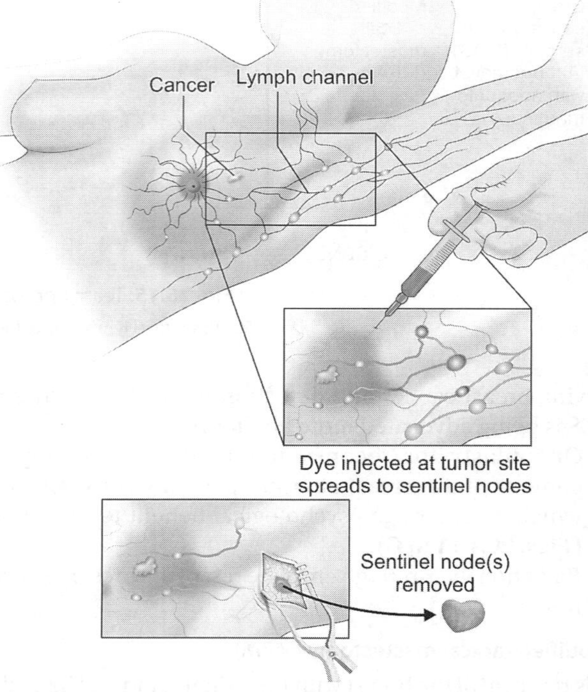

Fig. 26.18: Sentinel lymph node biopsy.

 **Clinical Pointer**

Reconstruction surgery after mastectomy is possible with Implants or autologous tissue.

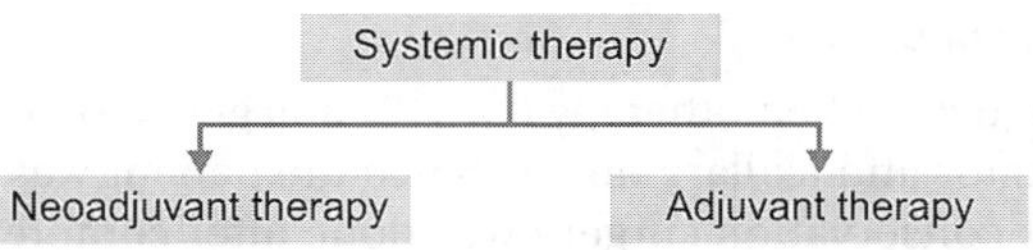

Fig. 26.19: Classification of systemic therapy.

Systemic Therapy

There is a major role of systemic therapy **(Fig. 26.19)** in the management of breast cancer. Depending on the stage, type, grade, receptors status, genetic and prognostic tests different systemic therapy is advised.

- Chemotherapy
- Targeted therapy
- Immunotherapy
- Endocrine therapy

Neoadjuvant therapy (NAT)

The therapy given preoperatively in large tumors and advanced stages of cancer to downsize the tumor, make it operable and preserve the breast is called neoadjuvant therapy.

Adjuvant therapy

The therapy given postoperatively is called adjuvant therapy.

Radiation Therapy

- Radiation therapy is usually given as the last in the sequence to irradiate the chest wall in advanced cases with large tumors, axillary involvement and where breast has been preserved. Many advances have been there in the machines and technique of radiation therapy also.
- There is External Beam therapy where the radiation is given externally or intraoperative radiation can be given in cases of breast preservation so as to avoid the complications of external therapy like skin irritation, pigmentation, etc.

BREAST CANCER AND PREGNANCY

Pregnancy-related breast cancer is rare. Many women have gone on to have healthy babies and live healthy lives after a diagnosis of breast cancer. Any breast cancer that is found during pregnancy, while breastfeeding, or within a year following delivery of a baby is considered a **pregnancy-related breast cancer**.

Treatment options are more complicated in women who are diagnosed to have breast cancer during pregnancy, as there needs to be a right balance between the treatment for cancer while protecting the baby. Pregnant women can safely get treatment for breast cancer, although the types of treatment used and the timing of treatment might be affected by the pregnancy. The treatment will depend on:

- Size of the tumor
- Location or site of the tumor
- Stage of the cancer
- Duration of pregnancy (trimester)
- Overall health
- Personal preferences

It is generally safe to have surgery for breast cancer in pregnancy. Chemotherapy seems to be safe for the baby if given in the second or third trimester of pregnancy, but it is not safe in the first trimester. Other breast cancer treatments, such as hormone therapy, targeted therapy, and radiation therapy, are more likely to cause adverse effects to the baby and are not usually given during pregnancy.

Ending the pregnancy is no longer routinely recommended when breast cancer is found. Still, this option may be discussed when looking at all the treatment choices available, especially for metastatic (stage IV) or aggressive cancers that may need treatment right away, such as inflammatory breast cancer.

During the First Trimester (First 12 weeks)

Surgery offered is usually a mastectomy in the first trimester of pregnancy. This is because not all women who have a mastectomy need radiotherapy, whereas radiotherapy is usually needed after breast-conserving surgery. Radiotherapy is generally not recommended at any time during pregnancy because of the risk of radiation to the baby. Chemotherapy is usually avoided during first trimester as it is unsafe for the baby as most of the development of the fetus occurs during this period.

During the Second Trimester (13–27 weeks)

If the diagnosis occurs in the second trimester breast-conserving surgery may be an option if chemotherapy has to be given. Radiation therapy then will be done after the baby is born, till then chemotherapy can be administered.

During the Third Trimester (28 weeks to delivery)

Breast-conserving surgery may be an option as radiotherapy can be given after the baby is born.

Surgery

- Modified radical mastectomy or breast conservation surgery can be done depending on the timing of pregnancy as stated above.
- Sentinel lymph node biopsy can be done by the Radionuclide dye injection. Blue dye is avoided as it is unsafe for the baby.

Breast Reconstruction

Breast reconstruction at the time of surgery (immediate reconstruction) is not usually offered during pregnancy. Reasons include a higher risk of bleeding during pregnancy and minimizing the time under general anesthetic. Breast reconstruction will generally be offered at a later date (delayed reconstruction).

Chemotherapy

Chemotherapy is generally not recommended in the first 12 weeks and after 35 weeks of pregnancy or within 3 weeks of delivery because it can lower the blood counts of the mother. This could cause bleeding and increase the chances of infection during birth. Holding off on chemotherapy for the last few weeks before delivery allows the mother's blood counts to return to normal before childbirth.

Radiation Therapy

Radiation therapy should not be given during pregnancy.

Breastfeeding

Breastfeeding may be possible for some women diagnosed during pregnancy after breast surgery, but not while having chemotherapy, radiotherapy, hormone or targeted therapy.

Breastfeeding is most successful from the other, non-treated breast.

ROLE OF A PHYSIOTHERAPIST IN BREAST CANCER MANAGEMENT

A physiotherapist plays a key role in management of breast cancer especially in prevention of a major side effect of lymphedema postoperatively after axillary dissection surgery.

- The upper limb physiotherapy should begin on the same evening of surgery and should be advised to be done frequently during the day, so as to prevent the occurrence of lymphedema.

Clinical Pointer

There is no other way to prevent lymphedema except for physiotherapy and it is important to explain to the patient that lymphedema is a consequence and not a complication of the surgery performed.

- Should lymphedema occur, the physiotherapist attains a rather more important role to manage it.

Summary

Breast cancer is the commonest cancer occurring in women worldwide and the incidence is rising. The age of occurrence is decreasing, hence younger women are getting breast cancer. With more women becoming aware and newer modalities of screening as well as diagnosing, more and more cases are diagnosed at early stage. The management of breast cancer has undergone a major paradigm shift from being more aggressive to conservative in order to preserve the breast and axilla, and prevent complications related to axillary dissection. The newer diagnostic modalities and understanding of the disease has helped develop newer molecules of systemic therapy to achieve higher cure rates, decrease the recurrence rates and mortality as well as improve the overall survival and quality of life.

CLINICAL EXAMPLES

Locally Advanced Cancer

A 35-year-old female presented with a 5 cm lump in the right breast and 2–3 axillary nodes on radiological examination. Core needle biopsy showed invasive ductal carcinoma grade 3, ER-PR-HER2-

Treatment Done

Neoadjuvant chemotherapy (NACT) was given to downsize the tumor and axillary nodes. Since the patient was young Breast conservation surgery was done after completion of NACT with axillary dissection. Radiation therapy was also given to the breast and axilla as breast was preserved and axillary nodes were found malignant. She was referred to a physiotherapist on the same day of surgery for her upper limb physiotherapy so as to avoid lymphedema and other complications. In the long-term follow up and checkups because of good physiotherapy she did not develop any limb side effects. Triple negative cancers have the worst prognosis amongst all breast cancers, hence a regular follow-up is a must in these cases.

Invasive Lobular Carcinoma

A 65-year-old female presented with diffuse lump in right breast. On mammography and sonography huge diffuse lump was found on right breast but also a small diffuse lump in the left breast. Hence, an MR mammogram was done, which showed bilateral lesions. Core needle biopsy on both sides showed invasive lobular carcinoma. The patient wanted bilateral mastectomy, ALND on right side and SLNB on left side followed by reconstruction by implants on both sides.

ALND with lymphedema and other arm issues

A 45-year-old female with 5 cm lump and axillary nodes positive with ER+PR+HER2-.

She opted for modified radical mastectomy and hence complete axillary lymph node dissection was done. Adjuvant chemotherapy was given followed by radiation therapy. She developed lymphedema soon after that. She was referred to physiotherapist for compression stockings, decompression and upper limb physiotherapy. The lymphedema reduced over a period of 4–5 months and with physiotherapy she maintained a good quality of life.

Review Questions

1. Explain the anatomy and physiology of breast.
2. Describe benign breast disease in detail.
3. Explain classification of breast cancer.
4. Mention the risk factors for occurrence of breast cancer.
5. What investigations should be done in a suspected case of breast cancer?
6. Explain staging of breast cancer.
7. Explain the various surgical procedures in breast cancer.
8. What is the team approach in management of breast cancer?

Bibliography

1. Alkabban FM, Ferguson T. Breast Cancer. In: StatPearls [Internet]. Treasure Island (FL): StatPearls Publishing; 2022. [Updated 2021 Aug 7]. Available from: https://www.ncbi.nlm.nih.gov/books/NBK482286/

2. Breast Cancer Expert Committee of National Cancer Quality Control Center; Health Management Professional Committee of Beijing Breast Cancer Prevention and Control Society. [Comprehensive management guideline for breast cancer follow-up and healthcare (2022 edition)]. Zhonghua Zhong Liu Za Zhi. 2022;44(1):1-28. Chinese. doi: 10.3760/cma.j.cn112152-20211029-00798. PMID: 35073646.
3. Das S. A Concise Textbook of Surgery, 11th edition. Kolkata, 2020. S Das Kolkata publishers. India.
4. Desantis CE, Ma J, Goding Sauer A, Newman LA, Jemal A. Breast cancer statistics, 2017, racial disparity in mortality by state. CA Cancer J Clin. 2017;67(6):439-48.
5. Ferley J, Soerjomataraml I, Ervik M, Dikshit R, Eser S. GLOBOCAN 2012 v1.0. Cancer Incidence and Mortality Worldwide: IARC Cancer Base No. 11. Lyon, France: International Agency for Research on Cancer; 2013.
6. Momenimovahed Z, Salehiniya H. Epidemiological characteristics of and risk factors for breast cancer in the world. Breast Cancer (Dove Med Press). 2019;11:151-64. doi: 10.2147/BCTT. S176070. PMID: 31040712; PMCID: PMC6462164.
7. O'Connell PR, McCaskie AW, Williams AS. Bailey & Love's Short Practice of Surgery, 27th edition. Florida. CRC Press Publishers. USA. 2018.
8. World Health Organization. Guidelines for management of breast cancer. EMRO Technical Publications Series 31. 2006.

Multiple Choice Questions (MCQs)

To test your understanding and recall of key concepts.

1. **Which artery primarily supplies blood to the breast?**
   A. Internal mammary artery
   B. Axillary artery
   C. Brachial artery
   D. Thoracic artery
2. **What is the significance of the 'axillary tail of Spence' in breast anatomy?**
   A. It contains the main blood supply of the breast
   B. It is the primary site for milk production
   C. Breast cancer can develop in the axillary tail
   D. It supports the pectoralis muscle
3. **The most common benign tumor in breast occurring in younger women is________.**
   A. Fibroadenoma B. Phyllodes tumor
   C. Hamartoma D. Sclerosing adenosis
4. **Why is breast-conserving surgery (BCS) commonly advocated in younger women?**
   A. It avoids the need for radiotherapy
   B. It provides psychological benefits by preserving the breast
   C. It eliminates the risk of recurrence
   D. It requires less follow-up
5. **Breast surgery involving removal of both the pectoral muscles is called as__________.**
   A. Radical mastectomy
   B. Modified radical mastectomy (MRM)
   C. Breast conservation surgery (BCS)
   D. Axillary lymph node surgery
6. **A 35-year-old patient with a painless lump in her breast undergoes core needle biopsy revealing ER+PR+HER2-. What systemic therapy is likely?**
   A. Targeted therapy
   B. Hormonal therapy
   C. Chemotherapy
   D. Radiation therapy
7. **Which diagnostic tool is most suitable for evaluating dense breast tissue in women under 40?**
   A. Mammography
   B. MRI
   C. Ultrasonography
   D. PET-C
8. **Which of the following is *not* a risk factor for the occurrence of breast cancer?**
   A. Internal or hormonal exposures
   B. Lifestyle factors
   C. Environmental factors
   D. Eating Habits
9. **The triple-negative breast cancer (TNBC) has a worse prognosis compared to hormone receptor-positive breast cancer because __________.**
   A. TNBC lacks targeted treatment options
   B. TNBC metastasizes less frequently
   C. TNBC is resistant to chemotherapy
   D. TNBC is associated with a low Ki-67 index
10. **An optimal treatment plan for a pregnant woman diagnosed with breast cancer in the second trimester would be __________.**
   A. Perform a mastectomy and start chemotherapy immediately
   B. Breast-conserving surgery with delayed radiation therapy after delivery
   C. Avoid surgery and administer hormonal therapy
   D. Perform reconstruction surgery during the same procedure
11. **Which of the following statements is true for lymph node biopsy?**
   A. Sentinel lymph node biopsy (SLNB) reduces complications, such as lymphedema while maintaining oncological safety
   B. SLNB is more invasive and causes more complications than axillary lymph node dissection
   C. SLNB is ineffective for detecting metastasis
   D. ALND is preferred due to fewer complications

ANSWERS

1. A	2. C	3. A	4. B	5. A
6. B	7. C	8. D	9. A	10. B
11. A				

Chapter 27

Gynecological Cancers

Ava Desai

LEARNING OBJECTIVES

At the end of the chapter, the reader will be able to:
- Describe the main types of gynecologic cancers.
- Discuss the symptoms, signs and diagnosis of common gynecologic cancers.
- Understand staging of gynecologic cancers.
- Learn about the preventive aspects if any and the management.
- Get a brief idea about the role of the physiotherapist in the management of gynecologic cancers.

CHAPTER OUTLINE

- Introduction
- Cervical cancer
- Endometrial cancer
- Malignant ovarian tumors
  - Epithelial ovarian cancer
  - Germ cell ovarian tumors
- Vulvar cancer
- Vaginal cancer
- Palliation in gynecologic cancer
- Role of the physiotherapist

INTRODUCTION

Gynecologic cancer includes all cancers originating in the female reproductive organs **(Fig. 27.1)**. The main types are mentioned in **(Box 27.1)**. They have different symptoms and signs. The main modalities of management include surgery, radiotherapy and chemotherapy, along with targeted therapy. Management, prognosis and survival depend to a large extent on stage at diagnosis and histological type.

Physiotherapy plays a very important adjunctive role at all times in the proper management and rehabilitation of women suffering from genital cancer.

CERVICAL CANCER

- Cancer of the uterine cervix was formerly the most common cancer in Indian women. Even now it ranks only second to breast cancer.
- Approximately 150,000 new cases are reported annually in India. Due to lack of screening, most are diagnosed in late

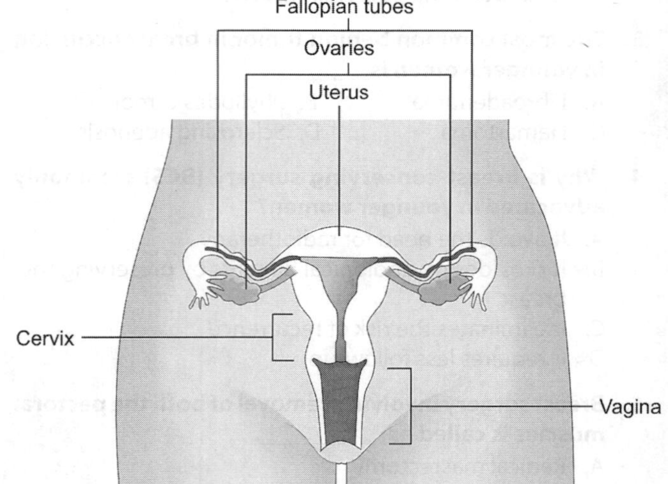

Fig. 27.1: Organs of the female reproductive system *(For color version, see Plate 8)*.

Box 27.1: Main types of gynecologic cancer.

- Cervical cancer
- Endometrial cancer
- Ovarian, fallopian tube and peritoneal cancer
- Vaginal cancer
- Vulvar cancer
- Gestational trophoblastic disease

stages resulting in about 76,000 deaths from this cancer yearly in India.

- On the other hand, *if detected early, cervical cancer is highly curable*. In developed countries mandatory screening has greatly reduced the number of cases and deaths.
- It is also *the only gynecologic cancer which can be detected in the preinvasive stage* and is amenable to both primary and secondary prevention.

Infection with high-risk types of human papilloma virus (HPV) is a 'necessary' cause of this cancer. Infection with HPV is common among sexually active individuals, and is usually cleared naturally. Cervical precancer and cancer occur over several years if the infection is not naturally cleared and persists in the cervical epithelium.

Preventive Aspects

Primary prevention: HPV vaccine, if given appropriately, can prevent about 80% of cervical cancers.

- The vaccine should not be taken if pregnant, but can be given if breastfeeding.

Secondary prevention: It can be done by detecting and treating preinvasive lesions.

- Regular screening of all women with Pap smear every three years; or with co-test (Pap + HPV) every 5 years,
  Pap smear is a screening method. It is a cytological examination of the exfoliated cells shed from the cervix. It is reported by the Bethesda System.
- Visual Inspection with Acetic acid (VIA) or with Lugol Iodine (VILI) for screening is an acceptable alternative to Pap smear in low-income countries
- Colposcopy and biopsy is indicated if the smear report is abnormal or if the cervix looks clinically suspicious. The colposcope is an instrument to examine the transformation zone of the cervix. If any abnormalities are seen, such as aceto-white epithelium or abnormal vascularity, a colposcopy directed punch biopsy of this area can be taken for proper diagnosis.

Education and awareness

- Condom use, safe sex and faithful partner to reduce the chances of HPV infection.
- Awareness regarding early symptoms.

Symptoms

No symptoms are seen in very early cases, hence all women, *even if asymptomatic,* must be screened regularly.

Early symptoms

- Vaginal discharge
- Irregular periods
- Abnormal vaginal bleeding—intermenstrual, postcoital or postmenopausal.

As the disease progresses

- Malodorous discharge
- Irregular, sometimes profuse bleeding
- Anemia due to continuous bleeding
- Severe lower abdominal pain or backache
- Urinary or fecal incontinence due to fistulae
- Lower limb edema may be a sign of nodal pressure on the iliac veins
- Symptoms due to metastatic disease, e.g., pain due to bony metastases
- Oliguria or anuria—involvement of the parametria can result in obstructive uropathy and ultimately renal failure—a common terminal event if the disease is untreated.

Signs

- General physical examination including palpation of supraclavicular and inguinal nodes.
- On speculum examination the cervical growth is assessed as is involvement of the vagina.
- Bimanual and rectal examination are essential to assess vaginal and parametrial involvement.

Diagnosis

- Biopsy of the cervical growth is the first step in diagnosis.
- The most common histopathological type is squamous cell carcinoma, followed by adenocarcinoma. Adenosquamous and clear cell are rarer types.
- Ultrasound, MRI, CT and PET CT scan are advised as required for further information regarding local extent and distant spread.

Clinical Pointer

FIGO Staging

The International Federation of Gynecology and Obstetrics, or FIGO, system is used to stage cancers. Four main stages are based on the results of a physical exam, imaging scans, and biopsies. The staging is based upon the local, regional and distant spread of the disease.

FIGO Staging in Cervical Cancer

Invasive cervical cancer spreads by direct extension into the parametrium, vagina, uterus, and adjacent organs, i.e. bladder and rectum. It also spreads along the lymphatic channels to the regional lymph nodes, namely, obturator, external iliac, internal iliac, and thence to the common iliac and para-aortic nodes. Distant metastasis to lungs, liver, and skeleton by the hematogenous route is a late phenomenon, as is intraperitoneal spread.

In cervical cancer, the FIGO stage is decided after clinical examination. Radiological assessment or biopsy may be used to assist in staging.

- **Stage 1:** The carcinoma is strictly confined to the cervix
- **Stage 2:** The carcinoma invades beyond the uterus, but has not extended onto the lower third of the vagina or to the pelvic wall
- **Stage 3:** The carcinoma involves the lower third of the vagina and/or extends to the pelvic wall and/or causes hydronephrosis or nonfunctioning kidney and/or involves pelvic and/or para-aortic lymph nodes
- **Stage 4:** The carcinoma has extended beyond the true pelvis or has involved (biopsy proven) the mucosa of the bladder or rectum.

Management of Cervical Intraepithelial Neoplasia (CIN) (Box 27.2)

CIN2/3 are preinvasive lesions. Their eradication will prevent invasive cancer. Management depends on the age and parity.

- In older women, hysterectomy is appropriate.
- In younger women or those desirous of children, conservative management with cryo, laser vaporization, knife conization or large loop conization (LEEP) of the transformation zone.
- Meticulous follow-up is advised to detect any recurrence.

Management of Invasive Cancer

Radiotherapy can be curative in all stages whereas surgery is indicated only in the earlier stages.

Surgery

See **Box 27.2**.

Radiation

- *Adjuvant radiotherapy* may be required after assessing the prognostic factors in the surgical specimen.
- *Concurrent chemoradiation:* If diagnosed in later stages, or even in early stages in a patient unfit for radical surgery, the treatment of choice is Radiotherapy. Weekly low dose cisplatin is given simultaneously to potentiate the effect of radiation.
- *Hemostatic radiation* is used as an emergency measure for severe bleeding.

Treatment of recurrence: It is individualized. Salvage radiation or chemotherapy may be required.

Pain relief and palliation: As many cases present in late stage, pain relief and palliation play a very important role in the management of cervical cancer.

Box 27.2: Management of cervical cancer.

- CIN 2/3: Hysterectomy/cryo/CO_2 laser/knife cone/Loop electrosurgical excision procedure (LEEP)
- Stage IA1: Hysterectomy
- Stage IA2: Hysterectomy + pelvic lymphadenectomy
- Stage IB1/IB2/IIA: Radical hysterectomy + pelvic lymphadenectomy or curative chemoradiation
- All other stages: Curative chemoradiation

 **Key Points**

Cervical cancer

- Second most common cancer in Indian women
- In India, most cases are in advanced stages with high morbidity and mortality
- Persistent infection with high risk HPV is one of the causes
- It is preventable but not prevented in our country
  - Primary prevention by HPV vaccine
  - Secondary prevention by detecting and eradicating precancer
  - Education and awareness of both doctors and public is necessary.
- Early symptoms include discharge, intermenstrual, postmenopausal or postcoital bleeding
- Management and prognosis depend on FIGO stage
  - Surgery indicated in early stages only
  - Radiotherapy + concomitant chemotherapy is the treatment of choice in advanced cases
  - Treatment of recurrence is individualized
  - Pain relief and palliation is integral part of management
- Survival depends mainly on stage of disease

Survival

It depends on the stage of the disease.

ENDOMETRIAL CANCER

Endometrial cancer is the most common uterine malignancy. Endometrial cancer is the most common gynecological cancer in developed countries. Uterine sarcomas are rare.

- It is usually seen in the perimenopausal age group.
- It may be seen in young women especially those undergoing treatment for polycystic ovaries (PCOS), infertility or those who are obese.
- The risk of endometrial cancer (type 1) increases with any factor producing unopposed estrogen, such as anovulatory cycles in PCOS, estrogen secreting tumors, estrogen hormone replacement therapy and obesity.
- Those endometrial cancers which are not estrogen dependent (type 2) have a worse prognosis.

Screening

- Unlike cervical cancer, screening is not recommended for all women.
- Women with family history, especially of Lynch syndrome, should have regular screening and endometrial biopsies along with tests for other cancers as advised, starting from a young age.

Symptoms

Endometrial cancer must be ruled out if any of the following symptoms are present:

- Postmenopausal bleeding or even mild spotting
- Postmenopausal watery or purulent discharge

- Perimenopausal heavy irregular or frequent periods,
- Younger premenopausal women with abnormal bleeding, especially if cycles are anovulatory.

Signs

- General physical examination must never be omitted.
- Abdominal examination is usually normal in early cases. If there is a large pyometra, a midline hypogastric mass may be felt.
- On speculum examination, the cervix, vagina and vulva should be carefully examined to look for any metastases.
- Bimanual palpation to assess uterus, adnexae and pelvis.

Diagnosis

- Endometrial aspiration biopsy in the outpatient department
- The most common histological type is endometrioid adenocarcinoma. Clear cell and serous carcinomas have a worse prognosis.
- Fractional curettage under anesthesia if office biopsy is technically not possible
- Radiological evaluation, such as ultrasound, MRI, CT and PET CT scan are advised as required for further information regarding local extent and distant spread.
- In any postmenopausal women with bleeding, if ultrasound reveals endometrial thickness more than 3–4 mm, it is considered abnormal and biopsy is warranted.
- MRI is particularly useful to look for myometrial invasion and cervical involvement.

FIGO Stage

In endometrial cancer, the final stage is decided after surgery and histopathological evaluation of the specimen, i.e., Surgico-pathological staging.

- **Stage 1:** Tumor confined to the corpus uteri
- **Stage 2:** Tumor invades cervical stroma, but does not extend beyond the uterus
- **Stage 3:** Local and/or regional spread of the tumor
- **Stage 4:** Tumor invades bladder and/or bowel mucosa, and/or distant metastases.

Management

Surgery

- Total hysterectomy and bilateral salpingo-oophorectomy is the cornerstone of treatment.
- Lymphadenectomy can be omitted in grade 1, endometrioid type, with no or less myometrial invasion.
- Lymphadenectomy is required for staging in grade 3 lesion, a high risk type.

Radiation

Adjuvant radiation: The need for postoperative adjuvant radiation is decided after assessing the prognostic factors in the histopathological report. Radiation decreases the local recurrence rate but has no effect on overall survival.

Chemotherapy

- Adjuvant chemotherapy may be considered with high-risk histological types

Hormone therapy

Progestational agents are often found to be useful in advanced or recurrent endometrial cancer.

Treatment of recurrence

It depends on the site of recurrence and previous treatment, e.g., a recurrence at the vaginal vault can be easily treated with radiation if she was previously treated with surgery alone.

Survival

The 5-year survival depends on stage, grade, and type of disease.

Key Points

Endometrial cancer

- Most common genital tract cancer in developed countries
- Common in perimenopausal age and presents with bleeding or discharge
- Also seen in young women with unopposed estrogen as in obesity, PCOS or infertility
- Type 2 endometrial cancer (high grade, serous, clear cell) is not estrogen dependent and have worse prognosis
- Early symptoms include abnormal periods, post-menopausal spotting, bleeding or discharge
- Management and prognosis depends on FIGO stage:
  - Surgery is the cornerstone of treatment
  - Adjuvant radiation decided after assessing prognostic factors
  - Chemotherapy and hormonal therapy indicated in certain situations
  - Treatment of recurrence individualized
  - Molecular classification is nowadays an important adjunct in management
- Survival depends mainly on stage

MALIGNANT OVARIAN TUMORS

- The most common malignant ovarian tumors are epithelial ovarian cancer including serous, mucinous, endometrioid, clear cell and transitional cell types.
- Non-epithelial malignant ovarian tumors are less common. Of these, germ cell tumors occur in young girls and women.
- Other rarer types include sex cord-stromal tumors and metastatic tumors.

Epithelial Ovarian Cancer

The term epithelial ovarian cancer (EOC) includes ovarian, fallopian tube and primary peritoneal cancer.

- More than two-thirds of patients present in advanced stages.
- Surgery for these cases is very challenging
- Many combination chemo and targeted therapies are required.

Clinical Pointer

Among all gynecologic cancers, epithelial ovarian cancer (EOC) is the most difficult to treat and has the highest fatality to case ratio.

Screening

Unlike cervical cancer, there is no single screening test for early detection.

- Screening for ovarian cancer is not recommended in the general population.
- For women at high risk, such as those with a strong family history, screening with transvaginal ultrasound, CA 125 and bimanual examination is recommended.

Prevention

- Oral contraceptive use for 5 years or more can reduce the risk of developing ovarian cancer substantially. It is the only proven method for prevention.
- In high-risk women with an inherited mutation, prophylactic salpingo-oophorectomy is recommended after childbirth is complete.

Symptoms

- EOC is known as the **"whispering disease"** as in the early stages there are only non-specific symptoms. The vague complaints may include "gassiness" or bloating, a frequent desire to pass urine, abdominal pain or constipation. If such complaints persist for more than a few weeks, the physician must have a high index of suspicion and suspect ovarian cancer.
- Usually, these non-specific symptoms go unreported and *most patients present in late stages* with complaints of abdominal distension, pain, anorexia, early satiety and weight loss.
- Some women present with large volume ascites and pleural effusion. Many patients have weight loss and are generally hypoproteinemic and debilitated.

Signs

- General examination may reveal metastatic nodes or a breast lump.
- The abdomen may be distended due to ascites or upper abdominal disease.
- Bimanual examination may reveal a fixed pelvic mass with irregular consistency or rectovaginal nodularity. However, the ovary may not be enlarged and still harbor disease.
- Hence, radiological investigation is very important in a suspected case of ovarian cancer.

Radiological Investigations

- Ultrasound, including transvaginal sonography, is an excellent tool to characterize ovarian and adnexal masses.
- MRI is the best option to characterize the nature of the lesion if the ultrasound findings are indeterminate
- CT scan and PET CT scan are useful to look for distant spread.

Tumor Markers

- The most commonly used tumor marker is CA 125. *However, it cannot be used alone as a diagnostic test for ovarian cancer as it has a low specificity and sensitivity.*
- HE4 is a relatively new marker.
- CA 19-9 and CEA are markers for gastrointestinal tumors, but may be raised in some ovarian tumors such as mucinous tumors and metastatic tumors.

FIGO Stage

FIGO stage is surgico-pathological and decided after surgery.

- **Stage 1:** Tumor confined to ovaries or fallopian tube(s)
- **Stage 2:** Tumor involves 1 or both ovaries or fallopian tubes with pelvic extension (below pelvic brim) or peritoneal cancer
- **Stage 3:** Tumor involves 1 or both ovaries or fallopian tubes, or peritoneal cancer, with cytologically or histologically confirmed spread to the peritoneum outside the pelvis and/or metastasis to the retroperitoneal lymph nodes
- **Stage 4:** Distant metastasis excluding peritoneal metastases

Management

Most women require surgery as well as combination chemotherapy and targeted therapy.

Surgery

The goals of surgery depend on the stage and extent of the disease

- **Staging surgery in apparently early cases:** When the disease is apparently early and seems confined only to the ovary there is a substantial chance that there is microscopic (invisible) spread to omentum, peritoneum, lymph nodes, etc. Hence after removing the ovarian tumor, opposite ovary and uterus, omentectomy, peritoneal biopsies and lymph node dissection must be done to rule out this occult spread. This will confirm the true extent and stage of the disease and allow tailored adjuvant therapy and prognosis.
- **Cytoreductive surgery (CRS) in advanced cases:** Ovarian cancer spreads via direct dissemination to many intraperitoneal areas, such as omentum, peritoneum, serosa of both small and large bowel, liver, spleen, etc. It also spreads to the retroperitoneal nodes.

In advanced stage ovarian cancer, *surgery can improve survival only if maximal cytoreduction of all visible disease is achieved* (i.e., there should be no visible disease after surgery (R0) or the residual should be <1 cm). This is called *optimal cytoreduction* and will benefit the patient. If more than this volume of disease is left behind after surgery, survival benefit is doubtful.

Surgery to achieve this optimal cytoreduction is very challenging. Surgical maneuvers, such as total peritonectomy, bowel resection, splenectomy, liver resection, etc., are often required. These surgeries must be carried out by a team of experienced oncologists preferably in high volume tertiary centers.

If after extensive preoperative assessment, the surgeon feels that R0 cytoreduction is feasible, then the patient is scheduled for **primary (upfront) cytoreductive surgery** followed by adjuvant chemotherapy. If on the other hand complete cytoreduction of all disease does not seem likely, then the patient is given neoadjuvant chemotherapy after which she is scheduled for **interval CRS surgery**. The timing of surgery - upfront or interval—is not as important as achieving optimal or complete cytoreduction.

- **Secondary CRS:** After a disease-free interval, if the cancer recurs in a solitary area accessible to surgery, it can be surgically removed before restarting chemotherapy.

Chemotherapy

Combination chemotherapy is required in all stages, except Stage Ia. Chemotherapy is given as **neoadjuvant** before interval CRS, or as **adjuvant** after surgery. Most ovarian cancers present in late stages and recurrences are very common. Many different regimes for **salvage** chemotherapy are used.

Survival

The most important prognostic factor is FIGO Stage. If properly staged and treated, 5-year survival for stage 1 is approximately 90%. However, most cases are diagnosed in late stages where survival rates fall.

Key Points

Epithelial ovarian cancer (EOC)

- EOC includes ovarian, fallopian tube and primary peritoneal cancers
- Usually presents in late stages, challenging to treat and among the deadliest cancers of the female genital tract
- Screening recommended for high risk women with family history
- Early symptoms non-specific, hence usually present in late stages
- Ultrasound and MRI very useful to characterize and differentiate adnexal lesions
- Management and prognosis depend on FIGO stage
- Staging surgery for apparently early ovarian confined disease
- Cytoreductive surgery (primary or interval) for advanced disease
- Combination chemotherapy as neoadjuvant or adjuvant required in almost all cases
- Targeted therapy improves results
- Recurrences are common, usually treated with salvage chemotherapy and less often surgery
- Survival mainly depends on stage

Germ Cell Ovarian Tumors

These rarer ovarian tumors occur in young girls or women under the age of 40 years.

- They include dysgerminoma, endodermal sinus tumor, immature teratoma, choriocarcinoma and mixed variety.
- They are usually unilateral and detected in the early stages.
- Besides CA 125, tumor markers to be sent are alpha fetoprotein, LDH and beta hCG.
- Though they are highly malignant and rapidly growing, there is an excellent cure rate with surgery and chemotherapy.
- In most cases fertility can also be preserved so that normal periods and child-bearing can be achieved.

VULVAR CANCER

Cancer of the vulva usually occurs in elderly women. However, younger women also develop this disease, usually due to HPV infection.

- The most common type is squamous cell carcinoma.
- As in cervical cancer, a preinvasive stage exists [vulvar intraepithelial neoplasia (VIN)].

Hence, any vulvar symptom or skin change must be carefully assessed for early detection.

Symptoms

Change in skin color, itching, burning, swelling, ulceration, sores or pain over the vulva must be reported immediately.

Signs

- General examination must include nodal areas. The inguinal region especially must be carefully palpated for enlarged or fixed nodes.
- Speculum examination and Pap smear to assess vaginal extension or cervical disease.
- Local examination may reveal an ulcer, nodule or suspicious skin change. Often lichen sclerosus co-exists in the surrounding skin and should be documented. Urethral and anal areas must be carefully examined to rule out extension.

Diagnosis

- An outpatient biopsy under local anesthesia usually suffices for diagnosis.
- Careful clinical examination and CT scan are used to determine local and distal extent of disease.

FIGO Stage

- **Stage 1:** Tumor confined to the vulva
- **Stage 2:** Tumor of any size with extension to lower one-third of the urethra, lower one-third of the vagina, lower one-third of the anus with negative nodes
- **Stage 3:** Tumor of any size with extension to upper part of adjacent perineal structures, or with any number of nonfixed, nonulcerated lymph node
- **Stage 4:** Tumor of any size fixed to bone, or fixed, ulcerated lymph node metastases, or distant metastases.

Treatment

- Surgery is the cornerstone of treatment.
- Radical vulvectomy with inguinofemoral node dissection is usually done.
- Surgery can be tailored and modified after assessing the disease extent.

- Adjuvant radiation and in some cases chemotherapy is sometimes necessary depending on the prognostic factors
- Neoadjuvant radiation or chemotherapy may be required before surgery if urethral or anal involvement is present.

VAGINAL CANCER

Primary vaginal cancer is less common. It is more often secondarily involved in cervical, vulvar or other cancers.

The most common type is squamous cell, followed by adenocarcinoma.

Symptoms

The common complaints are:
- Vaginal discharge
- Postmenopausal or postcoital bleeding
- Urinary symptoms.

Diagnosis

Biopsy, careful clinical examination, if necessary, under anesthesia, and radiological investigations will help determine extent of local and distal spread.

Treatment

- Radiation therapy, usually with concomitant chemotherapy, is the treatment of choice in most cases of primary vaginal cancer.
- Surgery has a limited role in selected cases only.

PALLIATION IN GYNECOLOGIC CANCER

Palliative care and pain relief is an integral and important part of cancer management.

Many cases of gynecologic cancer are advanced or recurrent and require pain relief, palliation of symptoms and sympathetic counseling of the patient and family.
- Intractable pain is an unfortunate late event. A pain relief specialist will prescribe analgesics in a systematic, stepladder (tiered) pattern. Nerve blocks are also used when indicated.
- In cervical and vaginal cancer, involvement of the parametria can result in obstructive uropathy and ultimately renal failure.
- Anterior or posterior infiltration of cervical or vaginal cancer may ultimately result in vesicovaginal or recto-vaginal fistulae. Urinary diversion with PCN, or colostomy may be required.
- Life-threatening hemorrhage requiring surgery (emergency internal iliac ligation/embolization) or hemostatic radiation may be required in cases, such as untreated cervical cancer or a vaginal nodule of choriocarcinoma.
- Many cases of advanced ovarian cancer develop intestinal obstruction and recurrent ascites, which is difficult to manage.
- Symptoms due to metastatic disease must be treated on merit, e.g., pain due to bone metastases, supraclavicular nodes, cerebral metastases may be palliated with radiation.

ROLE OF THE PHYSIOTHERAPIST

Physiotherapy is of utmost importance in the management of cancer patients and survivors. Even in cured patients, quality of life and functionality is often affected. Those with recurrent or advanced disease are enormously benefited by appropriate physical therapy. Some of the main areas where the physiotherapist's involvement is beneficial are:
- Preoperative chest physiotherapy and assessment of physical and nutritional status (prehabilitation)
- Postoperative chest physiotherapy, early mobilization and ambulation
- Many centers nowadays follow the ERAS (enhanced recovery after surgery) protocol. Prehabilitation and postoperative active physiotherapy play a very important role in early recovery and discharge from hospital.
- Perioperative prevention and management of deep vein thrombosis
- Lymphedema prevention and management
- Pelvic floor exercises for urinary problems
- Use of vaginal dilators after pelvic radiotherapy
- Advise regarding exercises, nutrition and other care at home
- Psychological support

Summary

Key points of the conditions are described at the end of each condition.

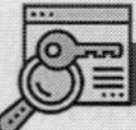

Review Questions

1. What are the common types of gynecological cancers?
2. Write a short note on prevention of cervical cancer.
3. Write a short note on endometrial cancer.
4. Write a short note on vulvar cancer.
5. Describe palliative therapy in gynecologic cancer.
6. What is the role of the physiotherapist in gynecologic cancer?

Bibliography

1. Balasubramaniam G, Gaidhani RH, Khan A, Saoba S, Mahantshetty U, Maheshwari A. Survival rate of cervical cancer from a study conducted in India. Indian J Med Sci 2021;73(2): 203-11.
2. Practical Gynecologic Oncology. Berek JS, Hacker NF (eds). Lippincott Williams and Wilkins, 2005.
3. Special Issue: FIGO Cancer Report 2021, Int J Gynecol Obstet. 2021;155(S1):1-134. Guest editors Sean Kehoe and Neerja Bhatla.

Multiple Choice Questions (MCQs)

To test your understanding and recall of key concepts.

1. **Which of the following is *true* for the FIGO staging in cervical cancer?**
   A. Stage 1: The carcinoma is not confined to the cervix
   B. Stage 2: The carcinoma invades beyond the lower third of the vagina or to the pelvic wall
   C. Stage 3: The carcinoma involves the lower third of the vagina and/or extends to the pelvic wall
   D. Stage 4: The carcinoma is confined to true pelvis
2. **What is the most common cause of cervical cancer?**
   A. Obesity
   B. Human papillomavirus (HPV) infection
   C. Chronic pelvic inflammatory disease (PID)
   D. Endometriosis
3. **Which histological type is most common in endometrial cancer?**
   A. Clear cell carcinoma
   B. Adenosquamous carcinoma
   C. Endometrioid adenocarcinoma
   D. Mucinous carcinoma
4. **Why is FIGO staging important in gynecological cancers?**
   A. It predicts the response of the patient to chemotherapy
   B. It determines local, regional, and distant spread for tailored treatment
   C. It identifies specific gene mutations that increase risk of cancer
   D. It ensures eligibility for radiation therapy for different stages of cancer
5. **Which gynecological cancer is also known as the "whispering disease"?**
   A. Epithelial ovarian cancer
   B. Breast cancer
   C. Uterine cancer
   D. Cervical cancer
6. **Which of the following is *not* a part of the the ERAS (enhanced recovery after surgery) protocol?**
   A. Perioperative prevention and management of deep vein thrombosis
   B. Obesity prevention
   C. Pelvic floor exercises for urinary problems
   D. Use of vaginal dilators after pelvic radiotherapy

ANSWERS

1. C	2. B	3. C	4. B	5. A
6. B				

Chapter 28

Cancer—General Physiotherapy

R Harihara Prakash

LEARNING OBJECTIVES

At the end of the chapter, the reader will be able to:

- Describe the various physical and psychological problems/complications faced by women due to cancer.
- Understand the general concept of physiotherapy as part of cancer management with special emphasis on breast cancer as an example.
- Use tools to assess the problems associated with cancer.
- Discuss the physiotherapy management for a cancer survivor.

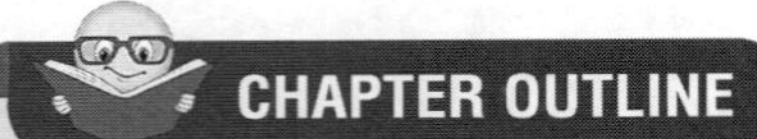

INTRODUCTION

Physical therapy has evolved in leaps and bounds over the years and it has opened avenues to offer services to various specialties and the rehabilitation of a cancer survivor is an expanding area of clinical practice that is not only most rewarding to patients, but also a very promising career pathway for physiotherapists.

Cancer rehabilitation especially with regards to women's health while addressing breast cancer or ovarian cancer needs innovative management, clinical expertise with research evidence and understanding patient preference. Owing to its complexity, rehabilitation of cancer and the secondary problems in women remains a challenging task and hence needs multimodal therapy addressing both physical and psychological issues.

The most commonly occurring cancers in women are:

- Cancer of the breast (chapter 26)
- Gynecological cancers (chapter 27)
- Colorectal cancer
- Lung cancer
- Skin cancer
- Thyroid cancer
- Lymphomas

Cancer treatment may include surgical removal, radiation therapy, and chemotherapy, depending on the type and stage of cancer. Once cancer is diagnosed, the primary goal is to stop the spread or to remove the cancer tissues using a single or the combination of all the above treatments. Most treatments involve chemotherapy, medical radiation therapy, or hormonal treatments. Weak immune system is the most common complication of cancer and cancer treatment. This can lead to frequent infection.

- Radiation therapy can be internal or external.
- Chemotherapy may be given by injection, by mouth, or through a catheter inserted into the abdomen (intraperitoneal).

These cancer treatments always have side effects. This can occur when the treatment affects the healthy cells. It may differ from person to person.

Box 28.1: Signs and symptoms associated with cancer.

- Easy fatiguability
- Lump or thickening of tissues that can be felt under the skin
- Weight fluctuations, either unintended loss or gain
- Skin changes, such as yellowing, darkening or redness of the skin, unhealed sores, or changes to existing moles in the body
- Changes in routine bowel or bladder habits
- Persistent cough
- Difficulty in breathing
- Difficulty in swallowing
- Hoarseness of voice
- Persistent indigestion or discomfort after eating
- Persistent, unexplained muscle and/or joint pain
- Persistent, unexplained raise in temperature or night sweats
- Unexplained bleeding

Breast cancer, being the most common cancer in women, the problems related to the cancer, postoperative symptoms/ complications and general physiotherapy management; will be discussed in this chapter taking breast cancer as an example.

PROBLEMS RELATED TO CANCER IN WOMEN

Signs and symptoms caused by cancer in women vary depending on which part of the body is affected.

Some general signs and symptoms associated with, but not specific to, cancer are shown in **Box 28.1**.

ROLE OF PHYSIOTHERAPY—GENERAL CONSIDERATIONS

The role of physiotherapy begins right from the pretreatment of cancer in the form of evaluating the problems of the patient which enables the therapist to establish a rapport with the patient. A brief assessment by the therapist which may include both physical and cognitive status of the patient followed by explaining the role of physiotherapy will provide ample opportunity for the patient to share the concerns and get clarifications for the same.

Assessment

The physiotherapy assessment (*see* Chapter 4: Assessment in Women's Health) should focus on the following:

- Functional status of the patient, assessing the difficulties in day-to-day life activities, such as grooming, overhead activities, bathing, etc.
- General mobility
- Muscle strength
- Overall health condition of the patient

The physical examination includes:

- Specific range of motion (ROM) of neck, shoulder, shoulder girdle and upper extremities for women with breast cancer
- Checking for hand dominance
- Changes in skin color and skin sensation
- Gross and fine motor skills
- Girth measurements on both the sides

By undertaking the presurgical assessment, the therapist has an opportunity to educate the patients about postoperative complications and play a role in their prevention. This will help the patients to understand the importance of early physiotherapy intervention which will in turn help in preventing further problems and postoperative complications. Moreover, readiness to undertake physiotherapy after the surgical intervention will increase and the patient will be compliant to physiotherapy care and will actively participate in the exercise program.

Physiotherapy for a patient who is posted, for example, for modified radical mastectomy (MRM) aims at keeping the upper extremity joints mobile including the shoulder girdle and maintaining the strength of the upper limb group of muscles including the chest muscles.

Postoperative Physiotherapy Goals

Short-term Goals

Physiotherapy aims at the following short-term goals:

- To prevent postsurgical edema
- To reduce postsurgical incisional pain
- To prevent of postsurgical joint stiffness
- To provide skin care
- To promote joint mobility

Long-term Goals

Physiotherapy is the mainstay of treatment and aims at the following long-term goals:

- To prevent and manage lymphedema
- To increase the reduced joint mobility
- To treat neuropathic and postural changes
- To improve the functional outcome
- To improve the quality of life

Postoperative Physiotherapy Intervention

To achieve the short-term goals, the physiotherapist works on the following areas:

Day 0

Positioning of the affected part

The patient who undergoes modified radical mastectomy (MRM) may be required to stay in bed for a few days; hence the upper limb positioning is important to prevent post-operative edema and stiffness. The affected side arm should be slightly abducted and flexed at the shoulder with the distal aspect of the limb elevated and supported **(Fig. 28.1)**. Care should be taken to rest the arm elevated while the patient is made to sit up. This type of elevation of the affected part helps in preventing fluid collection at the distal segment.

Periodic Girth Measurement

During MRM, as the procedure includes removal of axillary lymph nodes, there are high chances that the patient may develop lymphedema. As the saying goes 'prevention is better than cure', preventing lymphedema is much easier than managing it once it sets in. Hence careful monitoring of the limb is essential and periodical circumferential measurements of the whole limb starting from the axilla to the middle finger

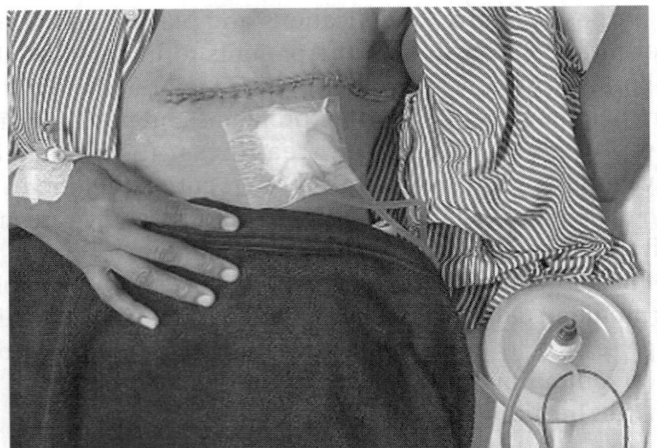

Fig. 28.1: Arm positioning of the affected side with drainage tube.

are required from day 1 of the surgery. The same should be documented. An example of the documentation sheet for the upper limb is given in **Table 28.1**. Calculation of lymphedema size and lymphedema reduction using girth measurements is discussed in Chapter 29: Cancer and Lymphedema.

From Day 1 to Day 3

Care of drain

In a typical surgical case, drain is inserted into the body nearer to the surgical site so as to remove excessive fluid which gets collected as a result of the surgery. Drain *in situ* reduces the risk of infection and hastens the rate of recovery.

- It is essential to be vigilant in taking care of the drain while in lying or during exercise sessions so that it does not get pulled out from its position.
- The drain should be kept sterile by using clean hands to handle it during positioning. The hands should be kept clean with soap and water.

This drain may be in place for one or two weeks or sometimes longer, depending on the fluid which gets drained out from the surgical site. As a routine, drains are removed when the fluid amount that drains is less than 30 mL per day. Patient should be well-educated about the importance of drain which is *in situ* and its care till it is removed.

Managing incisional pain

- The common complaint immediately after the surgery is pain at the incision site **(Fig. 28.2)** which can be managed by application of ice pack over the area of pain. The patient also complains of pain in and around the shoulder which can be addressed by the ice application **(Fig. 28.3)**.

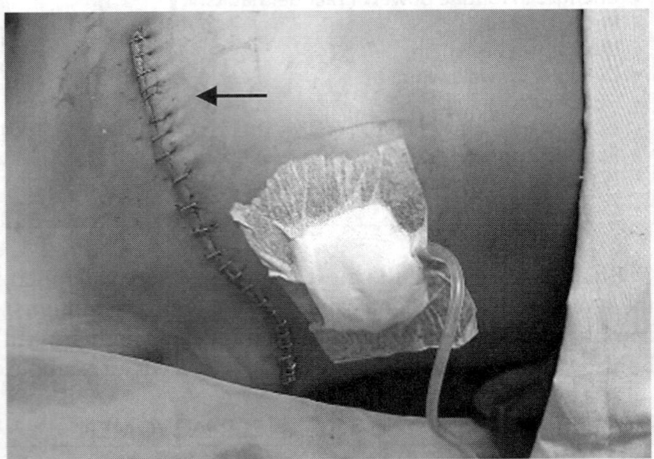

Fig. 28.2: Incision line of MRM.

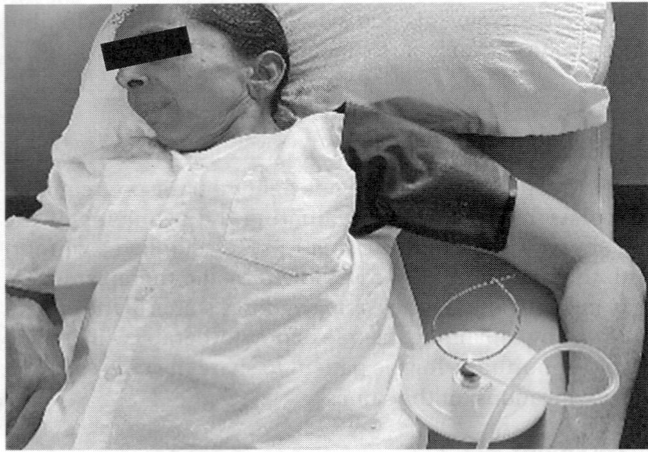

Fig. 28.3: Ice pack application to left shoulder.

Table 28.1: Upper limb edema measurement log.

Date/time																		
Site/Side	R	L	R	L	R	L	R	L	R	L	R	L	R	L	R	L	R	L
Axilla																		
9″ above elbow																		
6″ above elbow																		
3″ above elbow																		
Elbow																		
3″ below elbow																		
6″ below elbow																		
Wrist																		
Palmar crease																		
Middle finger																		

- Patient education and counseling can help in managing this type of pain.

Clinical Pointer

The therapist should assess and record the range of motion of the affected side shoulder **(Fig. 28.4)** using the goniometer.

- Gentle passive and active assisted range of motion exercises in both supine and if patient is comfortable in sitting position can be started **(Figs. 28.5A and B)**. While performing these exercises, therapist should be careful knowing the type and extent of incision and not traumatize the incision or jeopardize the healing process.
- As the days progress from day 2 to day 3, the therapist should encourage the patient to move up and about the bedside, maintaining the normal posture. Here, the therapist should be vigilant in monitoring the patient as they tend to keep the affected arm adducted with elbow flexed to 90° and supported by the unaffected limb. This pattern should be strictly discouraged as it may be detrimental making the shoulder joint and girdle prone to severe joint stiffness. If this problem is addressed at the beginning stage, the overall patient functional outcome will be better.
  The breathing pattern of the patient should be monitored by assessing the chest expansion at all the three levels. This will help the therapist to notice any chest complications which may arise during the hospital stay.

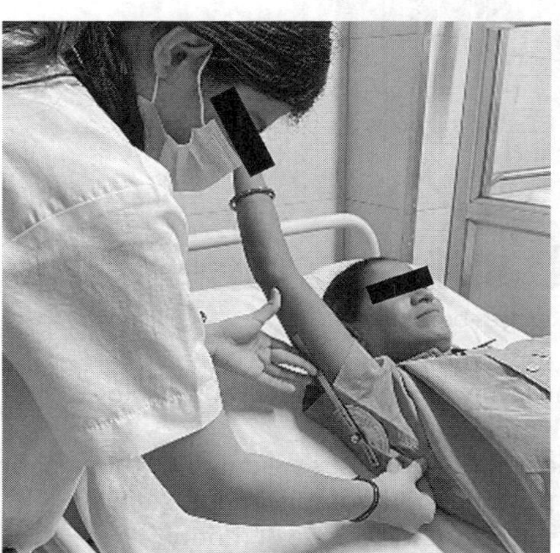

Fig. 28.4: Measuring ROM of shoulder joint of the affected side.

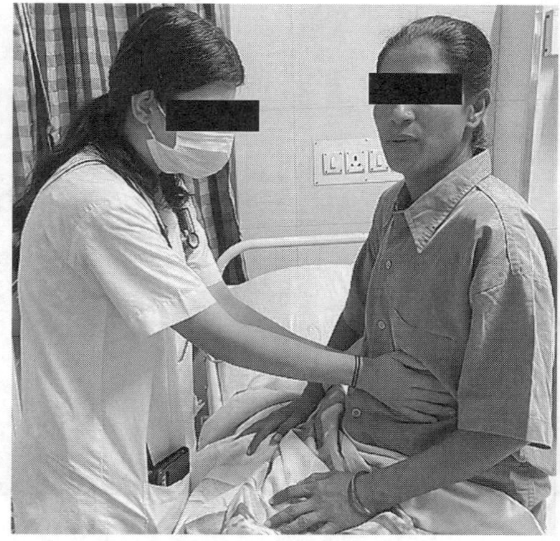

Fig. 28.6: Chest expansion exercise.

- Breathing exercises need to be started prophylactically to prevent any chest complications **(Fig. 28.6)**. These exercises can be done supervised twice a day and the patient and their caretaker should be advised to perform the exercises on their own at least 3 to 4 times a day.

Day 4 to 5

- Active and free exercises for the neck and shoulder that include shoulder rotation, shoulder shrugs, and shoulder bracing which are kept under patient tolerance level **(Figs. 28.7A to F)** can be started.

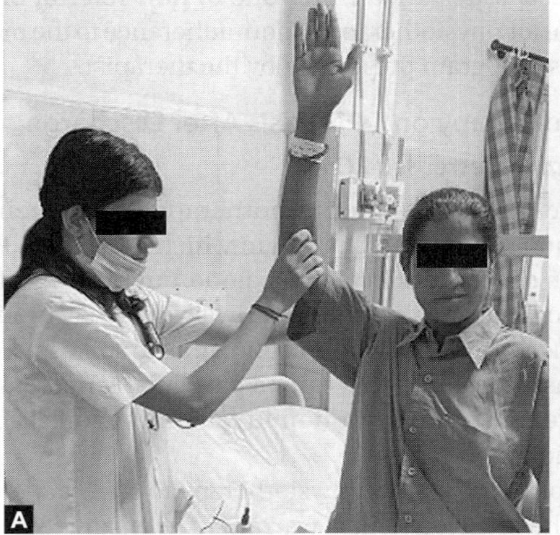

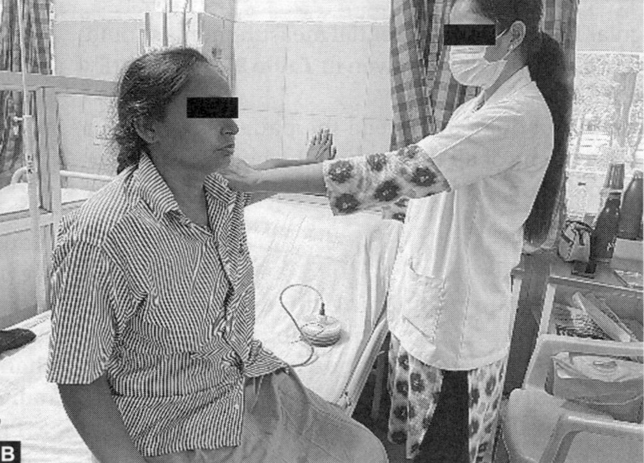

Figs. 28.5A and B: Active assisted shoulder ROM exercise of the affected side.

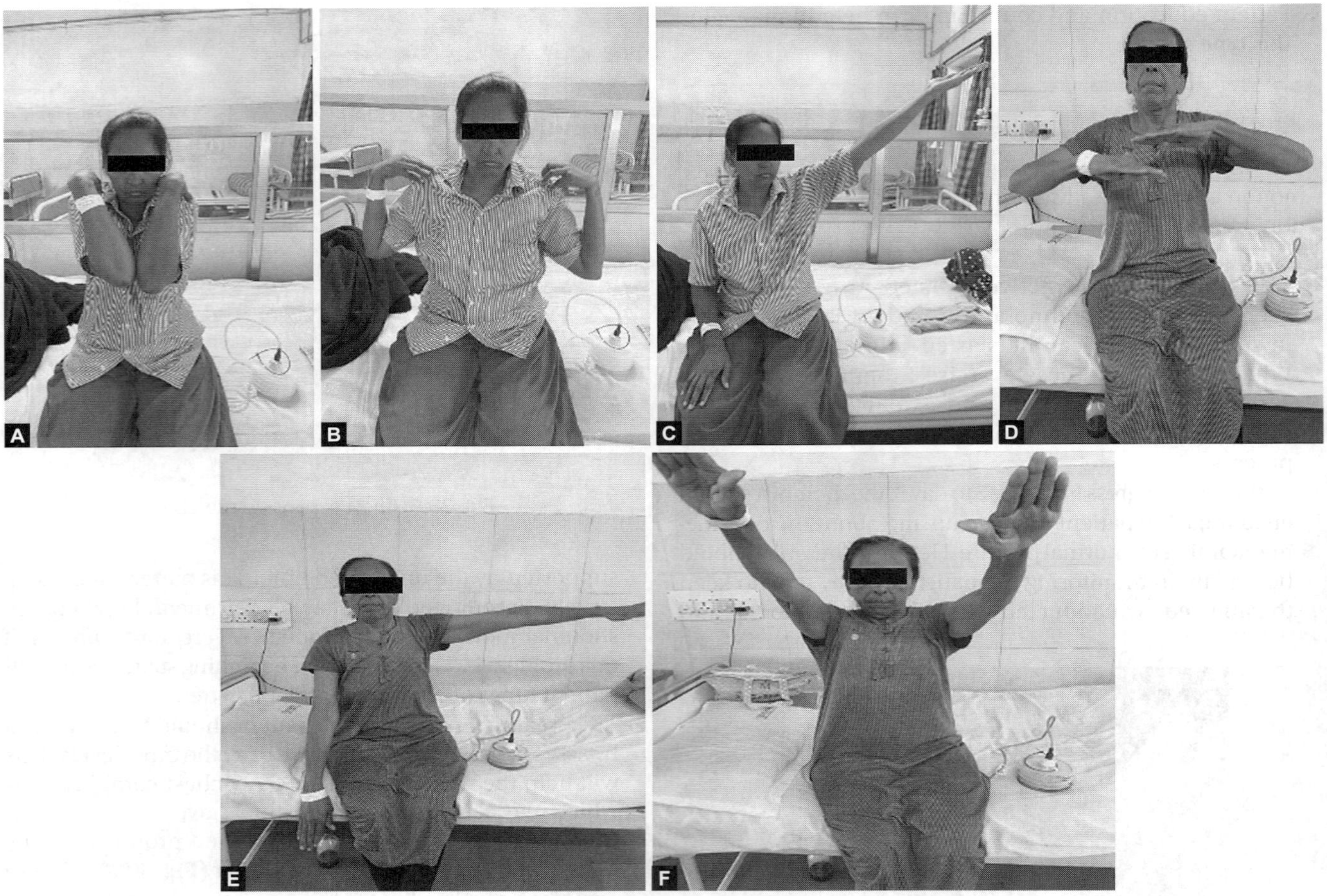

Figs. 28.7A to F: Shoulder free ROM exercises bedside.

Clinical Pointer

The patient should be educated that pain may be perceived while performing these exercises. Enough reassurance should be given during this period as patients may become apprehensive and stop performing the exercises which may become a strong reason for postoperative complications.

- The regular muscle circumferential measurements should be carried out as per the log given in **Table 28.1** to identify occurrence of lymphedema.
- The therapist should encourage the patient to perform active movements of all the parts of the body to enhance blood circulation and promote healing and prevent deconditioning.

On the Day of Discharge

A strict home program mentioning the exercise regime, frequency, skin care, girth measurement log should be given to the patient and follow-up appointments should be clearly mentioned in the discharge summary. They can be given an exercise diary to ensure exercise adherence till their follow up visit. Majority of the patients pass through uneventful course post discharge and do not require physiotherapy on regular basis once they achieve full ROM, muscle strength and no signs of lymphedema.

Physiotherapy becomes essential to those patients who develop postoperative complications, such as:

- Decreased shoulder range of motion
- Lymphedema of the affected side upper limb
- Hampered day to day functional activities

These issues arise either due to non-referral or delayed referral for physiotherapy or non-adherence to the mentioned exercise program prescribed by the therapist.

Physiotherapy on OPD Basis After Discharge

Managing Decreased ROM

Patients will visit the physiotherapy department with a common but treatable problem which is restricted range of motion of not the affected part alone, but majority of the time the proximal and distal joints as well. This may be either due to disuse or may be a complication due to soft tissue changes, such as adhesions. This can be particularly noted as fibrotic change that inhibits motion in patients who have received radiation therapy.

- Prior to the start of physiotherapy to such patients, X-ray of the involved joint is warranted to ensure joint integrity and to check the status of the bones.

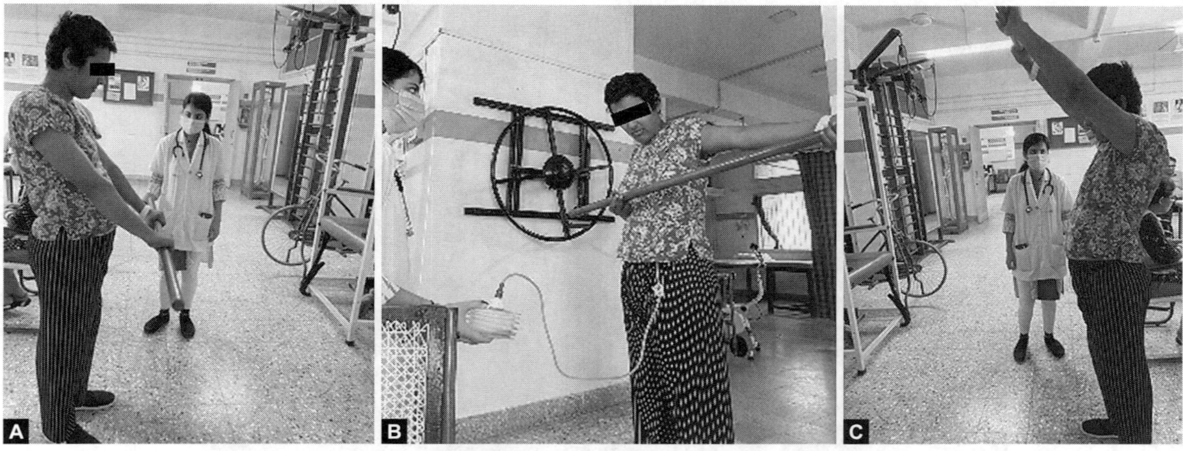

Figs. 28.8A to C: Wand exercises.

- Careful examination of the chest wall and axilla should be done to check for any adhesions which may be restricting the joint ROM.
- Prior to passive or active ROM exercises, application of deep friction massage can break the adhesions and can increase the circulation which can make the soft tissues supple.
- Gentle stretching of the soft tissues around the joint will be beneficial. Gentle joint mobilization if the bones are healthy, will aid in improving the joint ROM.
- Wand exercises **(Figs. 28.8A to C)**, wall ladder exercises **(Fig. 28.9)**, exercises can complement the approach in increasing the ROM of shoulder of the affected arm.

Lymphedema Management

This is one of the most common complications which can occur to a patient within a short time of the post-surgical intervention or sometimes as a late complication. Managing lymphedema needs specialized care.

- Application of elastic crepe bandage is the immediate line of action. The bandage should be worn in a figure of eight pattern and the pressure should be evenly increased from distal to proximal end **(Figs. 28.10A and B)**.
- Patient should be instructed to keep the limb always elevated.
- The patient should be taught to do hand pumping exercise with the crepe bandage on with the arm in elevated position which will aid in reducing the edema.
- Application of specialized techniques, such as manual lymphatic drainage (MLD) technique will result in excellent reduction in the swelling.

The primary aim of edema management is to detect at the early stage than to treat after it becomes a long standing complication. The early signs of edema include the following changes:

- Marked fullness in the arm due to increased interstitial fluid
- Color changes usually reddening
- Change in skin temperature.

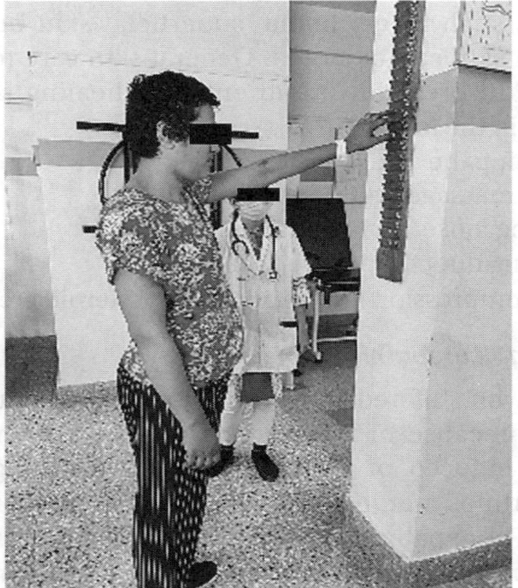

Fig. 28.9: Wall ladder exercises.

Once the above signs are noted, elevation of the arm is warranted immediately. Use of a soft ball to squeeze along with the application of elastocrepe bandage helps in reduction of the edema.

As mentioned earlier, circumferential measurements of both the extremities should be taken and recorded (*refer* **Table 28.1**). This procedure should be periodically repeated preferably by the same therapist at the same time of the day using the same inch tape. Patient can be advised to do contrast bath with hot and cold water by dipping the affected arm alternatively and also instructed to do pumping exercise with sponge or a smiley ball. This can be done two to three times a day.

For detailed management of Lymphedema, the reader can refer Chapter 29: Cancer and Lymphedema.

Skin Care

The patients may have wounds which would have been caused by delayed healing due to radiation therapy.

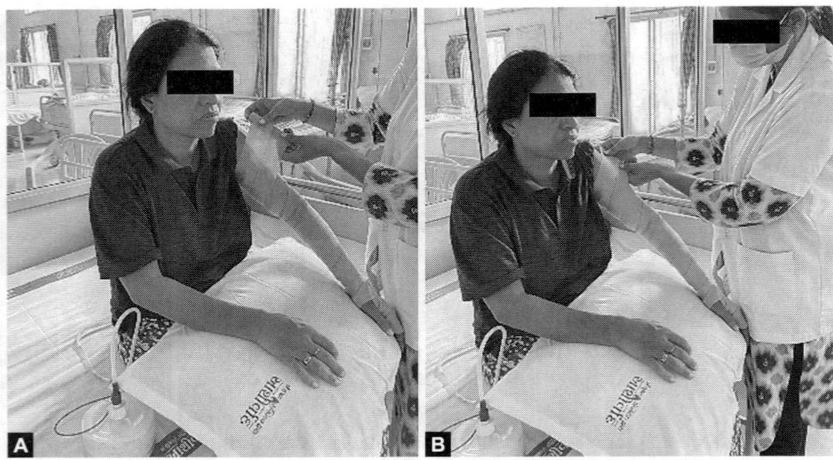

Figs. 28.10A and B: Application of elastocrepe bandage.

Changes, such as erythema, superficial skin break, and ulcerated skin can be noted. General skin care to prevent further skin breakdown and enhance healing should be provided in the form of:

- Cleansing the skin
- Tissue massage around the site
- Wearing loose, non-binding clothing
- Avoiding direct exposure to sun
- Cold compression and application of steroid cream

Managing Neuropathic Problems

Patients who suffered cancer may experience neuropathic changes because of injury to the nerve, which may be radiation induced, or a permanent damage during surgery, or sometimes nerve entrapments secondary to tissue fibrosis. These patients may experience symptoms, such as pain, altered sensation or sometime short-term sensory loss and weakness. If it is a temporary damage to the nerve, the symptoms may subside over time, may be six months to one year. Those who suffer a permanent damage to the nerve may have long-term problems leading to severe disability.

- These problems can be addressed with timely intervention, such as mobility exercise, release of adhesions, edema reduction.
- Transcutaneous electrical stimulation (TENS) may reduce the symptoms and can aid in functional activities.

Managing Postural Changes

Majority of the patients particularly who have undergone radical mastectomy tend to develop a typical asymmetrical posture. The initial asymmetry can be noted at the shoulder as compared to the uninvolved side. The shoulder may be held in a depressed, protracted position which can result in rotation and lateral flexion of the neck towards the affected side.

- This postural asymmetry can be easily managed by introducing chest expansion exercises, shoulder girdle exercises and posture correction in front of the mirror at an early stage.
- Emphasizing on postural education to the patient in the early stage helps preventing secondary changes.

Management of Cancer-associated Cachexia

Cancer-associated cachexia is acknowledged as a multi-factorial syndrome that is characterized by a continuous decrease in skeletal muscle mass, along with or without accompanying fat loss. Cancer causes the immune system to release certain chemicals called cytokines into the bloodstream which can cause inflammation that contributes to muscle mass reduction and fat loss. Cytokines speed up the body metabolism, which can make the patient lose calories faster and leads to extreme weight loss. This state of ill health is known as Cachexia. Evans et al. have defined cancer-associated cachexia as a minimum weight loss of at least 5% of body weight in less than or equal to one year in the presence of underlying illness, along with three of the following criteria:

- Decrease in muscle strength
- Fatigue
- Loss of appetite
- Decline in fat-free mass index
- Biochemical changes including increase in inflammatory markers (CRP >5.0 mg/l, IL-6 >4.0 pg/mL)
- Anemia (HGB <12 g/dL)
- Decreased serum albumin (Alb <3.2 g/dL)

Treatment of cancer cachexia needs a multidisciplinary approach and is considered palliative. Apart from pharmacological therapy, the treatment includes, nutritional supplement and a tailor made exercise protocol. Exercise in the beginning can prevent cachexia and can help in developing the muscle mass. Endurance exercises (a high number of repetitions performed over extended time periods against relatively low resistance) will be of greater benefit as compared to strength training (heavy weight with less repetitions). Combination of resistance and aerobic muscle training has been suggested to be incorporated into cachexia treatment programs. Exercise training is able to increase both strength and endurance in healthy conditions, depending on the type of exercise, and moreover, it has been proven to act as an excellent anabolic drive for skeletal muscle in combination with anabolic steroids or other muscle anabolic drugs.

Managing Cancer-related Fatigue

Cancer-related fatigue (CRF) is one of the most common symptoms experienced by patients which is chemotherapy and/or radiotherapy induced. As experiencing fatigue is subjective in nature, the National Comprehensive Cancer Network (NCCN) suggests patient self-reporting fatigue scale from *0 (no fatigue)* to *10 (severe fatigue)*. Multi-item tools to assess fatigue include:

- *Brief Fatigue Inventory*
- *The Cancer-related Fatigue Distress Scale.*

Management of fatigue is part of the continuum of cancer management. Patient education forms the base of fatigue management as it is due to chemotherapy and/or radiotherapy along with nutrition, hydration, and energy conservation exercises which can empower the patient to manage CRF. Physiotherapy is a safe and an effective method of treatment to manage fatigue. Techniques, such as massage, myofascial release (MFR), proprioceptive neuromuscular facilitation (PNF) and active exercises prove to be effective in reducing CRF in long term.

Cognitive behavioral therapy teaches patients to understand how thoughts can influence their feelings and behavior. CBT can also be utilized to manage pain associated with various oncologic diseases. CBT in the form of Memory and Attention Adaptation Training (MAAT) can assist cancer survivors develop adaptive skills to enhance daily cognitive performance and emotional coping strategy which might be affected with the disease process or chemotherapy. They are taught to recognize and identify thought patterns and behaviors when they occur and to use cognitive coping skills to modify them.

Promoting Functional Outcome and Quality of Life

Cancer being a life-threatening disease, cancer survivors suffer low quality of life (QoL) because of poor functional outcome. Patients may find difficulty in performing day to day activities, not due to physical problems alone, but also due to low psychological status, such as depression, anxiety, etc. There is a wide range of QoL tools which can measure the generic quality of patient's life (SF-36, Nottingham Health Profile) to cancer specific QoL tools, such as for example, Functional Assessment of Cancer Therapy.

- FACT-B for breast cancer
- FACT-G for general functional assessment
- FACT-br for brain tumors

They help to identify the various components, such as physical, emotional, cognitive and social levels of the patients. The nature of the physical therapists work, apart from managing the physical problems, provides a vehicle for patients to express their concerns, to ask questions regarding their problems, to verbalize their fears and to discuss their jobs, families and significant others. It is a privileged communication to which the therapist must respond in a positive but realistic manner, cautioning patients to expect the worst and to hope for the best because people are **survivors** by nature.

Simple alternative methods of adopting a regular meditation program, relaxation technique, aerobic exercise in the form of regular walking, engaging in day to day life affairs, such as cooking, bathing, cleaning house with short breaks in between, will integrate the patient into the routine activities as before and thereby improve the quality of life.

Summary

In this fast moving life with changing lifestyle, human beings suffer various diseases and one such life-threatening disease is cancer. The most common is the breast and cervical cancer in women worldwide and there is a steady increase in the number of people affected by this disease. Management of cancer needs a multi-disciplinary approach and physiotherapy has an important role. By nature, this physiotherapy profession deals with prevention, health promotion and rehabilitation. As part of the preoperative care, a physiotherapist role is to assess, educate and improve the overall physical condition of the patient by incorporating various joint mobility and muscle strengthening exercises. Physiotherapy has a definite role to manage postoperative, radiation induced pain and to prevent postoperative complications especially lymphedema. It also helps in combating the post-operative complications with advanced and innovative management thereby bringing back the lost functions of the patient and improving the quality of life.

CLINICAL EXAMPLE

A 37-year-old female has complaints of heaviness in the upper limb post her mastectomy. She complains of difficulty in lifting her arm while performing overhead activities. She feels physical asymmetry in her body while standing in front of the mirror and moreover, being in the early adulthood, cares for her external appearance. While talking to her, she expressed a lot of apprehension and fear about her future life.

- List down the problems faced by the patient.
- Write relevant examination/assessment on basis of complaints
- Write appropriate physiotherapy management with clinical reasoning.

Suggested Physiotherapy Management

- **Lymphedema management:** General and advanced techniques that includes arm elevation, application of crepe bandage, hand pumping exercise, massage and manual lymphatic drainage
- **Shoulder ROM exercises:** Active and active assisted exercises, use of equipment, such as wall ladder, shoulder wheel and pulley, shoulder joint mobilization. Use of any pain relieving modalities, such as TENS, cryopacks.

- **Posture correction:** Mirror biofeedback, posture correction exercises, regular stretching program and yogasanas
- **Education and counseling:** Cognitive behavioral therapy, relaxation techniques and meditation.

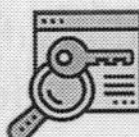

Review Questions

1. List the common cancer that affect women.
2. Explain the preoperative physiotherapy in cancer patient.
3. List down the common complications in breast cancer.
4. Discuss in detail the physiotherapy management for post-mastectomy patient.
5. Enlist the commonly used assessment and outcome measurement tools in cancer.

Bibliography

1. Aagaard P. Making muscles "stronger": exercise, nutrition, drugs. J Musculoskelet Neuronal Interact. 2004;4:165-74.
2. Argilés JM, Busquets S, López-Soriano FJ, Costelli P, Penna F. Are there any benefits of exercise training in cancer cachexia? J Cachexia Sarcopenia Muscle. 2012;3:73-6.
3. Charles L. McGarvey III. Physiotherapy for the Cancer Patient, Churchill Livingstone Inc.1990.
4. Ferlay J, Soerjomataram I, Dikshit R, Eser S, Mathers C, Rebelo M, et al. Cancer incidence and mortality worldwide: sources, methods and major patterns in GLOBOCAN 2012. Int J Cancer. 2015;136(5):E359-E86.
5. Kaarthigeyan K. Cervical cancer in India and HPV vaccination. Indian J Med Paediatr Oncol. 2012;33(1):7-12.
6. Kwekkeboom KL, Cherwin CH, Lee JW, Wanta B. Mind-body treatments for the pain-fatigue-sleep disturbance symptom cluster in persons with cancer. J Pain Symptom Manage. 2010;39 (1):126-38.
7. World Health Organization (WHO). Cancer prevention and control in the context of an integrated approach. Geneva: WHO; 2017. https://apps.who.int/iris/bitstream/handle/10665/275676/A70_R12en.pdf?sequence=1andisAllowed=y.
8. World Health Organization (WHO). International Agency for Research on Cancer. India factsheet. Lyon: IARC; 2018. https://gco.iarc.fr/today/data/factsheets/populations/356-india-fact-sheets.pdf.
9. World Health Organization (WHO). International Agency for Research on Cancer. Latest global cancer data: cancer burden rises to 18.1 million new cases and 9.6 million cancer deaths in 2018. Geneva; 2018. https://www.who.int/cancer/PRGlobocanFinal.pdf.

Multiple Choice Questions (MCQs)

To test your understanding and recall of key concepts.

1. What is the most common cancer affecting women worldwide?

A. Cervical cancer
B. Breast cancer
C. Ovarian cancer
D. Colorectal cancer

2. Why is periodic girth measurement important post-mastectomy?

A. To monitor muscle strength
B. To detect early signs of lymphedema
C. To evaluate joint flexibility
D. To check for postural asymmetry

3. How does a physiotherapist prevent postoperative joint stiffness after breast cancer surgery?

A. By prescribing TENS therapy
B. By encouraging the patient to perform active and assisted range of motion exercises
C. By using ice packs on the surgical site post surgery
4. D. By limiting physical activity of the involved shoulder post surgery

5. A 45-year-old woman post-mastectomy has difficulty lifting her arm overhead. What is the best initial intervention?

A. Start with weightlifting exercises
B. Apply a hot pack and begin shoulder stretching exercises
C. Use wall ladder and wand exercises for shoulder mobility
D. Perform electrical stimulation for muscle strengthening

6. A patient with cancer-related fatigue reports difficulty completing daily activities. Which physiotherapy strategy should be prioritized?

A. Strength training exercises
B. Relaxation techniques and aerobic exercises
C. Contrast baths and massage therapy
D. Joint mobilization and manipulation

7. Which of the following statements is correct with respect to the role of manual lymphatic drainage (MLD) in lymphedema management?

A. It promotes lymphatic fluid stagnation to reduce swelling
B. It improves lymph circulation and reduces fibrosis
C. It is effective only in stage III lymphedema
D. It eliminates the need for compression garments

8. A patient undergoing chemotherapy reports persistent fatigue and poor quality of life. Which tool can be used to assess her quality of life?

A. Nottingham health profile
B. Functional assessment of cancer therapy (FACT)
C. TNM staging system for cancer
D. Cancer care evaluation scale

ANSWERS

1. B	2. B	3. B	4. B	5. C
6. B	7. B	8. B		

Chapter 29

Cancer and Lymphedema

Nipa Atul Shah

LEARNING OBJECTIVES

At the end of the chapter, the reader will be able to:
- Understand the basics of lymphedema.
- Understand the contributing factors of lymphedema related to cancer.
- Describe the evaluation process of lymphedema.
- Describe the treatment of lymphedema—complete decongestive therapy (CDT).

CHAPTER OUTLINE

- Introduction
- Anatomy of lymphatic system
  - Function of the lymphatic system
  - Parts of the lymphatic system
  - Functions of lymph nodes
- Classification of lymphedema
- Prevalence of lymphedema in women after cancer
- Etiology and contributing factors of lymphedema
  - Etiology
  - Risk factors
- Stages of lymphedema
- Signs of lymphedema
- Evaluation
  - Demographic data
  - History
  - Examination
  - Measurement of limb lymphedema
  - Investigations
- Complications of lymphedema
- Lymphedema management
  - Complete decongestive therapy
  - Diet
  - Traveling with lymphedema
  - Pneumatic compression pump
  - Kinesiology taping
  - Low level LASER therapy
  - Extracorporeal shockwave therapy
  - Surgery for lymphedema

INTRODUCTION

Lymphedema is a very common and debilitating serious condition which may affect extremities, trunk, abdomen, head, neck and external genitalia. Failure of the lymphatic system (lymphatic vessels and lymph nodes are damaged, removed or impaired) leads to overloading of a body region with lymphatic fluid and subsequent development of swelling. Lymphedema is a progressive disorder characterized by abnormal accumulation of protein-rich fluid in the interstitial space.

This disease is often first noticed by the patient as heaviness of limb, followed by asymmetry or increased circumference of an extremity. As swelling slowly progresses, patients may have difficulty fitting into clothing. Once well established, lymphedema may cause the following problems:
- ❖ Fatigue related to the size and weight of the extremity
- ❖ Embarrassment in public
- ❖ Recurrent bacterial or fungal infections
- ❖ Pain
- ❖ Restricted range of motion (ROM)
- ❖ Severe impairment of daily activities

Ultimately, it may affect the quality of life of patients.

ANATOMY OF LYMPHATIC SYSTEM

Lymphatic system serves as an accessory route by which lymph fluid can flow from interstitial tissue into the bloodstream (venous circulation) **(Fig. 29.1)**.

Lymph fluid contains:
- Water
- Protein
- Long chain fatty tissue
- Cells

Function of the Lymphatic System

The lymphatic system works to drain those substances that cannot be drained directly by the blood stream and collect and transport lymph fluid from interstitial fluid to blood stream. Functions of lymphatic system are:
- Fluid regulation
- Immune surveillance
- Transport of large molecules

Parts of the Lymphatic System

The lymphatic system is made up of parts as shown in **Figure 29.2**.

Entry-point of Lymph to the Lymphatic System

- Lymphatic capillaries are located beneath the epidermis and cover the entire body surface to form **web-like networks** in the interstitial spaces. They absorb the lymph fluid into the lymphatic system from interstitial space.
- There is no pump, but the lymph moves via skeletal muscle action, respiratory movement, and contraction of smooth muscle in vessel walls.
- From the lymphatic vessels the lymph fluid moves to the regional lymph nodes which are very important structures of the lymphatic system **(Fig. 29.3)**.
- From lymph nodes, lymph travels via lymphatic vessels to the lymphatic trunk. The largest lymphatic trunk is thoracic duct which empties the lymphatic fluid into the venous angle (formed by internal jugular and subclavian veins).

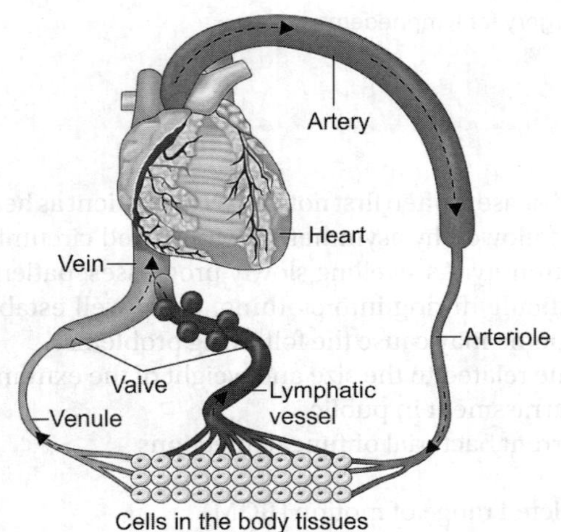

Fig. 29.1: Lymphatic system *(For color version, see Plate 8)*.

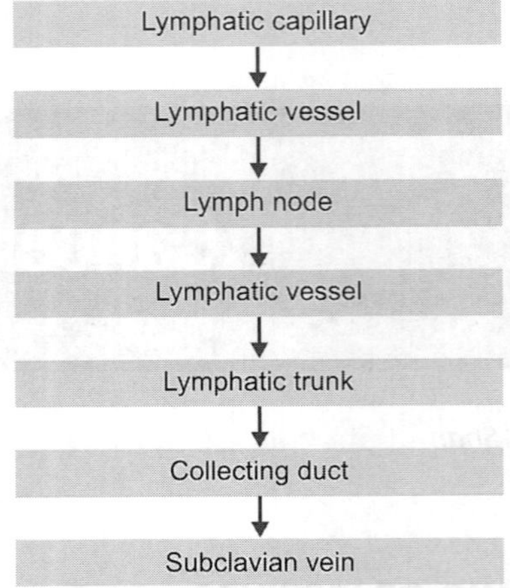

Fig. 29.2: Parts of the lymphatic system.

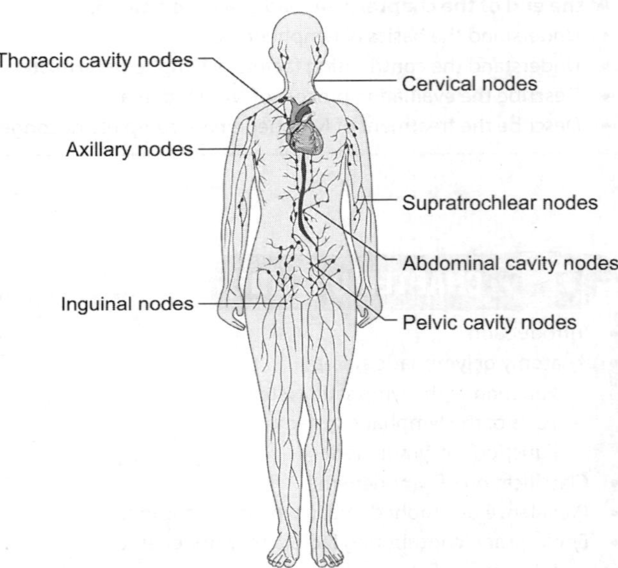

Fig. 29.3: Major lymph nodes in the body.

Functions of Lymph Nodes

- **Protective:** Filter the harmful material
- **Immune:** Produce antigen-stimulated lymphocytes
- Thickening of lymph fluid

CLASSIFICATION OF LYMPHEDEMA

- **Primary lymphedema** develops without any cause at different stages of life (mainly in lower limbs). It may be present at birth or can develop later in life but may be triggered by minor trauma, infection or immobility.
- **Secondary lymphedema** is much more common, develops after surgery or radiation therapy for various cancers, trauma, scarring, or infection of the lymphatic system.

 **Clinical Pointer**

Lymphedema can also be classified as mild (<20% increase in limb volume), moderate (20–40% increase in limb volume) or severe (>40% increase in limb volume).

This chapter will discuss about secondary lymphedema after cancer in women.

PREVALENCE OF LYMPHEDEMA IN WOMEN AFTER CANCER

Worldwide 140–250 million cases of lymphedema are estimated to exist, with filariasis (parasitic infection) being the most common cause, followed by breast cancer-related lymphedema (BCRL). Research data for the incidence of BCRL suggests that more than one in five women who survive breast cancer will develop arm lymphedema. Other gynecological cancers like cervical, endometrial, and vulvar have shown to have incidence risk of lower limb lymphedema between 5 to 49%. The incidence of lower limb lymphedema is even less documented than BCRL. Other less common conditions like genitourinary or head and neck cancers also develop lymphedema in women.

All patients who have undergone lymph node dissection in cancer treatment should be considered to be at a lifetime risk for developing lymphedema.

ETIOLOGY AND CONTRIBUTING FACTORS OF LYMPHEDEMA

Etiology

Surgery

- It is the most common cause for secondary lymphedema as cancer surgical procedures include the removal of adjacent lymph nodes. Lymph node dissection or lymphadenectomy involves dissection of lymph nodes and subsequent biopsy of the tissues to determine whether they are cancerous or noncancerous.
- Lymph nodes are the commonest sites for metastases of solid tumors. Many types of malignant tumors have a natural tendency to produce lymph node metastases at an early stage. Hence, lymph node dissection and biopsy become crucial to assess the spread of cancer. Since after lymph node dissection, there is accumulation of lymph in the interstitial tissues, it causes lymphedema.
- Lymphadenectomy can be regional or radical. Following are the most common sites of lymph nodes dissection:
  - Axillary lymph nodes (for breast cancer) **(Box 29.1)**
  - Inguinal lymph nodes (for anal and vulvar cancers)
  - Cervical lymph nodes (for head/neck cancers and thyroid cancers)
  - Retroperitoneal lymph nodes (for ovarian cancers)
- Removal of axillary lymph nodes leads to upper limb lymphedema, inguinal and retroperitoneal lymph nodes leads to lower limb lymphedema, whereas that of cervical lymph nodes leads to lymphedema of the face or neck.

Box 29.1: Axillary lymph nodes.

The axillary lymph nodes are divided into three levels:
1. Level I (low axilla)—located in lower part of the armpit
2. Level II (mid axilla)—located in middle part of the armpit
3. Level III (high axilla)—located in upper part of the armpit near the breastbone (sternum)

Radiation Therapy

Radiotherapy is given to destroy cancer cells that may remain after surgery. This may also damage normal cells and compromise the lymphatic system and may contribute to onset of lymphedema. Radiation can cause fibrosis in tissue which can affect lymph transportation and result in restricted range of motion of surrounding joints.

Chemotherapy

Chemotherapy is also one of the cancer treatments contributing to developing lymphedema.

Risk Factors

- Risk factors for development of breast cancer-related lymphedema include:
  - Axillary lymph node dissection
  - Lymphangitis
  - Infection
  - Obesity (body mass index ≥25 kg/m^2)
  - Duration of axillary drainage
  - Postoperative radiotherapy
- There is strong evidence that patients at risk of developing lymphedema should maintain a healthy weight or avoid weight gain and patients at risk of developing lymphedema as well those with lymphedema should undergo a supervised exercise regime to prevent lymphedema. There is insufficient evidence to support claims that limb constriction, elevation, heat/cold, or air travel can trigger lymphedema. There is also limited evidence to support venipuncture triggers lymphedema.

STAGES OF LYMPHEDEMA

Box 29.2 shows the stages of lymphedema according to International Society of Lymphology (ISL).

Box 29.2: Stages of lymphedema.

Stage 0: Latency stage: Subclinical stage with no swelling and normal tissue consistency. Person is at risk of developing lymphedema.

Stage I: Reversible stage: Edema is soft (pitting) and elevation reduces swelling.

Stage II: Spontaneously irreversible stage: Hardening of the tissue and lymphostatic fibrosis, Stemmer's sign positive (inability to lift the skin over finger or toe) with frequent infection.

Stage III: Lymphostatic elephantiasis: Extreme increase in volume with typical skin changes (papilloma, deep skin folds, warts), Stemmer's sign positive.

SIGNS OF LYMPHEDEMA

- Swelling of the arm or legs, which may include finger or toes **(Fig. 29.4)**
- Feeling of heaviness or tightness of skin may be first sign for lymphedema
- Difficulty in moving different joints of limb
- Thickening of the skin, with or without skin changes such as blister or warts
- Pain may or may not be present
- Fatigue

EVALUATION

Demographic Data

- Patient's name, age, gender
- Occupation
- Affected limb and dominant limb
- Date of surgery (if any)
- Number of radiations (if any)
- Chemotherapy sessions (if any)

History

- History of onset of lymphedema after surgery
- Lymphedema duration in months
- Pain history including site, side, intensity and increasing and decreasing factors
- Medical history including other associated comorbidities

Examination

- Posture
- Skin color
- Muscle atrophy
- Scar examination—adherent or nonadherent, healed or nonhealed
- Temperature

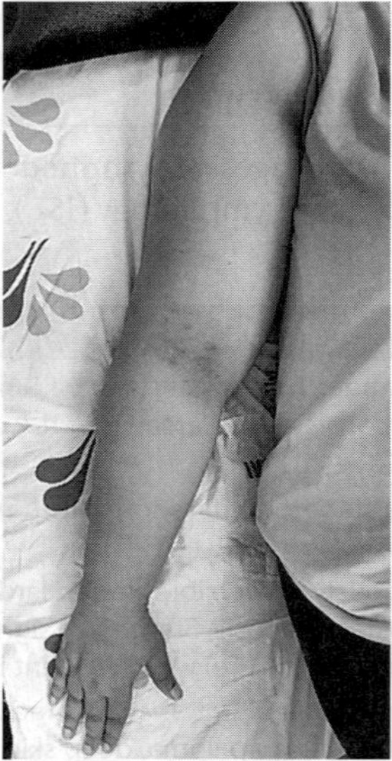

Fig. 29.4: Swelling of the entire upper extremity.

Box 29.3: Lymphedema and Breast Cancer Questionnaire (LBCQ)

It is an interview tool assessing indicators of lymphedema experience and symptom management strategies. It assesses patients' self-reported symptom management for 19 different symptoms like limitation of shoulder, elbow, wrist and hand movement, weakness in the arm or hand, aching, breast swelling, chest wall swelling, swelling with pitting, tenderness, blistering, heaviness, stiffness, numbness, rashes, firmness/tightness, raised temperature of the arm and redness. The subject is first questioned about the presence of these symptoms in the last 30 days or at any point in the last 365 days. If the symptoms are present, the subject is asked an open-ended question about how they manage that symptom. The LBCQ also includes questions about demographics and treatment history, and open-ended questions about treatment, disease course and symptom management.

- Sensory examination
- Range of motion of affected limb
- Muscle strength
- Presence of truncal lymphedema or genital lymphedema
- Pitting and presence of fibrosis
- Stemmer sign
- Lymphedema and Breast Cancer Questionnaire (LBCQ) **(Box 29.3)**

Measurement of Limb Lymphedema

Circumference Measurement

Arm circumference

Lymphedema is assessed by the arm circumference as follows **(Figs. 29.5A to C)**:

- It is measured at 7 symmetrical levels (metacarpophalangeal joints, radial styloid process, at 10, 20, 30 and 40 cm from the radial styloid process and over olecranon) of the affected and contralateral arm.
- The lymphedema size is expressed as the ratio of the total circumference of the affected and unaffected arm, and calculated according to the formula shown in **Box 29.4**.
- The degree of lymphedema reduction is calculated by the formula shown in **Box 29.5**.

Perometer

A perometer is a device that uses an array of optoelectronic infrared sensors for volume measurement. It is a rapid, hygienic and clinically applicable technique to monitor limb volumes even for routine assessment. It has relatively better accuracy than other techniques.

Water Plethysmography (Water Displacement Method)

It measures the volume of liquid displaced by the limb. It is a gold standard technique to measure limb volume. It, however, has hygiene issues.

Bioimpedance

Tissue resistance to flow of electrical current is used to measure limb volume. The disadvantage of this method is that it cannot be used in bilateral involvement.

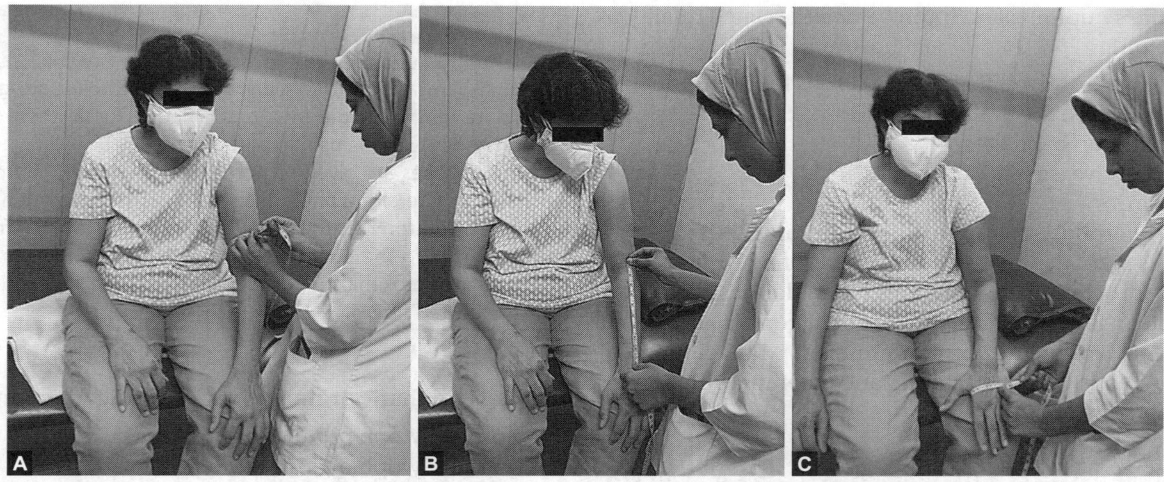

Figs. 29.5A to C: Measurement of limb circumference. (a) Arm circumference; (b) Locating landmarks; (c) Hand circumference.

Box 29.4: Formula to calculate lymphedema size.

$$\frac{\text{Total circumference of the affected arm} - \text{Total circumference of the unaffected arm}}{\text{Total circumference of the unaffected arm}} \times 100$$

0% indicates the same total circumferences of two arms

Box 29.5: Formula to calculate the degree of lymphedema reduction.

$$\frac{\text{Total circumference of the affected arm before treatment} - \text{Total circumference of the affected arm after treatment}}{\text{Total circumference of the affected arm before treatment} - \text{Total circumference of the unaffected arm}} \times 100$$

Investigations

Lymphangiogram

It is an old technique utilized to visualize lymphatics. A skin incision is made and direct cannulation of lymphatics is done. Since it is invasive, it carries the risk of infection, local inflammation, fibrosis, emboli and hypersensitivity reactions. It is more time consuming and painful. It has been abandoned to a great extent after the development of lymphoscintigraphy.

Lymphoscintigraphy

It is a gold standard imaging test used for functional evaluation of the lymphatic channels. A radiolabeled tracer is injected and the uptake into the lymph nodes is estimated. It is a simple, reproducible, credible, well-tolerated and objective method to diagnose the presence of lymphedema.

Ultrasound

It analyzes volumetric changes like thickness of epidermis, increase in subcutaneous layer, change in muscle mass, etc., along with structural changes like hyperechogenic dermis and hypoechogenic subcutaneous layer. It also helps in assessing soft tissue changes but does not provide any information about truncal anatomy of lymphatics. A duplex ultrasound is extremely useful in patients with lower limb swelling.

Computed Tomography (CT) Scan

It helps not just in confirming a diagnosis but also monitoring effect of treatment. Common CT findings in lymphedema include honeycomb appearance, increased fat density, thickening of calf skin, thickening of subcutaneous compartment and thickened perimuscular aponeurosis.

Magnetic Resonance Imaging (MRI)

MRI helps in differentiating between lymphedema, lipedema, and phlebedema. Features of lymphedema on MRI include a honeycomb pattern above the fascia between the subcutis and muscle, increased volume of subcutaneous tissue, circumferential edema and marked dermal thickening. It also shows typical features of angiosarcoma.

COMPLICATIONS OF LYMPHEDEMA

- Lymphangitis
- Lymphangio-adenitis
- Lymphorrhea (leaking of lymph fluid)
- Recurrent cellulitis
- Superficial bacterial and fungal infections
- Deep vein thrombosis
- Severe functional impairment
- Psychosocial dysfunction
- Cosmetic problems
- Complications following surgery include hematoma, seroma, skin necrosis and partial wound separation.

LYMPHEDEMA MANAGEMENT

Complete Decongestive Therapy (CDT or Vodder Technique)

It is the GOLD standard recommended management for Lymphedema. CDT is not a cure for lymphedema. It can help control the symptoms and improve health related quality of life (HRQoL).

Complete decongestive therapy (CDT) has four components:
1. Manual lymphatic drainage (MLD)
2. Compression bandages
3. Decongestive exercises
4. Skin care

CDT is a two-phase therapy as shown in **Table 29.1**.

In Phase I, patient has to consult a certified lymphedema therapist for active treatment which lasts as long as necessary/ until plateau is reached, then the patient continues phase II at home by following all components. Management of lymphedema is life-long maintenance therapy with regular follow-up visits.

Manual Lymph Drainage (MLD)

MLD is a gentle manual treatment that improves the activity of the lymphatic system. It also re-routes the lymph flow from **blocked areas** to healthy unaffected areas to the venous system.

- MLD strokes **(Fig. 29.6)** should be gentle in pressure. Too much pressure may result in lymphangiospasm and hyperemia.
- It has two phases—working phase and resting phase, with each stroke lasting for 1 second in the working phase and 5–7 repetitions in the same area. Direction of strokes depends on anatomy of lymphatic system. **Box 29.6** describes the technique of MLD for BCRL.

Table 29.1: Phases of CDT.

Phase I (treatment phase)	*Phase II (maintenance phase)*
MLD	Self MLD
Compression bandaging	Compression stocking during the day and bandaging at night
Self-care (skin/nail care) education	Self-care (skin/nail care) education
Decongestive exercises	Decongestive exercises

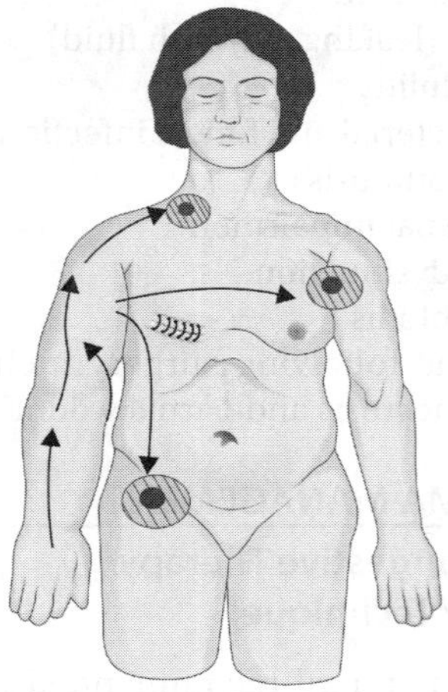

Fig. 29.6: Direction of strokes for MLD for BCRL.

Box 29.6: Technique of MLD for breast-cancer related lymphedema (BCRL).

Initial strokes are given to clear neck area. Strokes are given to stimulate venous angle in supraclavicular fossa, then cervical lymph nodes with the palmar part of hand.

Then strokes are given to normal lymph nodes (contralateral axillary, ipsilateral inguinal) followed by strokes to open up the channels (anastomoses) so that the fluid can be drained from the affected side to the unaffected side. Similarly, strokes are given from distal to proximal on the affected side of the limb and then to the unaffected side.

Manual lymphatic drainage has following functions:

- Improves lymph production
- Increases lymphangio-motorocity
- Improves lymph circulation
- Special techniques are used to break down fibrous connective tissue
- Promotes relaxation and has an analgesic effect

Compression

After MLD, compression therapy is given to prevent reaccumulation of evacuated lymph fluid and to improve efficiency of the muscle and joint pumps. It also provides support for tissues that have lost elasticity.

Types of compression depends on the phase of therapy:

- In Phase I, multilayered compression bandaging is given. Short stretch bandages are used which exert a high working pressure on the tissue and provide strong support during muscle contraction.
- In Phase II, compression stockings have to be worn throughout the patient's life after reduction of lymphedema for maintenance therapy during the day time.

Specific class (CC) of bandage is required for lymphedema:

- For upper extremity—CC II (30–40 mm of Hg seamless/ 23–32 mm of Hg seamed)
- For lower extremity—CC III (40–50 mm of Hg seamless/ 34–46 mm of Hg seamed)

Decongestive Exercises

Exercises are always performed with the bandages/ compression garment.

- Active ROM, stretching and strengthening exercises involving affected parts of lymphedema **(Figs. 29.7A to H)**
- Diaphragmatic breathing exercise
- Aerobic exercises **(Fig. 29.7I)** play a very important role for weight control and for lymphedema management, e.g., walking, cycling, swimming.

Importance of exercises

- Increase muscle pumping
- Increase lymph vessel activity and lymph transportation
- Increase venous and lymphatic return

The enthusiasm for exercise for lymphedema can be attributed to recent research findings:

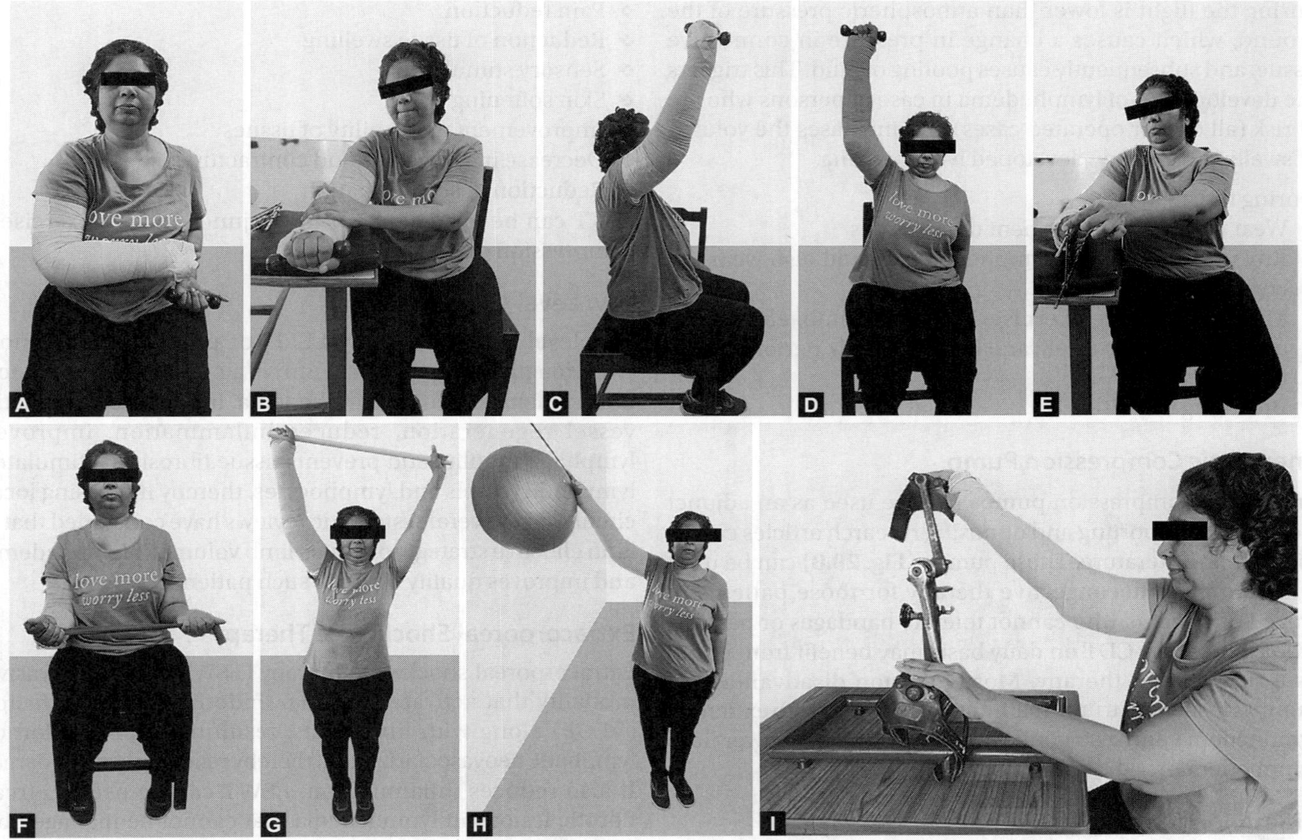

Figs. 29.7A to I: Exercises for lymphedema: (A) Strengthening of contralateral extremity; (B) Strengthening of wrist muscles; (C) Strengthening of shoulder muscles (lateral view); (D) Strengthening of shoulder muscles (anterior view); (E) Strengthening of finger muscles; (F) Strengthening of shoulder rotators; (G) Active assisted exercises of shoulder using wand; (H) Proprioceptive exercises using vestibular ball; (I) Aerobic exercises for upper extremity using arm ergometer.

- Exercise is safe, contrary to past beliefs
- Does not increase or exacerbate lymphedema
- Pain/tenderness may be reduced.

Box 29.7 shows some evidences regarding exercise for lymphedema.

Skin and Nail Care

Eliminate bacterial and fungal growth

- Use medicated powders, hydrocortisone cream, where indicated
- Bathe daily

Box 29.7: Evidence for use of exercises for lymphedema.

- **Resistance exercises:** Several systematic reviews have concluded that resistance exercises do not have a negative effect and they do not provoke or increase lymphedema. They are safe to use and produce significant strength gains in lymphedema patients. **Aerobic exercises:** Studies show that aerobic exercises like arm ergometry do not improve lymphedema status but can improve quality of life and function.
- **Aquatic therapy:** Aquatic therapy has been proven to improve functional capacity and quality of life in patients with lower limb lymphedema. It improves limb volume significantly immediately after the session in patients with breast cancer-related lymphedema.

Reduce the risk of infection

- Avoid injury, mosquito bite, itching
- Use low pH lotion
- Clean all injuries and consult a doctor immediately

Do's and Don'ts

- Avoid heat (no hot pack, sauna bath)
- Use caution while exercising
- No tight clothes, jewelery or band
- No venepunctures
- No blood pressure measurement on affected limb

Diet

No specific diet for lymphedema is followed but following suggestions can be kept in mind:

- Reducing water and/or protein intake is ineffective
- General recommendations:
  - Low caloric diet
  - Low sodium
  - High fiber
  - Vitamin rich diet

Traveling with Lymphedema

Air travel may be challenging for lymphedema patients and those who are at risk of lymphedema. The cabin pressure during the flight is lower than atmospheric pressure of the ground, which causes a change in pressure in connective tissue, and subsequently causes pooling of fluid. This triggers the development of lymphedema in case of persons who are at risk (all cancer operated cases) and increases the volume of swelling in already developed lymphedema.

During the flight:

- Wear compression garment or bandages
- Any person at risk of lymphedema should also wear the compression stocking
- **Muscle pumping exercise:** For upper limb, elevate the arm and squeeze a ball; and for lower limb, perform ankle toe movement
- Breathing exercises

Pneumatic Compression Pump

Pneumatic compression pumps may be used as an adjunct treatment. Supporting and opposing research articles can be found in the literature. These pumps **(Fig. 29.8)** can be used with complete decongestive therapy for those patients in stage I or patients who cannot tolerate bandages or patients who cannot take CDT on daily basis may benefit from pump as a supplement therapy. Most common disadvantage of pump is ipsilateral trunk quadrant gets swollen with extremity lymphedema and also genital swelling in case of lower limb lymphedema.

Kinesiology Taping

Kinesiology taping (KT) involves application of a relatively more elastic and thinner tape, made of 100% cotton, to the skin. The mechanism behind it, has not yet been fully understood. But it has been reported to facilitate myofascial release and reabsorption of lymphatic fluid in the adjacent tissues. It creates a pull on the superficial layers of skin, which creates space between the dermis and muscle. This relieves pressure on lymphatic channels and vessels and enhances lymphatic flow, resulting in better lymphatic drainage. Other effects of KT include:

- Relief of tissue fluid congestion
- Augmentation of blood and lymph circulation

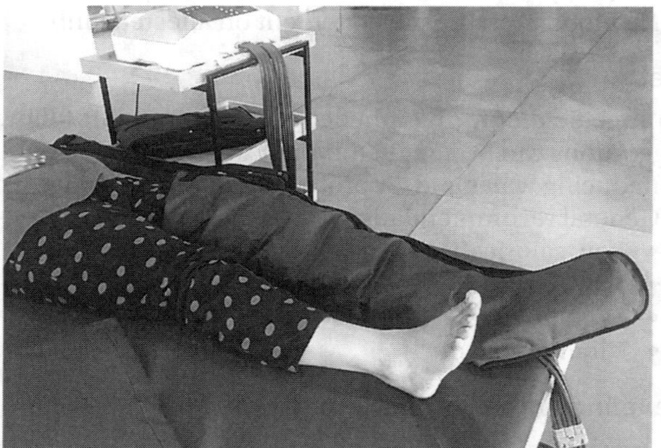

Fig. 29.8: Pneumatic compression device.

- Pain reduction
- Reduction of tissue swelling
- Sensory stimulation
- Skin softening
- Improvement of pliability of tissues
- Decrease in adhesions and contractures
- Reduction of scar formation

KT can be used alone or in conjunction with exercises, compression garments and CDT.

Low Level LASER Therapy

Low level LASER therapy (LLLT) or photobiomodulation (wavelength range 650–1000 nm) is a noninvasive approach for the management of lymphedema. It promotes lymphatic vessel regeneration, reduces inflammation, improves lymphatic motility and prevents tissue fibrosis. It stimulates lymphatic vessels and lymphocytes, thereby increasing local circulation. Several systematic reviews have concluded that it is an effective strategy to reduce limb volume in lymphedema and improves quality of life of such patients.

Extracorporeal Shockwave Therapy

Extracorporeal shockwave therapy (ESWT) is a noninvasive modality that activates vascular endothelial growth factor (VEGF) along with fibroblasts, resulting in promotion of lymphatic neovascularization, thereby relieving lymphedema. It also reduces inflammation. ESWT can be used to treat fibrotic lesions in lymphedema that cannot be managed by CDT alone. Hence, ESWT can be used as an adjuvant therapy with CDT. It has been proven to be a successful management strategy in stages 2 and 3 lymphedema.

Surgery for Lymphedema

Following surgeries are available for the management of lymphedema.

- Liposuction
- Lymphaticovenous anastomosis (lymphovenous bypass)
- Vascularized lymph node transfer surgery (lymphovenous transplant)
- Charles procedure to remove excess skin folds or papillomas after CDT or as an adjunct to CDT.

Summary

Lymphedema is abnormal accumulation of lymphatic fluid in interstitial tissues. It can be classified as primary or secondary. Secondary lymphedema is a common complication following surgical management of cancer. It is more prevalent in females undergoing radical mastectomy. There are four stages of lymphedema. Examination of lymphedema involves investigations like lymphoscintigraphy, ultrasound, etc. Limb volume measurements can be done using volumetric methods, perometry, bioimpedance analysis or limb circumference measurement. Management of lymphedema consists of complete decongestive therapy, pneumatic compression therapy, kinesiology taping, low level LASER therapy, extracorporeal shockwave therapy, etc. If it cannot be managed using these strategies then surgical management is considered.

CLINICAL EXAMPLE

Example 1

History and Examination

A 46-year-old female has undergone right-sided modified radical mastectomy followed by chemotherapy and radiotherapy. During radiotherapy, she started having heaviness in her arm as well as in the upper back. She was also having pain in upper chest and back and started developing tightness in upper chest tissues with difficulty in end range of shoulder movement. She is a working woman in corporate office. One day she found difficulty in wearing her blouse which did not fit on the right side, she was worried and consulted her physician and was sent to a lymphedema therapist.

The lymphedema therapist evaluated her in detail. Circumference measurement was taken and she was found to have a difference of 3 to 4 cm compared to unaffected side. She was diagnosed with lymphedema with truncal involvement.

Suggested Management

The therapist started complete decongestive therapy. Within three days, she got relief in pain and heaviness in chest and upper back. Every week, the therapist took circumference to see the progression. CDT was given for 3 weeks. Marked reduction in swelling was recorded.

When plateau was seen, patient was explained how to self-manage at home. Patient is doing self-manual lymphatic drainage, wearing compression stockings during day and bandages at night. She is also doing exercises with stocking and going for a walk for 30 minutes daily.

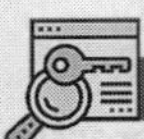

Review Questions

1. Describe anatomy and physiology of the lymphatic system in detail.
2. Explain the assessment of a patient affected with lymphedema in detail.
3. Explain lymphedema management in detail.
4. What are the possible risk factors leading to lymphedema?
5. Write short notes on:
   a. Surgical management of lymphedema
   b. Complete decongestive therapy
   c. Care to be taken by a patient with lymphedema
   d. Complications of lymphedema
   e. Manual lymphatic drainage

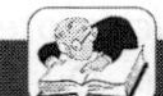

Bibliography

1. Ambroza C, Geigle PR. Aquatic exercise as a management tool for breast cancer-related lymphedema. Topics in Geriatric Rehabilitation. 2010;26 (2):120-27.
2. Ancukiewicz M, Russell TA, Otoole J, Specht M, Singer M, Kelada A, et al. Standardized method for quantification of developing lymphedema in patients treated for breast cancer. Int J Radiat Oncol Biol Phys. 2011;79(5):1436-43. doi: 10.1016/j.ijrobp.2010.01.001. Epub 2010 Jun 3. PMID: 20605339; PMCID: PMC2952286.
3. Bae H, Kim HJ. Clinical outcomes of extracorporeal shock wave therapy in patients with secondary lymphedema: a pilot study. Ann Rehabil Med. 2013;37(2):229-34. doi: 10.5535/arm.2013.37.2.229. Epub 2013 Apr 30. PMID: 23705118; PMCID: PMC3660484.
4. Baxter GD, Liu L, Petrich S, Gisselman AS, Chapple C, Anders JJ, et al. Low level laser therapy (Photobiomodulation therapy) for breast cancer-related lymphedema: a systematic review. BMC Cancer. 2017;17(1):833. doi: 10.1186/s12885-017-3852-x. PMID: 29216916; PMCID: PMC5719569.
5. Bojinović-Rodić D, Pjanić S, Popović T, Nožica-Radulović T. Factors influencing efficacy of complete decongestive treatment in patients with breast cancer-linked arm lymphoedema. Scr Med. 2021;52(2):132-7. DOI:10.5937/scriptamed52-3063.
6. Buchan J, Janda M, Box R, Schmitz K, Hayes S. A randomized trial on the effect of exercise mode on breast cancer-related lymphedema. Medicine and Science in Sports and Exercise. 2016;48(10):1866-74.
7. Cemal Y, Pusic A, Mehrara BJ. Preventative measures for lymphedema: separating fact from fiction. J Am Coll Surg. 2011;213(4):543-51. doi: 10.1016/j.jamcollsurg.2011.07.001. Epub 2011 Jul 28. PMID: 21802319; PMCID: PMC3652571.
8. Dionne A, Goulet S, Leone M, Comtois AS. Aquatic exercise training outcomes on functional capacity, quality of life, and lower limb lymphedema: pilot study. J Alternat Complement Med. 2018;24:9-10.
9. Foldi M, Foldi E, Kubik S. Textbook of Lymphology, 3rd edition. Elsevier; 2012.
10. Greene AK, Goss JA. Diagnosis and staging of lymphedema. Semin Plast Surg. 2018;32(1):12-16. doi: 10.1055/s-0038-1635117. Epub 2018 Apr 9. PMID: 29636648; PMCID: PMC5891654.
11. Hasenoehrl T, Palma S, Ramazanova D, et al. Resistance exercise and breast cancer–related lymphedema—a systematic review update and meta-analysis. Support Care Cancer. 2020;28:3593-3603. https://doi.org/10.1007/s00520-020-05521-x
12. Intermittent Pneumatic compression acts synergistically with manual lymphatic drainage in complex decongestive physiotherapy for breast cancer treatment related lymphedema. Lymphology. 2009;42(4):188-94.
13. Jørgensen MG, Toyserkani NM, Hansen FG, Bygum A, Sørensen JA. The impact of lymphedema on health-related quality of life up to 10 years after breast cancer treatment: NPJ. Breast Cancer. 2021;7:70. https://doi.org/10.1038/s41523-021-00276-y.
14. Keilani M, Hasenoehrl T, Neubauer M, et al. Resistance exercise and secondary lymphedema in breast cancer survivors—a systematic review. Support Care Cancer. 2016;24:1907-16. https://doi.org/10.1007/s00520-015-3068-z.
15. Kwan ML, Cohn JC, Armer JM, et al. Exercise in patients with lymphedema: a systematic review of the contemporary literature. J Cancer Surviv. 2011;5:320–36. https://doi.org/10.1007/s11764-011-0203-9.

16. Lee KW, Kim SB, Lee JH, Kim YS. Effects of extracorporeal shockwave therapy on improvements in lymphedema, Quality of life, and fibrous tissue in breast cancer-related lymphedema. Ann Rehabil Med. 2020;44(5):386-92. doi: 10.5535/arm.19213. Epub 2020 Sep 28. PMID: 32986941; PMCID: PMC7655225.
17. Louveau A, Smirnov I, Keyes TJ, et al. Structural and functional features of central nervous system lymphatic vessels, Nature. 2015;523(7560):337-41.
18. Malicka I, Rosseger A, Hanuszkiewicz J, Woźniewski M. Kinesiology taping reduces lymphedema of the upper extremity in women after breast cancer treatment: a pilot study. Prz Menopauzalny. 2014;13(4):221-6. doi: 10.5114/pm.2014.44997. Epub 2014 Sep 9. PMID: 26327858; PMCID: PMC4520367.
19. McKenzie DC, Kalda AL. Effect of upper extremity exercise on secondary lymphedema in breast cancer patients: A pilot study. J Clin Oncol. 2003;21:463-66.
20. Mulita F, Lotfollahzadeh S, Mukkamalla SKR. Lymph Node Dissection. In: StatPearls [Internet]. Treasure Island (FL): StatPearls Publishing; 2022. [Updated 2022 Jul 17]. Available from: https://www.ncbi.nlm.nih.gov/books/NBK564397/.
21. Nelson NL. Breast cancer-related lymphedema and resistance exercise: A systematic review. J Strength Cond Res. 2016;30(9):2656-65.
22. Norman SA, Localio AR, Potashnik SL, Simoes HA, Torpey Kallan MJ, Weber AL. Lymphedema in breast cancer survivors: incidence, degree, time course, treatment, and symptoms. J Clin Oncol. 2009;27(3):390-7. doi: 10.1200/JCO.2008.17.9291. Epub 2008 Dec 8.
23. Pekyavas NO, Tunay VB, Akbayrak T, Kaya S, Karatas M. Complex decongestive therapy and taping for patients with postmastectomy lymphedema: A randomized controlled study. Eur J Oncol Nurs. 2014;18(6):585-90.
24. Radina E, Armer J, Daunt D, Dusold J, Culbertson S. Self-reported management of breast cancer-related lymphoedema. J Lymphoedema. 2007;2(2):12-21. PMID: 20535235; PMCID: PMC2882024.
25. Scheer R. Compression garments for managing lymphoedema. J Lymphoedema. 2017;12 (1).
26. Sleigh BC, Manna B. Lymphedema. In: StatPearls [Internet]. Treasure Island (FL): StatPearls Publishing; 2022. [Updated 2022 May 29].. Available from: https://www.ncbi.nlm.nih.gov/books/NBK537239/.
27. Tantawy SA, Abdelbasset WK, Nambi G, Kamel DM. Comparative study between the effects of kinesio taping and pressure garment on secondary upper extremity lymphedema and quality of life following mastectomy: A randomized controlled trial. Integr Cancer Ther. 2019;18:1534735419847276. doi: 10.1177/1534735419847276. PMID: 31068019; PMCID: PMC6509974.
28. Tidhar D, Katz-Leurer M. Aqua lymphatic therapy in women who suffer from breast cancer treatment-related lymphedema: a randomized controlled study. Support Cancer care. 2009. DOI 10.1007/s00520-009-0669-4
29. Tiwari A, Cheng K, Button M, Myint F, Hamilton G. Differential diagnosis, investigation, and current treatment of lower limb lymphedema. Arch Surg. 2003;138(2):152-61. doi:10.1001/archsurg.138.2.152.
30. Turgay T, Denkçeken T. The effect of low-level laser therapy on quality of life in postmastectomy lymphedema patients. Biom Res Ther. 2020;7(9):3971-76. https:// doi.org/10.15419/bmrat.v7i9.628.
31. Ugur S, Arıcı C, Yaprak M, Mescı A, Arıcı GA, Dolay K, et al. Risk factors of breast cancer-related lymphedema. Lymphat Res Biol. 2013;11(2):72-5. doi: 10.1089/lrb.2013.0004. PMID: 23772716; PMCID: PMC3685313.
32. Zuther JE, Norton S. Lymphedema Management: The Comprehensive Guide for Practitioners. Fourth edition.

Multiple Choice Questions (MCQs)

To test your understanding and recall of key concepts.

1. What is the primary function of lymph nodes in the lymphatic system?

A. Transport of oxygen to tissues
B. Regulation of blood pressure
C. Filtration of harmful substances and immune surveillance
D. Synthesis of proteins

2. Which is the gold standard imaging test for evaluating lymphatic channels?

A. Ultrasound
B. Lymphoscintigraphy
C. Magnetic resonance imaging (MRI)
D. Computed tomography (CT)

3. Why is manual lymphatic drainage (MLD) used in the management of lymphedema?

A. To increase the production of white blood cells in the body
B. To stimulate lymph flow and reroute it from affected areas
C. To enhance arterial blood flow in the region
D. To reduce platelet aggregation

4. Which of the following is *true* regarding lymphedema?

A. Primary lymphedema occurs after surgery, while secondary lymphedema is congenital
B. Secondary lymphedema develops after trauma, surgery, or cancer treatment
C. Primary lymphedema affects only the lower limbs
D. Secondary lymphedema cannot be treated

5. A 48-year-old woman reports heaviness and swelling in her arm following breast cancer surgery. Which step should the lymphedema therapist prioritize?

A. Start resistance exercises immediately
B. Begin manual lymphatic drainage and compression bandaging
C. Perform venipuncture on the affected limb immediately
D. Recommend surgical lymph node removal by surgeon

6. In view of the risks associated with air travel for patients with lymphedema, what precaution is most critical during flights?

A. Reducing water intake on the day of flight
B. Wearing compression garments and performing muscle-pumping exercises
C. Taking diuretics before the flight
D. Avoiding breathing exercises

7. What is the clinical significance of Stemmer's sign in diagnosing lymphedema?

A. It confirms systemic infection in the body
B. It indicates advanced lymphedema with tissue fibrosis
C. It rules out secondary lymphedema in the limb
D. It identifies venous insufficiency in the limb

8. Which of the following is *not* a risk factor for development of breast cancer-related lymphedema:

A. Axillary lymph node dissection
B. Infection
C. Underweight patient (body mass index < 18.9 kg/m^2)
D. Postoperative radiotherapy

ANSWERS

1. C	2. B	3. B	4. B	5. B
6. B	7. B	8. C		

Section 6

Special Population

Section Outline

Chapter 30

Obesity in Women

Mariya P Jiandani

LEARNING OBJECTIVES

At the end of the chapter, the reader will be able to:
- Review prevalence of obesity in women.
- Describe various factors related to obesity in women.
- Understand role of estrogen and hormone replacement therapy.
- Describe health risks associated with obesity in women.
- Understand how to plan effective weight loss in obese women.

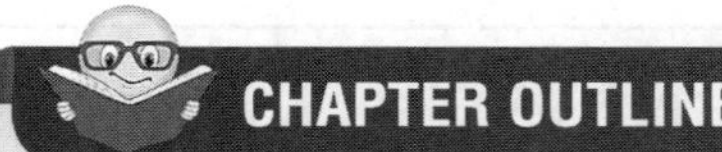

INTRODUCTION

India is witnessing an alarming increase in obese population to more than 30 million people. The problem is more acute among women than men. In the year 2019–2021, the prevalence of overweight or obesity has increased to 33% in urban areas and 20% in rural areas and economically 10% were in the lowest wealth quintile whereas 39% were in the highest wealth quintile.

With increasing age, the risk of increased waist hip ratio (WHR) increases. 65% of women aged 40–49 years have substantially increased WHR putting them to an increased risk of metabolic complications or disorders including:

- Diabetes
- Hypertension
- Dyslipidemia
- Cardiovascular disease
- Some cancers

Increased lifestyle unhealthy behaviors, increased physical inactivity and hormonal changes associated with menopause predisposes women to increased obesity risk.

ANTHROPOMETRIC MEASUREMENTS

Literature shows that high levels of adiposity are related to morbidity and mortality with recommendations of weight

Table 30.1: Classification of disease risk based on BMI and waist circumference.

BMI (kg/m²) ***Asian***	***Waist circumference Women[#] </=88 cm*** ***Risk category***	***Waist circumference cm (in)*** ***Cut off for Asians 80 cm***	***Risk category***
Underweight (<18.5)	-		
Normal (18.5–24.9) Asians (18.5–23)	-	<70 cm (27.5 in)	Very low
Overweight (25.0–29.9) Asians (23–27.5)	Increased	70–89 (28.5–35.0)	Low
Obesity, Class 1 (30.0–34.9) Asians (>/=27.5)	High	90–109 (35.5–43.0)	High
Obesity, Class 2 (35.0–39.9)	Very high	>110 (43.5)	Very high
Obesity, Class 3 (>/=40)	Extremely high		

[#]Dashes (-) indicate that no additional risk at these levels of BMI was assigned.

loss interventions for obese individuals. This is identified using body mass index (BMI) and/or waist circumference (WC) as both measures are strongly correlated with body fat and are simple to measure.

Body Mass Index

Body mass index (BMI) is calculated as weight in kilograms divided by height in meters squared and is often categorized for ease of interpretation. **Table 30.1** identifies the cut off points for BMI based on the relationship between BMI and mortality as given by the World Health Organization (WHO) and Asian references.

Waist Circumference

As abdominal adiposity may independently influence health outcomes, waist circumference (WC) and waist hip ratio (WHR) are recommended as they correlate with cardiovascular risk. **Table 30.2** highlights the risk associated with waist hip ratio.

- BMI, WC and WHR independently contribute to the prediction of non-abdominal, abdominal subcutaneous and visceral fat.
- The truncal fat includes fat over chest and abdomen both subcutaneous abdominal adipose tissue (SCAT) and intra-abdominal adipose tissue (IAAT), all of which are more in Asian Indians than in white Caucasians.
- Both BMI and WC should be used together (with equal importance) for population-and clinic-based metabolic and cardiovascular risk stratification.

Table 30.2: Risk associated with waist hip ratio.

	WHO	***Asian***
WHR by age	Very high risk	Carries disease risk
Young men	WHR >0.95	WHR: >0.9
Young women	WHR >0.86	WHR: >0.8
Men 60–69 years	WHR >1.03	
Women 60–69 years	WHR >0.90	

For children and adolescents, overweight and obesity are defined using age and sex specific nomograms for body mass index (BMI). Children with BMI equal to or exceeding the age-gender-specific 95th percentile are defined obese. Those with BMI equal to or exceeding the 85th but below 95th percentiles are defined as overweight and are at risk for obesity related comorbidities.

TYPES OF OBESITY

Android

In android (Apple type, **Fig. 30.1A**) type of obesity:

- The shoulders, face, arms, neck, chest and upper portion of the abdomen are bloated.
- The lower portion of the body, the hips, thighs and legs are thinner in proportion in comparison with the upper part.
- The vital organs affected will be mostly the heart, liver, kidneys and lungs.

Women who are under hormone treatment for their menstrual abnormalities or after childbirth, are more prone to this type of obesity. It occurs in females around menopause too, due to thyroid gland's functional disturbance.

Gynoid

In this type (Pear type, **Fig. 30.1B**):

- The lower part of the body has the extra flesh.
- The flesh is somewhat flabby in the abdomen, thighs, buttocks and legs.
- The face and neck mostly give a normal appearance.
- The vital organs affected mostly are the kidneys, uterus, intestines, bladder and bowels.

It is more common in females.

Barrel Type

Besides android and gynoid, there is one more type of obesity. Some people do not belong to any of the above two types of obesity.

- Their whole body from head to toe looks like a barrel.
- The fat tissues in their body hinder the movement of all the internal organs and consequently affect their brisk functioning.

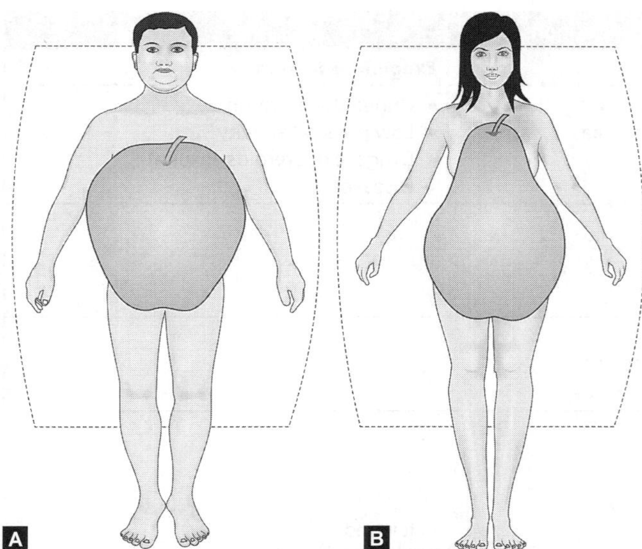

Figs. 30.1A and B: (A) Android obesity; (B) Gynoid obesity.

Middle Age Obesity

It is due to a reduction of physical activity and is usually seen around 40 years and above in females. The body slows down its metabolism and is more susceptible to stress. This can also fall within the period of pregnancy and menopause in women.

Gestational Obesity

This is the obesity that occurs during pregnancy. This is because it is a period associated with:
- Increased meals
- Changed food habits
- Periods of inactivity
- Leisure combined with physiological changes that promote increased fat deposition.

Factors Related to Obesity in Women

There are number of factors responsible for obesity which include environmental, lifestyle related, genetics, hormonal change and diseases.
- Single and polygenic **gene mutations** that occur naturally can produce obesity. Leptin deficiency has been documented in subsets of human obesity. Obesity has a familial tendency and if before 3 years of age the parent is obese it is a strong predictor of obesity in adulthood.
- Control of appetite and energy metabolism is a complex phenomenon influencing energy consumed and energy expended and occurs mainly in hypothalamus. This is controlled by **neuroendocrine interactions** where Leptin plays an important role. It is almost exclusively produced by the adipose tissue and acts centrally in the hypothalamus. Levels of Leptin and insulin in plasma have an inverse relationship in food intake. The major peptides that stimulate feeding are orexins A and B, which are secreted by the hypothalamus, and ghrelin, which is secreted by the stomach. Activation of specific neurons in arcuate, ventromedial and paraventricular nuclei triggers an orexigenic or anorexigenic effect, i.e., stimulating or reducing appetite. The expression of estrogen receptors, mainly ERα, occurs in this region. Activity of ghrelin the strongest orexigenic peptide, is reduced by estrogens. Hence a rapid decline in levels of estrogens would contribute significantly to an increase in appetite.
- **Food intake**: The Framingham nutrition study showed that in women high calorie diet, rich in fat, containing alcohol with less fiber and micronutrients used for 12 years increases the risk of abdominal obesity and metabolic syndrome 3–4 folds.
- **Puberty and menarche**: Various aspects of pubertal development are influenced by excess adiposity including timing of pubertal initiation and hormonal parameters during puberty. Early menarche is clearly associated with extent of obesity, with a two-fold increase in rate of early menarche associated with BMI greater than the 85th percentile. There appears to be associated a higher risk of psychological problems, risk-taking behavior, and future breast cancer with early puberty. Obesity during the pubertal transition may also promote the development of adolescent polycystic ovary syndrome (PCOS).
- **Parity and marital status**: Increasing age, parity and marriage, hormonal changes and less active lifestyle have also been associated with overweight among women. In addition, weight retained during pregnancy is often difficult for women to lose, even for obese women, contributing to increased BMI over time.
- **Menopause and obesity:** Menopause is associated with fear, anxiety and distressing symptoms such as hot flushes, mood disorders and sleep disturbances. An important concern of menopause is weight gain, usually central obesity. The main causes of changes in body composition associated with menopause are summarized in **Table 30.3**.

ROLE OF ESTROGEN

- Estrogens in women are responsible for fat accumulation in the subcutaneous tissue, especially in the gluteal and femoral regions. To cause a biological effect, estrogen connects with receptors ERα and ERβ.
- Estrogens increase fat oxidation in the skeletal muscles and inhibit hepatic and muscle lipogenesis. Lack of estrogens associated with menopause would result in a tendency for an increase in the visceral fat mass.
- Androgens promote the accumulation of abdominal fat. Therefore, relative hyperandrogenemia due to lack of estrogens results in unfavorable fat redistribution from gynoid to abdominal during menopause. Testosterone and androstenedione are aromatized to estrone (E1), estradiol (E2) and estriol (E3), leading to increased levels of these hormones in obese postmenopausal women than in nonobese subjects. In consequence, visceral fat mass increases during menopause by 44% and the mass of gynoid fat rises by approximately 32%.

Table 30.3: Main factors contributing to menopausal changes in body composition.

Genetic factors	*Hormonal factors*	*Exogenous factors*
• Genetic predisposition • Ethnicity • Epigenetic changes	• Rapid hypoestrogenemia • Relative hyperandrogenemia • Low SHBG* levels	• Unhealthy nutrition • Low physical activity • Drugs (e.g., steroids, insulin) • Diseases
↓		
• Increase in body weight • Increase and redistribution of fat mass (from gynoid to abdominal obesity) • Decrease in fat-free mass		

*SHBG: sex-hormone binding globulin

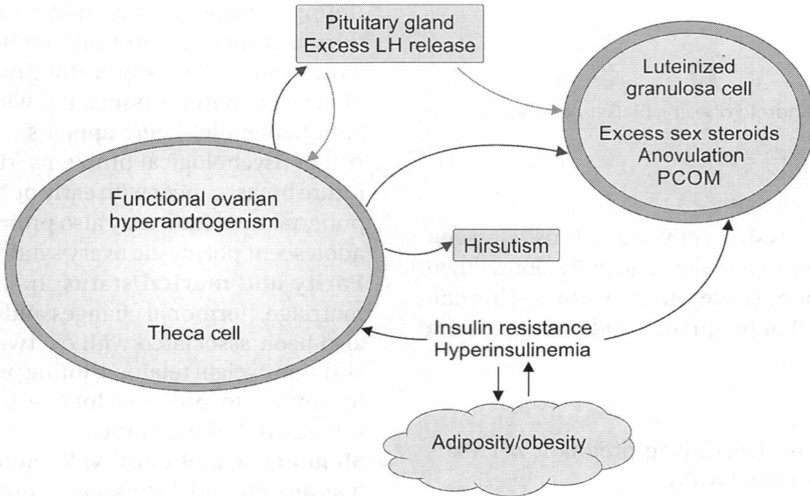

Fig. 30.2: Role of estrogen in obesity.
(PCOM: polycystic ovarian morphology; LH: luteinizing hormone)

- A decrease in the hepatic production of sex-hormone binding globulin (SHBG), which increases the bioavailability of androgens also contributes to development of central obesity. Postmenopausal women have a 4.88-fold higher risk of developing abdominal obesity compared to premenopausal women.
- Activation of α2A receptors results in the antilipolytic action and contributes to the accumulation of fat. The expression of α2A receptors is increased by estradiol in subcutaneous fat tissue in women and does not affect these receptors in the visceral fat.
- ERα receptors are involved in the beneficial effect of estrogens on adipose tissue distribution, glucose metabolism, and inflammation. ERα receptors can stimulate adrenergic β receptors in the visceral tissue, enhancing the process of lipolysis reducing abdominal fat mass.
- Fat tissue in obese women is the source of adipokines, the most important being leptin. Leptin inhibits appetite, acting centrally. Estrogens potentiate leptin action by increasing the expression and sensitivity of its receptors in the hypothalamus. An inverse correlation exists between the levels of estrogens and adiponectin, an important cytokine – opposite to leptin, increasing insulin sensitivity.
- Estrogens also inhibit the production of proinflammatory cytokines as IL-6 or tumor necrosis factor α (TNF-α) produced in fat tissue.

Figure 30.2 describes the role of estrogen in obesity.

ROLE OF HORMONE REPLACEMENT THERAPY

As lack of estrogen is of crucial significance to the development of obesity and initiates the action of other involved factors, substitution therapy with hormones, may help to prevent an increase in body weight and normalize metabolic disturbances.

- Hormonal replacement therapy [hormonal therapy of menopause (HTM)] reduces obesity, decreases abdominal fat mass (redistributes body fat), lowers the fasting glucose and insulin levels, improves blood lipid profile and, as a result, reduces cardiovascular risk.
- HTM irrespective of the route of administration (oral or transdermal) and whether a progestin component was

added to estrogens, caused an increase in fat-free mass, decrease in visceral fat, increase in insulin sensitivity, and decrease in LDL/HDL cholesterol ratio, and Lp(a), fibrinogen and plasminogen activator inhibitor (PAI) levels.

Evidence suggests treatment should begin during perimenopause or in the first few years after menopause. If initiated later, it may even be counterproductive and harmful. A word of caution exercised with higher E2 levels, not counterbalanced by progestins can lead to the following after the menopause:

- Massive bleeding in premenopausal women
- Risk of hyperplasia
- Endometrial cancer

HEALTH RISK OF OBESITY IN WOMEN

The burden of overweight and obesity on health are studied elaborately **(Fig. 30.3)**. Two-thirds of cardiovascular diseases are related to high BMI.

Child-bearing Age

- Among women of childbearing age, overweight and obesity have been associated with increased risk of non-communicable diseases (NCDs), pregnancy complications, cesarean section births, adverse birth outcomes, and infant mortality.
- Pregnancy complications include the risk of impaired glucose tolerance and gestational diabetes, miscarriage, preeclampsia, thromboembolism and maternal death. There are associations between maternal overweight and increased risk of intrapartum obstetric complications and risk of cesarean section births.
- Increased risk of shoulder dystocia, failure to progress, infant distress, higher risk of fetal death, stillbirth, congenital abnormality and previous cesarean deliveries are among many clinical factors which may lead to the decision to deliver an obese woman by cesarean section.
- Elevated BMI influences metabolic state, increases oxidative stress and inflammation, causes alterations in circulating inflammatory cytokines, hormones and metabolites, which are suggested to negatively affect gamete and embryo quality, early placental function and gene expression.

> **Clinical Pointer**
>
> A relatively small gain of 1 to 2 BMI units (kg/m^2) between pregnancies may increase the risk of gestational hypertension and gestational diabetes, even in women who are not overweight or obese. It also increases the likelihood of giving birth to a large baby.

- Relations between obesity and higher risk of preeclampsia, fetal growth restriction, or preterm birth can suggest that obesity is the cause of placental dysfunction.
- Offspring of obese mothers have up to 29% increased risk of hospital admission from cardiovascular disease and 35% increased risk of premature death in adulthood compared to offspring of normal BMI mothers.
- Obesity is also linked with infertility and polycystic ovarian disease.

Postmenopausal Risk

- Abdominal obesity is a key factor in the pathogenesis of insulin resistance and metabolic syndrome. Insulin sensitivity in postmenopausal women can lead to most severe metabolic disturbances—high postprandial glucose, hypertriglyceridemia, high C-reactive protein and

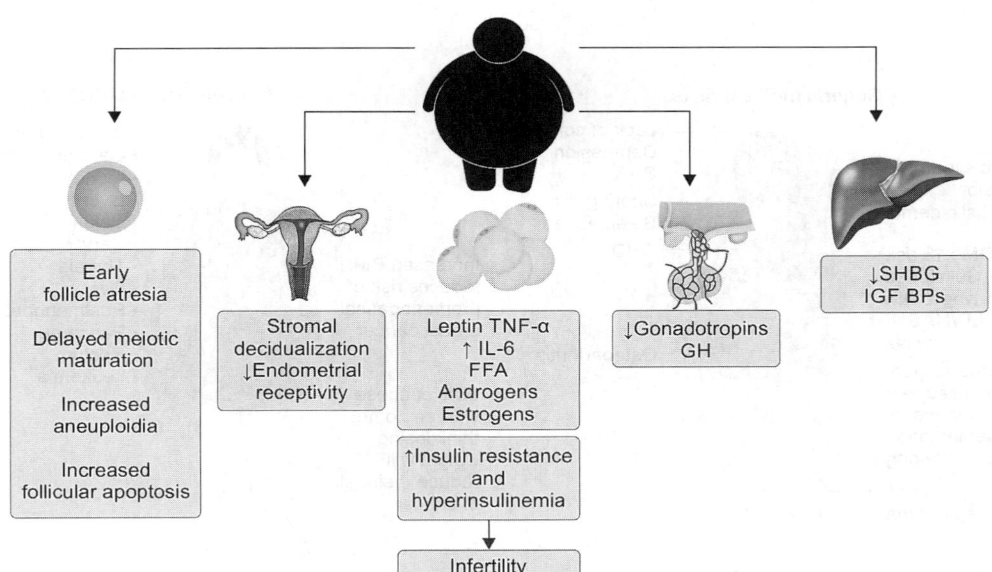

Fig. 30.3: Health risks with obesity *(For color version, see Plate 8)*.
(FFA: free fatty acids; GH: growth hormone; IGF BPs: insulin-like growth factor binding proteins; IL-6: interleukin 6; TNF: tumor necrosis factor; SHBG: sex hormone binding globulin)

interleukin 6 (IL-6) levels as well as low levels of Apo A1 gene and HDL cholesterol.

- Aromatase-derived estrogens do not have the protective status for insulin sensitivity and cardiovascular diseases, and there is increased risk of type 2 diabetes, hypertension, and dyslipidemia, and a higher rate of cardiovascular diseases in peri- and post-menopausal women.
- Hypertension is found more frequently in women after 55 years of age compared to men. Domination of vasoconstriction due to estrogen deficiency over vasodilatation effects can be a contributing factor due to decrease in prostacyclin and nitric oxide levels.
- Metabolic syndrome which ties together insulin resistance, visceral adiposity, dyslipidemia and hypertension, and is known to be interrelated is frequently seen postmenopausal.

A detailed representation of health risks during various life stages is presented in **Figure 30.4**.

MANAGEMENT OF OBESITY

Managing obesity is a community involvement. It is not one specialty or one individual approach but a holistic approach beginning with parent's involvement early in life, mothers taking care of themselves during pregnancy, community schools and work environment providing facilities for right nutrition and adequate physical exercise or activity, education, counseling forums and support groups. **Figures 30.5 and 30.6** highlight approaches toward weight control. Considerations for therapeutic drugs and bariatric surgery are outside the scope of this chapter.

Parental Education

- Parents, especially mothers have a habit of force-feeding children. If they are the only child or precious baby, the child is not only overfed but protected and may not have adequate physical activity.

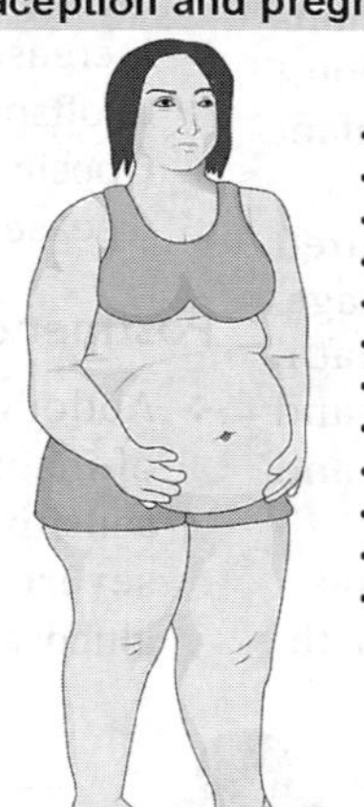

Fig. 30.4: Health risk during various life stages.
(CHC: combined hormonal contraception; CKD: chronic kidney disease; DVT: deep vein thrombosis; DM: diabetes mellitus; IVF: in-vitro fertilization; NAFD: nonalcoholic fatty liver disease; NASH: nonalcoholic steatohepatitis; PE: preeclampsia; BMI: body mass index; CVA: cerebrovascular accident; CHD: coronary heart disease)

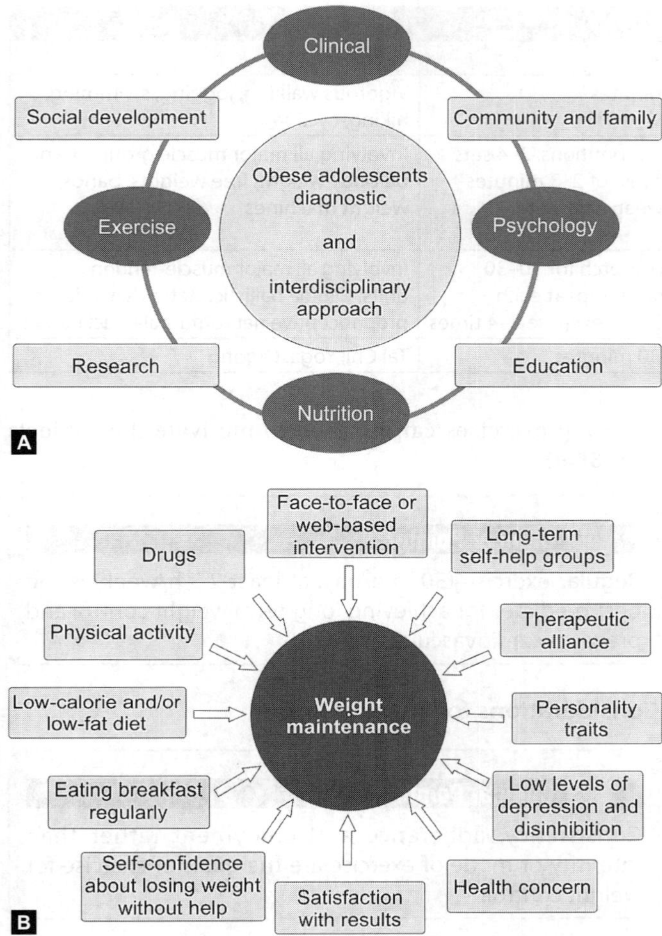

Figs. 30.5A and B: Approaches toward weight control.

- ❖ Parental involvement has been identified as an important determinant influencing young girls to be physically active. Daughters' weight status was affected by mothers' feeding practices. Mothers often exert influence over their daughters' dietary intake, which has been shown to negatively impact self-control over energy intake. It is important for the parents to be made aware and educated especially if genetics play a role in the family.
- ❖ Nutrition education in children in the form of games, colorful platter having fruits and veggies of all colors in a plate, educating about nutrient values and calories early and developing and encouraging hobbies that lead to caloric expenditure.

Involvement of Family

Efforts to achieve and maintain weight loss are more successful with family involvement. Positive eating behavior changes last longer if interventions are aimed at family rather than individuals' attitudes and habits.

Involvement of School and Workplace

- ❖ Schools and educational authorities need to include food and their nutrient and caloric values in the syllabus. Schools should be encouraged to provide healthy meals. Nutritional information at the point of choosing food and drinks should be provided.
- ❖ Workplace and school should promote healthy meals in canteen.
- ❖ Schools should encourage physical activity, have recreation rooms and provide incentives to be in healthy zones.

Physical Activity

- ❖ Exercise habits added to diet help to promote greater weight loss. Behavior that includes healthy eating and more intense physical activity in women in menopause is effective in reducing body weight, in particular the fat mass, whereas fat-free mass is maintained.
- ❖ Recommendations of scientific societies in respect of lifestyle in the menopause emphasize the importance of combining diet with exercise. Limited physical activity during this time accelerates the progress of aging and increases the cardiovascular and osteoporosis risk.

Exercise Prescription for Obesity

- ❖ Minimum weekly volume of 150 minutes of aerobic conditioning for fitness improvement
- ❖ For long-term weight loss and for prevention of weight regain in obese individuals exercise duration should progress to 250–300 minutes per week.
- ❖ The consensus concerning intensity is that moderate-intensity exercise at 55 to 69% of maximum heart rate is appropriate for the management of body weight rather than activity of more vigorous intensity.
- ❖ Obese persons may benefit from a resistance training program, which improves muscular strength and favorably affects functional tasks.
- ❖ Resistance training may also stimulate an increase in fat free mass. However, resistance training does not seem to affect energy expenditure or absolute weight loss.

The FITT Principle

In order to provide safe exercise guidelines, women with a low-risk pregnancy should be utilizing prescribed exercises in accordance with the FITT principle, characterized by the frequency, intensity, time and the type of the activity, i.e., modality of exercise. The suggested FITT guidelines by the ACSM as shown in **Table 30.4** are:

- ❖ Frequency:
  - Aerobic: At least 3–5 days a week, and preferably all days in the week.
  - Resistance: 2–3 days per week (non-consecutive).
  - Flexibility: At least 2–3 days of daily stretching per week.
- ❖ Intensity:
  - Aerobic: Moderate intensity (40–60% VO_2 reserve or 60–80% VO_2 max).
    - Exercise within target heart rate zones, dependent on the age and fitness level of the pregnant woman.
    - Rating of RPE (12–14 on a scale of 6–20)
    - "Talk test" to monitor exercise intensity.

Table 30.4: Principles of exercise prescription for obesity.

	Frequency	*Intensity*	*Time*	*Type*
Cardiorespiratory	5 days/week	Moderate	30 minutes	Vigorous walking, jogging, swimming, hiking, cycling
Strength	2–3 days/week	60–70% of one-rep max for novice, 40–50% of one-rep max for older person or sedentary person	8–12 repetitions, 2–4 sets with rest of 2–3 minutes between each set	Involving all major muscle groups. Can be body weight, free weights, bands, weight machines
Flexibility	2–3 days/week	Stretch to point of feeling tightness	Hold stretch for 10–30 seconds, repeat each flexibility exercise 2–4 times	Involving all major muscle-tendon units. Can be ballistic, static, dynamic, or proprioceptive neuromuscular facilitation
Balance	2–3 days/week	Has not been determined	20–30 minutes	Tai Chi, Yoga, Qigong

- Time:
  - Aerobic:
    - At least 15 minutes a day and gradually increasing to at least 30 minutes a day. This progression would result in total of 150 minutes per week of accumulated physical activity.
    - Vigorous intensity 75 minutes per week.
  - Resistance: 1–3 sets depending on level of experience (major muscle groups)
  - Flexibility: 10–30 seconds (static).
- Type:
  - Aerobic:
    - Physical activity that use the large muscle groups, with dynamic and rhythmic movement (per example walking, stationary cycling, swimming, group exercise) **(Figs. 30.6A to C)**.
    - A variety of weight-bearing and non-weight-bearing activities, well tolerated.
  - Resistance: A variety of free weight, machine, and body weight exercises, well tolerated **(Fig. 30.7)**.
  - Flexibility: Active, passive, and dynamic stretch exercises that target each muscle-tendon unit **(Figs. 30.8A to E)**

Group exercises can be used to motivate the subjects **(Fig. 30.9)**.

Clinical Pointer

Regular exercise (30 min/day, at least 2.5 h/week) is the best predictor for achieving long-term weight control and prevents cardiovascular events.

Considerations for Energy Output

Clinical Pointer

Consistency, adherence and enjoyment rather than intensity or mode of exercise are the goals of exercise for weight control.

Physical activity in the form of daily chores or a programmed exercise protocol, both use calories.

- Simple bodily movements that promote activities of daily living, especially walking in sunlight, help to augment and adhere to the circadian cycle, with emphasis on not assuming a sedentary, sitting or lying position in the daytime.

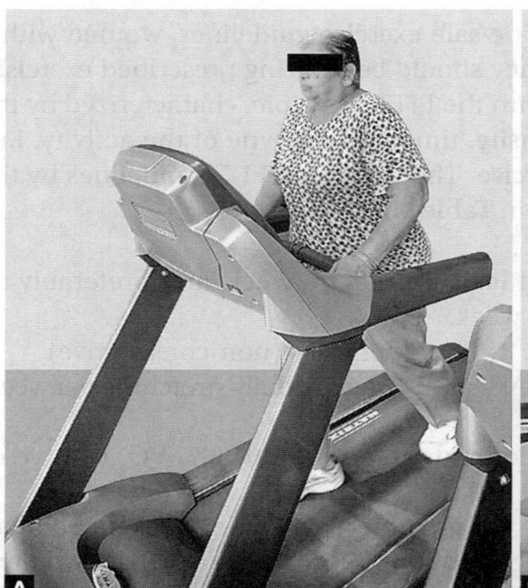

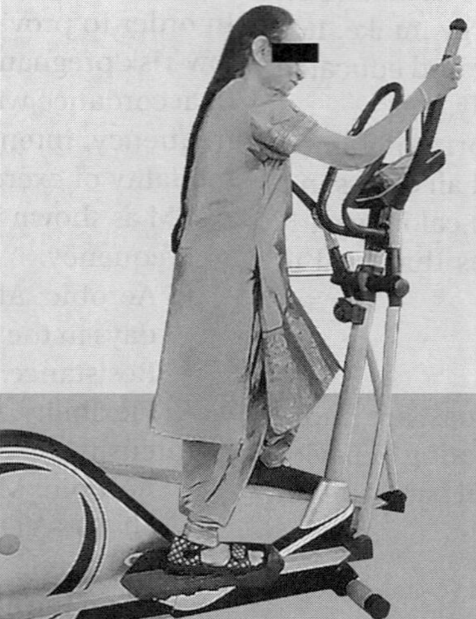

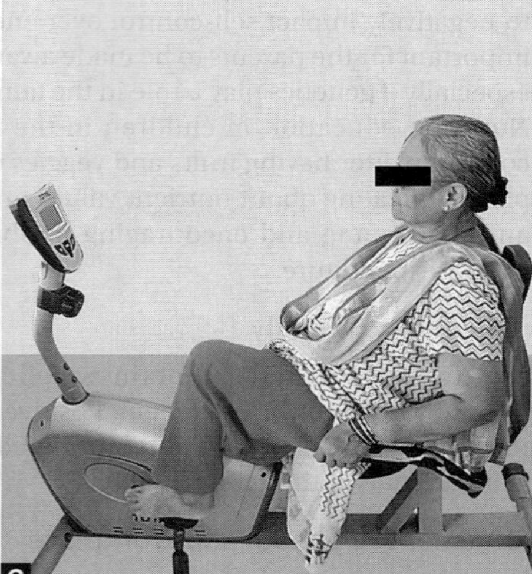

Figs. 30.6A to C: Aerobic exercises. (A) Treadmill walking; (B) Cross trainer; (C) Cycling.

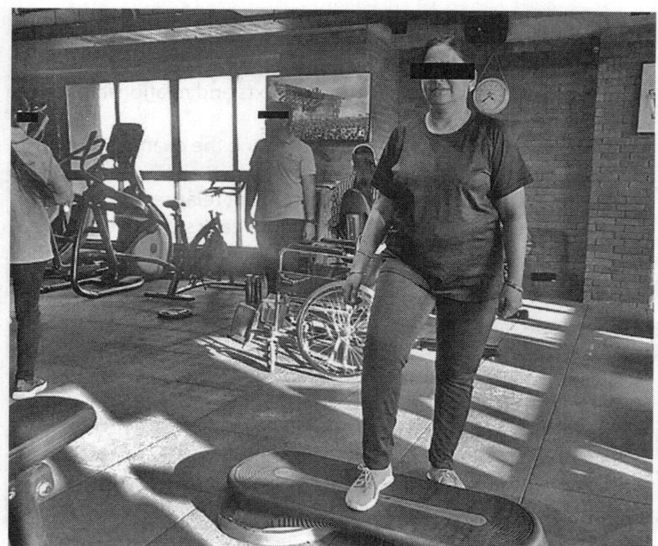

Fig. 30.7: Body weight resistance training.

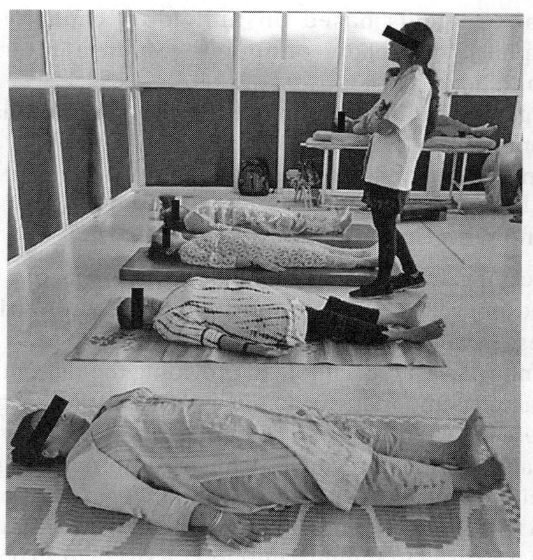

Fig. 30.9: Group exercises.

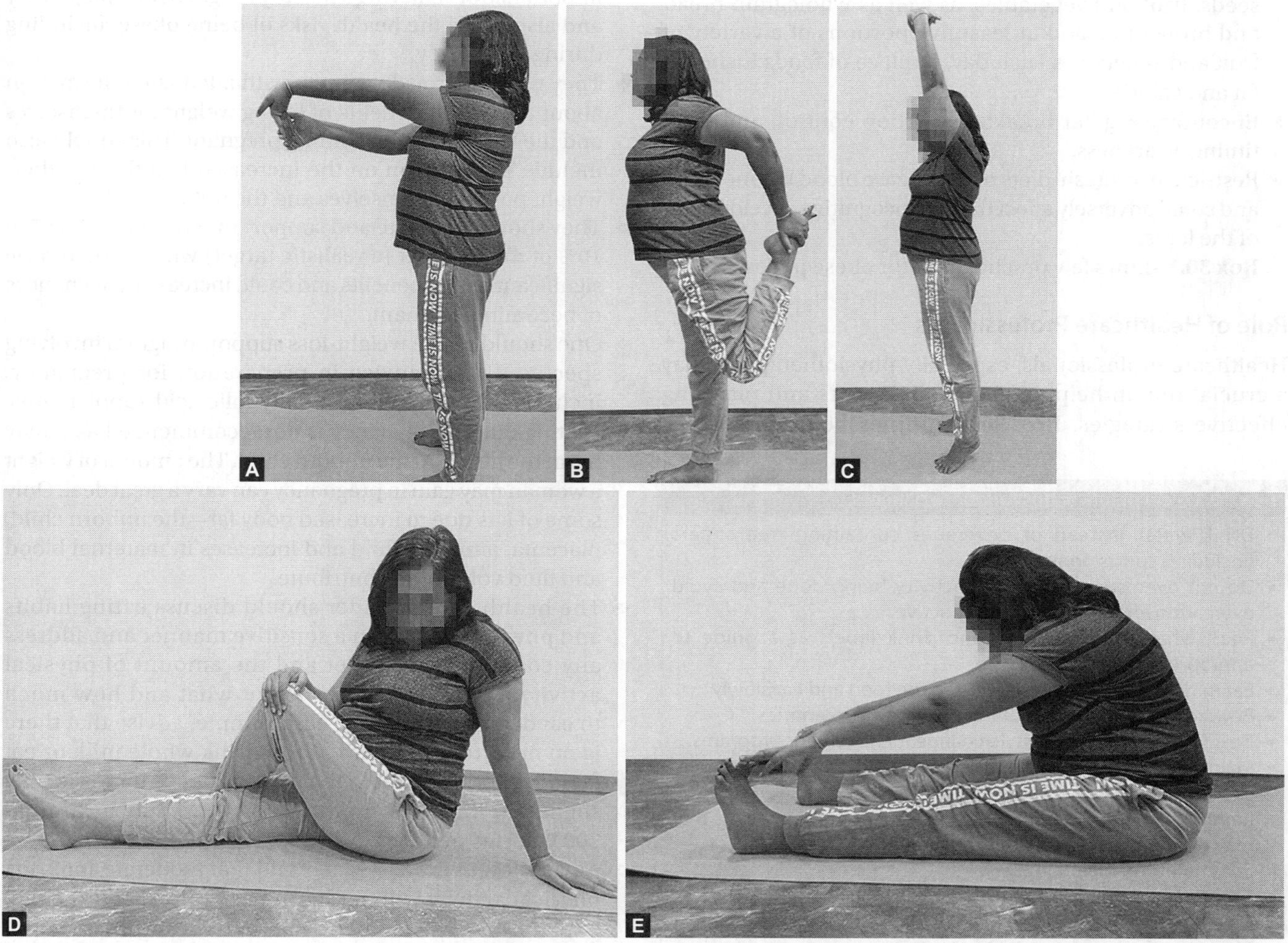

Figs. 30.8A to E: Flexibility exercises. (A) Stretching long finger flexors; (B) Stretching rectus femoris; (C) General whole body stretching; (D) Stretching piriformis; (E) Stretching calf and hamstrings.

- Realistic goals based on individual capacity with emphasis on steady continuous response in terms of health benefits.
- Target weight loss can be 5–10% of weight in initial 3–6 months.
- Choose activities that match lifestyle and schedule.

Dealing with Gestational Obesity

It is weight gain during pregnancy. The myth that one needs to feed oneself more is responsible for disproportionate increase in weight.

- Family plays a crucial role in providing the right nutrient intake. It is important to monitor weight and prevent getting obese before, during and after pregnancy.
- Healthy American women who are a normal weight for their height (BMI 18.5 to 24.9) should gain 11.5 to 16 kg (25 to 35 pounds) during pregnancy. Overweight women (BMI 25 to 29.9) should gain 7 to 11.5 kg (15 to 25 pounds) and obese women (BMI greater than 30) should only put on 5 to 9 kg (11 to 20 pounds).
- Eat fiber-rich foods such as oats, beans, peas, lentils, grains, seeds, fruit and vegetables, as well as wholegrain bread and brown rice and at least five portions of a variety of fruit and vegetables each day, in place of foods higher in fat and calories.
- Encourage regular breakfast, portion control, and meal timing awareness.
- Restrictive or 'crash' diets may increase blood ketone levels and could adversely affect the neurocognitive development of the fetus.

  Box 30.1 shows few practical tips for obese patients.

Role of Healthcare Professionals

Healthcare professionals, especially physiotherapists, play a crucial role in helping change behaviors and planning effective strategies. **Box 30.2** outlines behavior change strategies and **Box 30.3** outlines effective weight loss program.

Box 30.1: Few practical tips for obese patients.

- Drink water instead of beverages containing free sugars (including sports drinks).
- Do not overestimate physical activity being done and avoid overeating after being physically active.
- Read what you eat—food and drink labels as a guide to appropriate portion sizes.
- Eat mindfully—decorate, smell, see the food and eat slowly.
- Beware—even healthy is unhealthy in large quantities.
- Be informed—about lifestyle change management programs.
- Maintain reward and cheat diary and avoid giving 'sweet treats' as a reward or giving them regularly as gifts.
- Identify barriers—recognize personal and family behaviors that may be acting as barriers to change needs.
- Self-monitor—maintain diary.
- Choose the right activity.
- Develop a positive influence—family and friends are key sources of support for healthy weight management.

Box 30.2: Evidence-based behavior change strategy.

- Understand: The women's health-related behavior.
- Recognize: How women's social contexts and relationships may affect their behavior.
- Identify: Situations that might undermine the changes women are trying to make.
- Plan: 'If–then' coping strategies to prevent relapse.
- Help: Plan women's changes in terms of easy steps over time, feel positive about the benefits of health-enhancing behaviors and changing their behaviors

Box 30.3: Effective weight loss program.

- Find why someone might find it difficult to lose weight
- Tailor to individual needs and choices
- Be sensitive to the person's weight concerns
- Balance on healthy diet and regular physical activity
- Expect realistically to lose no more than 0.5–1 kg (1–2 lb) a week
- Identify and address barriers to change

- Healthcare professionals should educate women about importance of achieving a healthy weight before pregnancy and also stress the health risks of being obese, including during pregnancy.
- They need to provide women with adequate information about the health benefits of losing weight for themselves and the baby before becoming pregnant. This should also include information on the increased health risks their weight poses to themselves and the unborn child.
- They should motivate and support the women to lose 5 to 10% of their weight (a realistic target) which would have significant health benefits and could increase their chances of becoming pregnant.
- One should offer a weight-loss support program involving specific dietary advice in preparation for pregnancy, including the need to take daily folic acid supplements. Dieting during pregnancy is not recommended as it may harm the health of the unborn child. The amount of weight a woman may gain in pregnancy can vary a great deal. Only some of it is due to increased body fat—the unborn child, placenta, amniotic fluid and increases in maternal blood and fluid volume all contribute.
- The health care provider should discuss eating habits and physical activity in a sensitive manner and address any concerns about diet and the amount of physical activity. Dispel any myths about what and how much to eat during pregnancy. For example, advise that there is no need to 'eat for two' or to drink whole milk or eat fat laden foods. Explain that energy needs increase only slightly in the last 3 months (and then only by around 200 calories per day).
- Advise how to exercise safely and that moderate-intensity physical activity will not harm her or her unborn child. Explain to those women who would find this level of physical activity difficult that it is important not to be

sedentary, as far as possible. Encourage them to start walking and to build physical activity into daily life, for example, by taking the stairs instead of the lift, standing or walking rather than sitting for long periods.

- Do not weigh women repeatedly during pregnancy as a matter of routine. Only weigh again if clinical management can be influenced or if nutrition is a concern.

Post-delivery

- 6–8-week postnatal check is an opportunity to discuss weight. It is important to ask women who are overweight, obese or who have concerns about their weight if they would like any further advice and support now or later.
- During the postnatal check within the next 6 months a clear, tailored, up-to-date and timely advice on how to lose weight safely after childbirth should be provided.
- Benefits of a healthy diet and regular physical activity should be discussed, acknowledging the woman's role in the societal context, within the family and support systems. Advice on healthy eating and physical activity should be tailored as per the circumstances taking into considerations:
  - Demands of childcare
  - Older children
  - Level of fatigue
  - Postnatal impairments such as pelvic floor muscle weakness or backache.
- If pregnancy and delivery are uncomplicated, a mild exercise program consisting of walking, pelvic floor exercises and stretching may begin immediately. But the lady should not resume high-impact activity too soon after giving birth.
- Breastfeeding should be encouraged educating that a healthy diet and regular, moderate-intensity physical activity and gradual weight loss will not adversely affect the ability to breastfeed or the quantity or quality of breast milk. Women who exclusively breastfeed their infants for the first 6 months may require around an additional 330 calories a day which will be derived from fat stores. Though breastfeeding is often recommended as a strategy for promoting weight loss, findings from studies are mixed.
- Lack of sleep and a range of physical and psychological problems, such as backache, urinary and fecal incontinence, depression and fatigue, are common post-pregnancy and may impact on a woman's ability to be physically active and therefore, her ability to manage her weight. Women may also resume smoking and drinking alcohol. These habits may also affect their weight. Hence, they need to be adequately counseled.
- While planning to have a second child, weight management will help to achieve a healthy weight when they next become pregnant—and help prevent incremental weight gain over successive pregnancies.

Summary

Obesity is a growing health concern with complex interaction of various physiological, psychological, genetic and cultural factors. Obesity in women poses a risk not only in child-bearing age with adverse maternal and fetal outcome but also during menopause. Hormone therapy during menopause is a mix of benefits and risks. Effective approach of weight loss program needs to be dealt sensitively with a balance of diet and exercise which can be followed on long-term basis. It is important to change the behavior of not just the woman but the whole family to achieve positive outcome. There may be a number of psychological, emotional and social issues linked to weight management which need to be identified and addressed.

CLINICAL EXAMPLE

Assessment

Mrs Dixit, 48/F, housewife resides on ground floor, fair socio-economic status.

She was apparently alright 4 years back when she experienced irregularity in menses with pain and discomfort during menses for which investigations were done which showed leiomyoma of uterus, following which abdominal hysterectomy was done. After surgery her weight gradually increased by 10 kg.

After 2–3 months post-hysterectomy patient had symptoms of anxiety and fatigue after which she was diagnosed with borderline essential hypertension for which Losartan was started. She is also complaining of knee pain more on right side with visual analog scale (VAS) of 2/10 which is aggravated since last 3 weeks.

- No history of childhood obesity or any significant family comorbidity.
- Personal addictions of tobacco chewing—15–20 years, gave up for 5 years
- Nil cardiac or other systems involvement
- Obstetric history - 3 sons
  - 1st - normal delivery—stillbirth
  - 2nd and 3rd—cesarean section, age of youngest child—27 years
- **Diet history:** She is consuming 3 meals a day + takes tea 2/day with total calorie intake of 1,762 kcal/day
- **Exercise test:** Max workload - 7.1 MET, minor ST changes. Stress test is negative moderate tolerance.
  - 6 MWT: 450 meters
  - Adequate ionotropic and chronotropic response
- **Anthropometric parameters:**
  - Height—149 cm
  - Weight—69.8 kg
  - BMI—31.4 kg/m^2
  - Total body fat—40.4%, visceral fat—15
  - Basal metabolic rate—1365

- Abdominal circumference—104.2 cm
- Waist hip ratio—0.92

❖ **X-ray knee:** Suggestive of early degenerative changes.
❖ **Cardiac risk analysis:** (Framingham study in 1991) low-risk category which is 3% compared to healthy adult
❖ Impact of weight on quality of life (IWQOL - LIFE):
- Score
  - Physical functioning—31/55
  - Self-esteem—15/35
  - Social life—11/20
  - Public distress—6/25
  - Total—74/155

Contextual Factors

Contextual factors related to the example are described in **Table 30.5**.

Suggested Physiotherapy Management

Patient Education

❖ Educate about her condition and make her understand the need for weight reduction.
❖ Need of regular medicines for hypertension and regular follow-ups.
❖ Needs of regular exercise and diet control and interaction of various factors.
❖ Impact of weight on knee and exercises.

Short-term Goals

Knee care

❖ Use of hot packs for pain relief.
❖ Muscle activation and strengthening.

Weight reduction

❖ Caloric balance to reduce the total input.
❖ Exercise program and physical activity chart.
❖ Aerobic exercise training:
- As the patient is hypertensive avoid isometric exercise.
- The exercise regime should have regular periods of warm-up, conditioning and cool down.

Table 30.5: Contextual factors.

Environmental	*Facilitator*	*Barrier*
Social	Good family support	
Physical	House lives on ground floor	
Attitudinal	Positive outlook towards treatment Takes proper care of diet	
Personal	Co-operative Motivated	• Hypertension since 4 years • Menopausal due to hysterectomy since 4 years • Tobacco chewing - 15–20 years, gave up since 5 years

  - Warm up: 5–10 minutes
    - It is used to increase the circulation of all the muscles.
    - It is done to avoid abnormal cardiac effects.
  - Endurance training: Progressively increase the number of repetitions of exercises and volume to improve the endurance.
  - Cool down: Gradually reduces the intensity of exercises. It includes mat exercises, Shavasana and relaxation technique. Duration 10–15 minutes.

Long-term Goals

❖ Regular monitoring of hypertension and diet control
❖ Improve cardiac conditioning of the patient using various breathing exercises and thoracic expansion exercises
❖ Regular exercises for maintenance of the weight loss achieved
❖ Group therapy to improve social interactions of the patient.

Review Questions

1. What are the factors responsible for obesity in women?
2. Enumerate the maternal and fetal outcomes of obese pregnant lady.
3. What is the role of estrogen and write a note on hormone replacement therapy?
4. Discuss postmenopausal obesity.
5. What is the role of physiotherapist as a healthcare professional in management of obesity?
6. What advice should be given during and after childbirth in an obese women?

Bibliography

1. American College of Sports Medicine. ACSM's guidelines for exercise testing and prescription, 10th edition. Wolters Kluwer/ Lippincott Williams & Wilkins. American College of Sports Medicine-ACSM. 2018.
2. Catalano P, deMouzon SH. Maternal obesity and metabolic risk to the offspring: why lifestyle interventions may have not achieved the desired outcomes. Int J Obes (Lond). 2015;39(4): 642-9.
3. Catalano PM, Shankar K. Obesity and pregnancy: Mechanisms of short-term and long-term adverse consequences for mother and child. BMJ. 2017;356:j1.
4. Christiansen PK, Skjøth MM, Rothmann MJ, et al. Lifestyle interventions to maternal weight loss after birth: a systematic review. Syst Rev. 2019;8:327.
5. Donnelly JE, Blair SN, Jakicic JM, Manore MM, Rankin JW, Smith BK. American College of Sports Medicine. American College of Sports Medicine position stand: appropriate physical activity intervention strategies for weight loss and prevention of weight regain for adults. Med Sci Sports Exerc. 2009;41(2): 459-71.
6. Franks S. Polycystic ovary syndrome in adolescents. Int J Obes (Lond). 2008;32:1035-41.

7. Gaillard R, Durmus B, Hofman A, Mackenbach JP, Steegers EA, Jaddoe VW. Risk factors and outcomes of maternal obesity and excessive weight gain during pregnancy. Obesity (Silver Spring). 2013;21(5):1046-55. https://doi.org/10.1002/oby. 20088.
8. Gaur K, Keshri K, Joe W. Does living in slums or non-slums influence women's nutritional status? Evidence from Indian mega-cities. Soc Sci Med. 2013;77:137-46.
9. Golub MS, Collman GW, Foster PM, Kimmel CA, Rajpert-De Meyts E, Reiter EO, et al. Public health implications of altered puberty timing. Pediatrics. 2008;121(Suppl 3):S218–230.
10. Hong Y, Ory MG, Lee C, et al. Summary of the American College of Sports Medicine exercise recommendations for adults in the US. Walking and neighborhood environments for obese and overweight patients: perspectives from family physicians. Fam Med. 2012;44:336-41.
11. International Institute for Population Sciences. National Family Health Survey (NFHS-3), 2005–06: India. V. I. Mumbai: International Institute for Population Sciences; 2007:540.
12. Kalra S, Unnikrishnan AG. Obesity in India: The weight of the nation. J Med Nutr Nutraceuticals. 2012;1(1).
13. Kozakowski J, Gietka-Czernel M, Leszczyńska D, Majos A. Obesity in menopause—our negligence or an unfortunate inevitability? Prz Menopauzalny. 2017;16(2):61-65. doi: 10.5114/pm.2017.68594. Epub 2017 Jun 30. PMID: 28721132; PMCID: PMC5509974
14. Lean MEJ, Han TS, Morrison CE. Waist circumference as a measure for indicating need for weight management. BMJ. 1995;311:158-61 [PMC free article] [PubMed].
15. Maternal obesity and intrapartum obstetric complications among pregnant women: retrospective cohort analysis from medical birth registry in northern Tanzania. Obes Sci Pract. 2020;6(2):171–80. https://doi.org/10.1002/osp4.395.
16. Mishra A, Srivastavs U. Obesity and dyslipidemia in South Asians. Nutrients. 2013;5(7):2708-33.
17. Mottola MF. Components of exercise prescription and pregnancy. Clin Obstet Gynecol. 2016;59(3):552-58. doi:10.1097/GRF.0000000000000207.
18. Mwanamsangu AH, Mahande MJ, Mazuguni FS, et al. Maternal obesity and intrapartum obstetric complications among pregnant women: Retrospective cohort analysis from medical birth registry in Northern Tanzania. Obes Sci Pract. 2020;6:171-80. https://doi.org/10.1002/osp4.395.
19. National Institute for Health and Clinical Excellence. Obesity: Guidance on the prevention, identification, assessment and management of overweight and obesity in adults and children. NICE clinical guidance 43. 2006.
20. Ostbye T, Peterson BL, Krause KM, Swamy GK, Lovelady CA. Predictors of postpartum weight change among overweight and obese women: results from the active mothers postpartum study. J Women's Health (Larchmt). 2012;21(2):215-22. https://doi.org/10.1089/jwh.2011.2947.
21. Pescatello L, Arena R, Riebe D, Thompson PD, et al. Exercise prescription for healthy population with special consideration and environmental considerations. Clin Obstet Gynecol. 2014;59(3):552-58.
22. Roberts JM, Bodnar LM, Patrick TE, Powers RW. The role of obesity in preeclampsia. Pregnancy hypertens. 2011;1(1):6-16. https://doi.org/10.1016/j.preghy.2010.10.013 PMID: 21532964.
23. World Health Organization. Obesity: Preventing and managing the global epidemic. Report of a WHO consultation. World Health Organization Technical Report Series. 2000;894:1-253. [PubMed]

Multiple Choice Questions (MCQs)

To test your understanding and recall of key concepts.

1. **What is the waist circumference cutoff for high cardiovascular risk in Asian women?**
   A. 75 cm
   B. 80 cm
   C. 85 cm
   D. 90 cm
2. **Which type of obesity is associated with fat accumulation primarily in the upper body?**
   A. Gynoid
   B. Android
   C. Barrel type
   D. Middle-age obesity
3. **Why does menopause increase the risk of abdominal obesity?**
   A. Increased levels of estrogen
   B. Decline in estrogen and relative hyperandrogenemia
   C. Reduced calorie consumption
   D. Enhanced fat oxidation
4. **Which health condition is most commonly associated with obesity in postmenopausal women?**
   A. Hypoglycemia
   B. Cardiovascular disease
   C. Osteoporosis
   D. Alzheimer's disease
5. **A postmenopausal woman experiences central obesity and mild hypertension. Which type of exercise would be best for her condition?**
   A. High-intensity resistance training
   B. Moderate-intensity aerobic exercises
   C. Flexibility exercises only
   D. Isometric exercises
6. **Why is abdominal obesity considered as a significant risk factor for metabolic syndrome?**
   A. It enhances insulin sensitivity and promotes fat loss
   B. It leads to increased visceral fat, insulin resistance, and inflammation
   C. It reduces the levels of androgens and estrogen
   D. It improves cholesterol metabolism in the body
7. **What is the relationship between leptin and estrogen in obesity?**
   A. Estrogens potentiate leptin action by increasing the expression and sensitivity
   B. Estrogens suppress leptin action by decreasing the expression and sensitivity
   C. Leptin inhibits the effects of estrogen on fat distribution
   D. Leptin and estrogen work independently in appetite regulation

8. A 35-year-old woman with a BMI of 28 kg/m² and a waist circumference of 88 cm reports fatigue, irregular menstrual cycles, and recent weight gain. She has a sedentary lifestyle and consumes a high-calorie diet with low fiber. Her laboratory results show mildly elevated fasting glucose and triglycerides. What would be the first step in managing her condition?

A. Recommend hormone replacement therapy
B. Initiate a high-intensity interval training (HIIT) program
C. Begin a low-calorie, high-fiber diet combined with moderate-intensity aerobic exercises
D. Prescribe medication for triglycerides and glucose control

9. A 50-year-old woman, postmenopausal, presents with central obesity (waist circumference of 95 cm) and a diagnosis of metabolic syndrome. Her Bone Mineral density is –2. Which combination of interventions is most appropriate for addressing her overall health?

A. High-protein diet, weightlifting, hormone replacement therapy and dietary supplements
B. Moderate-intensity aerobic exercise, resistance training, and dietary adjustments with calcium and vitamin D supplementation
C. Low-calorie diet, flexibility exercises, pharmacological management of metabolic syndrome and dietary supplements
D. Exclusive focus on weight reduction through a very low-calorie diet

ANSWERS

1. B	2. B	3. B	4. B	5. B
6. B	7. A	8. C	9. B	

Chapter 31

Women's Health in Sports

Preetha Ramachandra, Kiransha R Velingkar

LEARNING OBJECTIVES

At the end of the chapter, the reader will be able to:

- Understand with evidence-based information regarding the challenges faced by female athletes throughout their lifespan beginning from menstrual disturbances during adolescence.
- Know about the hurdles during pregnancy.
- Learn about the issues related to urinary incontinence.
- Understand the complications associated with menopause.

CHAPTER OUTLINE

INTRODUCTION

The participation of women in recreational and professional sports has increased markedly, thus requiring more knowledge on the influence of sports on women's health. Sex has been identified as a major determinant of athletic performance due to existing anatomical and physiological differences between males and females, such as height, weight, body fat, aerobic capacity, anaerobic threshold, and hormonal fluctuations.

The musculoskeletal differences existing between both the sexes like narrower pelvis, increased VMO hypertrophy, wider femoral notch, genu varum, medial tibial torsion in males compared to wider pelvis, less developed VMO, narrow femoral notch, genu valgum, and lateral tibial torsion in females, predisposes females at greater risk for developing anterior cruciate ligament injury, patellofemoral pain syndrome, medial tibial stress syndrome, and injuries to the spine.

Additionally, relative maximal oxygen uptake (VO_2 max) for untrained women typically averages 15–30% below scores for men. In trained women, the difference becomes less, but women still present with a 10–15% lower VO_2 max. The difference in aerobic capacity is attributed to lower oxygen carrying capacity, lower blood volume, fewer red blood cells, lower hemoglobin content, smaller heart, lower stroke volume, and smaller muscle fiber area in women compared to men. Furthermore, the most recognized factor to explain the sex difference in performance is the concentration of circulating testosterone, which is 10 to 15 times higher in men than in women. However, higher rate of testosterone in females leads to symptoms of hyperandrogenism like infertility, obesity, hirsutism, and hormonal imbalances.

The existing contrast between men and women makes it necessary to formulate a tailored assessment and exercises guideline in female athlete to improvise on their

Box 31.1: Low energy availability.

In the Female Athlete Triad, LEA is how much energy remains after body functions. LEA may occur with or without an eating disorder. EA is calculated by taking the dietary energy intake (in kilocalories) and subtracting the energy (in kilocalories) expended during exercise.

sport performance while maintaining physical and mental wellbeing. In this chapter we describe the influence of exercise and sport on women's health across the lifespan.

MENSTRUAL DISTURBANCES AND FEMALE ATHLETES

Participation in sports has physiologic, psychologic, and social benefits, however, the Female Athlete Triad (FAT) has always been a well-known negative effect of female participation in sports. The term FAT was first coined by the American College of Sports Medicine in 1992, as the interrelated condition including disordered eating, amenorrhea, and osteoporosis which was then updated in 2007, to reflect the interdependence of low energy availability (LEA) (with or without eating disorders) with amenorrhea, decreased bone mineral density, and osteoporosis, which may result in the non-simultaneous occurrence of the clinical symptoms. However, in 2014, the International Olympic Committee replaced FAT and reported the syndrome as relative energy deficiency in sport (RED-S), which highlighted the impact of low energy availability on the human body and recognized FAT as one of the outcomes of LEA **(Box 31.1)** in the RED-S model.

Amenorrhea is the most common menstrual abnormality in a female athlete.

- Primary amenorrhea refers to a delay in the age of menarche (no menses by age 15 years in the presence of normal secondary sexual development or within 5 years after breast development if that occurs before the age of 10 years)
- Secondary amenorrhea is a loss of menses after menarche.

Other types of menstrual irregularities include anovulation, luteal phase deficiency, and oligomenorrhea.

The etiology of exercise-associated menstrual cycle irregularity appears to be related to 'energy drain'—the phenomenon of a calorie deficit. Restricted energy availability as a result of reduced energy intake and/or increased energy expenditure leads to low leptin levels and stimulates compensatory mechanisms, such as weight loss, metabolic hormone alterations, or energy conservation that subsequently cause central suppression of reproductive function and concomitant hypoestrogenism.

Clinical Pointer

The major complications of exercise-associated menstrual cycle irregularity include reduced fertility, and decreased bone mass.

Box 31.2: Common eating disorders in athletes.

- Anorexia nervosa is linked to an unfounded fear of fatness that may be related to family or societal pressures to be thin. The person with anorexia may use a variety of techniques to remain thin, including starvation, exercise, and laxatives.
- Bulimia nervosa is characterized by episodes of binge eating followed by compensatory behaviors such as self-induced vomiting usually for the preventing weight gain.

Sports and Eating Disorders

A study conducted on 1600 students aged between 15 and 25 years of age in South India, reported 26.06% participants were prone to eating disorders. Female athletes are at risk of developing eating disorders due to pressure to maintain a low body weight along with poor guidance about nutrition and weight loss from the athletic community. The two common eating disorders affecting female or male athletes are anorexia nervosa and bulimia **(Box 31.2)**.

Warning signs of anorexia nervosa are rapid weight loss, mood swings, excessive exercise, and avoiding food-related activities, whereas, bulimia displays the signs of noticeable weight loss, depressive mood, excessive concern about weight, bathroom visits after meals, and strict dieting followed by binge eating **(Fig. 31.1)**.

Clinical Pointer

Anorexia Athletica is a term used by some researchers to describe a disordered eating pattern seen in the female athlete who has an intense fear of gaining weight, even though she is underweight.

Although maintaining an optimal body composition for the competition is important to achieve athletic success, eating disorders are not an appropriate means of weight loss. Therefore, trainers, athletes, and coaches need to recognize the warning signals of eating disorders and be prepared to assist the athlete in obtaining the appropriate help. The Female Athlete Triad Consensus Panel Screening Questions and diagnostic tests like complete blood count, hormonal levels, and dual-energy X-ray absorptiometry (DEXA) should be used during athletes' preparticipation evaluation to prevent athlete triad.

Female Hormones and Injury Risk

Exercises or sports-associated injuries may affect the injured athlete's quality of life or career. One way to avoid these injuries is through identifying risk factors which then could be addressed with corresponding interventions. Studies state that some exercise-induced injuries are more common in women than in men, suggesting that female sex is itself a risk factor.

- Anterior cruciate ligament (ACL) injuries are more prevalent in women than in men. Additionally, several studies have concluded that there is decreased relative risk of ACL tear during the luteal phase. Lefevre, et al.

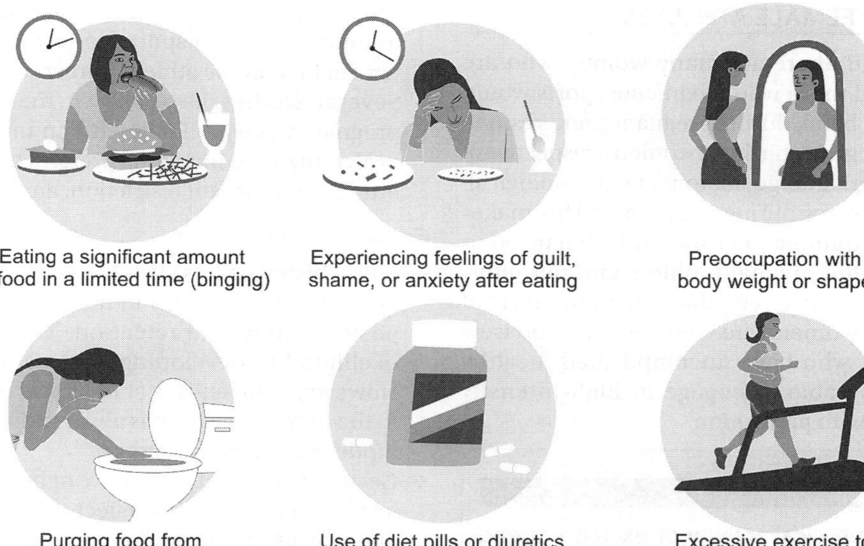

Fig. 31.1: Common signs and symptoms of bulimia.

concluded that female skiers should take special care during the preovulatory phase of the menstrual cycle as this phase associates with ACL rupture. The popular explanation for the statistical correlation between the preovulatory phase and injury peak is directly linked to high estrogen levels which causes mechanical weakness of ligaments, which would then—in turn—increase the likelihood of ACL injuries.

- Additionally, two meta-analyses have concluded, that knee laxity varies within the menstrual cycle, with the highest laxity occurring during ovulation, followed by the luteal phase and the lowest laxity occurring in the follicular phase. However, both meta-analyses concluded, that periods of increased laxity were not associated with an increased prevalence of ACL ruptures, thus suggesting that there is no direct link between hormonal effects on ACL injuries and hormonal effects on knee laxity.
- Adding on, studies found postural control impairment in women who suffered premenstrual symptoms thus increasing the postural sway in the luteal phase, when symptoms like discomfort and pain were particularly prevalent, while sway values stayed stable throughout the menstrual cycle in women without premenstrual symptoms. The postural sway in women with premenstrual symptoms may be related to changes in kinesthesia, as these women also detected greater passive movement in the knee.

Monitoring of Menstrual Cycle Phases in Elite Sports

- The use of routine menstrual cycle (MC) phase monitoring in elite sports is becoming increasingly widespread.
- Elite sporting organizations, like Chelsea Football Club and the United States Women's National Soccer and Swimming Teams, have recently begun using a smartphone app to track athletes' MCs. This app is used by players to record when menstruation and various menstrual symptoms occur which can be accessed by the coaches and support staff to identify any changes in an athlete's performance during the various phases of the MC.
- A study conducted on 15 elite female rugby players to explore the athlete's past and present experiences and perceptions of the menstrual cycle in relation to its impact on sporting performance showed that almost all athletes (93%) reported menstrual cycle-related symptoms. Among these 33% perceived heavy menstrual bleeding and 67% considered these symptoms impaired their performance. Furthermore, two-thirds of these athletes self-medicated to alleviate symptoms.
- The effect of MC phase on strength was examined in both dominant and non-dominant limbs in two studies. There was a significant increase in dominant handgrip strength in the late follicular phase and there were significant, but unspecified, differences between phases in non-dominant handgrip strength. The non-dominant hamstring to quadriceps strength ratio was significantly decreased in the follicular phase compared to the luteal phase but there was no change in the strength ratio of the dominant limb.

Prevention Strategies Towards the Triad

- Educating the female athlete, coaches, and caregivers
- Making the resources freely available
- Checking the required nutrition intake
- Encouraging programs to improvise athlete's self-esteem, and promoting a positive training environment
- Breaking taboos and myths
- Practicing adequate rest intervals
- Formulation of tailored exercises regimen
- Consumption of vitamin D and calcium to prevent loss of bone mineral density
- Monitoring the menstrual cycles
- Practicing a holistic approach

PREGNANCY AND FEMALE ATHLETES

In the current scenario, there are many women who are interested in sports and those who are in elite sports would prefer to avoid a career break during pregnancy and resume their sports careers after giving birth. All women irrespective of their sports background undergo anatomical, physiological, and biomechanical changes during pregnancy. This makes it important that their training load should be balanced to meet the demands of the pregnant athlete and her fetus. Although there is no evidence regarding the upper level of safe exercise intensity, women who were regular exercisers before pregnancy and who have uncomplicated, healthy pregnancies should be able to engage in high-intensity exercise programs, yet with precaution.

Clinical Pointer

A moderate level of physical activity or exercise during pregnancy is always considered safe for pregnancy.

In the first trimester of pregnancy, nausea and vomiting can interfere with athletic participation. As pregnancy proceeds further than 14 weeks, some of the physiological changes, such as weight gain, ligament laxity, and changes in balance and posture will affect athletic training and performance.

Specific exercise precautions after the 14th week include:
- Avoiding training and competition in the supine (lying on the back) position
- Avoiding the Valsalva maneuver
- Avoiding activities with a high-risk of falling

Thus, it is advisable to develop individually tailored exercise prescription for pregnant athletes so that they do not cross the threshold beyond which the fetal parameters get compromised.

Clinical Issues during Pregnancy and Postpartum which can Impact the Performance of Athletes

Nausea and Vomiting

- Severe nausea and vomiting are associated with reduced food and water intake which can lead to dehydration with signs of postural hypotension and tachycardia.
- Dietary support and adequate fluid intake are central to management.
- Some evidence suggest that women with a high intake of fatty foods have a higher risk of hyperemesis gravidarum and that low-energy high-protein diets are associated with a reduction of nausea and vomiting in pregnancy, compared with a diet high in carbohydrates. Women may also benefit from frequent small meals.

Mental Health and Well-being

- It is assumed that the athletes engaged in sports may not suffer from mental health issues. But studies have proven that female athletes undergo more mental health issues than male athletes.
- These symptoms may be aggravated during pregnancy due to injury, failure in sports performance, and involuntary termination of the athletic career.
- Several studies have shown that depression during pregnancy is associated with an increased risk for poor birth outcomes, including preterm birth, low birth weight, intrauterine growth restriction, and preeclampsia.

Gestational Weight Gain

- Elite athletes are less likely to gain weight during pregnancy and they are less likely to develop fetal macrosomia and postpartum weight retention. This in turn, reduces the likelihood of developing chronic diseases later in life. However, if the fetus is at the lower end of the birth chart in the third trimester, it is always advisable to provide only moderate-intensity exercise.
- Gestational weight gain above or below the recommended levels can have adverse effects on both mother and fetus and may be of concern for pregnancy outcomes as well as for a return to sport.
- Reduced gestational weight gain is associated with preterm birth and difficulty to initiate breastfeeding. Greater gestational weight gain is associated with increased risk of gestational diabetes mellitus and hypertensive disorders, prolonged labor, caesarean section, macrosomia, and large for gestational age infants, as well as postpartum weight retention and later overweight/obesity. Hence, there must be an adequate balance between calorie intake and physical activity so that it does not interfere with the growth of the fetus.

Eating Disorders during Pregnancy

- Eating disorders are common among athletes compared to non-athletes as athletes are under constant performance pressure and stress of improving their results.
- The pregnant athlete with a past or current eating disorder should be considered as being at higher risk of pregnancy complications, such as hypertension, miscarriage, difficult labor, premature delivery, and intrauterine growth restriction. Hence, it is essential to monitor her for meal plans, training load, and continuous monitoring of maternal and fetal health.
- The involvement of a multidisciplinary team (which includes a nutritionist, a psychiatrist, maternal-fetal medicine specialist) emphasizes early recognition and treatment of symptoms, meal planning, training regimen adjustments, and evaluation of maternal or fetal consequences of malnutrition.

Stress Fractures

- A previous study has reported that stress fractures are common among athletes in the postpartum period. There could be multiple contributing factors for this which include:
  - A sudden increase in the training load in the postpartum period
  - Insufficient strength training during and early postpartum

- Inadequate intake of calcium and vitamin D3 during pregnancy and while breastfeeding during postpartum

- This indicates that much of a focus is essential in improving bone health, such as optimal energy intake, calcium, and Vitamin D3 intake and focus must be given to strength training and weight-bearing exercise during the breastfeeding phase among elite athletes.

Measuring Performance During Pregnancy

Owing to transient fetal bradycardia at >90% of VO_2 max, it is not advisable to conduct the test in research settings. An alternative to VO_2 max testing during pregnancy is to predict target heart rates (HR) for training from VO_2 peak tests or to predict VO_2 max from submaximal testing. Target HR ranges do exist based on age that was calculated from fit women at 16–20 weeks of pregnancy who had a VO_2 peak of >27.2 mL/kg/min (women aged 20–29 years) and >26.1 mL/kg/min (women aged 30–39 years). The target HR ranges were based on 60–80% of measured VO_2 peak values and are listed as 145–160 bpm (women aged 20–29 years) and 140–156 bpm (women aged 30–39 years). Testing with ventilatory analyses (e.g., expiratory volume/VO_2) is often used to determine target zones for distance and interval training in elite athletes, and could provide pregnant women with an alternative form of submaximal exercise testing. If an elite athlete wished to continue training based on ventilatory threshold test results, she can be assured that during mild or moderate exercise the RER (respiratory exchange ratio) is not significantly different in pregnant women than in non-pregnant women.

Previous research has reported that the Borg Rating of perceived exertion (RPE) does not correlate with maternal heart rate during pregnancy. The heart rate predicted from RPE was underestimated during walking, aerobic classes, and circuit training in the second trimester. Similar results were reported in the third trimester while cycling and while aerobic classes. Hence in a pregnant athlete, it is advisable to measure the heart rate directly and RPE must not be used as the only measure to determine exercise intensity from the second trimester.

Strength Training

- Light to moderate weight training is not associated with any adverse health effects during pregnancy.
- Previous research has reported greater strength gains in women who performed strength training twice a week for 12 weeks. However, heavy strength training in pregnancy may lead to the Valsalva maneuver which may lead to increased blood pressure and intra-abdominal pressure which can reduce the blood supply to the fetus. This can also put excessive pressure on the pelvic floor support which may increase the risk of urinary or fecal incontinence and pelvic organ prolapse.
- Avoiding the Valsalva maneuver by exhaling with an open airway also seems prudent. In the absence of studies on elite athletes, International Olympic Committee (IOC) agreed that female athletes may consider refraining from repetitive heavy lifting efforts in the first trimester of pregnancy to avoid the potential risk of miscarriage. However, as IOC emphasized, these recommendations are based on low-quality evidence.

Flexibility Training

- Owing to the excessive ligament laxity due to hormonal changes during pregnancy, overstretching must be avoided as joints may be lax and may have instability.
- When running or cycling, rocky terrains or unstable grounds should be avoided, since the joints are laxer in pregnancy, and ankle sprains and other injuries may occur.

Training Volume

- It has been stated that competitive athletes maintain a more strenuous training regimen than less active women throughout pregnancy, more quickly resume training postpartum and that giving birth results in a positive performance effect.
- Recent studies have shown that most recreational and competitive runners voluntarily reduce their training volume in the first, second and third trimesters compared with prepregnancy levels and fewer than one-third continue to run during the third trimester. The reasons for this may be commonly reported complaints during these periods, such as nausea and fatigue in the first trimester and musculoskeletal complaints and constipation in the third trimester.

Specific Considerations and Safety Issues Regarding Exercise During Pregnancy

Since competitive athletes tend to maintain a more strenuous training schedule throughout pregnancy and resume high-intensity postpartum training sooner as compared to other pregnant women, they require frequent and closer supervision. Such athletes should pay particular attention to avoiding hyperthermia, maintaining proper hydration, and sustaining adequate caloric intake to prevent weight loss, which may adversely affect fetal growth.

Hydration and Urinary Incontinence

Although pregnant women are advised to drink water before, during, and after exercise, they experience urinary incontinence during exercise because of mechanical and anatomical changes. Thus, there are considerations to take into account to minimize urinary incontinence related to exercise, such as:

- Voiding before activity
- Avoiding breath holding
- Avoiding Valsalva maneuver during exercise
- Practicing pelvic muscle-strengthening exercises
- Minimizing high-impact activities when incontinence symptoms appeared
- Using an external pad during exercise

Falls and Injury

High-risk sports can be divided into:

- Those with risk of trauma (sports leading to collision or sudden deceleration)
- Those with physiological risk factors

Maternal trauma could lead to abruption of the placenta which can lead to acute or chronic fetal hypoxia or death. A few examples of contact high-risk sports are downhill ski racing, pole vaulting, equestrian activities, or sports with a high potential for contact, such as ice hockey, soccer, basketball etc. In relation to physiological risk, pregnant women should refrain from diving, because the fetus is not protected from decompression problems and is at risk of malformation and gas embolism after decompression disease.

The US guidelines include some activities (i.e., racket sports or running) as safe if pregnant women usually practice this prior to pregnancy. From a practical point of view, it would be valuable to develop guidelines on the adaptation of exercises to the different needs of pregnant women and action to minimize the risk of participating in various sports activities during pregnancy. This would allow women to self-assess the benefits and risks of a particular physical activity so that they can make informed decisions about participation.

Clinical Pointer

Fieril, et al. report that modifying the type of exercise, altering exercise goals, and being extra attentive during the performance are recommended strategies to overcome exercise barriers in pregnancy. Hence, in the absence of medical contraindications, the decision to stop or continue particular sports activities should be based on the assessment of a woman's individual abilities, skills, previous experience, and sense of security and comfort related to performing this activity.

Nausea and Dizziness

- While performing physical activity, it is necessary to avoid the Valsalva maneuver, prolonged isometric contraction, and motionless standing.
- In view of the supine hypotensive syndrome, it is necessary to avoid physical activity in the supine position after week 16 of pregnancy. Due to the weight of the growing fetus, exertion or prolonged periods in the supine position may reduce venous return and cardiac output.

Heat, Humidity, and Environment

- Pregnant women should avoid exercising in a hot humid environment, be well hydrated at all times, and dress appropriately to avoid heat stress.
- Prolonged exercise should be performed in a thermo-neutral environment or in controlled environmental conditions (air conditioning) with close attention paid to proper hydration and caloric intake.
- Pregnant women are quite sensitive to smell. Exercise should be performed in a clean environment, avoiding air pollution and bad smell settings.

Sportswear and Shoes

- Pregnant women should wear comfortable and proper exercise footwear that gives strong ankle and arch support and provides impact-absorbing features, especially during weight-bearing activities and outdoor activities.
- Sportswear should be light and comfortable and allow perspiration. Moreover, it should be seamless, due to the increased sensitivity of the skin.

URINARY INCONTINENCE AND FEMALE ATHLETES

Urinary incontinence (UI) may be a barrier to women's participation in sports and fitness activities. Therefore, it may be a threat to women's health, self-esteem, and well-being.

- Previous literature has reported that female athletes in comparison to non-athletes had a larger mean diameter of the puborectalis muscle, a greater descent of the bladder neck, and a larger urogenital hiatus area during the Valsalva maneuver which could be associated with UI.
- High-impact activities that involve increased intra-abdominal pressure can damage the pelvic floor muscles in long term, decreasing the strength of the pelvic floor muscles and increasing the risk of stress urinary incontinence.
- Muscular fatigue due to over activation of Type II fibers and its inability to maintain the muscle tone of pelvic floor muscles could also affect the continence mechanism.

The cross-sectional areas and thickness of the levator ani and puborectalis were measured by Kruger, et al. using magnetic resonance imaging (MRI) and were found to be increased in women who participated in long-term, high-impact sports, and exercise. High-impact training results in thicker muscles that may compensate for greater muscle distensibility. Reasons could be that those who are involved in high-impact sports already have stronger and thicker PFMs, or due to differences in connective tissue or muscle biomechanics that may be a consequence of high-impact training. Women with stress incontinence have less collagen concentration in their skin and periurethral tissue, and a decreased ratio of type I to type III collagen. Moreover, high-impact varsity athletes with increased foot arch flexibility had less urinary incontinence, possibly because of the better shock-absorbing capacity of their lower extremities. In conclusion, two opposing hypotheses exist on the effect of exercise on PFMs, with a possible mixed effect of both mechanisms on the athletes' urinary incontinence.

It has been reported that women use vaginal tampons to prevent urine leakage during high-impact activity or use pads or panty liners due to urine leakage. Urinary incontinence during physical activity may compel them to stop practicing and or limit their exercising. Others change their sport modality, choosing walking as their primary activity to reduce urinary leakage. Coping strategies used by the athletes during the training included using protective pads, frequent toilet visits, and limited fluid intake.

Pelvic floor dysfunctions can have a huge impact on an athlete's life. Athletes who are involved in high-impact exercise must be advised about pelvic floor dysfunctions and their prevention.

Prevalence

- A recent systematic review has reported that the prevalence rate of urinary incontinence to be 28% to 29.6% among female athletes compared to non-athletes. Another meta-analysis has reported that the mean prevalence of UI is 36.1% (95% CI 26.5% –46.8%), ranging from 19.4% to 76% among all-level female athletes.

- Professional female athletes have thrice the risk of developing urinary incontinence compared to inactive women.
- A recent study about the prevalence of urinary incontinence among sports women mentioned that 91% of female athletes reported about urine leakage during training. They also reported that the activities which triggered leakage of urine were rotation, running, jumping and lifting weights.
- Among specific sports, 80% of female athletes who played rugby reported urinary incontinence followed by the swimmers. The intermittent bursts of high-intensity exercise, running and bruising involved in rugby may increase the force on the pelvic floor. The torsion and rotation movements among swimmers may increase the incidence of urinary incontinence. Another proposed explanation for the cause of urinary incontinence in swimmers is that reduced training volume of increased intensity may induce fatigue and hence the electrical activity level of the pelvic floor muscles in female athletes.
- Another review has shown a prevalence rate of UI of 75.6% in volleyball, 72.7% for trampolining, 50% for indoor soccer, 45.5% for cross-country skiers and runners, 44% for running, 34.8% for basketball, 20.8% for athletics and 20% for handball athletes. Urgency urinary incontinence was most apparent in cyclists and football (soccer) players.
- Athletes reported urine loss more frequently during the end of the training session and the second part of the competition, suggesting that pelvic floor muscular endurance is required. Ree, et al. found that there was short-term fatigue of the PFMs in women with stress urinary incontinence following 90 min of strenuous physical exercise. This indicates that muscular fatigue due to lack of muscle endurance can also result in urinary incontinence.

Risk Factors

- Risk factors associated with urinary incontinence **(Fig. 31.2)** are:
  - Constipation
  - Family history of urinary incontinence

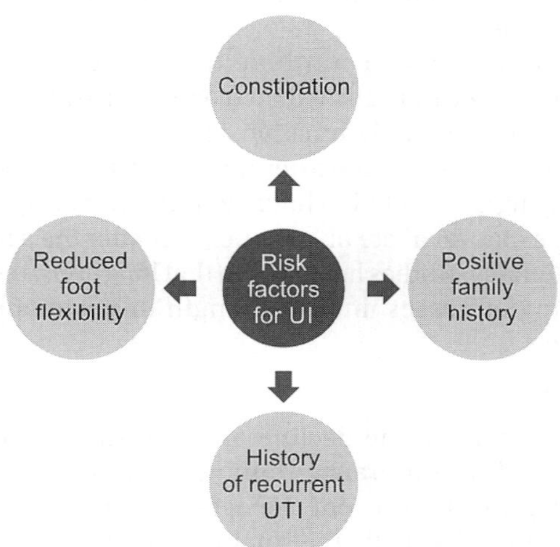

Fig. 31.2: Risk factors associated with urinary incontinence. (UI: urinary incontinence; UTI: urinary tract infections)

  - History of recurrent urinary tract infections
  - Decreased foot flexibility
- Eating disorders in athletes are also considered to be a risk factor for both stress and urgency urinary incontinence owing to reduced estrogen levels. Another explanation for eating disorders being a causative factor for urinary incontinence is that they may result in a lack of energy and nutrition needed to build and strengthen muscles, ligaments, and fascia. Eating disorders may involve repetitive induced vomiting which can increase the intra-abdominal pressure and weaken the pelvic floor muscles. In addition to this, high-impact sports are likely to generate higher intra-abdominal pressures, leading to pelvic floor muscle weakness, morphological and functional changes in ligaments and connective tissue, or an increased diameter of the levator hiatus. Therefore, the general belief that physically fit women have a stronger pelvic floor due to regular exercise preventing the development of UI should be questioned further.
- Another interesting finding is that more athletes experienced leakage during training rather than competition (95.2% vs. 51.2%), possibly because of higher catecholamine levels during the competition that act on the urethral α-receptors to maintain its closure.

Prevention and Management of Urinary Incontinence in Female Athletes

The prevalence of urinary incontinence is higher in athletes as compared to non-athletic women.

Pelvic floor physiotherapy as a treatment for urinary incontinence in elite female athletes, former elite female athletes, and pregnant athletes who engage in regular aerobic activity, is found to be beneficial in reducing the symptoms of incontinence.

- Treatment of urinary incontinence in athletes must start by keeping a check on the contributing factors, such as eating disorders, genital atrophy, smoking, obesity, and reduction of caffeine and alcohol consumption.
- Female athletes with urinary incontinence should avoid excessive fluid consumption before training and competition but care must be taken to avoid dehydration. They should be instructed to void shortly before training sessions and competitions.
- A model has been proposed by Heath, et al. for screening and treatment of stress urinary incontinence in female athletes. It consists of a set of questions for screening a nulliparous female athlete who is post-pubescent and trains for more than 8 hours a week for stress urinary incontinence. The initial screening questions include if the athlete is involved in high-impact activities, such as jumping, running, landing, etc., and if they have a past or current history of disordered eating. The presence of one or both factors indicates that they need to be further screened and the questions asked as a part of a comprehensive interview include—Do you experience urinary leakage during regular activity? or Do you have involuntary leakage of urine on effort, exertion, sneezing, or coughing? Or Do you experience urine leakage during training or sports activity and if so how often? If the screening

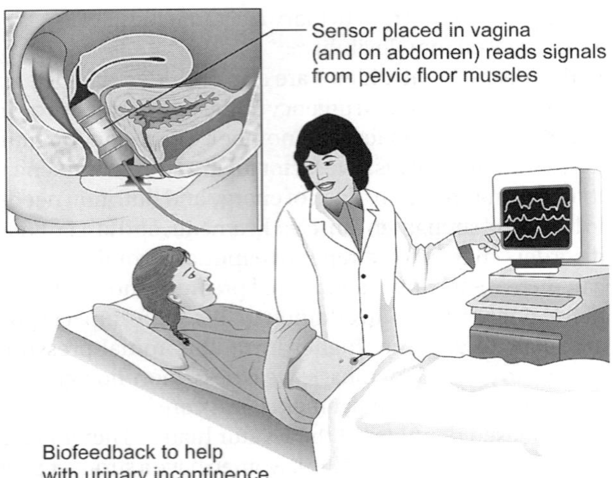

Fig. 31.3: EMG biofeedback for pelvic floor muscles.

questions indicate that they have symptoms of stress urinary incontinence, they should be referred to a Women's Health Physiotherapist for further screening and potential treatment.

- Pelvic floor muscle training (PFMT) is an important component for both prevention and treatment of urinary incontinence, and it has no known side effects and is considered the first line of treatment for all types of urinary incontinence especially stress urinary incontinence. Biofeedback in the form of vaginal and anal surface electromyography **(Fig. 31.3)**, manometers, and dynamometers can be an adjunct to PFMT as it helps to improve awareness of muscle function and to improve patient's motivation during training.
- Emphasis should be given to precontraction of pelvic floor muscles before any activity which involves an increase in intra-abdominal pressure to prevent urethral descent and leakage during exertion. The goal is to provoke a quick, strong, and well-defined PFM contraction before and during the rise in intra-abdominal pressure, known as 'the Knack'.
- The use of biofeedback techniques includes training in different positions and PFM contraction while performing real physical activities.
- Surgery must be considered only if the conservative therapy fails or its causes have been evaluated thoroughly or if the degree of incontinence severely bothers the athlete. Common surgical treatments include pubovaginal sling procedures, retropubic suspension, and periurethral injections. However, surgery is inappropriate in young women, including elite athletes, who are continent during regular daily activities and have incontinence only during exercise and sport.

Urinary incontinence is frequent and troublesome among exercising women and athletes leading to poor quality of life owing to comprised performance, feelings of concern, frustration and embarrassment of experiencing urinary leakage during the competition and is highly under-reported. High-impact sports and eating disorders increase the risk for urinary incontinence. Non-athletic women should be encouraged to participate in mild to moderate exercise activities that improve their general health and may even improve urinary incontinence. Urogynecological assessment is advised in competitive athletes and pelvic floor muscle training should be the first-line of treatment for urinary incontinence in women, and should probably be incorporated into athletes' training programs. It is very important to sensitize all the professionals (physiotherapists, coaches, fitness instructors and sports doctors) involved to timely detect or prevent urinary incontinence.

MENOPAUSE AND FEMALE ATHLETES

Menopause is a physiological phase that is characterized by the permanent cessation of menstrual cycle due to loss of ovarian follicular function. Perimenopause is a time period that begins with the first onset of menstrual irregularity and ends after 1 year of amenorrhea. There are two stages to the perimenopause or menopausal transition: the early transition, where cycles are mostly regular, with relatively few interruptions, and the late transition, where amenorrhea becomes more prolonged and lasts for at least 60 days, up to the Final menstrual period (FMP). During menopausal transitions women experience various physical, psychological, and social changes that may affect their quality of life and wellbeing.

Some of the signs and symptoms experienced during this period are hot flushes, night sweats, palpitations, impaired cognition, sarcopenia, osteoporosis, stress fractures, vaginal dryness, decreased libido, sleep disturbance, and depression. There are a growing number of people over the age of 50 that compete in competitive athletic events. These "masters athletes" represent an interesting subgroup of older adults because they possess unique physiological characteristics that could be termed "exceptionally successful aging". In the following text, we describe the age-related changes which have a negative effect on performance.

Muscular Strength

- Age-related sarcopenia occurs due to both a decrease in fiber size and a decrease in the number of fibers present in the muscle.
- Number of factors contribute to sarcopenia, including inactivity, free radical-mediated damage (oxidative stress) to muscle fibers, inflammation, and decreases in anabolic hormones, such as testosterone. The rate of muscle loss with aging is variable, but both men and women tend to lose muscle mass at a rate of 1–2% per year after the age of 50.
- Additionally, studies have shown that long-term resistance training increases muscle strength in postmenopausal women.

Endurance

- Aging results in the decline of VO_2 max, which can be increased by endurance training. However, endurance training cannot prevent the age-related decline in VO_2 max, but individuals that maintain endurance training programs throughout the life span tend to sustain higher VO_2 compared to sedentary individuals.

- Studies indicate that the age-related decline in VO_2 max occurs due to a decrease in both maximal cardiac output and a decline in the maximal arterio-venous oxygen difference.
- Physical activity guidelines recommend 60 min or more physical activity daily, with muscle and bone strengthening to improve or maintain VO_2 max levels.

Osteoporosis

- A growing concern for a female athlete is osteoporosis, which happens due to estrogen deficiency and inadequate calcium intake. Being a major concern, its complications include fractures that have a high rate of morbidity and mortality.
- It is important to reduce the loss of bone prior to or at the time of menopause. A variety of moderate-impact exercises and strength training has been shown to reduce the rate of loss of bone mass in the postmenopausal period.
- Studies state that exercise along with calcium intake is needed to retain calcium balance in postmenopausal women because of increased urinary calcium losses associated with low estrogen levels. The recommended daily intake of calcium in postmenopausal women is 1200 mg per day. However, evidence from a recent Cochrane review states that calcium supplementation alone has a small positive effect on bone density. Similarly, Vitamin D is also important for bone health. Oral vitamin D supplementation of 700–800 IU/day appears to reduce the risk of hip and any non-vertebral fractures in ambulatory or institutionalized elderly persons.

Exercise Guidelines

- A comprehensive pre-exercise evaluation and a tailored training program are necessary for menopausal/postmenopausal women.
- Thorough history and examination should be performed, paying close attention to risk factors and signs and symptoms of menopausal transition phase.
- The major risk factors in this population are related to cardiovascular disorders, and musculoskeletal injuries.
- Examination, such as hemoglobin, glucose, electrolyte, cholesterol levels, Electrocardiography (ECG/EKG) should be performed prior to commencing an exercise program. The American College of Sports Medicine has formulated assessment and treatment guidelines for older adults and individuals with osteoporosis.
- A cross-sectional observational study conducted in 2013 concluded that a moderate level of physical activity was associated with reduced psychosocial and physical menopause symptoms in perimenopausal Korean women. Additionally, walking for more than 6 months improves femoral neck bone mineral density in menopausal women as analyzed in 10 different trials.
- Balance training is an important aspect of rehabilitation in enhancing sports performance and rehabilitation. In addition to muscle changes associated with aging, several diseases interfere with balance by affecting the sensory, neurological, cognitive, and musculoskeletal functions of the elderly. While balance training generally means exercise on unstable surfaces, a more specific program has been developed by Dr. Vladimir Janda named, "Sensorimotor Training" (SMT) **(Box 31.3)**.
- Plyometric training and agility training **(Fig. 31.4)** help in improving bone mineral density which in turn helps in preventing osteoporosis.

Box 31.3: Sensorimotor training.

- Sensorimotor training (SMT) can be characterized as a progressive balance training program using labile surfaces to elicit automatic postural stabilization.
- The older athlete should progress through three stages of SMT: Static, Dynamic, and Functional. Within each stage, individuals progress through exercises in different postures, progressive BOS, and learn to challenge the COG.
- SMT improves proprioception, strength, and postural stability in a variety of lower extremity conditions, including ankle instability and anterior cruciate ligament (ACL)/knee instability. In fact, SMT has been shown to be more effective than traditional rehabilitation at improving function and muscle reaction in ACL reconstruction rehabilitation.

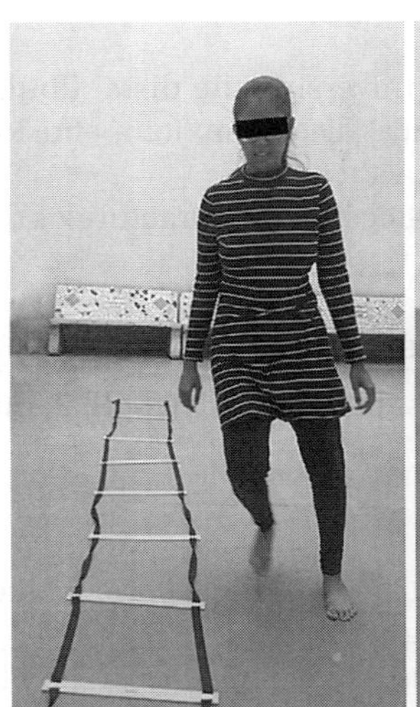
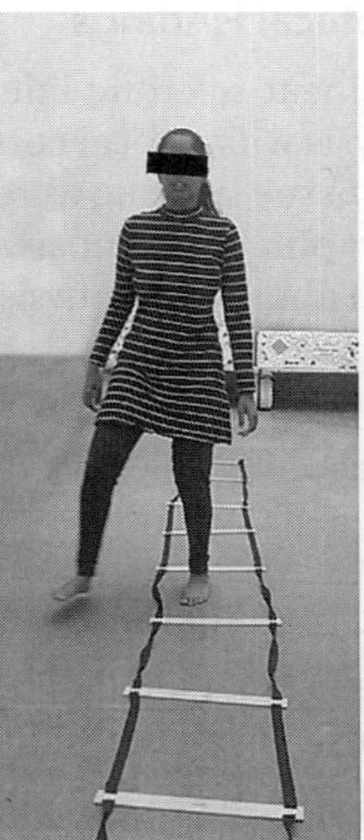
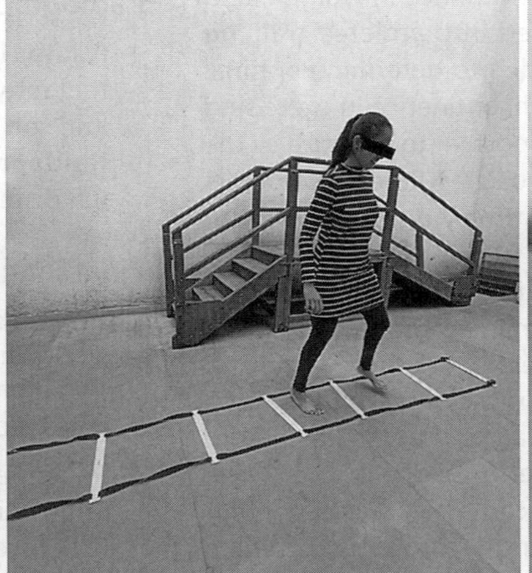
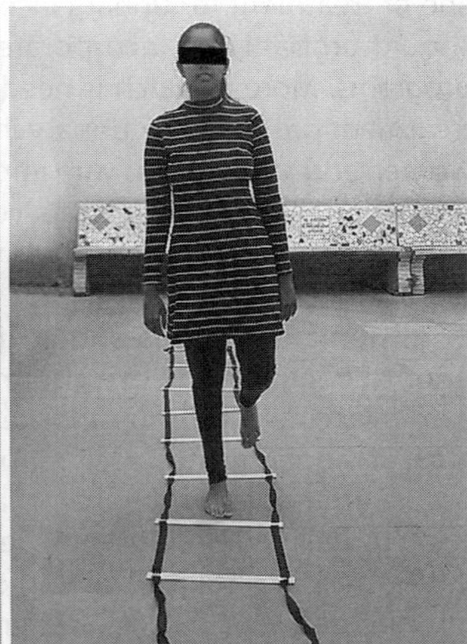

Fig. 31.4: Agility training.

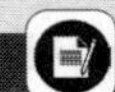

Summary

The Female Athlete Triad is a common medical condition in a physically active female involving three components: (1) low energy availability with or without disordered eating (2) menstrual dysfunctions, and (3) low bone mineral density. The menstrual phases have an effect on the female athlete's performance. Therefore, tracking the phases will help in improving performance and minimizing injuries. Exercising women may have decreased incidence of dysmenorrhea due to exercise-related hormonal effects on the lining of the uterus or increased endorphin levels. Joint laxity, hormonal imbalance, limb size, limb alignments predispose females towards anterior cruciate ligament rupture rather than males.

Women who were regular exercisers before pregnancy and who have uncomplicated, healthy pregnancies should be able to engage in high-intensity exercise programs, yet with precaution. A moderate level of physical activity or exercise during pregnancy is always considered safe for pregnancy. Clinical complications associated with pregnancy can have an impact on athlete's performance. Safety considerations must be followed to prevent associated complications during pregnancy.

Urinary incontinence is frequent and troublesome among exercising women and athletes leading to poor quality of life owing to comprised performance, feelings of concern, frustration, and embarrassment of experiencing urinary leakage during the competition and is highly under-reported. High-impact sports and eating disorders increase the risk for urinary incontinence. Non-athletic women should be encouraged to participate in mild to moderate exercise activities that improve their general health and may even improve urinary incontinence. Urogynecological assessment is advised in competitive athletes and pelvic floor muscle training should be the first line of treatment for urinary incontinence in women, and should probably be incorporated into athletes' training programs. More research is needed to determine optimal treatment protocols for urinary incontinence in exercising women and athletes. It is very important to sensitize all the professionals (physiotherapists, coaches, fitness instructors and sports doctors) involved to timely detect or prevent urinary incontinence.

All female athletes should gain medical clearance prior to beginning an exercise training program to avoid cardiovascular and musculoskeletal-related symptoms. Most of the age-related decline in muscle mass and strength occurs after age 50. The major factor that results in age-related decline in endurance performance is a decrease in VO_2 max. Resistance training can assist in maintaining muscle mass and muscular strength throughout the life span.

CLINICAL EXAMPLE

An 18-year-old young female runner reports left-sided lateral ankle pain for about three weeks. No history of trauma or any other specific mechanism of injury was reported.

History

- **History of present illness:** Resumed running for 6 km, four times a week after a long break. Reports consulting a gynecologist two years back for amenorrhea, treated with calcium and vitamin D.
- Current menstrual history suggests infrequent cycles with more than 45 days of amenorrhea.
- **Medical history/surgical history/systemic evaluation:** No abnormality detected
- **Dietary history:** Irregular diet regime, patient extremely conscious of gaining weight, poor body image.

Pain Examination

- **Site of pain:** Lateral aspect of the left ankle proximal to the lateral malleolus.
- **Type of pain:** "Sharp" directly over the lateral malleolus.
- **Progress:** Steady increase since a week
- **Aggravating factors:** Full weight-bearing ambulation (walking and running) as well as during the toe-off phase of ambulation
- **Relieving factors:** Rest, termination of aggravating activity (walk/run), cryotherapy, and pain killers (NSAIDs).

Physical Examination

- Mild local edema, no ecchymosis/deformity/scar
- **Body mass index (BMI):** 17 kg/m^2
- **Mobility:** AROM and PROM the left ankle show decrease in range of dorsiflexion and inversion due to pain.
- **Special tests:** Anterior drawer test (test for the cruciate ligaments), malleolar squeeze are positive for pain but no associated laxity.

Radiographical Findings

- A faint linear sclerotic line traversing the distal fibular metaphysis with a focal cortical distortion. Joint effusion and soft tissue swelling were also noted.
- **Radiographical diagnosis:** Recent stress fracture of the left distal fibular metaphysis.

Final Diagnosis: Female Athlete Triad

Clinical reasoning: Recent stress fracture and hypothalamic amenorrhea.

Suggested Management

- Patient education on diet (to increase her caloric intake) and counseling for body image correction
- **Fracture management:** Conservative (rest, ice, rehabilitation, manual therapy, and temporary cessation of running for three weeks).

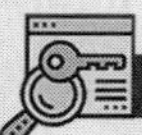

Review Questions

1. Describe female athlete triad.
2. Differentiate between anorexia nervosa and bulimia.
3. Elaborate on the influence of female hormones on sports injuries.
4. Write a note on preventive measures that can be taken towards female athletic triad.
5. Mention the precautions to be taken while prescribing exercises to a female athlete after the 14th week of gestation.
6. Explain the clinical issues during pregnancy and postpartum which can impact the performance of athletes.
7. Elaborate on the specific training considerations and safety issues regarding exercise during pregnancy.
8. Discuss the hypotheses regarding the effect of high-impact activities on the pelvic floor muscles.
9. Elaborate on the risk factors associated with urinary incontinence.
10. Explain the role of physiotherapy in the prevention and management of urinary incontinence in female athletes.
11. Describe the age-related changes that occur in women and its influence on sports performance.
12. Write a note on sensorimotor training.
13. Write an essay on influence of exercise and sport on women's health across the lifespan.

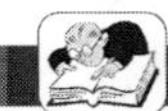

Bibliography

1. American College of Sports Medicine. ACSM's Guidelines for Exercise Testing and Prescription, 9th edition. Philadelphia: Lippincott Williams & Wilkins; 2013.
2. Beals KA, Meyer NL. Female athlete triad update. Clin J Sport Med. 2017;26:69-89.
3. Bo K, Artal R, Barakat R, et al. Exercise and pregnancy in recreational and elite athletes: 2016 evidence summary from the IOC expert group meeting, Lausanne—Part 1. Br J Sports Med. 2016;50:571-89.
4. Bo K, Morkved S. Exercise and pelvic floor dysfunction in women. Best Pract Res Clin Obstet Gynaecol. 2021;74:81-91.
5. Bo K, Sundgot-Borgen J. Stress and urge urinary incontinence in elite athletes and controls. Med Sci Sports Exerc. 2001;33:1797-1802.
6. Bo K. Pelvic floor muscle training in prevention and treatment of urinary incontinence: evidence update. Curr Opin Obstet Gynecol. 2014;26:404-10.
7. Carmichael MA, Thomson RL, Moran LJ, Wycherley TP. Menstrual cycle phase and athletic performance: narrative review. Int J Environ Res Public Health. 2021;18:1667.
8. Carvalhais A, Natal R, Bo K. High-level sport and urinary incontinence in elite athletes. Br J Sports Med. 2018;52:1586-91.
9. Da Roza T, Brandao S, Mascarenhas T, Jorge RN, Duarte JA. Training volume and urinary leakage in trampolinists. Clin J Sport Med. 2015;25:270-75.
10. De Souza MJ, Koltun KJ, Etter CV, Southmayd EA. Current status and future directions of the female athlete triad. Curr Osteoporos Rep. 2017;15:577-87.
11. De Souza MJ, Nattiv A, Joy E, et al. Female Athlete Triad Coalition consensus statement on treatment and return to play. Br J Sports Med. 2014;48:289-309.
12. De Souza MJ, Williams NI. Energy deficiency as a contributing factor for bone loss in amenorrheic athletes. Curr Sports Med Rep. 2005;4:38-44.
13. Eliasson K, Larsson T, Mattsson E. Stress incontinence in nulliparous elite trampolinists. Scand J Med Sci Sports. 2002;12:106-10.
14. Erdener U, Budgett R. Exercise and pregnancy: advice for competitive and elite athletes. Br J Sports Med. 2016;50:567-70.
15. FIGO Committee on Women's Health and Well-Being. Physical activity and women's health. Int J Gynaecol Obstet. 2022;157:303-09.
16. Findlay RJ, Macrae EH, Whyte IY, Easton C, Forrest LJ. Menstrual cycle and performance in elite rugby players. Br J Sports Med. 2020;54:1108-13.
17. Gordon CM. Clinical practice: functional hypothalamic amenorrhea. N Engl J Med. 2010;363:365-73.
18. Guirro EC, Borin LC, Nunes FR. Pelvic-floor muscle pressure in female athletes. PM R. 2013;5:189-193.
19. Heath A, Folan S, Ripa B, et al. Stress urinary incontinence in female athletes. J Womens Health Phys Ther. 2014;38:104-09.
20. Herzberg SD, Motu'apuaka ML, Lambert W, et al. Menstrual cycle and contraceptives on ACL injuries: meta-analysis. Orthop J Sports Med. 2017;5:2325967117718781.
21. Hewett TE, Zazulak BT, Myer GD. Effects of menstrual cycle on ACL injury risk: systematic review. Am J Sports Med. 2007;35:659-68.
22. Koutedakis Y, Jamurtas A. The dancer as a performing athlete: physiological considerations. Sports Med. 2004;34:651-61.
23. Kruger JA, Dietz HP, Murphy BA. Pelvic-floor function in elite nulliparous athletes. Ultrasound Obstet Gynecol. 2007;30:81-85.
24. LeFevre N, Bohu Y, Klouche S, Lecocq J, Herman S. ACL tear during menstrual cycle in female skiers. Orthop Traumatol Surg Res. 2013;99:571-75.
25. Loucks AB, Kiens B, Wright HH. Energy availability in athletes. J Sports Sci. 2011;29(Suppl 1):S7-S15.
26. Matzkin E, Curry EJ, Whitlock K. The female athlete triad: past, present and future. J Am Acad Orthop Surg. 2015;23:424-32.
27. Miller CA, Golden NH. Eating disorders: clinical presentation, epidemiology, and prognosis. Nutr Clin Pract. 2010;25:110-15.
28. Moore K, Dumoulin C, Bradley C, et al. Adult conservative management. In: Abrams P, Cardozo L, Khoury S, (eds). Incontinence, 5th edition. Paris: International Consultation on Incontinence; 2013. p. 1101-227.
29. Mottola MF, Davenport MH, Brun CR, et al. VO_2 peak prediction and exercise prescription for pregnant women. Med Sci Sports Exerc. 2006;38:1389-95.
30. Mountjoy M, Sundgot-Borgen J, Burke L, et al. IOC consensus statement on relative energy deficiency in sport (RED-S): 2018 update. Br J Sports Med. 2018;52:687-97.
31. Narici MV, Maffulli N. Sarcopenia: characteristics, mechanisms and significance. Br Med Bull. 2010;95:139-59.
32. Nattiv A, Agostini R, Drinkwater B, Yeager KK. The female athlete triad.
33. Nygaard I, DeLancey JOL, Arnsdorf L, Murphy E. Exercise and incontinence. Obstet Gynecol. 1990;75:848-51.
34. Otis CL, Drinkwater B, Johnson M, Loucks A, Wilmore J. ACSM position stand: the female athlete triad. Med Sci Sports Exerc. 1997;29(Suppl 5):i-ix.

35. O'Neill ME, Cooper KA, Mills CM, et al. Accuracy of Borg's ratings of perceived exertion in pregnancy. Br J Sports Med. 1992;26:121-24.
36. Petrov Fieril K, Fagevik Olsen M, Glantz A, Larsson M. Experiences of exercise during pregnancy among women performing resistance training. Phys Ther. 2014;94:1135-43.
37. Pires T, Pires P, Moreira H, Viana R. Urinary incontinence in high-impact sport athletes: systematic review and meta-analysis. J Hum Kinet. 2020;73:279-88.
38. RCOG. Exercise in Pregnancy. Scientific Impact Paper No. 64. London: Royal College of Obstetricians and Gynaecologists; 2020.
39. Ree ML, Nygaard IE, Bo K. Muscular fatigue in pelvic floor muscles after strenuous activity. Acta Obstet Gynecol Scand. 2007;86:870-876.
40. Reis AO, Camara CNS, Santos SG, Dias TS. Pelvic-floor contraction capacity in volleyball and basketball athletes. Rev Bras Med Esporte. 2011;17:97-101.
41. Somerson JS, Isby IJ, Hagen MS, Kweon CY, Gee AO. Menstrual cycle and ACL rupture: meta-analysis. JBJS Rev. 2019;7:e2.
42. Sorrigueta-Hernandez A, Padilla-Fernandez BY, Marquez-Sanchez MT, et al. Benefits of physiotherapy on urinary incontinence in high-performance female athletes: meta-analysis. J Clin Med. 2020;9:3240.
43. Stice E, Marti CN, Rohde P. Course of DSM-5 eating disorders: 8-year prospective study. J Abnorm Psychol. 2013;122:445-457.
44. Sundgot-Borgen J, Torstveit MK. Eating disorders in elite athletes vs general population. Clin J Sport Med. 2004;14:25-32.
45. Tanaka H, Seals DR. Endurance exercise performance in masters athletes: mechanisms of decline. J Physiol. 2008;586:55-63.
46. Teixeira RV, Colla C, Sbruzzi G, Mallmann A, Paiva LL. Prevalence of urinary incontinence in female athletes: a systematic review and meta-analysis. Int Urogynecol J. 2018;29:1717-25.
47. Walden M, Hagglund M, Werner J, Ekstrand J. Epidemiology of ACL injury in football: gender-related review. Knee Surg Sports Traumatol Arthrosc. 2011;19:3-10.
48. WHO. Global recommendations on physical activity for health. Geneva: World Health Organization; 2010.
49. Wojtys EM, Huston LJ, Boynton MD, Spindler KP, Lindenfeld TN. The effect of the menstrual cycle on anterior cruciate ligament injuries in women as determined by hormone levels. Am J Sports Med. 2002;30:182-8.
50. Zazulak BT, Paterno M, Myer GD, Romani WA, Hewett TE. Menstrual cycle effects on anterior knee laxity: systematic review. Sports Med. 2006;36:847-62.

Multiple Choice Questions (MCQs)

To test your understanding and recall of key concepts.

1. **Which of the following is a part of the Female Athlete Triad?**
   A. Hyperglycemia
   B. Amenorrhea
   C. Hyperlipidemia
   D. Hypokalemia

2. **What is the recommended daily calcium intake for postmenopausal women?**
   A. 800 mg
   B. 1000 mg
   C. 1200 mg
   D. 1500 mg

3. **Why are female athletes at higher risk for ACL injuries during certain menstrual phases?**
   A. Increased testosterone levels
   B. High estrogen levels causing ligament laxity
   C. Decreased progesterone levels
   D. Reduced oxygen uptake

4. **An 18-year-old athlete with irregular menses and a stress fracture is diagnosed with the Female Athlete Triad. What is the first step in management?**
   A. Prescribe NSAIDs
   B. Initiate physical therapy
   C. Address caloric intake and body image concerns
   D. Recommend surgery for the stress fracture

5. **A pregnant athlete in her second trimester wants to continue high-intensity training. Which precaution should be advised?**
   A. Avoid exercising in a supine position
   B. Reduce daily water intake
   C. Perform strength training with heavy weights
   D. Train in hot, humid conditions

6. **What explains the higher prevalence of urinary incontinence in female athletes compared to non-athletes?**
   A. Lower muscle strength
   B. Increased collagen density
   C. High-impact sports causing pelvic floor weakness
   D. Reduced training intensity

7. **Which of the following is associated with an exercise-associated menstrual cycle irregularity ?**
   A. Calorie excess
   B. Excess energy availability
   C. High leptin levels
   D. Central suppression of reproductive function

8. **Which of the following is *not* a common sign and symptom of bulimia?**
   A. Eating less in more time
   B. Experiencing guilt
   C. Preoccupied with body weight
   D. Purging of food

9. **Which of the following is *not* a risk factor associated with urinary incontinence in athletes?**
   A. Constipation
   B. Family history of urinary incontinence
   C. History of recurrent urinary tract infections
   D. Increased foot flexibility

ANSWERS

1. B	2. C	3. B	4. C	5. A
6. C	7. D	8. A	9. D	

Chapter **32**

Women at Workplace

Reena Kumari, Parul R Agarwal

LEARNING OBJECTIVES

At the end of the chapter, the reader will be able to:
- Understand the general ergonomic risk factors at workplace and pathophysiology leading to injury.
- Know the work-related musculoskeletal disorders in women and factors predisposing women to injuries at work.
- Provide ergonomic management and recommendation for worksite wellness for women.
- Know the protective provisions for women employees for safeguarding the interest of women and the various statutes that Indian Government has for the same.

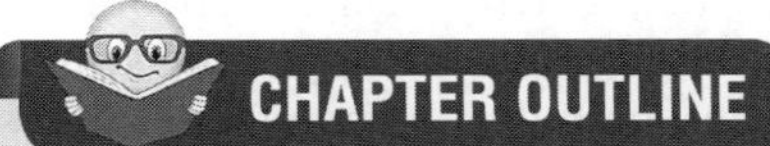

INTRODUCTION

There is steady increase in female workforce in professional technical and managerial work. Globally, working women account for 47.7% which has been slowed down from 50.9% in 2019. Due to difference in biological and physiological characteristics, women are at increasing risk for musculoskeletal disorders especially when insufficient attention is paid to the design of work, workstation, equipment and environment. In addition, women also spend hours on domestic work which increases with the number of children and dependents in the family which add to the existing risk for musculoskeletal disorders. Gender-based division of labor has lots of variability across society and culture. Additionally at workplace during their careers also they face disparity in job status in terms of poorly paid work which adds on to the psychological stress.

GENERAL ERGONOMIC RISK FACTORS AT WORKPLACE AND PATHOPHYSIOLOGY FOR INJURY

Ergonomics is the application of scientific information concerning human beings to the design of objects, system and environments for human use. Working practices and work area which are efficient and not harmful have long-term effect on health which reduces sickness absence, labor turnover and increases the productivity. An ideal and ergonomically safe workplace increases the worker's productivity, performance, health and safety.

Work may affect the health when:
- Workers are exposed to some injurious agents like toxic chemicals
- Work is performed under adverse environmental conditions, e.g., heat, cold, noise, etc. (e.g., women working

in gruh udyogs in hot environment or constant noise of machines)
- Work involves overexertion or cumulative overuse of musculoskeletal or other body structures
- Work may be psychologically stressful because it is mentally or emotionally demanding
- Work involves high-risk of accident injury like construction work, mining
- Work may promote unhealthy lifestyle like obesity in sedentary workers, etc.

Work-related Disorders

Employment or work can influence our lives in a positive way as a source of income and social benefits but on the other hand, it can have a negative influence on workers' physical, mental and psychosocial state of health. Work-related disorders are of multiple etiologies in which work is significant contributory factor in some or all cases. Musculoskeletal disorders (MSDs) are injuries and illnesses that affect muscles, nerves, tendons, ligaments, joints, spinal discs, skin, subcutaneous tissues, blood vessels, and bones. Many names have been used for musculoskeletal disorders as shown in **Box 32.1**.

"Work-related musculoskeletal disorders (WMSDs/WRMSDs) are the musculoskeletal disorders to which the work environment and the performance of work contribute significantly". Unlike various occupational diseases that originate due to exposure to particular hazardous agents, most WRMSDs are termed as work related because their work conditions are a major contributing factor for the development or exacerbation. Various studies have revealed the high prevalence of musculoskeletal disorders among females as compared to male. Healthcare professionals (more than 90%), desk workers (more than 70%), cultivators (more than 50%) and homemakers are at more risk in developing work-related musculoskeletal disorders. The majority of women suffer from upper body musculoskeletal symptoms including shoulders, neck and lower back. The gender difference in symptoms, in terms of occurrence and severity may be explained by repetitive work, equipments with poor ergonomic designs at work and less opportunity to relax and exercise outside the work.

This gender difference has been exacerbated by parenthood in early stages of life. The sex segregation of women in to sedentary lifestyle, repetitive and routine work, persisting gender balance at domestic as well at work are the interlinking factors that explain the gender difference in musculoskeletal disorders.

Hormonal disturbances and postural stress due to women health conditions also affect women's physical health.

Box 32.1: Names used for musculoskeletal disorders.

- Cumulative trauma disorders
- Overuse syndrome
- Repetitive strain injuries
- Repetitive stress injuries
- Occupational overuse syndrome

Ergonomics

Ergonomics is the science of matching the job to the worker and product to the user. An effective match is one which optimizes the working efficiency, performance, productivity, health and safety, comfort and ease of use.

Ergonomic Risk Factors at Workplace

There can be multiple risk factors present at workplace which can expose the women for various musculoskeletal disorders due to job-related components or poorly designed workplace. Some female-dominated professions require lifting heavy loads and adopting faulty postures, while office work requires high level of static muscular contractions. At workstations females have to use the tools that were designed for men. Thus all the issues—force, poor posture, static muscular contractions and repetitions are the risk factors for musculoskeletal disorders. Researchers believe the combination of biomechanical, physiological and psychological factors contribute to musculoskeletal disorders.

Main risk factors for work-related illness causing musculoskeletal disorder can be categorized under one or combination of the following.

Force

An inescapable force, i.e., gravity acts on all our body segments all the time. The surface of supporting structure (floor, chair, armrest, etc.) provides the equal and opposite reaction force so that no movement occurs. All our body tissues do not accept pressure equally well. The fat pad on the heel of the foot is especially adapted to accept high levels of pressure while standing and walking and ischial tuberosity of pelvis gets conditioned to bear weight while sitting. However, coccyx of spine quickly becomes painful when exposed to high pressure during slouched sitting, similarly tip of elbow easily becomes irritated while leaning on table or desk when height of table is too low or too high **(Fig. 32.1)**.

Depending on the postures, these forces can become considerable and result in unwanted physiological

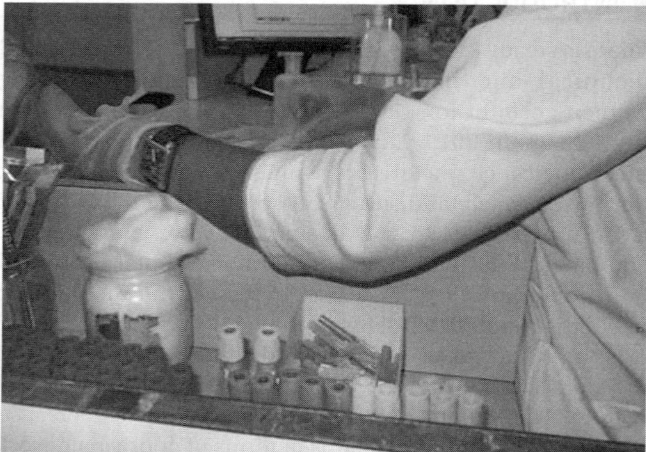

Fig. 32.1: Prolonged contact stress on wrist.

consequences. Some of the job components where force can negatively impact the musculoskeletal system are:

- Excessive heavy lifting and/or lowering
- Excessive heavy pushing and/or pulling
- Long distance carrying
- Wide grasping or pinching grips

Repetition

Tissue microtrauma occurs due to repetitive tasks leading to inflammation, followed by fibrosis and other structural changes in the tissue. Task which requires similar motion every few seconds causes repetition and there may be observed signs of fatigue.

During fine movement, the muscles/tendons and articular joints of the thumb, hand and wrist are exposed to highly repetitive motion and loading and there is greater risk of tendinitis in workers performing highly repetitive forceful tasks. It has been reported that 90% of pipette users, who continuously use pipettes for more than an hour on a daily basis, had more of hand and elbow disorders. Also, rapid stereotypical repetitive, nearly simultaneous fine motor movements can degrade the sensory representation of the hand and may lead to a loss of normal motor control of a targeted task, commonly referred to as focal hand dystonia or occupational hand cramps. Repetitive movement during keyboard use showing various muscle activities during typing has been evaluated through electromyography (EMG) suggesting that MSDs in the upper extremities are related to excessive repetitive musculoskeletal loading.

Inappropriate Posture

Postures away from neutral position cause prolonged low level muscle contractions and changes in intervertebral disc pressures. Incorrect working posture while using computer or while lifting load which is physically demanding in healthcare professions like physiotherapy and nursing may result in WRMSD. Static muscle work is a condition in which muscle or group of muscles contracts for sustained period. This causes localized muscle fatigue and increases the risk of musculoskeletal disorders. It has been observed that prolonged computer task over a period of time leads to frequent use of forward neck posture. Sustained forward flexed posture of the spine may increase cervical compression loading and this posture if associated with prolonged sitting could aggravate the neck pain. Studies also have reported that awkward and extreme postures are one of the most common risk factors for musculoskeletal disorders.

Some of the workstation designs which can cause adoption of inappropriate posture are **(Figs. 32.2 and 32.3)**:

- Work surface too high or low
- Location of materials which promote reaching in awkward positions
- Table/bench lacking adequate leg space
- Equipment/table placing limb or torso on sharp edges
- Chair lacking adequate/adjustable seat height

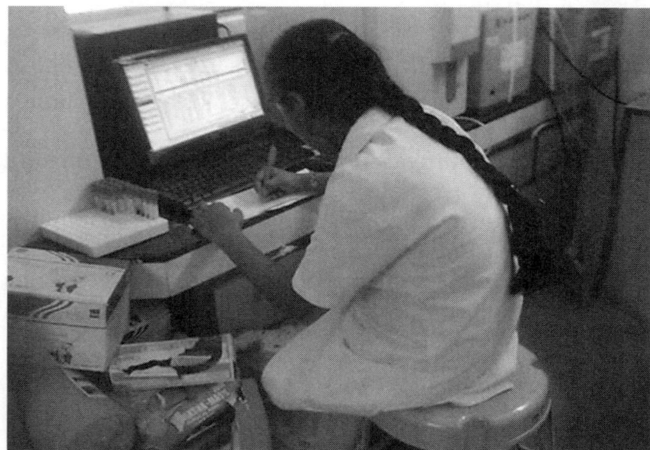

Fig. 32.2: Computer workstation illustrating awkward posture due to inappropriate seating.

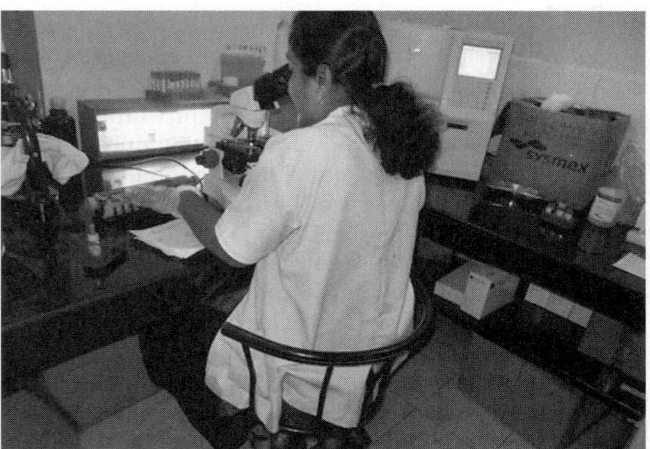

Fig. 32.3: Microscope workstation illustrating the absence of leg space and use of elevated shoulder while viewing microscope.

It has been reported that ulnar deviation of the wrist greater than 20° was associated with musculoskeletal symptoms and downward head tilt was associated with increased discomfort and clinical abnormality. Greater keyboard height and working with hands and forearm supported is found to be associated with decreased musculoskeletal discomfort in the neck, shoulder and forearm.

Trapezius myalgia is most commonly associated with static work in front of a visual display unit (VDU) with a fixed posture. An investigation showed that presence of neck flexion greater than 20° while working in VDU can predict the presence or absence of neck pain.

Environmental risk factors at workplace which can cause MSDs are:

- Room temperature/equipment too hot or cold
- Lighting too bright/dim, glares making vision difficult
- Noisy area
- Work area lacking adequate sitting/standing surface

WORK-RELATED MUSCULOSKELETAL DISORDERS IN WOMEN

Common work-related illness and musculoskeletal disorders in women due to work are:
- Visual and neurovascular problems such as tension headache and eyestrain
- Stress-related symptoms such as insomnia, irritability, menstrual disturbance
- Musculoskeletal disorders such as supraspinatus tendinitis
- Thoracic outlet syndrome
- Lateral epicondylitis
- Carpal tunnel syndrome
- Trigger finger
- Tension neck
- Occupational cramps
- Lower back pain

Vulnerability to Risk for Injury During Pregnancy and During Aging

Workplace risk factors can have magnified effect on women at various stages of life.
- During pregnancy, several changes in women's body like hormonal changes, postural variation due to weight gain, shift of line of gravity, fluid retention account for musculoskeletal pain especially in third trimester.
- Evidence has reported significant increase in hand, wrist, neck, low back, knee, ankle and foot pain during pregnancy. The enlarging gravid uterus accompanying compensatory lumbar lordosis and shift of center of gravity may increase strain on ligaments, bones, muscles of lumbar region. The relaxed abdominal wall muscles (mainly rectus), due to effect of hormonal changes, may not be able to maintain posture; as a result, compensation happens and paraspinal muscles are forced to undertake the whole function and get fatigued causing low back pain. Lower extremity also has to absorb extra force due to alteration in mechanics causing hip pain as a result of increased mechanical load. Additionally, symphysis pubis diastasis or dysfunction and sacroiliitis are also occasional causes of hip pain during pregnancy.
- Other musculoskeletal problems women usually encounter during pregnancy are carpal tunnel syndrome which is attributed to hormonal changes (increased relaxin level), fluid accumulation, nerve hypersensitivity and glucose level fluctuation. This causes wrist pain which becomes disabling for women, especially at workplace, where fine movements are needed like keyboard operation, medical laboratory professionals, etc.
- Pedal edema as the pregnancy advances is one of the contributory factors for musculoskeletal pain which could be due to reduced muscle activity in lower extremity leading to accumulation of fluid extravasation in the extracellular space and gravity-dependent position of lower extremity for long time. Women at workplace during third trimester experience this very often where they have to work in cramped space and jobs demanding prolonged standing or sitting position without feet support.

As the woman approaches menopausal phase, changes in body hormone like estrogen also affect the health of women.
- There is a rapid decrease in muscle mass and strength, making them prone to muscle injuries, aches and pain.
- Some of the workplace and job demands add to the impact of aging or postmenopausal symptoms and make women more prone to injury.
- Not only skeletal muscle but even pelvic floor muscles are impacted during menopause and underlying weakness in their pelvic floor muscles often existing from obstetric injury during childbirth or chronic history of constipation, coughing can make them prone to develop urinary or fecal incontinence relating to pelvic floor weakness. In such situation, having inappropriate toilet facilities at workplace can affect the psychology of the working women and affect performance at workplace.
- Additionally, estrogen regulates production of cortisol a stress hormone which is increased as the estrogen levels drop down. These higher levels of cortisol can cause muscle to become tense and painful making women more sensitive to pain.
- Estrogen deficiency also decreases the collagen content of connective tissue, resulting in muscle injury and tendinopathies. So, workplace demanding sudden changes in body position, reaching activities, etc., makes them prone to musculoskeletal injury.
- Osteoporosis is another physiological change happening due to decreased estrogen level during menopause leading to loss of bone density and making them prone to fracture.

ERGONOMIC MANAGEMENT AND RECOMMENDATION FOR WORKSITE WELLNESS

Work-related disorders can be prevented by certain modifications and advice **(Figs. 32.4 and 32.5)**.

Solution to Postural Problems

- Avoid forward inclination of head and neck by adjusting visual demands
- Avoid forward inclination of trunk
- Avoid use of upper limb in raised position
- Avoid twisted or asymmetrical postures
- Wherever possible, keep joints within middle third of their range of motion
- Provide an adequate backrest in all seats
- Whenever muscle forces must be exerted, limb should be in the position of greatest strength and good posture principle must not be compromised.

Solution to Inappropriate Working Height

The optimal working height is the one which minimizes the static muscle loading, maintains ideal posture and minimizes the degree of effort for performance of that activity.
- For tasks requiring hand manipulation involving moderate degree of force and precision, height should be between 50 mm to 100 mm below elbow height.
- For lighter and delicate tasks like writing, working height table can be from 50 mm to 100 mm above elbow height with wrist in supported position preferably.

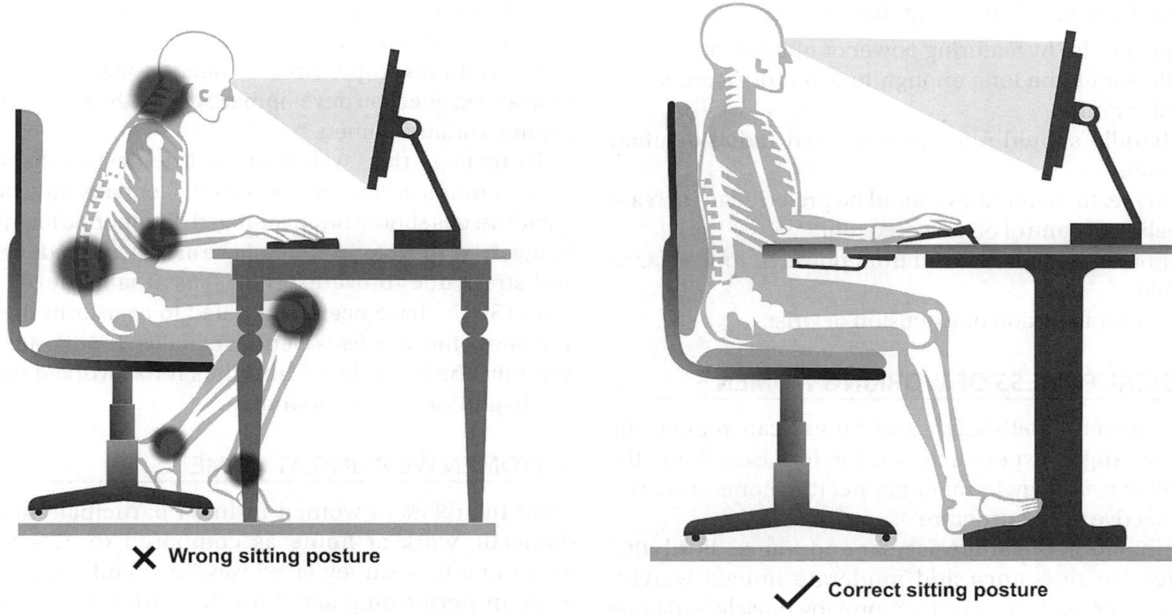

Fig. 32.4: Incorrect and correct computer workstations.

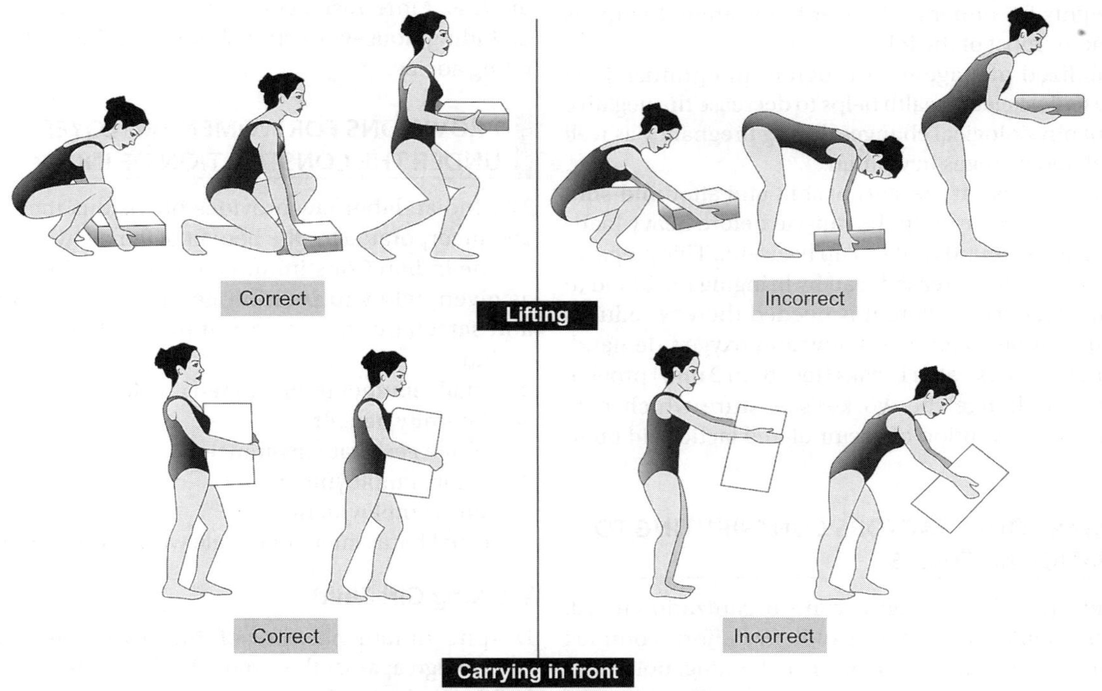

Fig. 32.5: Incorrect and correct lifting techniques.

- For heavier tasks requiring downward force on work objects, the working table height should be from 100 mm to 250 mm below elbow height.
- For lifting and handling tasks, the height can be from knuckle to little above elbow height.
- For two handed pushing and pulling tasks, recommended height is little below elbow height.

Solution to Lifting and Handling Tasks

- Proper body mechanics must be followed while lifting and handling weights.
- Use of mechanical aids wherever possible.
- Loads to be handled must be checked for their stability, proper grip and handles.

Solution to Repetitive Tasks Using Hand Tools

- Design handles by featuring power or oblique grip.
- Handle should be long enough to avoid pressure to the base of thumb.
- Tool handle should not cause marked radial or ulnar deviation.
- Properly textured handles should be preferred to increase the feeling of control on powered tool.
- Vibration should be reduced from powered tool as far as possible.
- Avoid extreme flexion or extension of wrist.

PHYSICAL FITNESS OF WORKING WOMEN

Women's general well-being and fitness can reduce the amount of fatigue experienced on the job. Exercise is the most effective strategy to maintain healthy bones, muscles and connective tissue structure.

- A combination of cardiovascular endurance, flexibility, progressive resistance and moderate impact weight-bearing exercise can assist in improving muscle and bone health.
- A steady moderate exercise program of 30 min per day that includes walking at comfortable speed and using light weights for upper and lower body strengthening is sufficient for most of the jobs.
- Individualized management program to optimize long term musculoskeletal health helps to decrease the negative impact of physiological changes during pregnancy as well as age related changes in women.
- Stretching exercise at the start of shift and after mid-shift break in order to warm up the muscle before heavy loads or intensive task is undertaken can be useful. This prepares the muscle for the increased load by bringing the blood to active muscles even before it is needed thereby reduces the mismatch between blood flow and oxygen demand. Intermittent short stretch breaks (less than 2 min) provide a chance to change the worker's posture which may contribute to prevention of accumulated lactic acid build up.

ORGANIZATIONAL FACTORS CONTRIBUTING TO OCCUPATIONAL STRESS

Management policies as well certain organizational risk factors such as job requirements of heavy effort, complex task and environmental factors like heat, lighting, noise and vibration can increase the stress at workplace. The design of a good job must not include only ergonomically designed workplaces and equipment but organizational factors too that affect the workers' performance and reduce the occupational stress. There is strong interconnection between the management policies and the extent to which they influence the workers' ability to work well without excessive stress.

Factors related to job control such as skill levels, perceived job importance and factors related to communication such as peer pressure, management policies, inadequate communication between departments, too many responsibilities to perform all needed task. All these can have added effect on development of health-related ailments among working women.

To manage this, system should be designed such that the communications are enhanced, feedback on workplace quality issues should be encouraged. Ergonomic team should be involved. Job rotations should be included to reduce fatigue and stress due to overexertion. Sustainable development goals (SDGs) have been designated to transform the world, and one of the policies is Gender Equality. It works upon, "No one must be left behind" and thus it has worked upon the health and well-being of woman.

WOMEN WORKING AT HOME

More than 90% of women in India participate in unpaid domestic work at home as compared to 27% of men. According to a survey, a housewife spends 97 hours per week in performing activities like lifting heavy children and groceries and performing tasks like cooking, cleaning, washing and other household activities. Prolonged work hours lead to musculoskeletal problems and associated distress. More researches are required on domestic labor including housework and childcare using ergonomics and lifting advice.

PROVISIONS FOR WOMEN EMPLOYEES UNDER THE CONSTITUTION OF INDIA

The Indian labor law provides provisions that are enacted and incorporated for the benefit of female workers.

The Indian Constitution contains number of provisions as given below to prohibit gender-based discrimination and safeguard the interest of the working woman. These include:

- Equal remuneration for men and female workers
- Maternity benefit
- Employees' State Insurance
- Factory employment
- Mines employment
- Sexual harassment of female workers at workplace

Working Girl Child

Despite Indian network of 700 organizations called as "Campaign against the child labor" and efforts of NGOs like NJBB (Nav Jeevan Bala Bhawan), girl child labor is preferred as it is found to be stable and less demanding. Working areas of girl child labor include dangerous industries, agriculture areas, in street and at home, generally as hidden child labor. School going children carry heavy school bags on one shoulder and may indulge in sports activities. Abnormal loading and posture, overuse of muscles and lack of awareness towards health may lead to mechanical back pain, painful scoliosis, neurological entrapment and systemic findings.

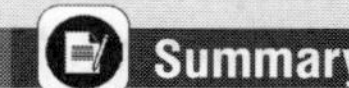

Summary

Women's perspective towards career and to support in economic necessities has shown the significant rise of female population of all the ages in workforce. Force, repetitions, inappropriate posture and lifting heavy loads at the workplace as well at domestic front has contributed to increase in musculoskeletal disorders. Development of all the work sites including furniture, tools, devices and environment, taking into consideration women's health issues should be done. They must be designed in sophisticated manner to help in prevention of musculoskeletal problems due to ergonomic hazards. Women should be recommended to follow principles of ergonomics in their daily practice taking regular restbreaks and in between stretches and exercise to reduce the risk of work-related musculoskeletal disorders.

CLINICAL EXAMPLE

Female physiotherapists, the healthcare professionals are susceptible to develop musculoskeletal injuries because of their nature of work due to:

- Repeated handling of patients
- When transferring or repositioning patients
- Working in extremely awkward positions

Lifting becomes more difficult by the increasing weight of patients to be lifted due to the obesity epidemic and an increasing number of elderly people who require assistance with daily living activities leading to backpain. Upper extremity musculature is more affected because of application of manipulation and mobilization techniques especially the thumb. Chest physiotherapy, percussion techniques cause strain in hand and wrist muscles. Correct ergonomic set ups including appropriate heights of couches and chair, efficient stretches, frequent breaks and back support should be followed.

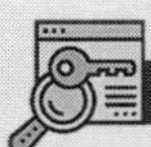

Review Questions

1. Why are women more prone to develop work-related musculoskeletal disorders?
2. Discuss about the work-related musculoskeletal disorders in detail considering the women's health.
3. Write about the ergonomic management and recommendations for worksite wellness.
4. Write about the vulnerability to injury during pregnancy and old age.
5. Write about the Government measures taken for health of a woman at workplace.

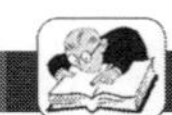

Bibliography

1. Agrawal PR, Maiya AG, Kamath V, Kamath A. Musculoskeletal disorders among medical laboratory professionals—a prevalence study; 2014.
2. Agrawal PR. Work-related musculoskeletal disorders in medical laboratory professionals. Mahi Publication; 2021.
3. Bridger RS. Introduction to ergonomics, 3rd edition. CRC Press; 2008.
4. Bureau of Labor Statistics. 2003. Total recordable cases—Injuries and illnesses. Bureau of Labor Statistics; 2003.
5. Deasy and Lasswell. Designing Places for People. New York: Watson-Guptill Publication; 1990.
6. Horton R. GBD 2010: understanding disease, injury, and risk. Lancet. 2012;380(9859):2053-4. Epub 2012/12/19.
7. Silverstein B, Clark R. Interventions to reduce work-related musculoskeletal disorders. J Electromyogr Kinesiol. 2004;14(1):135-52. Epub 2004/02/05.
8. Stephen Pheasant. Ergonomics, work and health. Aspen Publisher. USA. ISBN 0-87189-320-7.
9. Woolf AD, Pfleger B. Burden of major musculoskeletal conditions. Bulletin of the World Health Organization. 2003;81(9):646-56.

Multiple Choice Questions (MCQs)

To test your understanding and recall of key concepts.

1. What is the main ergonomic risk factor for women working in sedentary jobs?
   A. Static muscle work
   B. Environmental temperature
   C. Sedentary lifestyle
   D. Hormonal imbalance

2. Which musculoskeletal disorder is commonly associated with static work at a visual display unit?
   A. Lateral epicondylitis
   B. Trapezius myalgia
   C. Thoracic outlet syndrome
   D. Carpal tunnel syndrome

3. What is the optimal working height for tasks involving light precision work?
   A. Below knuckle height
   B. 50–100 mm below elbow height
   C. 50–100 mm above elbow height
   D. At shoulder height

4. How does menopause increase vulnerability to workplace injuries?
   A. By reducing muscle mass and strength due to hormonal changes
   B. By causing fluid retention in the lower extremities
   C. By increasing flexibility of joints
   D. By promoting estrogen-induced bone growth

5. A pregnant woman working in an office reports wrist pain due to prolonged typing. Which ergonomic modification would you recommend?
   A. Using a wrist support and adjusting keyboard height
   B. Switching to handwritten tasks
   C. Encouraging the use of an exercise ball instead of a chair
   D. Replacing her workstation with standing desks

6. Analyze why static muscle work contributes to musculoskeletal disorders.

A. It increases oxygen supply to muscles
B. It causes lactic acid build-up and localized fatigue
C. It improves fatigue over time
D. It increases repetitive strain injuries

7. Which factor is a major contributor to ergonomic risk during the third trimester of pregnancy?

A. Decreased blood circulation in upper extremities
B. Increased weight and shift of the center of gravity
C. Reduced production of relaxin hormone
D. High bone density

8. A postmenopausal employee with osteoporosis needs ergonomic adjustments to prevent injuries. What modifications would you suggest?

A. Provide high chairs and require tasks involving frequent bending
B. Incorporate standing desks and lifting aids to reduce spinal strain
C. Focus on seated work only and eliminate movement breaks
D. Remove all weight-bearing tasks from her job

ANSWERS

1. A	2. B	3. C	4. A	5. A
6. B	7. B	8. B		

Section 7

Application of Yoga in Women's Health

Section Outline

Chapter **33**

Yoga—Concepts

✍ *Mohammed Sabir Shaikh*

LEARNING OBJECTIVES

At the end of the chapter, the reader will be able to:

- Understand concepts of Yoga.
- Establish Yoga as a unique entity different from exercise or therapy.
- Understand the history and various deviations in Yoga.
- Define and classify Yoga as mentioned in scriptures.
- Understand the very important aspect of Ashtanga Yoga (eight-fold path).
- Know how Yoga is not a therapy but a way life leading to healing.

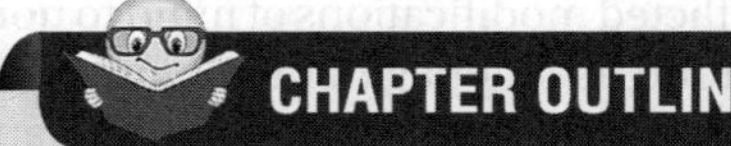

- Introduction
  - History of Yoga
- Definition of Yoga in various scriptures
- Classification of Yoga (classical approach)
  - Bhavana Yoga
  - Prana Samyama Yoga
- The eight-fold path of Patanjali
  - Yama and Niyama
  - Asana (psychosomatic posture)
  - Pranayama (expansion of breath)
  - Pratyahara (withdrawal of senses)
  - Dharana (concentration)
  - Dhyana (meditation)
  - Samadhi
- Textual understanding of Yoga as a therapy
- Yogic concept of health and disease
  - Human nature and various aspects of its existence

INTRODUCTION

Yoga is an ancient Indian spiritual science belonging to the earlier system of Indian philosophy (Bharatiya Tattva jnana). Yoga is an art and science of healthy living which focuses on bringing harmony between mind and body **(Fig. 33.1)**.

The word 'Yoga' is derived from the Sanskrit root verb 'Yuj,' which literally means 'to yoke' or 'to join' or 'to unite.' As per Yoga texts or scriptures the practice of Yoga leads to the union of individual consciousness (Soul/Atma) with the Universal Consciousness (Supreme Soul/Paramatma), indicating a perfect harmony between the mind, body and soul. One who experiences this oneness of existence is said to be in the state of Yoga, and is termed as a Yogi. A Yogi is the one who has attained a state of freedom (Mukti, Nirvana or Moksha). Thus, the aim of Yoga is self-realization, to overcome all kinds

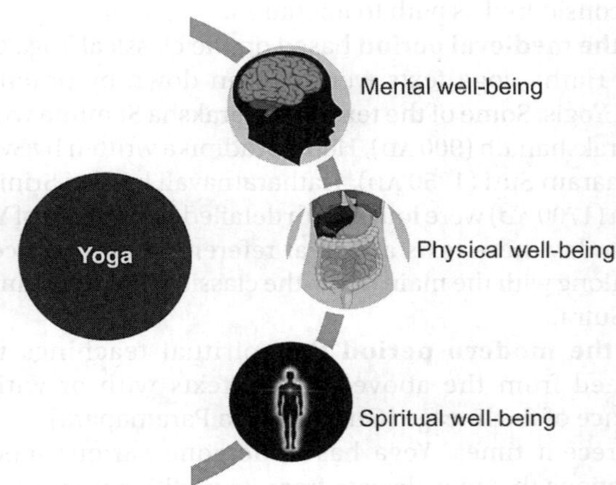

Fig. 33.1: Yoga: Harmony between the mind, body and soul.

of sufferings leading to 'the state of liberation' (Moksha) or 'freedom' (Kaivalya).

The main objective of Yoga is living life with the purpose of freedom and attaining health by bringing harmony in all walks of Life. "Yoga" also refers to an inner science comprising of a variety of practical methods and means through which every human being can realize this union and achieve mastery over their destiny. Yoga has proved itself by catering to both material and spiritual upliftment of humanity. The basic human values are inculcated through Yoga Sadhana (disciplined practice of Yoga).

Health is one of the primary concerns of the modern world where every day scientists are carrying out various researches to tackle innumerable diseases and ailments. Yoga plays a very vital role here as a complementary and alternative medicine (CAM).

History of Yoga

History of Yoga can be traced back to pre-Vedic times to Harappa and Indus valley civilization where seals of Hindu God Lord Shiva meditating in Yoga pose were found during excavation. Broadly the history can be divided in four periods, viz. the Vedic period, the classical period, the medieval period and the modern period.

During the vedic and classical period all the spiritual teachings were transmitted orally from the Guru (Preceptor/Master) to Shishya (disciple/student) in an ashrama known as Guru-shishya Parampara (lineage). The spiritual teachings were the teachings of Vedas (Rigved, Yajurved, Samaved, and Atharvaveda). One can find the mention about Yoga and its practices in these Vedic literature (1500-3000 BC) which also elaborate upon about the purpose and its applications.

Based on the teachings of Vedas where the information about Yoga lay scattered, the classical Yoga texts came into existence. Yoga texts like Bhagavad Gita (600 BC), Yoga Vasishta (500 BC), The Patanjali's Yoga Sutra (200 BC) were compiled by great Vedic scholars like Veda Vyasa, Sage Valmiki and Sage Patanjali respectively. Many other types of Yoga like Jnana Yoga (Yoga of wisdom), Karma Yoga (Yoga of action/deeds), Bhakti Yoga (Yoga of love and devotion) and Raja Yoga (Royal Yoga/Ashtanga Yoga) also exist. All the paths were considered as path to liberation.

In the medieval period based on the classical Yoga texts, many Hatha yoga texts were written down by practicing Hatha Yogis. Some of the texts like Goraksha Samhita written by Gorakshanath (900 AD), Hathapradipika written by Swami Swatmaram Suri (1350 AD), Hatharatnavali by Shri Srinivasa Bhatta (1700 AD) were found with detailed knowledge of Yoga. Even today these texts are great references for practices of Yoga along with the main one—the classical text of Patanjali's Yoga Sutra.

In the modern period the spiritual teachings were obtained from the above various texts with or without guidance of the lineage (Guru-shishya Paramapara).

In recent times, Yoga has undergone various modern adaptations that may deviate from its traditional essence. To name a few there is a concept of Hot Yoga, which is practiced in a forty degree Celsius plus room and yogic practices are performed in a perspiring environment. There is a concept of Power Yoga in which Yoga is done to the exertion of an exercise leading to fatigue, again contradicting the principle of relaxation in action or action in relaxation.

DEFINITION OF YOGA IN VARIOUS SCRIPTURES

Yoga as explained in various scriptures has been found to be the goal as well as means to reach the goal (self realization). It has been defined in different manners in different scriptures like Upanishads and Yoga texts.

- **"Samatvam Yoga uchyate" (Bhagavad Gita II/48):** According to Bhagavad Gita, Yoga is the state of equanimity in which a person remains unaffected by different situations such as success and failure, attachment and aversion in life. This equanimous state of mind leads to freedom from the imbalances of mind and helps to make an individual stable and peaceful.
- **"Yogah karmasu kaushalam" (Bhagavad Gita 2.50):** Dexterity in skill is Yoga. Selfless work without any expectation, done like worship without expecting any result (non-attachment) is Yoga. Bhagavad-Gita emphasizes 'awareness in action' that too without any expectation of fruits leading to efficient and skillful outcome.
- **Yogah cittavritti Nirodhah (Patanjali Yoga Sutra I.2):** Cessation of modification of mind stuff is Yoga. It is re-channelization of afflicted modifications of mind to non-afflicted. Also understood as stoppage of fluctuations or ripples of thoughts in mind (i.e., towards integration and harmony) is Yoga.
- **Yogah manah prashamana upayaha (Yoga Vasistha):** Yoga is a means for quietening the mind.
- **Tam yogamiti manyante sthiram indriya dharanam (Kathopanishad 2.6.11):** Restraint of senses leading to stability of mind is considered to be Yoga.
- By restraining or controlling the senses which leads to a focused state of the mind is Yoga. (Shvetashvatara Upanishad 2.8)

Above mentioned definitions of Yoga highlight the 'Means' aspect of Yoga which consists of Practical and Methodical aspects of Yoga in the form of various techniques or methods like Asana, Pranayama, etc., leading towards the accomplishment of union or integration, i.e., the 'Goal' aspect of Yoga. The value of Yoga as a method mentioned above (here in the form of definitions) has been practiced in some form or the other by the yogis according to their own temperament throughout the history in the name of various forms or dimensions of Yoga.

CLASSIFICATION OF YOGA (CLASSICAL APPROACH)

Classically, Yoga is broadly classified into two as shown in **Table 33.1**.

Bhavana Yoga

- **Jnana Yoga:** It is the path of knowledge and wisdom. This involves intense mental discipline. The student (sadhaka)

Table 33.1: Classification of Yoga.

Type	*Description*
Bhavana Yoga	It consists of developing a particular attitude in oneself and towards world. The Yoga schools coming under this group are—Jnana Yoga, Bhakti Yoga and Karma Yoga.
Prana Samyama Yoga	It consists of attainment of highest realization through control over Prana (energy/ breath flow). The Yoga schools coming under this group are—Mantra Yoga, Hatha Yoga, Laya Yoga and Raja Yoga.

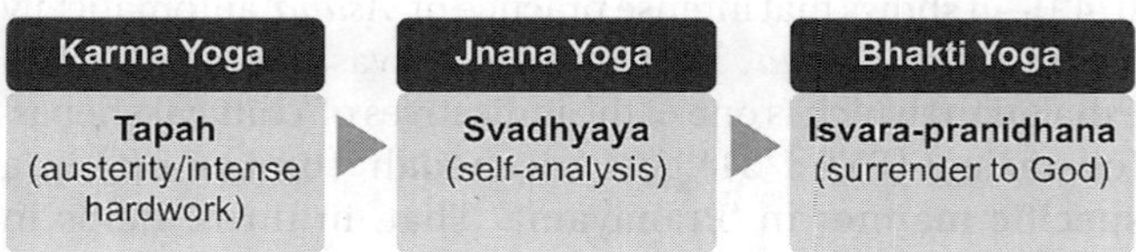

Fig. 33.2: Yogas in the practice of Kriya-yoga.

learns to discriminate between the real and the unreal, between finite and the infinite.

- **Bhakti Yoga:** Bhakti Yoga is Yoga of devotion. This path is the way of love and devotion. It is a path of self-surrender, of devoting and dedicating all resources, in attaining the ultimate reality.
- **Karma Yoga:** The path teaches us to do our own duties in life selflessly, dedicating the fruits of our action to mankind. Practicing this aspect of yoga helps us to live in the world without being distressed. The gems of Karma Yoga are available in one of the important systems of Indian philosophy known as Mimamsa Philosophy. This Karma Yoga is known as Nishkama Karma Yoga in Bhagavad Gita.

In Patanjali Yoga Sutras, we get a profound combination of *jnana-bhakti-karma*-Yogas in the practice of ***Kriya-yoga*** **(Fig. 33.2)** as explained in its second chapter, wherein:

Tapas, svadhyaya and isvarapranidhana have been a part and parcel of one's life right from the ancient times. But the objectives or motivations differed from one individual to another, often conditioned by the passage of time. So, when these practices are directed with the sole objective of attaining Samadhibhavana (i.e., to develop an inner ambience of spiritual absorption) by weakening the powerful grip of *Kleshas,* i.e., afflictions or miseries, it is known as *Kriya-yoga.*

Prana Samyama Yoga

- **Mantra Yoga:** Mantra yoga involves chanting of certain sounds called mantras which are traditionally transmitted to the students and are used as an object of concentration and meditation. Defined as *Mananat trayate iti Mantra*—that which protects the mind is a mantra, as a result of repeated recitation, mantra makes one free from evil thought, ensues good thoughts leading to no thoughts. Mantras are based on the theory of esoteric sounds and have esoteric relationship with the various energy centers in human body.
- **Hatha Yoga:** Most important practice (sadhana) system and directly related with control over respiration therefore, a balance between *Ha* (masculine energy) and *Tha* (feminine energy) is called Hatha Yoga. Hatha Yoga is the most followed system which recognizes fundamentally *Asana, Kumbhaka, Mudra and Nadanusandhana (Antaranga Yoga)* as limbs of Hatha Yoga. *Ha* and *Tha* balance is facilitated when one undergoes various practices such as *Shatkarma* (cleansing practices) and *Nadishodhana* (cleansing of energy channels). Traditionally the Hatha School recognizes eight varieties of *Pranayama* (breath manipulation/*Kumbhakas*). Some traditions apply recitation of Pranava (Om) or Bija Mantra in the course of controlled inhalation, retention and exhalation.
- **Laya Yoga:** Etymologically it means complete absorption. It includes the essence of Mantra Yoga, practice of Pranayama and attention of mind on one point inside the body. It can be *Chakras* (energy centers) or even *Bhrumadhya* (center of eyebrows), *Nasagra* (tip of the nose) or *Jihvagra* (tip of the tongue). Laya proceeds with control over five sense organs—which is usually known as *Pratyahara* (withdrawal of senses). Concentration on various *Chakras* result into arousal of Kundalini (Psychic energy) which passes through the seven *Chakras* and reaches to *Sahasrara* (universal energy centre) and unites with *Shiva* (Supreme Consciousness). This is called Maha laya.
- **Raja Yoga:** It is a state of Yogic attainment. *Raja Yoga* is also known synonym of *Samadhi*. Patanjali's *Ashtanga Yoga* (eight-fold path Yoga) has been identified as Raja Yoga. It is interesting that Patanjali's Ashtanga Yoga is the root for almost every variety of Yoga and can be practiced by a person of any faith and thus seems very much relevant to the modern society.

Let us briefly understand the classical eight-fold path of Patanjali along with the missing aspect of yoga in contemporary times **(Fig. 33.3)**.

THE EIGHT-FOLD PATH OF PATANJALI

The Yoga Sutra of Patanjali is divided into four chapters. Its field of action is to refine the activities of *chitta* (the psyche)

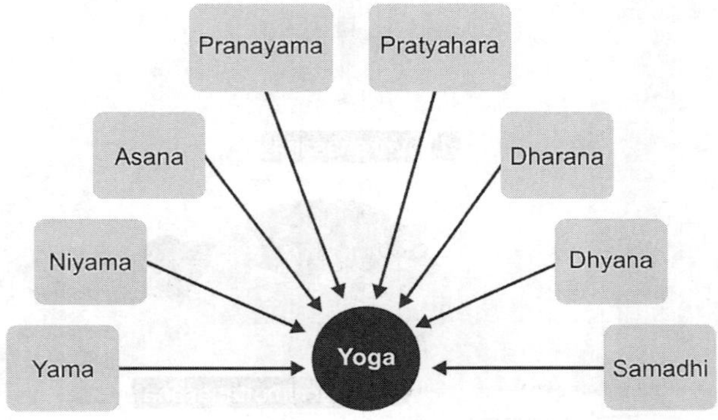

Fig. 33.3: Eight limbs of Yoga.

and thereby get absolute mastery over it. Thus, keeping this theme in mind, Patanjali defines Yoga as-"chitta - vritti - nirodha". It does not mean that a student of Yoga becomes a 'mind-less' being, rather he is in 'Complete awareness' with a transformed mind which due to its transparent (*sattvika*) pure nature can function to actualize the Self, as well as, the nonself. This state can be achieved through dedicated and determined practice (*abhyasa*) and absolute detachment (*vairagya*).

Yama and Niyama

Patanjali, as well as, all above mentioned schools of yoga develop a process of self-transformation wherein purity of moral **Yamas** (self-restraints) and ethical **Niyamas** (self-observations) is the foundation and is considered to be indispensable for this journey. One cannot allow themself to be impure, indisciplined, untruthful and harmful to others and at the same time try to practice Yoga. Thus, one has to be rooted in goodness, purity, truthfulness, self-reliance, patience and perseverance, sincerity and honesty, contentment and in selfless services.

Asana (Psychosomatic Posture)

Patanjali defines Asana as 'sthirasukhamasanam' (PYS II/46) 'steady and comfortable posture' which is accepted as the characteristics, as well as, the technique of an 'Asana' and as a consequence of this interpretation, the next verse (P.Y.S.II/47) provides the technique of a posture. Unfortunately, this has lost its significance in *Asana* practice, i.e., effortlessness (*prayatnashaithilya*) and engrossment with infinite (*Ananta samapatti*) is hardly observed. Thereby *'Asana'* is generally taken to be meant for solely the physical body or body positioning.

Few examples of Asanas from Hatha Yoga texts **(Fig. 33.4)**:
1. Vrikshasana
2. Paschimottanasana
3. Dhanurasana
4. Matsyendrasana
5. Matsyasana

Pranayama (Expansion of Breath)

Patanjali has given emphasis on silencing the activities of chitta (mind stuff) by way of prolonging and silencing the process of breathing activities to stand still. *'tasminsati shvasaprashvasayor gati-vicchedah pranayamah'* (PYS II/49)—it shows that intense practice of *'Asana'* automatically leads to *'Pranayama'*. The 'shvasa-prashvasa' (inhalation and exhalation) which is one of the indicatives of 'chittavikshepas' (obstacles) (PYS I/31) gets 'vicchedah' (broken off) in a specific manner in 'Pranayama'. That, in turns, helps in removing all dark coverings (ignorance) of consciousness (PYS II/52) and mind becomes fit instrument to enter into the field of *Dharana* (i.e., concentration) (PYS II/53). This aspect of pranayama, in contemporary times, is neglected and used only for overcoming a few disorders.

In Hatha yoga, when *nadis* (psychic channels) are purified by the regular practices of Pranayama, Prana (psychic energy) is made to enter into the ultimate path towards consciousness (*Sushmana*) with the help of various practices of Hatha Yoga (like bandhas and mudras, etc.) and moves upward leading to the state of Manonmani (Self-realization), the highest level of Yogic Consciousness (HP II/41-42). Unfortunately, this aspect of Pranayama (*Kumbhaka*) is often under-emphasized in contemporary practice.

Few examples of Pranayama from Hatha Yoga texts **(Fig. 33.5)**.

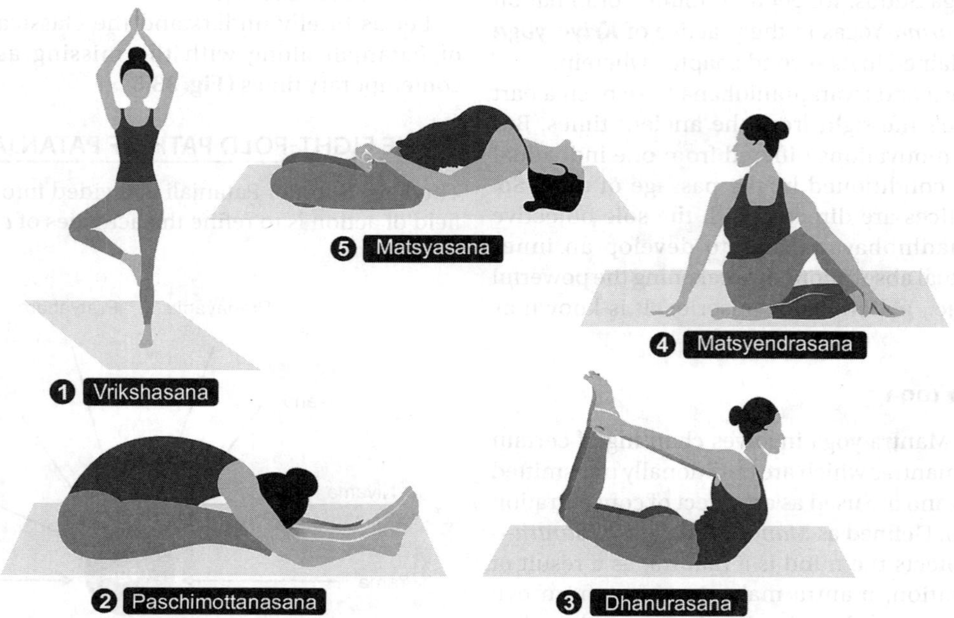

Fig. 33.4: (1) Vrikshasana; (2) Paschimottanasana; (3) Dhanurasana; (4) Matsyendrasana; (5) Matsyasana.

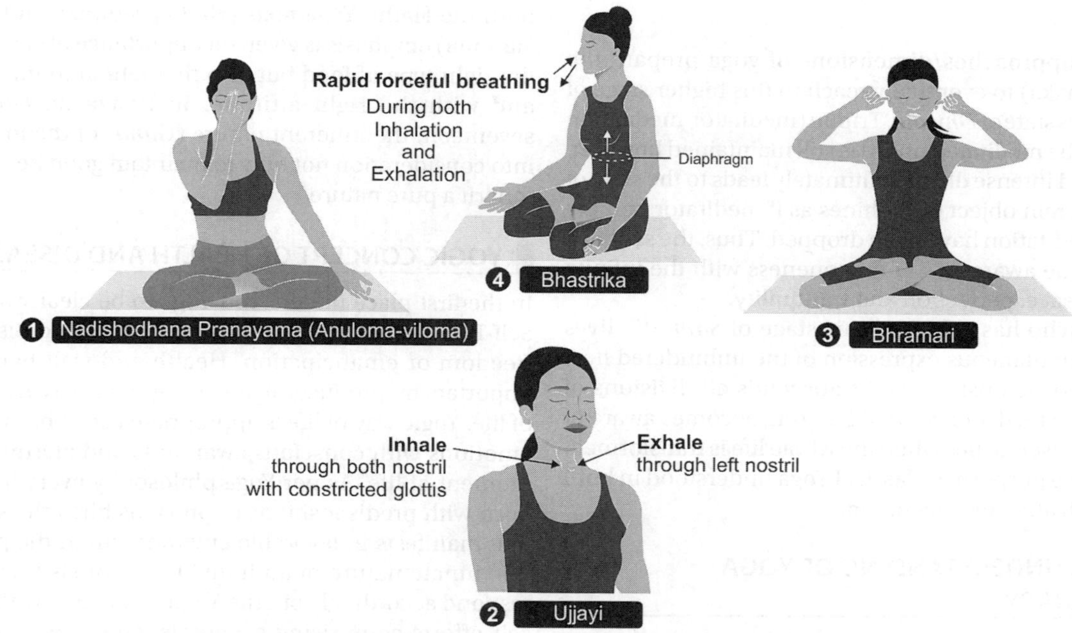

Fig. 33.5: (1) Nadishodhana Pranayama (Anuloma-viloma); (2) Ujjayi; (3) Bhramari; (4) Bhastrika.

1. Nadishodhana Pranayama (Anuloma-Viloma)
2. Ujjayi
3. Bhramari
4. Bhastrika

Pratyahara (Withdrawal of Senses)

Whenever we interact in the outer world our mind constantly goes on gathering sensations of external world through senses and mind reacts to them. If one wants to remove such distractions of mind then one should develop a mental ability to let go its involvement with external sensations leading to internalized consciousness.

Practice of Pratyahara senses withdrawal: Shanmukhi Mudra **(Fig. 33.6)**.

Dharana (Concentration)

In this stage, mind develops an ability to cultivate its scattered focusing power on an object of concentration through willful consistent practice. When this unbroken concentration process is continued then this concentration culminates into *Dhyana* (yogic meditation).

Dhyana (Meditation)

It is an uninterrupted flow of consciousness towards a chosen object. When consciousness expands to its still higher stages it is termed as *samapatti*—a complete fusion into the chosen object and then it goes beyond conscious and subconscious levels and assumes the super conscious flow and there arises a *Prajna* (wisdom) known as *Ritambhara* (intuitive wisdom).

Practice of Dhyana

See **Fig. 33.7**.

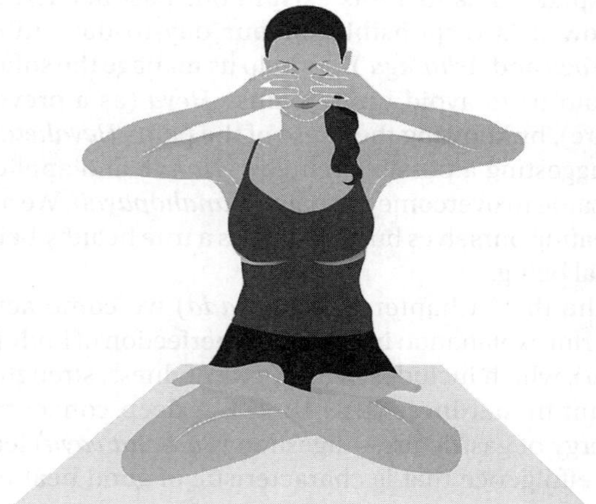

Fig. 33.6: Shanmukhi Mudra.

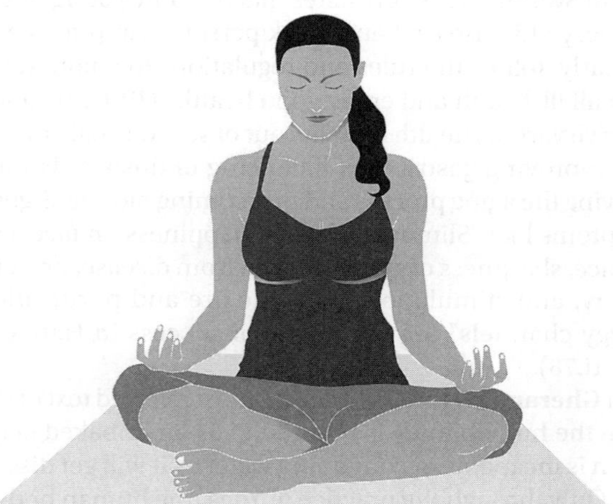

Fig. 33.7: Dhyana (Meditation).

Samadhi

All classical approaches/dimensions of yoga prepare the student (sadhaka) to eventually reach to this higher stage of *Dhyana*. In this state of *Dhyana*, Triputi (meditator, meditation and object to be meditated upon) is still maintained however, prolonged and intense dhyana ultimately leads to the state of *Samadhi* wherein object only shines as if meditator and the process of meditation have been dropped. Thus, the sadhaka regains the true awareness of that oneness with the infinite and attains peace, perfection and tranquility.

A person who has achieved this stage of *Samadhi* lives their life as spontaneous expression of the unhindered flow of supreme consciousness and transcends all divisions of culture, caste, creed and color. When one becomes aware of the infinite consciousness then the whole life is transformed, that is what the purpose of classical Yoga understood in both senses—unification or integration.

TEXTUAL UNDERSTANDING OF YOGA AS A THERAPY

In the second chapter (*Sadhana pada*)of **Patanjali Yoga Sutra**, the concept of *Klesha* (afflictions/ miseries/pain) is well explained as its roots exist in our past deeds/actions and how it is responsible for our day-to-day suffering. *Kriya Yoga* and *Ashtanga Yoga* help us manage the sufferings and train us to avoid future pains -*Heya* (as a preventive measure), by knowing the cause of the pain -*Heyahetuh* and also suggesting a possible remedy -*Hanah* and application of the same to overcome the pain -*Hanahopayah*. We are not just treating ourselves but evolving as a true healthy being - a spiritual being.

In the third Chapter (*Vibhutipada*) we come across a wonderful explanation in relation to perfection of body (*Kaya sampat*), which includes beauty, gracefulness, strength, and adamantine hardness (PYS III-47). A deep concentration on energy of gastric fire—digestion (*Samana vayu*) leads to bright effulgence that is characteristic of good health (PYS III-41).

In the Hatha Yoga text of **Hathapradipika,** the author Swami Swatmarama Suri states that not only young but even old, very old, diseased and weak persons can practice Yoga regularly, follow the rules and regulations to attain freedom from all ill-health and enjoy good health (HP-I.64). One can observe various health benefits out of several yogic practices like improving gastric fire, balancing of doshas (Humors), delaying the aging process and overcoming old age. Signs and symptoms like "Slimness of body, happiness on face, clarity of voice, sharpness of eyes, freedom from disease, preserving vitality, and stimulation of gastric fire and purification of energy channels" are the marks of success in Hatha Yoga (HP- II.78).

In **Gheranda Samhita**, another most referred text of Hatha Yoga, the human body is referred to as an unbaked clay pot which is incapable of containing water as it will get dissolved in it. Only through the practice of Yoga, the human body gets baked (strengthened) to hold the divine Soul (GhS-I.8). In both the Hatha Yoga texts (Hathapradipika and Gheranda Samhita) emphasis is given on importance of eating not only the right type of food but also the right amount (*Mitahara*) and with the right attitude. In Bhagavad Gita chapter seventeen, the inherent nature (*Guna*) of the food is taken into consideration not only to maintain good health but also inherit a pure nature.

YOGIC CONCEPT OF HEALTH AND DISEASE

In the first place understand Yoga to be clearly a science of Self-Realization (Moksha Shastra). The final goal is liberation, freedom or emancipation. Health and well-being are just important by-products of practicing Yoga or living a Yogic way of life. Yogic way of life is appropriate use of body, mind and emotions with conscious awareness and alertness at every moment of life. As per Yoga philosophy every individual is born with predispositions of previous birth the seed karma that manifests in favorable environment in the present life. The innate nature of an individual propels them to act or respond accordingly but the Yogic education with dedicated self-efforts comprising of morals, ethics, posture, breath-work and other discipline help to maintain and sustain the state of health.

Human Nature and Various Aspects of its Existence

In Taittiriya Upanishad an ancient vedic scripture the nature of human existence is explained in the form of five-fold system known as *Panchakosha*. Another way of understanding the nature of human existence is *Trisharira* —the three-fold system. Yoga accepts these systems which help us understand our multidimensional real human nature which helps us understand our body at various levels.

The **Panchakosha** (five-fold sheath/layer) system considers a human being to exist on many levels at one time. Each of the layers represents a unique understanding of energy and vibrations. These layers are interdependent and respond to a change simultaneously. They can be explained as:

- **Annamaya Kosha (the physical sheath):** It is the grossest layer—the physical body which we can experience through our senses. Our gross body which is made up of different cells, tissues, bones and muscles is sustained by proper supply of energy and nutrients through food (anna), proper exercise, proper excretion, hygiene, rest and sleep.
- **Pranamaya Kosha (the pranic/vital energy body):** Subtler than the physical body, the prana (life energy) keeps the gross body alive by flowing through the nadis (channels) reaching out to every cell as per the need in different situations of living life. If there is any obstacle occurring in the path of flow of prana it results in imbalance or disease in the physical body.
- **Manomaya Kosha (the mental body):** It is a subtler layer than the pranic/vital body. The mind which works on the feeds from the senses leading to various thoughts and impressions has a great influence on Pranamaya and Annamaya Kosha with the emotions bringing considerable

changes to our breathing and heart rate. Such prolonged effect of emotions on the grosser layers leads to various disorders.

- **Vijnanamaya Kosha (the intellectual body):** Subtler than the mental body the intellectual body comprises wisdom and discriminating agency, a higher conscience which is responsible for discerning good and bad. This layer is highly concerned with the state of homeostasis.
- **Anandamaya Kosha (the blissful body):** It relates to the subtlest true nature of our existence. Anandamaya kosha is the ultimate connectivity with the self beyond the mind, body, intellect getting detached from the influence of other layers. It leads to freedom or liberation (*moksha*).

The **Trisharira** comprises of *Sthula* (gross), *Sukshma* (Subtle) and *Karana* (causal). The gross body is made up of *Saptadhatus* (seven substances), they are *rasa* (chyme), *rakta* (blood), *mamsa* (flesh), *meda* (fat), *majja* (bone-marrow), *asthi* (bone) and *shukra* (semen). Yoga and Ayurveda understand the importance of *saptadhatu* as well as the *Tridosha* (three humors). The balance of seven substances and three humors (*vata, pitta and kapha*) are vital for good health. The harmony of *Prana* (vital energy) and the stability of *Nadis* (energy channels) and the proper functioning of *Chakras* (energy centres), all contribute to better health. The *chakras* can be corelated to psycho-neuro-immuno-endocrine axis.

Tridosha concept is common to all systems of traditional Indian medicine. It can be understood as functional ability of *Panchamahabhuta* (the five basic elements) and *Triguna* (innate quality of nature). Health is the outcome of balanced *tridosha* and disease is imbalance of the same.

In the modern world people are facing many types of diseases and disorders mostly due to wrong living lifestyle which needs to be corrected by every individual themselves. To live a healthy life, it is important to do daily routine as advocated for a healthy life. Yoga as mentioned earlier is a way of life that gives lot of importance to proper and healthy lifestyle. The main aspects of it are as follows:

- **Aahar**: A healthy diet which is full of nourishment with adequate intake of water. The sattvic diet includes a balanced portion of fresh fruits, green salads, sprouts, cereals, wheat, rice, green leafy vegetables, etc. The fresh food is prepared with love and affection.
- **Vihar**: A proper approach towards daily routine work, avoiding too much exertion and doing justice to recreational activities with enthusiasm. Observing proper relaxation at mental and physical level. A balanced and healthy communication with people in the society without being self-centered and easily get involved with the nature and other activities for universal wellbeing.
- **Aachar**: A behavioral approach towards understanding the importance of health by doing exercises or practicing Yoga on a regular basis to maintain overall physical and mental health to ensure the vital functioning of cardio-respiratory health.
- **Vichar**: Observation of social conduct and self-discipline (Yama-Niyama) leading to right thoughts and right attitude towards life is important for health and wellbeing. Moral and ethical thinking also leads to discipline in spirituality.

Summary

Yoga is an ancient wisdom, a philosophical way of life leading to self-realization (salvation). It is based on Samkhya-philosophy—theory of dualism (Purusha and Prakriti) comprising of consciousness and matter. With regular practice of true Yoga an individual develops a state of clarity (Jnana Yoga) towards reality (the Ultimate Truth—Supreme Consciousness).

Yoga therapy is treatment of an individual as a whole, a holistic approach in the form of physical, mental, emotional and spiritual interventions leading to realization of truth. A disease or an ailment is not looked upon as a problem rather a reason to bring changes in our lifestyle, in our thinking, in our approach towards life. The whole concept of disease or our sufferings in Yoga is to know our actions, their results, overcoming expectations and attachments and realize that happiness and sufferings in material world are one and same that leads to sufferings.

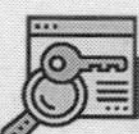

Review Questions

1. How is Yoga defined in various scriptures?
2. What is the classification of Yoga?
3. What are the eight steps in Yoga?
4. Write a short note on textual understanding of Yoga therapy.
5. Write a short note on the yogic concept of health and disease.

Bibliography

1. Ananda B. Bhavanani Yoga Chikitsa: Application of Yoga as a Therapy. Pudecherry, India: Divyananda Creations; 2013.
2. BR Sharma Notes on Yoga: Classical and Contemporary Perspective. Lonavala, India: Kaivalyadhama; 2006.
3. Swami Digambarji Hathapradipika of Swatmaram. Lonavala, India: Kaivalyadhama; 1990.

Multiple Choice Questions (MCQs)

To test your understanding and recall of key concepts.

1. **What is the literal meaning of the word "Yoga"?**

   A. Meditation 2. Union
   3. Exercise 4. Awareness

2. **Which scripture defines Yoga as "Yogah cittavritti nirodhah"?**

   A. Bhagavad Gita B. Patanjali Yoga Sutra
   C. Yoga Vasistha D. Kathopanishad

3. According to Patanjali, what are the three components of Kriya Yoga?

A. Pranayama, Dharana, Dhyana
B. Yama, Niyama, Samadhi
C. Tapas, Svadhyaya, Ishvarapranidhana
D. Asana, Pranayama, Pratyahara

4. Why is yoga referred to as a "science of self-realization"?

A. It promotes physical fitness in an individual
B. It aims to unify individual and universal consciousness
C. It is based on ancient philosophical cultures and traditions
D. It focuses on relaxation techniques

5. Evaluate the following scenario: A practitioner wishes to address emotional imbalances using Yoga. Which approach is most appropriate?

A. Focus solely on asanas like Vrikshasana and Paschimottanasana
B. Combine meditation (Dhyana) with controlled breathing (Pranayama)
C. Engage in vigorous physical activities like Power Yoga
D. Practice withdrawal of senses (Pratyahara) exclusively

6. Which Yogic principle best addresses the imbalance caused by over-reliance on sensory stimuli?

A. Asana
B. Dharana
C. Pratyahara
D. Samadhi

7. Imagine a scenario wherein a practitioner wishes to address emotional imbalances using Yoga. Which approach is most appropriate?

A. Focus solely on asanas like Vrikshasana and Paschimottanasana
B. Combine meditation (Dhyana) with controlled breathing (Pranayama)
C. Engage in vigorous physical activities like Power Yoga
D. Practice withdrawal of senses (Pratyahara) exclusively

ANSWERS

1. B	2. B	3. C	4. B	5. B
6. C	7. B			

Chapter 34

Yoga for Women's Health

Anuprita Thakur

LEARNING OBJECTIVES

At the end of the chapter, the reader will be able to:

- Understand the role of Yoga in the various phases of woman's life.
- Understand the Yogic practices to be followed in special physiological and pathological conditions.

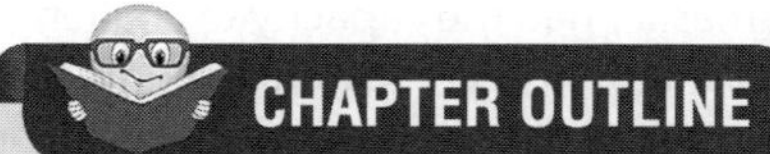

- Introduction
- General Yoga practices
  - Suryanamaskar
  - Asanas
  - Pranayama and Kriyas
  - Trataka
- Yoga in adolescence
  - Menstrual disorders
  - Polycystic ovarian syndrome
- Yoga in adulthood and middle ages
  - Prenatal Yoga
  - Postnatal Yoga
- Yoga in the transitional phase
- Yoga in elderly women

INTRODUCTION

From the beginning of puberty to menopause, a woman's body undergoes a great deal of physical and mental change that makes her prone to various physical, emotional, and psychological problems. Yoga offers a balance of body and mind and helps to revitalize and prepare the woman to deal with these problems. Practice of Yoga, thus, is beneficial to a woman in every stage of her life.

General guidelines to be followed while practicing Yogic techniques are shown in **Box 34.1**.

GENERAL YOGA PRACTICES

Table 34.1 shows some general practices that may be followed by any woman, right from an adolescent girl to a woman in any phase of life.

The detailed description of the technique of every practice and their individual contraindications are beyond the scope of this chapter and can be referred to from relevant sources.

Table 34.1: General Yoga practices that may be followed by any woman.

Asanas	Suryanamaskar **Siting:** Padmasana, Vajrasana, Malasana, Bhadrasana, Ardha Matsyendrasana, Paschimotanasana, Gomukhasana, Chakkichalasana **Supine:** Pavanamuktasana, Sethubandhasana, ViparitKarni mudra, Halasana **Prone:** Bhujangasana, Shalabhasna, Dhanurasana **Standing:** Tadasana, Vrikshasana, Virbhadrasana 1 and 2, Padahastasana, Trikonasana, Utkatasana Shavasana
Pranayama and Kriyas	Kapalbhatti, Anulomvilom, Bhrahmari, Bhastrika, Sitali
Dhyana	Om chanting, Trataka

Suryanamaskar

Suryanamaskar or sun salutation **(Fig. 34.1)** is a sequence of 12 linked asanas wherein each asana is performed with recitation of a 'beej' mantra and is coordinated with the

Box 34.1: General guidelines to be followed while practicing Yogic techniques.

- Yoga should be practiced in a quiet, calm and well ventilated place using a yoga mat or blanket on the floor.
- Clothing should be such that it facilitates the easy flow of movements.
- Yogic practices should be done on empty stomach or after a light snack. A gap of 4 to 4.5 hours should be maintained between full meal and Yoga practice.
- Avoid Yoga practice after heavy physical activity or sports or maintain a gap of at least half an hour between the two.
- There is no specific time to practice Yoga, however morning time is preferred, whenever possible, as it is said to energize and refresh your day.
- Avoid practicing yogic techniques during any illness or exhaustion. However, practices that give peace and relaxation can be continued.
- Asanas and pranayama can be continued during menstruation while avoiding certain practices (mentioned below).
- Yoga can be practiced from the 1st trimester of pregnancy, provided the woman has practiced yoga before. Otherwise it can be started from the 2nd trimester.
- It is recommended that a trained yoga teacher should be consulted for practice of Yoga, especially during pregnancy or in case of any health problem.
- Warm up or stretching exercises are recommended before the practice of asanas.
- Each Yogic practice has its own set of contraindications/ limitations that should be paid attention to.
- Generally Yogic practices are done in the following sequence: warm-up followed by asanas, pranayama, mudras and bandhas and ending the session with meditation and relaxation. However this sequence is not rigid and necessary sequence may be followed as per one's own requirement.
- Yogic practices should be performed in a slow, relaxed manner with continuous awareness of the body posture and breathing pattern. The body parts should be relaxed once the final posture is achieved and the concentration should be on breathing.
- While performing asanas, it is recommended to maintain the final posture for a longer duration rather than repeating the practice for more number of rounds.
- Rest can be taken in between two practices to relax the body instead of practicing the techniques non-stop.
- The practice of asanas should be started with easy postures and gradually progress to the difficult ones as one's body permits.
- Pranayama is known to bestow many health benefits if performed correctly. Thus the correct practice of Pranayama is mandatory.
- Breathing should always be done through the nose and no holding of breath should be practiced, unless specified.
- Yogic practices should be done as per one's own capacity; there should not be any competitive attitude during the practice of Yoga.
- A general Yoga practice can be followed by everyone; however a customized practice depending on one's own body needs would yield better results.

breathing. It involves movement of all body segments and thus can serve as a favorable model for whole body exercise.

Suryanamaskar can be very useful as a mobility exercise in both, children and adults. It has been observed that Suryanamaskar moves the spine and lower limbs through a large range of alternate flexion and extension movements. Thus, it can be effectively used in stretching of muscles and other soft tissues.

Research Pointer

- A study conducted in overweight/obese adults compared various forms of exercises such as circuit training, treadmill walking and Suryanamaskar for weight management and improvement in physical fitness. The study observed that all the three forms of exercises had similar beneficial effect of reducing weight and improving fitness with Suryanamaskar having added benefit in increasing the flexibility.
- This finding was supported by another study which showed an increase in muscular strength and endurance and positive change in body composition after 24 weeks of Suryanamaskar practice. It is thus recommended that Suryanamaskar can provide an economical and complete fitness regime without the need of any equipment or added space. Thus depending on the speed and repetitions performed, Suryanamaskar can also be effectively used to improve the cardiovascular endurance.
- A study assessing the kinematics of Suryanamaskar stated that Suryanamaskar had the capacity to challenge the postural mechanisms to a greater extent as compared to walking and thus recommended its use in training postural control in people with impaired balance.

The additional benefits of Suryanamaskar are that it helps to increase the lung capacity and improve the function of the digestive system.

Point to be Noted

- The ideal time for practice of Suryanamaskar is preferably in the morning.
- Women with back problems, hernia or who have undergone any recent surgery, should consult the doctor before practicing Suryanamaskar.
- Pregnant women should avoid the practice of Suryanamaskar.

Asanas

Asanas **(Fig. 34.2)** have a general benefit of improving the flexibility and muscle strength. The additional benefits of asanas lie in enhancing digestion, improving balance and coordination, improving the hormonal balance and blood circulation, etc.

- **Sitting asanas** improve the flexibility of the lower limb muscles and joints. They form the basis for the practice of Pranayama.
- **Supine asanas** allow relaxation and relief from weight bearing activities, stretch the back and hip muscles and aid in strengthening the anterior muscles like abdominals.
- The **forward bend asanas** from sitting or supine aid in digestion and relieve from symptoms like constipation.

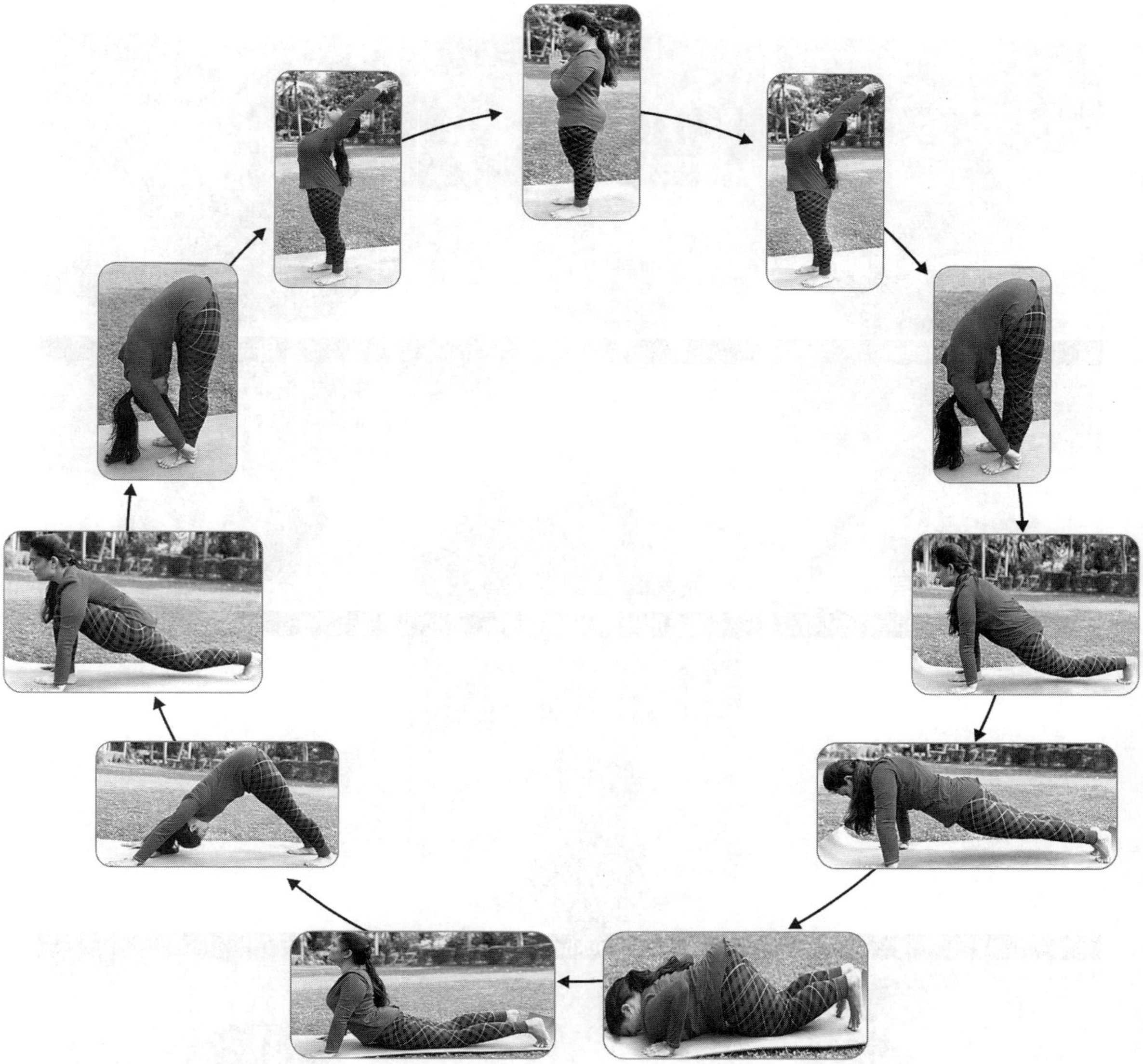

Fig. 34.1: Suryanamaskara.

- **Prone asanas** are useful in strengthening of back and hip extensors especially when forward flexion is to be avoided.
- The forward, prone and twisting asanas help in improving the spinal mobility.
- **Standing asanas** help in improving the sense of balance, improve the blood circulation in the lower limbs especially the calf due to strong contraction of the gastrocnemius.

Clinical Pointer

Though the benefits of asanas are numerous, general caution should be heeded while performing certain asanas. For example forward bending asanas to be avoided in cases of severe back pain, pelvic inflammatory disease (PID), spondylosis, balancing asanas in standing should be avoided in case of balance issues or should be done with the help of support.

Pranayama and Kriyas

Kriyas are the cleansing practices that are generally performed prior to the practice of Pranayama **(Fig. 34.3)**. Certain kriyas help in cleansing the digestive and respiratory systems. Pranayama improves the capacity of the lungs and also aids in promoting relaxation.

Trataka

Trataka is a meditation technique that involves focusing the eyes intently on a candle flame.

Research Pointer

Many studies have reported an improvement in various cognitive domains such as memory, attention, and concentration, etc., following practice of Trataka in adolescents, adults and elderly subjects.

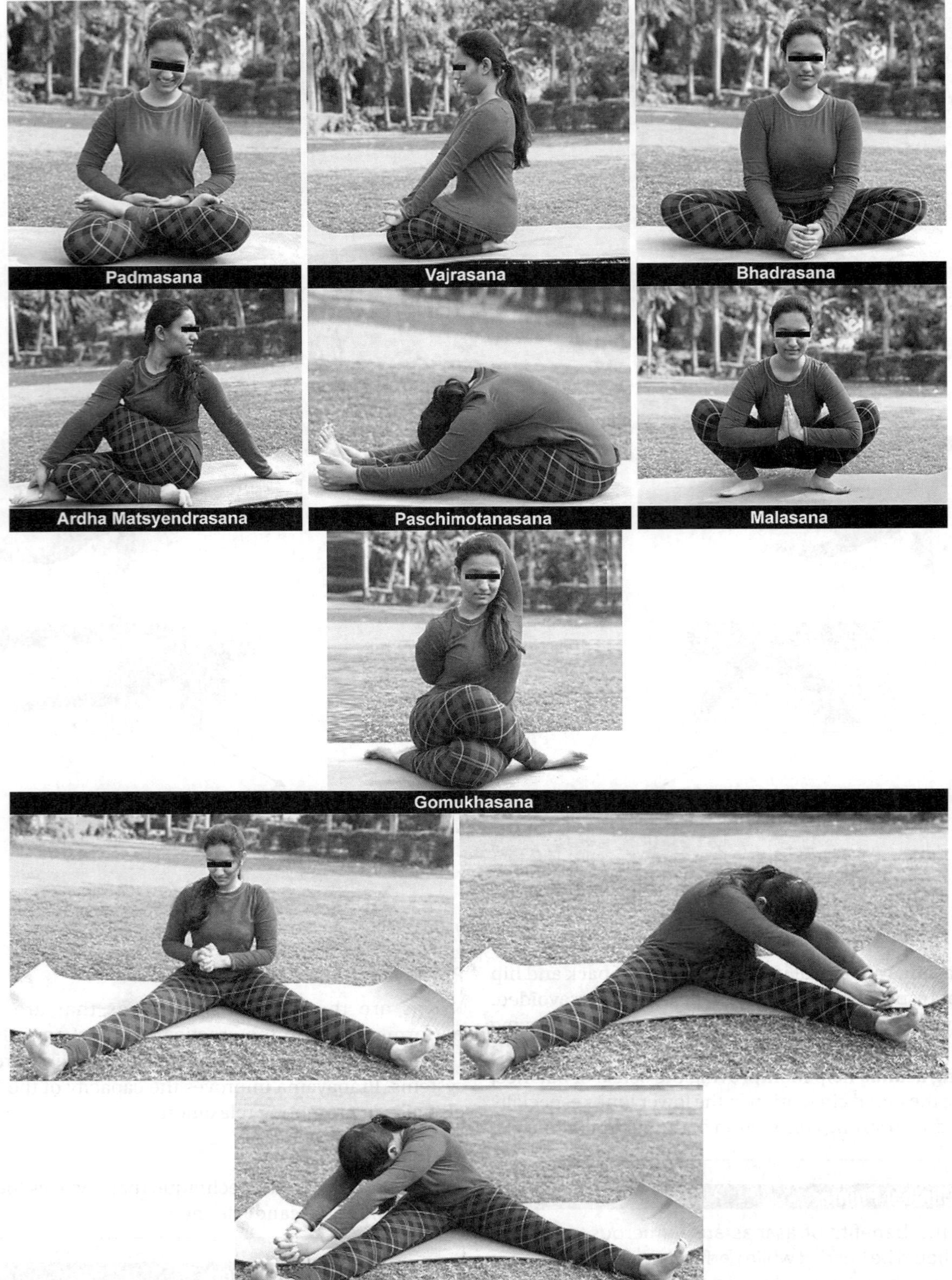
Padmasana
Vajrasana
Bhadrasana
Ardha Matsyendrasana
Paschimotanasana
Malasana
Gomukhasana
Chakki chalanasana

Fig. 34.2

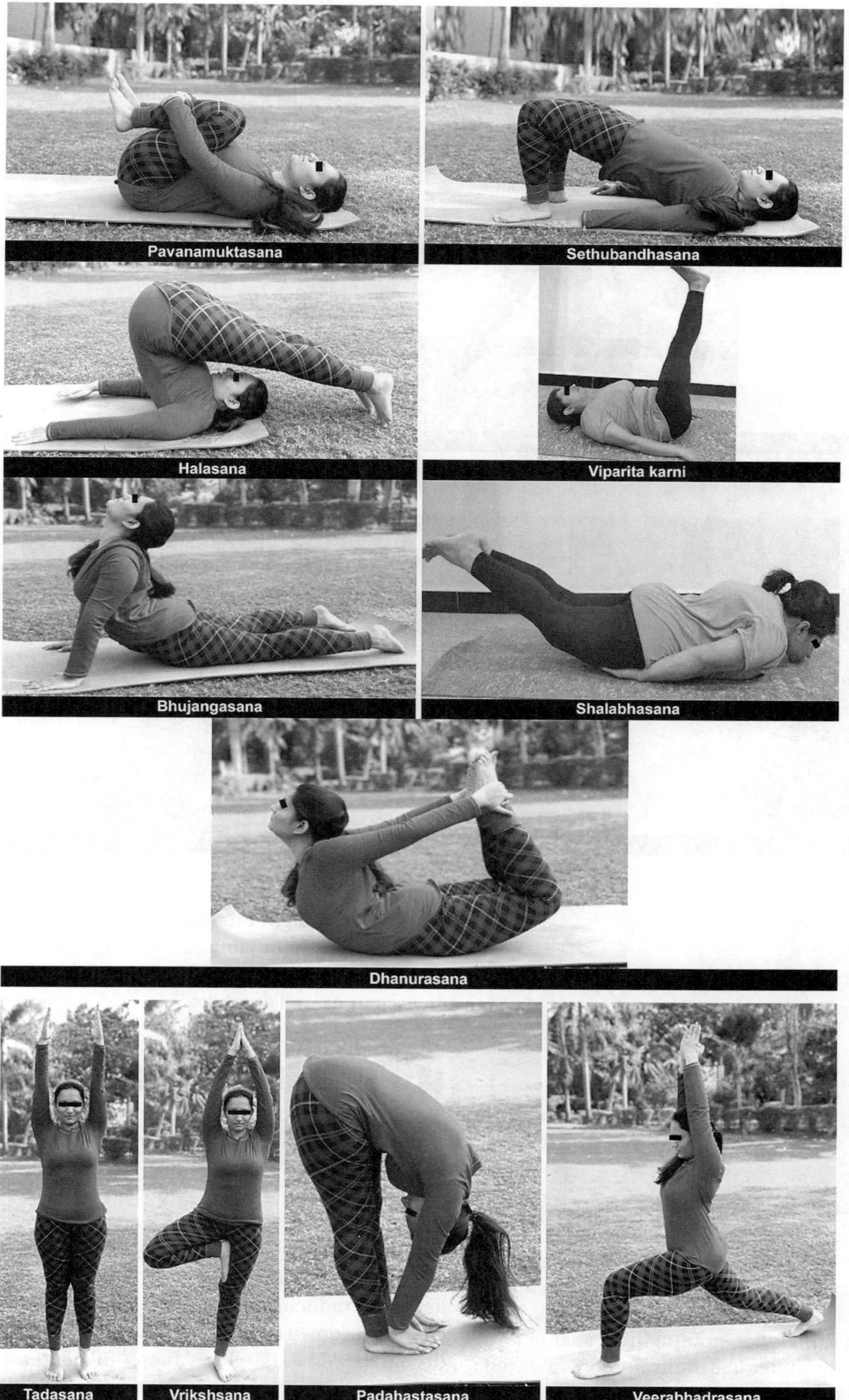
Pavanamuktasana
Sethubandhasana
Halasana
Viparita karni
Bhujangasana
Shalabhasana
Dhanurasana
Tadasana
Vrikshsana
Padahastasana
Veerabhadrasana

Fig. 34.2

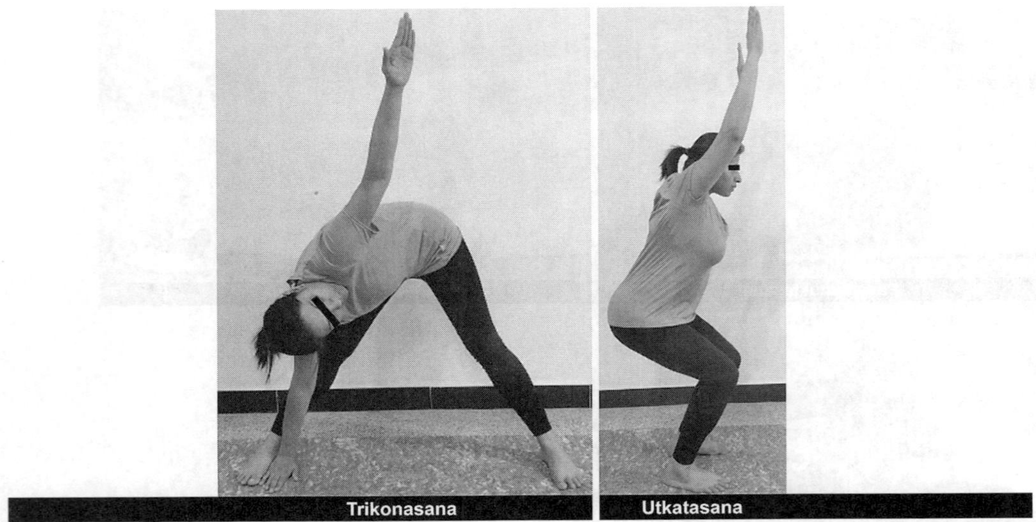

Fig. 34.2: Various asanas in different postures.

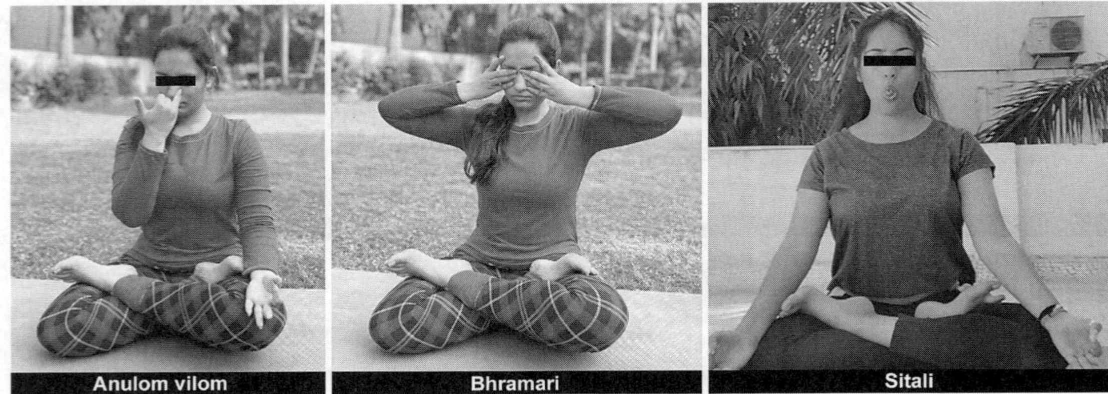

Fig. 34.3: Pranayama.

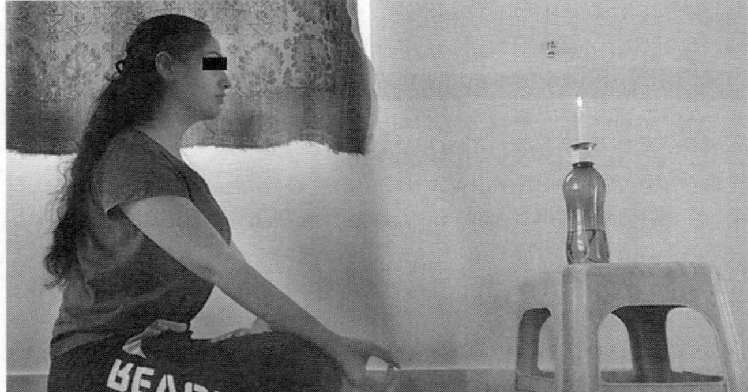

Fig. 34.4: Trataka.

Trataka **(Fig. 34.4)** is generally practiced in two stages:

1. A preparatory first stage that includes eye exercises.
2. A second stage that includes unblinkingly gazing at a candle flame for 2–3 minutes in a dimly lit room followed by visualizing the flame between the eyebrows with closed eyes. The second stage is repeated 2–3 times.

Trataka helps to reduce mind-wandering and thus enhance focus. A theory about Trataka suggests that the practice in dim light increases release of melatonin which in turn positively influences learning and memory. Thus, Trataka can be useful in improving memory and attention in adolescents as well as adults.

 **Point to be Noted**

Trataka is not recommended in people with serious eye disorders such as glaucoma or in people with psychiatric problems such as schizophrenia.

Apart from all these general benefits, Yogic practices are also known to be of assistance in regulating hormonal balance, controlling the blood pressure and especially effective in reducing stress. The hypothesized mechanism of action is the down regulation of the hypothalamus-pituitary-adrenal (HPA) axis which helps in decreasing cortisol levels which are known to induce stress. Additionally Yogic practices are also proven to shift the nervous system function from sympathetic to parasympathetic, thus helping the body to enter a state of relaxation.

YOGA IN ADOLESCENCE

A woman first experiences changes in her physical and mental state when she enters adolescence as this is the first phase of major hormonal changes occurring in her body. As discussed in Chapter 8: Adolescence, Puberty and Menarche, these pubertal hormones lead to physical as well psychological changes such as mood swings, fluctuating energy levels, etc. As a result of this, the adolescent girls often do not understand how to deal with these changes and this may add to their stress.

Practice of Yogic techniques like asanas, pranayama, meditation etc. can aid in achieving physical and emotional balance and thus help the adolescent girls to deal with this stress in a better manner.

The practice of Yoga in this age will not only help develop a healthy menstrual cycle but will also help to deal with the psychological changes occurring in this age.

 **Research Pointer**

- Studies show an improvement in physical, emotional, cognitive function (attention, working memory, executive function, etc.) and psychosocial well-being (self-image, confidence, etc.) in adolescents following Yogic practices.
- A study done in adolescents reported a reduction in anger, fatigue and depression after the practice of Yoga and thus the authors recommended inclusion of school – based Yoga practices to improve psycho-social well-being to promote long term outcomes for youth.
- Yoga also helps to improve the flexibility, develop good posture, manage weight, maintain hormonal balance, etc.

 **Point to be Noted**

- Studies have shown that intense practice of asanas can impede skeletal growth and affect the natural growth pattern, especially in the age group of 10 to 12 years. Thus a prudent approach with respect to the type, intensity and duration of practice of yogasanas is recommended in adolescence.
- During menstruation, the normal practices of Yoga can be continued. However certain practices may be avoided. Asanas that include inversions such as Halasana can lead to vascular congestion and increased menstrual bleeding. Other asanas that involve backward bends (e.g., Dhanurasana), twists (e.g., ArdhaMatsyendrasana) and standing asanas that put a pressure on the abdomen and pelvic region should also be avoided as these asanas can be exerting on the body during this period. Kriyas and Pranayama techniques like Bhastrika, Kapalbhati should also be avoided as these also exert excessive pressure on the abdomen and cause bleeding irregularities. It is also wise to avoid practice of the various Bandhas during menstruation.

Menstrual Disorders

As a result of unhealthy food habits, lack of adequate physical activity, stress, etc., menstrual disorders may be quite common in adolescent girls and women of reproductive age. Regular practice of Yoga is beneficial in the treatment of these disorders. Some practices are especially beneficial as they regulate the blood flow in these menstrual disorders and thus can be stressed upon more.

- For example, Bhadrasana, Virasana **(FIg. 34.5A)** and Suptavirasana **(Fig. 34.5B)** can help manage dysmenorrhea. Uttanasana and Paschimottanasana can aid in controlling excessive menstrual blood flow in menorrhagia.

Polycystic Ovarian Syndrome

Polycystic ovarian syndrome (PCOS) is a result of hormonal imbalance which is caused due to several factors such as diet, genetics, improper food habits, sedentary lifestyle, lack of physical activity, etc. This can further lead to stress, anxiety, depression and other psychological disorders.

Studies have shown a hyper-responsive HPA (hypothalamus-pituitary-adrenal) axis, increased sympathetic activation and enhanced heart rate activity in patients with PCOS which increases the overall stress response and is associated with depression, being overweight and increased risk of cardiovascular disease and diabetes.

Yoga is considered as one of the best complementary therapies in the treatment of PCOS as:

- It combats the root cause of PCOS, i.e., stress and obesity.
- Practice of various Yogic techniques help in balancing the sympathetic overdrive and reducing levels of stress hormones in the body.

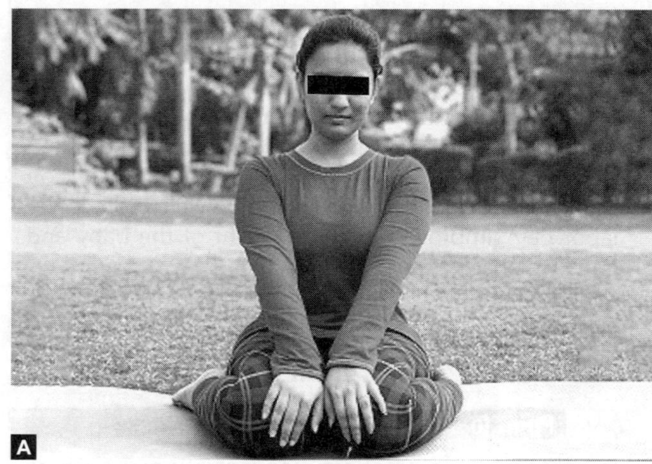

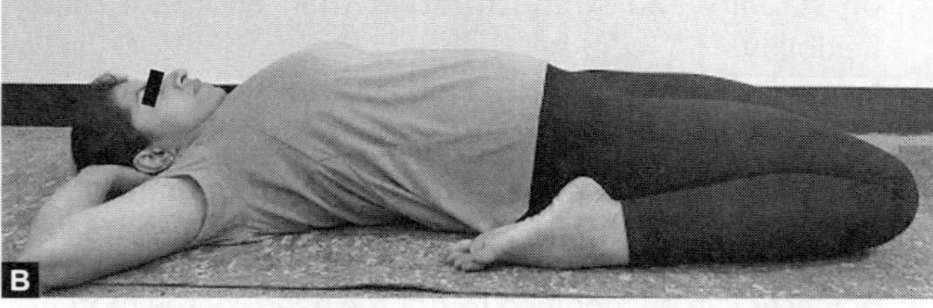

Figs. 34.5A and B: (A) Virasana; (B) Suptavirasana.

- The breathing techniques bring about relaxation and thus take care of emotional disturbances and increased heart rate while the practice of asanas help in managing the body weight, improving pelvic blood flow to reproductive organs and regulating hormonal imbalance.
- Practice of yoga nidra helps to restore the healthy sleep pattern.

Women with PCOS issues can perform all the practices mentioned earlier with emphasis on the following practices:

- Suryanamaskar
- Bhadrasana
- Chakkichalanasana
- Pranayama
- Om chanting

YOGA IN ADULTHOOD AND MIDDLE AGES

An adult woman often needs to multitask to be able to manage her home and career, in addition to the bodily and hormonal changes that she faces during menstruation and pregnancy. Yoga in this phase of life can help to bring about a physical and mental harmony and thus optimize her productivity.

Prenatal Yoga

Pregnancy is a very important condition in this phase of life of most women. It is a state in which a woman undergoes definite physiological and psychological changes. The common problems that a pregnant woman faces during pregnancy include physical issues such as fatigue, increased heart rate, pedal edema, ligament laxity, postural changes and psychological issues such as depression, nervousness, etc.

Research Pointer

- Yoga is reported to improve sleep patterns, reduce stress and anxiety, strengthen the uterine and spinal muscles and decrease low back pain in pregnant women.
- In addition, practice of Yoga during pregnancy has also shown to decrease chances of preterm labor, shorten labor stages, aid in normal delivery by relieving tension around the cervix by opening the pelvic region, lower labor pain, improve the birth weight of the baby and enhance post-delivery recovery.
- Yoga is adaptable, customizable and low-impact and thus can be considered as a safe activity for pregnant women.

Point to be Noted

- In prenatal Yoga practices, concentration should be on stability and strength rather than endurance and flexibility.
- Props like chair, wall, etc., can be used whenever needed as support while performing asanas.
- Avoid asanas in prone position or asanas that include deep forward bends, twists, inversions or techniques like Kapalbhati as they put pressure on the abdomen. These practices can be modified to suit the needs of the mother.

Following practices can be stressed upon in the prenatal phase:

- Asanas **(Fig. 34.6):**
  - Sukhasana
  - Paschhimotanasana
  - Marjarsana
  - Virbhadrasana 1 and 2
  - Tadasana
  - Utkatasana
  - Malasana
  - Adhomukhshvanasana
  - Anandabalasana
  - Viparitkarni (against the wall)
  - Konasana
  - Shavasana
- Pranayama and Kriya:
  - Anulomvilom
  - Bhrahmari
- Relaxation:
  - Yoga nidra
  - Om chanting

Postnatal Yoga

Postnatal Yoga helps a woman to recover quickly post-delivery. Yoga practice in the postnatal period benefits the woman by:

- Relaxing the muscles
- Restoring the strength of pelvic floor muscles
- Improving posture
- Enhancing mood
- Decreasing incidence of postpartum depression

Research Pointer

Studies have reported an increase in milk production as a result of increased release of prolactin and oxytocin due to the relaxation and calming effect provided by Yogic practices.

Postnatally, Yoga can be started after 6 weeks of vaginal delivery and after 8 weeks following cesarean delivery.

Following practices are recommended in the postnatal period:

- **Asanas:**
  - Tadasana
  - Parvatasana
  - Bhadrasana
  - Hastapadasana
  - Marjarasana
  - Anandabalasana
  - Veerbhadrasana
  - Utkatasana
  - Shavasana
- **Pranayam and Kriya:**
  - Anulomvilom
  - Kapalbhati
  - Bhrahmari
- **Relaxation:**
  - Yoga nidra
  - Om chanting

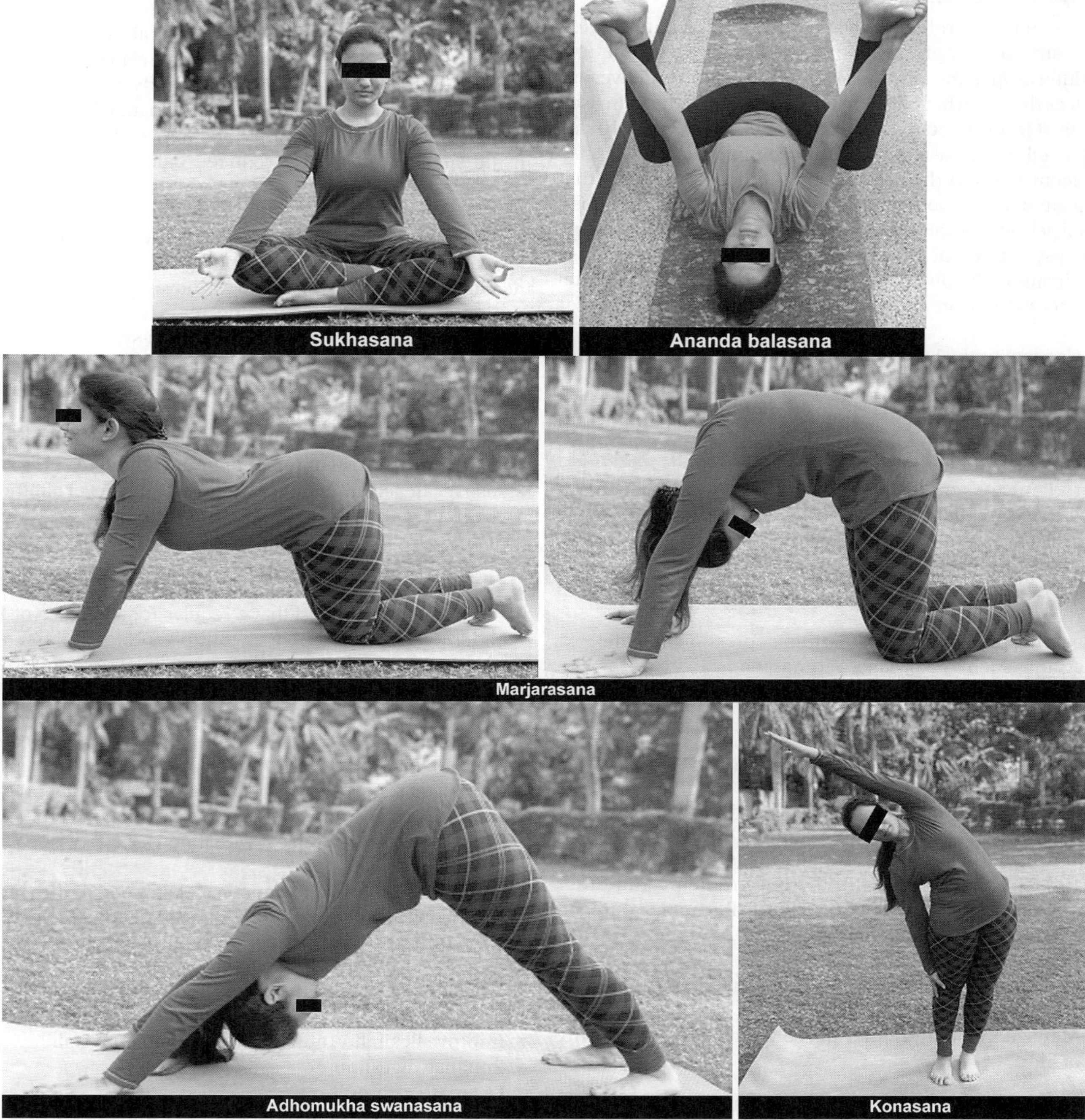

Fig. 34.6: Asanas that can be performed in prenatal period.

Point to be Noted

- Consult the gynecologist before starting the Yoga practices.
- Avoid or stop the practice of Yoga when experiencing excessive pain or bleeding.
- Check for diastasis recti before the practice of Yoga.
- It is advisable to avoid the practice of certain asanas immediately in the postnatal period: Suryanamaskar, Naukasana, Trikonasana, as these asanas can be exerting to the recovering mother, prone asanas such as Bhujangasana, etc., as they may be uncomfortable with the breasts filled with milk.

Postpartum Depression

One common problem observed in the postnatal period is postpartum depression (PPD). This can occur due to a sudden drop in the placental estrogen levels after delivery as well as the disturbance in the HPA axis leading the increased cortisol levels which is associated with stress. A study also reported a decrease in gamma aminobutyric acid (GABA) concentration in the cerebrospinal fluid postdelivery that contributes to mood disturbances and anxiety in the post-natal period. The treatment of PPD involves pharmacotherapy and psychotherapy. However, because of the side effects of medications involved and stigma associated with mental health, many women may defer from taking treatment for PPD.

Consequently, Yoga can serve as a great complementary alternative in the treatment of PPD.

Research Pointer

Studies have reported a reduction in cortisol production by down-regulation of the HPA axis and a correction in the GABA levels through stimulation of vagus nerve, both of which can help to reduce postpartum depression and improve the well-being and quality of life in women.

Suggested practices for postpartum depression include:
- Asanas such as Balasana, Padmasana
- Pranayama such as Bhrahmari
- Om chanting

YOGA IN THE TRANSITIONAL PHASE

This is the phase wherein a woman experiences menopause and some unpleasant changes and symptoms associated with it such as weight gain, mood swings, hot flushes, sleep disorders, fatigue and pain, thyroid problems and other chronic ailments like osteoporosis due to fluctuating estrogen levels. Yoga in this phase of life helps to:
- Balance the hormones
- "Helps maintain weight, digestive health, and emotional stability."
- Manage mood and inner peace to attain a good quality of life.

Research Pointer

- A 12 weeks yoga practice session reduced menopausal, stress and depression symptoms in postmenopausal women while increasing their quality of life scores.
- Meditation was observed to increase plasma melatonin levels that resulted in improved sleep quality while Pranayama and relaxation techniques mitigated mild to moderate hot flushes in postmenopausal women.
- Yoga also helped to decrease the physiological and psychological risk factors related to cardiovascular disease.

YOGA IN ELDERLY WOMEN

Aging results in slow and steady physical and functional impairment of the organ systems. It is associated with a lot of changes in the various systems of our body. Changes in the nervous system include reduction in brain function resulting in loss of memory and cognitive abilities, along with decline in the special senses and reduced balance control. The musculoskeletal system shows changes such as decrease in muscle and bone mass resulting in reduced muscle strength and bone fragility with limited mobility. Cardiac output decreases with an increase in blood pressure and increased incidence of atherosclerosis and cardiovascular disease. The respiratory system also shows a decrease in overall function. Changes are also observed in other organ systems resulting in slowing of digestion, sleep disorders, etc.
- For older women, Yoga serves as a safe and effective way to enhance their physical and mental health.
- Yoga has an advantage of being low-impact and thus useful in women with osteoporosis or limited mobility.
- Also it can accommodate women with any level of fitness or physical ability.

Research Pointer

- Studies have reported that a regular Yoga practice of 1 hour per day is effective in controlling blood pressure in hypertensive patients. This is mediated through the restoration of baroreceptor sensitivity and regulation of the autonomic nervous function.
- Long-term practice of yoga also resulted in reduction of serum cholesterol levels, number of angina episodes and improved exercise tolerance, indicating a retardation of progression and improvement in regression of coronary atherosclerosis in patients with coronary artery disease (CAD).
- Yoga was also found to improve balance and reduce the fear of fall in elderly and thus is recommended as one of the strategies in fall prevention in the elderly.

The benefits of yoga in the elderly women are many. Yoga helps to:
- Improve flexibility, muscle strength and joint stability
- Enhance digestion
- Decrease insomnia
- Improve memory and other cognitive functions
- Decrease the risk of depression and act as a mood booster to improve the overall sense of well-being.

Point to be Noted

- It is advisable to practice Yoga under a trained teacher rather than practicing unsupervised.
- Start slow and let the body get adjusted to the daily routine practices before starting/adding any new practices.
- Perform adequate warm-up before the actual practice.

- An elderly woman may practice the same asanas as those performed by a younger woman. However, in the elderly woman, focus can be on repeating a pose than holding the same pose for a longer period of time.
- Use of support from chair or wall is recommended while performing asanas that can challenge balance.

Disclaimer

Yoga is a way of life, wherein greater benefits are reaped by following all the Ashtangas. This chapter has just covered some parts of Ashtangas, i.e., Asana, Pranayama and Dhyana.

Summary

The benefits of Yoga range from improving the function of reproductive system, helping during and after pregnancy to giving a complete workout for the mind and body. Yoga, thus serves as a complete complementary health package for women in all age groups.

ACKNOWLEDGMENTS

I would like to express my gratitude towards Ms Bhavya Amin, Ms Dwiti Soni and Ms Archana Thakur for modeling for the various yogic poses in this chapter.

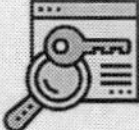

Review Questions

1. Describe the role of yoga in the pre- and postnatal phases.
2. Explain the benefits of Yoga in the various phases of a woman's life.

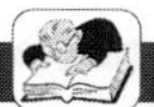

Bibliography

1. Abadibavil D, Sharifi N, Dashti S, FathiNajafi T. Effects of yoga in pregnancy on postpartum depression: A systematic review. Modern Care Journal. 2021; 18(S2): e115237.
2. Amarya S, Singh K, Sabharwal M. In: G. D'Onofrio, A. Greco, & D. Sancarlo (Eds.). Ageing Process and Physiological Changes. Gerontology; 2018.
3. Babbar S, Parks-Savage A, Chauhan S. Yoga during pregnancy: a review. American Journal of Perinatology. 2012;29(6):459-64.
4. Bhutkar M, Bhutkar P, Taware G, Surdi A. How effective is sun salutation in improving muscle strength, general body endurance and body composition? Asian Journal of Sports Medicine. 2011;2(4):259-66.
5. Boybay K, Yayan E. Effect of postpartum yoga on breastfeeding self-efficacy and Maternal Attachment in Primiparous Mothers. Breastfeeding Medicine. 2022;17(4):311-17.
6. Brown K, Koziol J, LotzMn. A Yoga-based exercise program to reduce the risk of falls in seniors: A pilot and feasibility study. Journal of Alternative and Complementary Medicine. 2008;14(5):454-57.
7. Buttner M, Brock R, O'Hara M, Stuart S. Efficacy of yoga for depressed postpartum women: A randomized controlled trial. Complementary Therapies in Clinical Practice. 2015;21(2):94-100.
8. Chikako H. Yoga for menopausal women. Journal of Yoga & Physical Therapy. 2018; 8: 285.
9. Curtis K, Weinrib A, Katz J. Systematic review of yoga for pregnant women: current status and future directions. Evidence-Based Complementary and Alternative Medicine. 2012:715942.
10. Felver C, Butzer B, Olson K, Smith I, Khalsa S. Yoga in public school improves adolescent mood and affect. Contemporary School Psychology. 2015;19(3):184-92.
11. Jahdi F, Sheikhan F, Haghani H, Sharifi B, Ghaseminejad A, Khodarahmian M, et al. Yoga during pregnancy: The effects on labor pain and delivery outcomes (A randomized controlled trial). Complementary Therapies in Clinical Practice. 2017;27:1-4.
12. Jakhotia K, Shimpi A, Rairikar S, Mhendale P, Hatekar R, Shyam A, et al. Suryanamaskar: An equivalent approach towards management of physical fitness in obese females. International Journal of Yoga. 2015;8(1):27-36.
13. Jorge M, Santaella D, Pontes I, Shiramizu V, Nascimento E, Cabral A, et al. Hatha Yoga practice decreases menopause symptoms and improves quality of life: A randomized controlled trial. Complementary Therapies in Medicine. 2016;26:128-35.
14. Keay L, Praveen D, Salam A, Rajasekhar K, Tiedemann A, Thomas V, et al. A mixed methods evaluation of yoga as a fall prevention strategy for older people in India. Pilot Feasibility Study. 2018;1;4:74.
15. Kulkarni K, Hiremath T, Swamidas S, Kottursheti I. An overview on yoga alongside its benefits in menarche and menopause. International Ayurvedic Medical Journal {online}. 2021:2225-2231.
16. Mahajan A, Reddy K, Sachdeva U. Lipid profile of coronary risk subjects following yogic lifestyle intervention. Indian Heart Journal. 1999;51(1):37-40.
17. Mallick T, Kulkarni R. The effect of Trataka, a yogic visual concentration practice, on critical flicker fusion. Journal of Alternative and Complementary Medicine. 2010; 16 (12):1265-67.
18. Manchanda S, Narang R, Reddy K, Sachdeva U, Prabhakaran D, Dharmanand S, et al. Retardation of coronary atherosclerosis with yoga lifestyle intervention. Journal of Association of Physicians India. 2000;48(7):687-94.
19. Mandal D, Ray U, Ghosh P. Differences in skeletal growth pattern of yoga practicing adolescent girls: A cross-sectional study. Journal of Ayurveda and Integrative Medicine. 2022;13:100550.
20. Mohyadin E, Ghorashi Z, Molamomanaei Z. The effect of practicing yoga during pregnancy on labor stages length, anxiety and pain: a randomized controlled trial. Journal of Complementary and Integrative Medicine. 2020;19;18(2):413-17.
21. Mullerpatan R, Agarwal B, Shetty T, Nehete G, Narasipura O. Kinematics of Suryanamaskar using three-dimensional motion capture. International Journal of Yoga. 2019;12(2):124-31.
22. Murugesan R, Govindarajulu N, Bera TK. Effect of selected yogic practices on the management of hypertension. Indian Journal of Physiology and Pharmacology. 2000;44(2):207-10.
23. Patil A, Vaidya R, Pathak S, Chauhan S, Surve S, Kokate P, et al. Yoga Therapy: The fourth dimension in the multidisciplinary management of women with polycystic ovary syndrome, a narrative review. The Indian Practitioner. 2018;71(4):45-51.
24. Raghavendra B, Singh P. Immediate effect of yogic visual concentration on cognitive performance. Journal of Traditional and Complementary Medicine. 2015; 6(1): 34-6.

25. Ram N, Venkatram P, Raghuram N, Ram A. Effect of holistic yoga program on anxiety symptoms in adolescent girls with polycystic ovarian syndrome: A randomized control trial. International Journal of Yoga. 2012;5(2):112-7.
26. Satyapriya M, Nagarathna R, Padmalatha V, Nagendra HR. Effect of integrated yoga on anxiety, depression & well being in normal pregnancy. Complement Therapies in Clinical Practice. 2013;19(4):230-6.
27. Selvaraj V, Jain V, Fabiola D, Sekar P, Babu A. Impact of yoga and exercises on polycystic ovarian syndrome risk among adolescent schoolgirls in South India Health Science Reports. 2020; 4: 3(4):e212.
28. Sengupta P. Health Impacts of Yoga and Pranayama: A State-of-the-Art Review. International Journal of Preventive Medicine. 2012;3(7):444-58.
29. Sethi J, Nagendra H, Tikhe S. Yoga improves attention and self-esteem in underprivileged girl student. Journal of Education and Health Promotion. 2013;2:55.
30. Shamanthakamani N, Raghuram N, Narendran V, Gunasheela S, Nagendra H. Efficacy of yoga on pregnancy outcome. Journal of Alternative and Complementary Medicine. 2005;11(2):237-44.
31. Sherlee J, David A. Effectiveness of yogic visual concentration (Trataka) on cognitive performance and anxiety among adolescents. Journal of Complementary and Integrative Medicine. 2020;17(3).
32. Shujuan Hu, Tao Xu, Xianwang Wang. Yoga as an exercise prescription for the pregnancy or postpartum period: recent advances and perspective. Yangtze Medicine. 2021;5(3): 157-70.
33. Swathi P, Bhat R, Saoji A. Effect of Trataka (Yogic Visual Concentration) on the performance in the corsi-block tapping task: a repeated measures study. Frontiers in Psychology. 2021;12:773049.
34. Talwadkar S, Jagannathan A, Raghuram N. Effect of trataka on cognitive functions in the elderly. International Journal of Yoga. 2014; 7(2): 96-103.
35. Thakur D, Singh S, Tripathi M, Lufang. Effect of yoga on polycystic ovarian syndrome: A systematic review. Journal of Bodywork and Movement Therapies. 2021; 27: 281-86.
36. Vaze N, Joshi S. Yoga and menopausal transition. Journal of Midlife Health. 2010;1(2):56-8.
37. Vhavle SP, Rao R, Manjunath NK. Comparison of yoga versus physical exercise on executive function, attention, and working memory in adolescent schoolchildren: A randomized controlled trial. International Journal of Yoga. 2019;12(2):172-73.

Multiple Choice Questions (MCQs)

To test your understanding and recall of key concepts.

1. **What is the recommended time to practice Suryanamaskar for maximum benefits?**
   A. Afternoon
   B. Evening
   C. Morning
   D. Night
2. **Which Yogic practice involves focusing on a candle flame to improve cognitive functions?**
   A. Pranayama
   B. Trataka
   C. Suryanamaskar
   D. Viparit Karni
3. **Why are forward-bending asanas contraindicated during menstruation?**
   A. They may cause vascular congestion and increased bleeding
   B. They may reduce pelvic flexibility
   C. They may restrict blood circulation to the lower limbs
   D. They maybe too physically exerting
4. **How does Yoga help manage polycystic ovarian syndrome (PCOS)?**
   A. By increasing estrogen levels and decreasing progesterone levels
   B. By reducing cortisol levels and balancing the HPA axis
   C. By improving testosterone secretion
   D. By stimulating rapid weight loss
5. **A pregnant woman has complains of back pain and is referred for safe Yoga practices. Which of the following should be recommended?**
   A. Tadasana and Marjariasana
   B. Bhujangasana and Halasana
   C. Kapalbhati and Naukasana
   D. Paschimotanasana and Uttanasana
6. **A postmenopausal woman wants to reduce the risk of osteoporosis and improve balance. Which combination of Yoga practices would be most beneficial?**
   A. Utkatasana and Shavasana
   B. Tadasana and Viparitkarni
   C. Trikonasana and Veerbhadrasana
   D. Naukasana and Kapalbhati
7. **Evaluate the following scenario: A woman in her first trimester wants to start Yoga but has no prior experience. What advice should be given?**
   A. Begin with intense Asanas like Suryanamaskar to build endurance
   B. Avoid Yoga completely until after delivery
   C. Start with basic poses and progress under the supervision of a trained Physiotherapist/Instructor
   D. Focus only on Trataka for cognitive benefits
8. **While designing a safe Yoga regimen for an elderly woman with reduced balance and mild osteoporosis, which elements should be included?**
   A. Balancing poses without support, Kapalbhati, and Trikonasana
   B. Supported poses like Tadasana and gentle Pranayama
   C. Intense practices to improve flexibility quickly
   D. Focus on prone poses to strengthen back muscles

ANSWERS

1. C	2. B	3. A	4. B	5. A
6. C	7. C	8. B		

Section 8

Newer Concepts

Section Outline

Chapter **35**

Evidence-based Practice in Women's Health

Sakshi P Arora, Waqar M Naqvi

LEARNING OBJECTIVES

At the end of the chapter, the reader will be able to:

- Understand the concept of evidence-based practice.
- Identify and explore evidence-based practice.
- Learn the different models to implicate evidence-based practice.
- Perceive the five-step process in evidence-based practice.
- Comprehend the key examination strategies expected to find evidences.
- Recognize different degrees of evidence and their comparing clinical approach methods.
- Assess the reliability, validity, and applicability on the basis of evidence.

CHAPTER OUTLINE

INTRODUCTION

This chapter advances the basic, critical, reflective, objective, and scientific approach of Physiotherapy (PT) to women's health. Practicing Physiotherapists irrespective of traditional or advanced settings must undertake the strong extensive practice in women's health and should implicate this knowledge to an assortment of phases that a woman goes through during her fertile age.

PT focuses on the treatment implication of mobility which assists in restoring, maximizing, and maintaining physical function, strength, motion, and independence for a complete well-being.

A complete evaluation and well formulated exercise protocol is required by a physiotherapist to restrain health problems in females throughout life. Various techniques and exercises are available which are specific to conditions like training of muscles, pattern of recruitment of muscles, strengthening of PFM, endurance training, mobility, strength, and flexibility training, mobility with movements, soft tissue mobilization, electrical modalities like therapeutic ultrasound (US), stimulation, etc., for reducing stiffness and pain.

The content in this chapter focuses on the expression of understanding and exploring the concept of evidence-based practice. The clinical experience of the therapist helps in ruling out the diagnosis right but the therapeutic specifications prioritize the patient's preference on gains from therapeutic knowledge and the research evidences build a fundamental proof of efficacy of the therapeutic procedure in the condition. Integrating the concerns, the evidence-based practice is recognized using different models. The methods to locate and apply key evidences with corresponding clinical category has been briefly described while mandating evidence-based on validity, reliability, and applicability.

CONCEPT OF EVIDENCE-BASED PRACTICE

Evidenced-based practice (EBP) is applying or implementation of systematic findings obtained through research into day-to-day practice of care which ultimately enhances the benefits of decisions made clinically. EBP basically includes integration of the relevant literature with the clinical findings and improve its application with skills according to the unique requirement of patient and their preferences personally. Bringing EBP into practice means limiting all the outdated therapeutic processes and opting for scientifically supported and effective methods meeting requirements of each patient. Physiotherapists applying EBP in daily practice must use their skills for assessing the applicability of recent advances in certain population of patients.

As physiotherapists, therapeutic care of the patient should raise the query about the implication of evidence in day-to-day practice. For instance, if there was a patient of dysmenorrhea, the line of treatment to be followed would be nonsteroidal anti-inflammatory drug for pain reduction but as physiotherapy progresses the therapeutic implication puts forth an evidence of reduced pain during menses following isometric contraction of pelvic floor muscles. The researchers identify the research question, test the validity and applicability of therapeutic muscle training and explore an effective evidence which is favorable for patient's preference as shown in **Figure 35.1**.

The steps to follow EBP as described in **Figure 35.2** and **Table 35.1** are:

1. Ask a valid question to the patient specifying their activities of daily living (ADLs) as the foremost important goal of physiotherapy is accomplishing independent ADLs. The question should be raised for the application of the existing technique in terms of the extent of effect obtained and the application of updated evidence in terms of the availability of technique and instruments for its effective application.

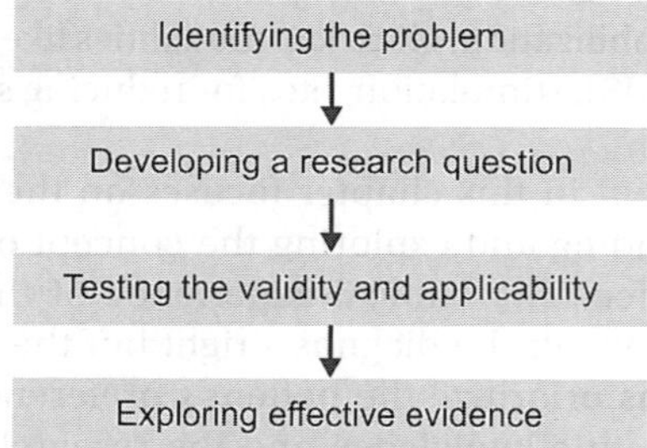

Fig. 35.1: Identified concept of evidence-based practice.

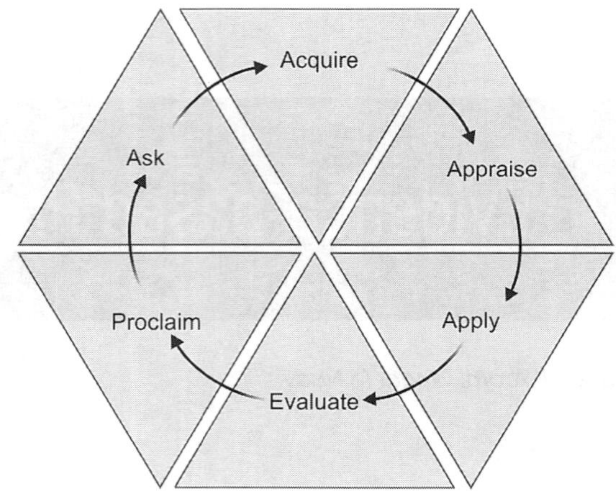

Fig. 35.2: Steps to follow the process of evidence-based practice.

Table 35.1: Key points to understand the concept of evidence-based practice.

Ask	Patient's preference and therapist's availability of resources
Acquire	Search for the valid associated literature
Appraise	Sort, review, and criticize valid and feasible literature
Apply	Integrate the updated technique with the patient's preference
Evaluate	Assess the outcome of the applied technique
Proclaim	Disseminate the results obtained

2. Acquire the condition and goal-oriented evidence. Formulate the question for implication and use the associated keywords for conducting a literature search.
3. Appraise the associated literature by thoroughly critiquing the findings implying itself with the patient's preferences.
4. Apply the findings of literature to the patient's finding and integrate the evidence with the therapeutic techniques, patient preference, and therapeutic expertise.
5. Evaluate the pre and post-treatment findings to review the implication of the research evidence using different valid and feasible outcome measures.
6. Proclaim the results obtained and summarize the effectiveness of the research evidence in a specific condition considering the supportive data and practice feasibility.

Identify and Explore Evidence-based Practice

EBP is about exploring the applicability of literature into decision-making and clinical practice **(Fig. 35.3)**. The goal of EBP is to utilize the relevant and effective evidences leading to decision as per patient requirement. As the availability of evidences evolve from research, EBP evolves from clinical skills expertly enhanced with research. It covers the clinical expertise of a physiotherapist with the preference of the patient. The EBP application benefits can be categorized using following factors for maximum outcomes:

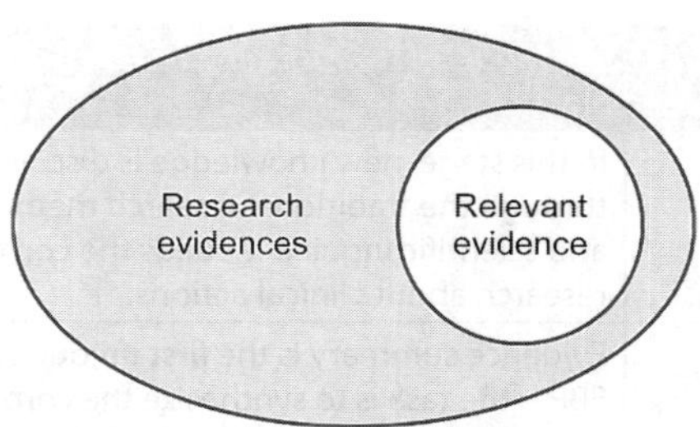

Fig. 35.3: Exploring and identifying the relevant evidence.

- Specific condition or outcome associated keywords
- Searching valid databases
- Considering the limitation of the application of the conclusive results of literature
- Exploring the effectiveness of the therapeutic assessment, intervention, and outcomes in similar population.

Clinical Experience Specification

During a patient encounter, the clinician goes through a thorough history of the present illness and past history for ruling out the causative factor of the diseased condition. It is recommended that the therapist go through a wide range of questions while turning their implicit knowledge gaps into explicit questions. **Table 35.2** and **Figure 35.4** show the clinical steps to be followed in clinical work.

Table 35.2: Clinical steps followed in the six aspects of clinical work.

Clinical evidence	Gather positive clinical findings and interpret them properly
Diagnosis	Follow a thorough physical and diagnostic assessment to derive the diagnosis
Prognosis	Identify the extent of injury and the duration and efficacy of the intervention applied
Therapy	Apply scientifically more effective treatment for prolonged efficacy
Prevention	Screen the limitation and reduce the risk factors
Education	Explore the EBP for rooting an effective concept in the clinical setting

Patient Preference Specification

The patient's preference of well-being is a key part of the evidence-based process **(Fig. 35.5)**. As described till now, the guiding principle of EBP refers to the patient-centered aims and goals of the treatment. The most applicable literature shall correspond to the outcomes expected by the patient from the treatment. The formulation and incorporation of the treatment methodologies shall prioritize the cultural considerations, needs, and values of the patient while working on the application of associated evidence.

Research Evidence Specification

Research is a rigorous assessment of the validity, reliability, and feasibility of the novel assessment techniques, interventions, and outcome measures in different conditions and populations. These findings encompass an all-dimension coverage of the applicability of research which is supported or contrasted by similar studies formulating the limitation of the application on the grounds of the available literature. The research evidence specifies the barriers, limitations, and the future scope for exploring and implicating the best expected outcome of the novelty.

DIFFERENT MODELS TO IMPLICATE EVIDENCE-BASED PRACTICE

Stetler's Model

The Stetler model of implication of research **(Table 35.3)**:

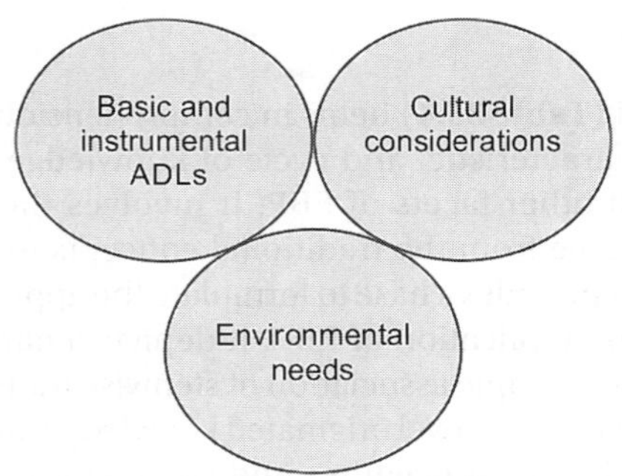

Fig. 35.5: Patient-centered specifications of EBP.

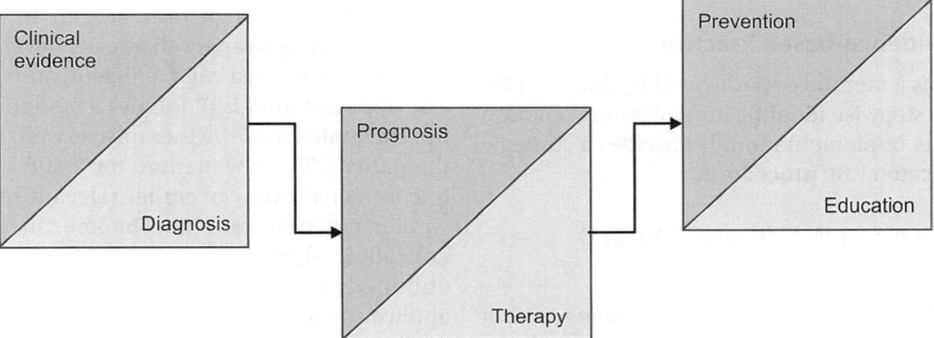

Fig. 35.4: Stepwise six clinical aspects of evidence-based practice.

Table 35.3: Five phases of Stetler's model.	
Phase I: Preparation	Purpose, context and sources of research evidence
Phase II: Validation	Credibility of findings and potential for/detailed qualifiers of application
Phase III: Comparative evaluation/decision making	Comparative evaluation/decision making—synthesis and decisions/recommendations per criteria of applicability
Phase IV: Translation/application	Translation/application—operational definition of use/actions for change
Phase V: Evaluation	Evaluation

Salient Features

- Assists therapists to evaluate the utility of the findings of the research along with available relevant literature that can be implied in clinical practice.
- Assesses the utility of an evidence to enroute changes at the organizational level and at therapist level.
- Enhances the critical and reflective application of evidences.
- Sets usage of research as its base and first step as evidence-informed practice.
- Paves a pathway to link the association of research utility with evidence-informed practice.
- Thus, as per the Stetler model, summation of research with evidence-informed practice demonstrates the applicability of evidence.

ACE Star

This model **(Table 35.4)** helps in comprehension of nature, pattern, characteristic, and cycle of knowledge which are linked with other facets of EBP. It involves the evolution of care ranging from the traditional concepts to the recent advances. It provides a base to formulate the approaches and processes of implication of EBP. It depicts a parsimonious implication of simple association of stepwise transformation of knowledge into a novel originated knowledge into practice. It includes known procedures and enhances the authentic applicability of EBP. It utilizes the proven scientific literature with the norms of EBP and provides a base for assessing and implementing the formally accepted literature in EBP.

Iowa Model of Evidence-based Practice

It was established as a method or pathway **(Fig. 35.6)** to EBP demonstrating the stepwise identification of issues, solution for research, and its implementation. It provides a strategic guidance for implicated EBP procedure.

THE 5-STEP PROCESS IN EVIDENCE-BASED PRACTICE

1. **Ask:** Phrasing the requirement of information in terms of causation, diagnosis, prevention, therapy, and prognosis into a valid outcome.

Table 35.4: ACE Star Model of transforming research evidence into evidence-based practice.	
Discovery research	In this stage, new knowledge is discovered through the traditional research methodologies and scientific inquiry. It builds the corpus of research about clinical actions.
Evidence summary	Evidence summary is the first unique step in EBP—the task is to synthesize the corpus of research knowledge into a single, meaningful statement of the state of the application.
Translation to guidelines	The transformation of evidence summaries into actual practice requires two stages: translation of evidence into practice recommendations and integration into practice.
Practice integration	This step involves changing both individual and organizational practices through formal and informal channels. Major aspects addressed in this stage are factors that affect individual and organizational rate of adoption of innovation and factors that affect integration of the change into sustainable systems.
Process/outcome evaluation	In EBP, a broad array of endpoints and outcomes are evaluated. These include evaluation of the impact of EBP on patient health outcomes, provider and patient satisfaction, efficacy, efficiency, economic analysis, and health status impact.

2. **Find supportive literature as evidence:** Tracing the valid literature in terms of effective outcome.
3. **Critically review and appraise the evidence:** Appraisal of the literature obtained for validity and reliability, applicability and impact.
4. **Integrate reviewed evidence with clinical expertise and patient's preference:** Critical analysis of evidence should integrate its efficacy with an expert skill and preference of the patient in terms of personal and instrumental requirements.
5. **Evaluate:** Assessing the efficiency and effectiveness in implementing the first four steps to improve the outcome for the next encounter.

NAVIGATION AND MAPPING TO LOCATE EVIDENCE

EBP is the use of prior research in a systematic and transparent way to apply an already developed evidence into clinical practice in a valid, efficient, and accessible manner. The application of EBP follows a systematic module as per the convenience of the therapist as well as the preference of the patient. The key method for justifying the outcomes is to conduct a review of earlier relevant studies and shortlist similar outcome criteria. The shortlisted data should be critically analyzed and reviewed for integrating the evidence obtained. The obtained evidence is then evaluated on application to the patient's preference.

This section highlights some opportunities and challenges in applying EBP to physiotherapy practice with specific

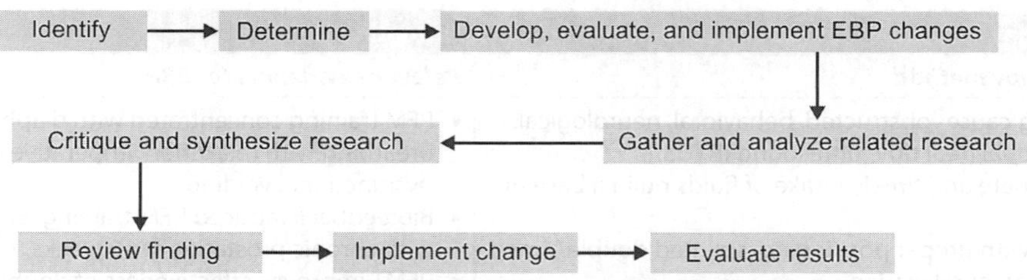

Fig. 35.6: Steps of the Iowa model for evidence-based practice.

conditions. A transparent and systematic approach is required to prove and bring an optimally utilized EBP design into practice.

EVIDENCES AND THEIR CURRENT CLINICAL REVIEW CLASSIFICATIONS

Stress Urinary Incontinence

Table 35.5 shows the traditional physiotherapy method and evidences for stress urinary incontinence.

Overactive Bladder Syndrome

Table 35.6 shows the traditional physiotherapy method and evidences for overactive bladder syndrome.

Overflow Incontinence

Table 35.7 shows the traditional physiotherapy method and evidences for overflow incontinence.

RELIABILITY, VALIDITY, AND APPLICABILITY ON THE BASIS OF EVIDENCE

Evidences obtained vary widely in terms of using appropriate outcome measures. For shortlisting the more implicit finding, validity of the outcome is referred. It basically determines the consistency of the results obtained so as to uniformly derive the conclusion of the research question. More substantial design of research, methods, and techniques guarantees that the review of results is unbiased and outcomes are more pertinent. Predisposition alludes to purposeful and unexpected errors in the review configuration, research techniques, data assortment, and results reported during a research.

Reliability of the outcome determines the best possible way to reduce the possible errors for consistent results. It demands a thorough perspicacity of bias categories, precariousness of error, and the influences of these biases on results of a research project. Implementation is demonstrated as per

Table 35.5: Traditional physiotherapy method and evidences for stress urinary incontinence.

Traditional physiotherapy method	*Relevant evidences for EBP*
• Education on pelvic floor muscle (PFM) anatomy and physiology, role of PFM, pathophysiology, identification of risk factors. • Fluid and dietary modification, fibrous or laxative supplements to prevent straining-splinting, defecation dynamics • Exercise modification to lower the impact on PFM. • Pelvic floor muscle training to improve endurance, strength, co-activation, and timing of contraction of lower abdominals added on with or without biofeedback (RTUS, EMG) or 'The Knack' • Bladder neck support with tampon/contiform/pessary • Weight loss	• Therapist supervised and guided PFM training protocol are found to be more effective as compared to self-administered programs. • Losing weight is to be considered a first line treatment to reduce prevalence of urinary incontinence. • Applying PFM training is more beneficial than no training or placebo training for women. • Vaginal cones and E-stim have positive impact on urinary incontinence but PFM training is a more effective method of treatment.

Table 35.6: Traditional physiotherapy method and evidences for overactive bladder syndrome.

Traditional physiotherapy method	*Relevant evidences for EBP*
• Education • Postvoid residual—determine cause • Check/treat bowel dysfunction • Fluid modification/timing • PFM with obliterated trigger points • Improve endurance and strength with urethral lift or closure • Rectified technique of co-activation of muscle (lower abdominal wall) using pattern of motor control for bracing of upper abdominal wall improving altered activation pattern. • Calming and retraining of bladder • Neuromodulation/transcutaneous electrical nerve stimulation (TENS) • Weight loss	• Applying PFM training is more beneficial than no training or placebo training for women and should be considered as primary method of treatment for all age women. • Training of bladder has an immediate impact. • Bladder and PFM training are to be considered as primary methods for treating conservatively. • Training bladder musculature could be equivalent to administration of antimuscarinic drug for overactive detrusor muscle with comparatively negligible side effects. • Training of PFM is more effective then administration of oxybutynin drug.

Table 35.7: Traditional physiotherapy method and evidences for overflow incontinence.

Traditional physiotherapy method	*Relevant evidences for EBP*
• Determine underlying cause–obstructed, behavioral, neurological. • Pre and postvoid residual [real time ultrasound (RTUS)]. • Education on appropriate and timely intake of fluids build a base of good bladder habits. • Dynamics of voiding with proper positioning, splinted double/timed voids, nullified straining or relaxation. • Training of PFM as per evaluation findings. • PFM compression combined sequence of breathing with visual feedbacks for affected relaxation. • Normalize resting tone, decrease pain. • Attain complete or consistent PFM relaxation. • Strengthening and training for underactive muscles. • Diaphragmatic breathing exercises for strategic relaxation.	• PFM training concentrated with diaphragmatic pattern of breathing with relaxation: imperative effects in children with dysfunctional voiding. • Biofeedback induced PFM training: Enhances strength in men with chronic prostatitis at 10 weeks. • PFMT improves effectiveness of double voids—in women with recurrent urinary tract infection (UTI). • PFMT with electrotherapeutic modality.

the applicability to a certain clinical setting and requirement of patient. This is where clinical expertise and professional judgement play a key role while implementing EBP.

Therefore, EBP is considered as a crystal category framework for constructing and putting forth summarized evidences which offers a stepwise systematic perspective for building recommendations in the clinical settings. It is referred to as the most accepted tool for assessing and implementing the evidence quality. It assists in assessing the intensity of requirement of patients, recognition and appraisal of key elements which directs the recommendation strength and direction which ultimately vitalizes the decision-making.

Summary

The main aim of women's health physiotherapy is to assess and plan a specific therapeutic line of treatment according to the different conditions and preferences per se for women of all age groups, using therapeutic skilled knowledge and clinical findings. Various physiological and hormonal alterations have an impact on social, psychological, and physical well-being of an individual. The methods to locate and apply key evidences with corresponding clinical category has been briefly described while mandating evidence-based on validity, reliability, and applicability. EBP is considered as a crystal category framework for constructing and putting forth the summarized evidences which offers a stepwise systematic perspective for building recommendations in the clinical settings. It is referred to as the most accepted tool for assessing and implementing the evidence quality. It assists in assessing the intensity of requirement of patients, recognition and appraisal of key elements which directs the recommendation strength and direction which ultimately vitalizes the decision-making.

CLINICAL EXAMPLES

- Ms V, a 33-year-old pregnant woman was referred with a diagnosis of "low back pain," that became severe at 22-weeks' gestation. She reports left lumbar/thoracic, right anterior rib/pectoral, and cervical symptoms, which are worsening as the pregnancy progresses. Pain is severely limiting her daily activities both at home and in the community. She has difficulty climbing stairs, grocery shopping, doing laundry, and other household chores. She is awakened at night by pain and also reports lower extremity numbness at night. She is a single mother of a 6-year-old son. Pertinent medical history includes: weight gain of 10 kg with her previous pregnancy; C-section delivery. No systemic medical conditions or medications other than prenatal vitamins.
  - Identify the short-term and long-term goals for the least complications.
  - Formulate a management plan and support it with the recent advances to follow evidence-based practice.
  - Correlate the recent advances with valid rationale supporting it.
- Mrs W, a 69-year-old woman with an 11-year history of menopause. She experiences low strength and endurance while performing her activities of daily living. She was a bank employee before retirement. She often complains of neck and upper back pain disturbing her sleep and is more in intensity during the nights. She also reports constipation and straining for evacuation. She is much less active with social and community activities as a result of this problem.
  - Identify the short-term and long-term goals.
  - Formulate a management plan and support it with the recent advances as per the Iowa Model of Evidence-Based Practice.
  - Correlate the recent advances with valid rationale supporting it.

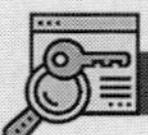

Review Questions

1. Describe the concept of evidence-based practice.
2. Write a short note on identifying and exploring evidence-based practice.
3. Describe any two models of evidence-based practice.
4. Write a brief explanation on the research methods needed to locate evidence.
5. Distinguish between various levels of evidence and corresponding clinical evidences of labor.

Bibliography

1. AlKetbi H, Hegazy F, Alnaqbi A, Shousha T. Evidence-based practice by physiotherapists in UAE: Investigating behavior, attitudes, awareness, knowledge and barriers. PLoS ONE. 2021;16(6):e0253215.
2. Alqahtani MM, Kashoo FZ, Ahmad F. Current scenario of evidence-based practice and rationale of preferred approach in stroke rehabilitation among physiotherapists in Saudi Arabia: A cross-sectional survey. Saudi J Health Sci. 2018;7(1):53.
3. Burns A. LibGuides: Cabarrus College of Health Sciences Library: IOWA Model [Internet]. [cited 2022 Jul 31]. Available from: https://cabarruscollege.libguides.com/c.php?g=465666&p=5283295
4. da Silva TM, Costa L da CM, Garcia AN, Costa LOP. What do physical therapists think about evidence-based practice? A systematic review. Man Ther. 2015;20(3):388-401.
5. Duff J, Cullen L, Hanrahan K, Steelman V. Determinants of an evidence-based practice environment: an interpretive description. Implement Sci Commun. 2020;1(1):85.
6. Dumoulin C, Cacciari LP, Hay-Smith EJC. Pelvic floor muscle training versus no treatment, or inactive control treatments, for urinary incontinence in women. Cochrane Database Syst Rev. 2018;2018(10):CD005654.
7. Fernández-Domínguez JC, De Pedro-Gómez JE, Jiménez-López R, Romero-Franco N, Bays Moneo AB, Oliva-Pascual-Vaca Á, et al. Physiotherapists' evidence-based practice profiles by HS-EBP questionnaire in Spain: A cross-sectional normative study. PLoS One. 2022;17(6):e0269460.
8. Frantz JM, Rowe M. Developing reflection and research skills through blogging in an evidence-based practice postgraduate physiotherapy module. Afr J Health Prof Educ. 2013;5(1):3-7.
9. Ghaderi F, Oskouei AE. Physiotherapy for women with stress urinary incontinence: A review article. J Phys Ther Sci. 2014;26(9):1493-9.
10. Kang H, Hong GRS. Effect of muscle strength training on urinary incontinence and physical function: a randomized controlled trial in long-term care facilities. J Korean Acad Nurs. 2015;45(1):35-45.
11. Purnell M. Health Library: Evidence-Based Practice: 5 steps of Evidence Based Practice - Overview [Internet]. [cited 2022 Jul 31]. Available from: https://library.health.nt.gov.au/EBP/overview
12. Richardson PE. David Sackett and the birth of evidence based medicine: how to practice and teach EBM. BMJ. 2015;350.
13. Rivera CE. Core and lumbopelvic stabilization in runners. Phys Med Rehabil Clin N Am. 2016;27(1):319-37.
14. Sampath KK, Darlow B, Tumilty S, Shillito W, Hanses M, Devan H, et al. Barriers and facilitators experienced by osteopaths in implementing a biopsychosocial (BPS) framework of care when managing people with musculoskeletal pain—a mixed methods systematic review. BMC Health Serv Res. 2021;21(1):695.
15. Segal NA, Williams GN, Davis MC, Wallace RB, Mikesky AE. Efficacy of blood flow-restricted, low-load resistance training in women with risk factors for symptomatic knee osteoarthritis. PM R. 2015;7(4):376-84.
16. Stetler model of evidence-based practice | NCCMT [Internet]. [cited 2022 Jul 31]. Available from: https://www.nccmt.ca/knowledge-repositories/search/83
17. Worum H, Lillekroken D, Roaldsen KS, Ahlsen B, Bergland A. Physiotherapists' perceptions of challenges facing evidence-based practice and the importance of environmental empowerment in fall prevention in the municipality—a qualitative study. BMC Geriatr. 2020;20(1):432.

Multiple Choice Questions (MCQs)

To test your understanding and recall of key concepts.

1. A 50-year-old woman with overactive bladder syndrome shows limited response to conservative management. According to the Iowa model, which is the next logical step?

A. Perform a surgical evaluation
B. Recommend antimuscarinic medication immediately
C. Conduct a literature review to identify additional effective interventions
D. Cease all ongoing interventions and refer to a urologist

2. Which exercise is most appropriate for a patient with stress urinary incontinence?

A. High-impact aerobic exercises
B. Pelvic floor muscle training with "The Knack" technique
C. Heavy weightlifting to improve core strength
D. Static stretching of the pelvic floor muscles

3. Which of the following aspect is NOT a key part of patient-centered evidence-based practice?

A. Patient preferences
B. Clinical expertise
C. Research evidence
D. Physician's preferences

4. A 60-year-old male with chronic pelvic pain syndrome (CPPS) presents with high pelvic floor muscle tone and significant stress levels. His past treatments with medication and physical therapy, focusing on strengthening have been ineffective. Based on the latest evidence, what is the most appropriate course of action?

A. Switch to biofeedback and relaxation-focused pelvic floor physical therapy
B. Introduce high-intensity interval training for general physical conditioning
C. Implement a surgical intervention to address the pain source
D. Continue existing strengthening exercises and add electrical stimulation

5. A physiotherapy department is considering integrating evidence-based practice more systematically. According to the ACE Star Model, which step is most critical for translating evidence summaries into clinical practice?

A. Practice integration through education and formal adoption of guidelines
B. Discovery research to establish new clinical knowledge
C. Process/outcome evaluation to measure patient satisfaction
D. Validation of findings through comparative trials

ANSWERS

1. C	2. B	3. D	4. A	5. A

Chapter 36

Male Pelvic Floor Physical Therapy

✍ *Smita Amit Mehta*

LEARNING OBJECTIVES

At the end of the chapter, the reader will be able to:

- Understand male pelvic floor (PF) structures and their contribution to PF dysfunction.
- Apply differential diagnosis in male PF dysfunction.
- Gain awareness of contributing factors to male PF dysfunction.
- Describe musculoskeletal treatment approach for male PF dysfunction.

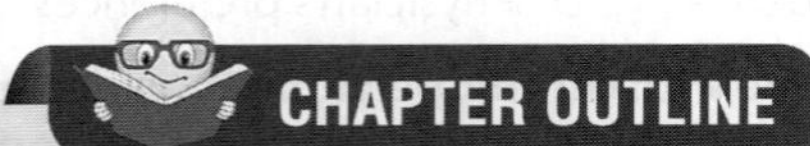

CHAPTER OUTLINE

- Introduction
- Anatomy and physiology of the male pelvis
  - Relevant anatomy/physiology
  - Male reproductive system
  - Male sexual function
  - Nerve supply
  - Blood supply
  - Pelvic floor muscles in males
- Common male pelvic floor conditions
  - Pelvic floor function related conditions
  - Pain related conditions
  - Other pelvic floor conditions
- Physical therapy evaluation and examination
  - History
  - Examination
- Physical therapy treatment
  - Physical therapy management

INTRODUCTION

Anyone who has pelvic floor (PF), can have PF dysfunction. The dysfunction can occur at any age and in any gender. Though PF conditions/dysfunctions are more common in women, men can also have PF conditions. PF issues can:

- Reduce function
- Lower the quality of life
- Negatively affect self-esteem
- Cause sleep disturbances
- Increase chances of anxiety/depression
- Increase chances of falls (related to nocturia)

This chapter is the introduction to male pelvic floor physical therapy (PFPT) and goal is to improve awareness regarding these conditions. Internal PF muscle assessment and manual therapy requires in-person training.

ANATOMY AND PHYSIOLOGY OF THE MALE PELVIS

Relevant Anatomy/Physiology

For detailed information please refer to anatomy textbook.

Skeletal Anatomy

Male pelvic cavity is longer, narrower and with tighter fascia compared to female pelvic cavity.

Male urinary system consists of kidneys, ureters, bladder, urethra, and penis **(Fig. 36.1)**.

- Male urethra is longer (18–20 cm) than female urethra (3–4 cm). Longer urethra helps with continence. Male urethra is part of urologic and reproductive system. It extends from bladder neck to glans penis. It passes through prostate and the penile shaft. Prostatic urethra angulates at about 35°.

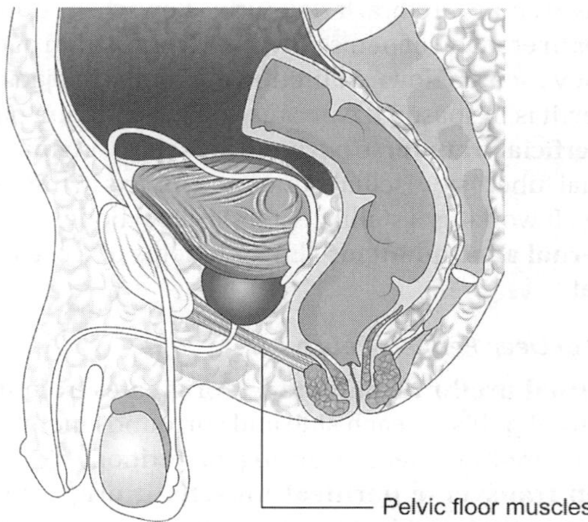

Fig. 36.1: Male urinary system *(For color version, see Plate 9)*.

- The detrusor muscle (bladder wall) is thicker in male as greater pressure is needed to empty the bladder through the longer urethra. Prostate gland provides continence but when enlarged, can cause urethral restrictions. Anatomical variations, lower urinary tract cells difference, sex hormones difference in both sexes influence the PF function.

Male urinary continence mechanism is maintained by detrusor, trigone and urethral sphincter muscles.

Sphincter Mechanisms

- **Proximal urethral sphincter:** Internal or bladder neck or Rhabdo sphincter-bladder neck continues as prostatic urethra. In females, the bladder neck and urethra are connected to anterior vaginal wall, making area mobile and subject to injury.
- **Distal urethral sphincter:** External sphincter

Urothelium: Inner lining of urinary system plays important role in immunity and acts as sensory organ. It transmits physical and chemical stresses to afferent nerves and hence plays important role in overactive bladder syndrome, painful bladder syndrome (interstitial cystitis) and bacterial infection. Shorter urethra and effect of estrogen on urothelium makes female more susceptible to urinary tract infections and men are less prone to urinary tract infection.

Male Reproductive System

It consists of the scrotum, testes, spermatic cord, epididymis, ductus deference, ejaculatory ducts, seminal vesicles, Cowper's glands, prostate, urethra, penis.

Besides containing erectile tissues, penis also gives way to urethra. Urethra is the common pathway for sperm, sperm related secretions and urine.

Primary function of prostate glands

- Produce portion of content of semen
- Assist in ejaculation of semen
- Act as a muscular valve

Male Sexual Function

Pelvic floor muscle plays an important role in male sexual cycle. The male superficial pelvic floor musculature (bulbocavernosus and ischiocavernosus) works together to create increased intracavernous pressure by limiting venous return, resulting in an erection. Ejaculation is created by rhythmic contractions of the bulbocavernosus muscle.

Phases of Sexual Cycle

- **Erection:**
  - *Excitement phase:* Stimuli such as visual, olfactory or imaginative can activate arousal. Sacral parasympathetic system gets activated and causes vasodilation. Superficial perineal muscles contract to keep blood in penis. Erection is vascular but it is maintained by superficial PF muscles.
  - *Plateau phase:* Besides increased blood flow, parasympathetic system stimulates secretion from seminal vesicles, prostate, and Cowper's glands.
- **Ejaculation-orgasm phase:** Rhythmic contraction of smooth muscles causes seminal emission. It depends on sympathetic nerve supply. Rhythmic contraction of superficial perineal muscle contraction ejects semen.
- **Ejaculation:** Semen is expelled through the penis.

Male testicles start inside the abdomen and descend from the abdominal cavity to the scrotum through the inguinal canal. Inguinal hernia is more common in males than females. If that area does not close well or if it is weak then it can cause hernia. Female inguinal canal is stronger due to surrounding ligaments. Activities that increase intra-abdominal pressure like heavy lifting, coughing, sports activities can lead to hernia.

Autonomic nervous system and superficial pelvic floor muscles play important role in sexual cycle.

Nerve Supply

- **Autonomic nervous system:** Sympathetic from T10-L2 and parasympathetic from S2–4.
- **Somatic nerves:** Pudendal nerve (S2–4) for pelvic floor muscles. It has three branches—inferior rectal, perineal and dorsal nerve of penis.
- **Ilioinguinal nerve (L1):** It is a motor and sensory nerve. Motor supply to abdominals and sensory supply to lower abdomen, proximal medial thigh, lumbar skin, base of penis and scrotum. Adhesions or scars from hernia repair, inguinal hernia, appendectomy, malalignment, heavy lifting and prolonged coughing can cause dysfunction.
- **Iliohypogastric nerve (T12 and L1):** It is a motor and sensory nerve. Motor innervation is for lower abdomen area and sensory supply is to pubic area. Dysfunction causes are same as for ilioinguinal nerve.
- **Genitofemoral nerve (L1 and L2):** It is a motor and sensory nerve. Motor supply is to cremaster muscle, sensory supply is to the scrotum, femoral triangle and upper medial thigh. Adhesions/scars in hernia repair, appendectomy, psoas abscess, tight clothing and bicycling can cause dysfunction.

- Testicle nerve supply is from T10-L2, so it is important to consider thoracic-lumbar junction area for source of scrotum pain. Scrotum is continuation of anterior abdominal wall with continuation of fascia of abdomen and pelvic cavity. Anterior abdominal wall is another source of pain in scrotum area.

Pudendal neuralgia: Prolonged cycling, constipation, certain sports, fall on buttocks, fitness exercises, pelvic radiation, entrapment in scar adhesions can cause dysfunction. Symptoms may include ejaculatory pain, unilateral or bilateral scrotal/testicular pain, perianal, rectal pressure or "golf ball sensation in rectum" and pain in suprapubic area. Centralization of symptoms is observed with chronicity.

Blood Supply

In males, pelvic blood supply is through internal iliac artery, external iliac artery and femoral artery. Dorsal artery is a branch of pudendal artery which is the branch of internal iliac artery. Dorsal artery of penis is important for blood flow for sexual function.

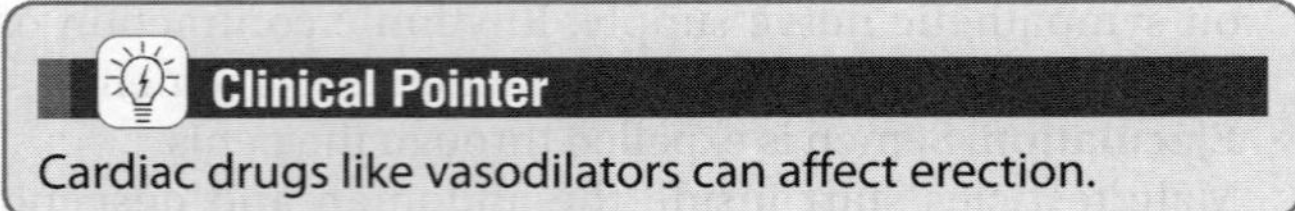

Pelvic Floor Muscles in Males

Figure 36.2 shows the pelvic floor muscles in males.

Layer 1 or Superficial

- **Ischiocavernosus:** It originates from ischial tuberosity, ramus and inserts in crus of penis. It is also known as "Erector penis" as it helps with penile rigidity.
- **Bulbospongiosus or bulbocavernosus:** It originates from perineal body, midline raphe and inserts in perineal membrane, corpus cavernosum. It relaxes during voiding, helps to empty urethra. It stops urine flow when contracts. It helps in erection of penis. Rhythmic contraction of it helps to move semen down in urethra and helps in ejaculation. When it is in spasm, it can cause postejaculation pain.
- **Superficial transverse perineal muscle:** It originates from ischial tuberosity, ischial ramus and inserts in the perineal body. It works as a stabilizer for perineal body.
- **External anal sphincter (EAS):** It helps to close the anal canal.

Layer 2 or Deep Perineal Pouch

- **External urethral sphincter:** It originates from inferior ramus of pubis on each side and surrounds membranous part of urethra. It relaxes during micturition.
- **Deep transverse perineal muscle:** It originates from ischial ramus and inserts on perineal body. It stabilizes perineal body along with superficial transverse perineal muscle.

Layer 3 or Pelvic Diaphragm

- **Levator ani (pubococcygeus/puborectalis, iliococcygeus, ischiococcygeus):** It originates from posterior aspect of pubic bone, tendinous arch, ischial spine and inserts on perineal membrane, perineal body, sides of anal canal and anococcygeal ligament. Deep pelvic diaphragm muscles support pelvic organs, maintain anorectal angle and external anal sphincter. During defecation, puborectalis relaxes.
- **Coccygeus:** It originates from ischial spine, sacrospinous ligament and inserts on lateral part of coccyx, sacral border. It helps to support pelvic organs, pulls coccyx forward.
- **Hip rotators** (obturator internus and piriformis) form pelvic walls.

PF Muscle Functions

- **Provide continence:** Bladder/bowel continence
- **Support pelvic organs:** Bladder and rectum
- Dynamic stabilization of spine

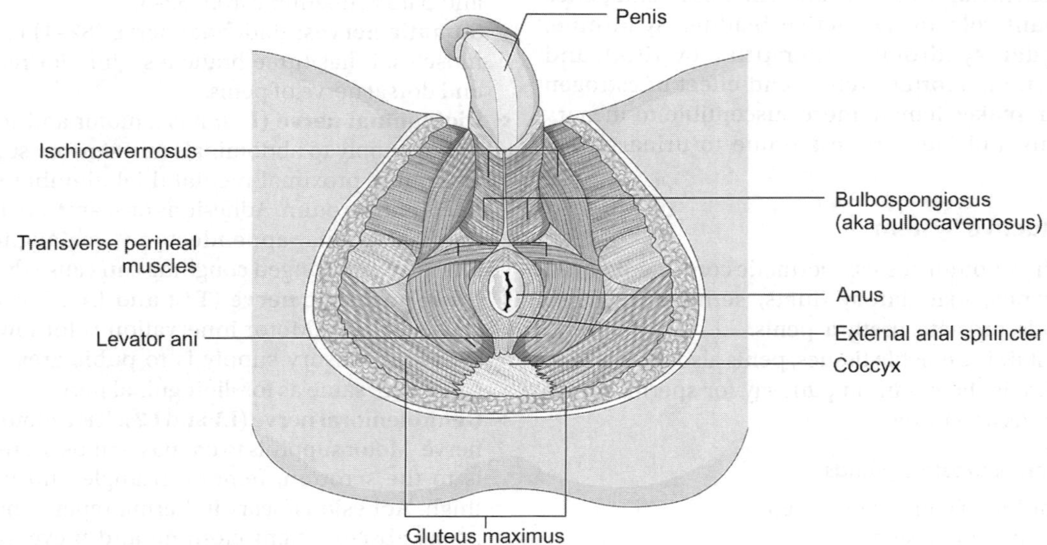

Fig. 36.2: Pelvic floor muscles in males *(For color version, see Plate 9)*.

- Muscular pumping action provided by them helps to move lymph and venous blood from the pelvic area
- **Sexual function:** Play important role during male sexual cycle.

COMMON MALE PELVIC FLOOR CONDITIONS

They can be broadly divided as function related, pain related and other conditions.

Pelvic Floor Function Related Conditions

- **Bladder conditions:** Incontinence, increased urgency/frequency, postvoid dribble, nocturia, dysuria, hesitancy, reduced flow, and strain to urinate
- **Bowel related:** Constipation, fecal urgency, fecal smearing, fecal incontinence, flatulence incontinence
- **Sexual dysfunction:** Erectile dysfunction, premature ejaculation, inability to gain or maintain erection.

Erectile dysfunction can be organic (vascular, neurologic, hormonal, or smooth muscle dysfunction), psychogenic or mixed.

Factors Influencing Pelvic Floor Functional Conditions

- **Habits and lifestyle:** Poor water intake, excessive bladder irritants intake, smoking, alcohol, artificial sweeteners, poor posture, poor body mechanics, habits of clenching/grinding teeth, work related voiding restrictions. PF tightness is seen in those who have habits of clenching/tightening teeth due to fascial connection.
- **Pelvic floor muscle dyssynergia:** Hypertonic or hypotonic
- Weak abdominals, weak multifidus, weak hip muscles.
- **Decreased use of diaphragm:** Diaphragm is the driving force in pelvic floor conditions. Pelvic floor lifts up during exhalation and moves down (relaxes) during inhalation due to their myofascial connection.
- Chronic straining in subjects with constipation may cause leakage due to weakened pelvic floor.
- Paradoxical cough mechanism/Valsalva increases downward pressure on PF.
- **Nerve damage:** Pudendal, Ilioinguinal, genitofemoral nerves
- Muscle guarding/tender points in psoas, obturator internus, piriformis, and abdominal wall
- **Pelvic abdominal surgeries/cancer:** Cancers in prostate/bladder/gastrointestinal (GI) system like prostatectomy, chemotherapy, radiation. Sometimes following surgeries like inguinal hernia repair, vasectomy and transurethral resection of the prostate (TURP)
- **Referred pain/visceral pain:** Hip pathology, surrounding organs
- **Certain medical conditions and comorbidities:** Diabetes, arthritis, lung conditions, obesity, hypertension, multiple sclerosis, Parkinson's disease, gastroparesis, space occupying lesions, anxiety, depression, recurrent infections, irritable bowel syndrome
- Certain medications like antihistamines, muscle relaxants, pain medications, iron supplements
- Sexual trauma
- **Coccyx injury:** Coccyx provides attachment to multiple PF muscles, ligaments and tendons
- Major life events or trauma can be the cause for the sudden change in PF functions in preteens and teenagers.

Urinary Incontinence (UI)

The prevalence of UI is less in men than women. UI worsens steadily as age advances.

Common types of urinary incontinence

- **Stress UI:** Involuntary leakage of urine with exertion. Stress UI is seen in case of prostate or other surgeries in the area, trauma, nerve injury, or pelvic floor and other core muscle weakness.
- **Urge UI:** Uncontrollable urge to urinate. Urge UI is more common.
- **Mixed UI:** Both stress and urge UI
- **Functional UI:** Not able to make it to void on time. One does need mobility, strength, balance, dexterity, and cognition to sense the urge and respond in time
- **Overflow UI:** Unable to empty the bladder completely followed by UI without urge
- **Overactive bladder (OAB):** Urgency and increased frequency with or without urge UI.

Bowel Concerns

Common complaints are constipation, fecal/flatulence incontinence, fecal urgency, fecal seepage, hemorrhoids, and fissures. Constipation can be due to poor diet, inadequate water intake, certain medication, frequent ignoring the urge to defecate, PF dyssynergia. Puborectalis muscle provides continence by maintaining anorectal angle. It has to relax during defecation, during dyssynergia it tightens up instead of relaxing **(Fig. 36.3)**.

Causes for fecal incontinence are multifactorial

- Pelvic floor weakness
- Sphincter damage
- PF dysfunction
- Constipation

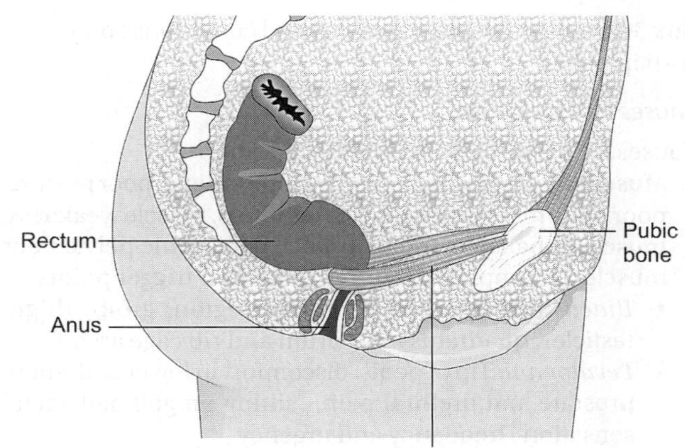

Fig. 36.3: Male anatomy for defecation.

- Diarrhea
- Neurological conditions
- Cognitive impairments
- Dementia
- Mobility/balance issues
- Poor dexterity
- Obesity
- Smoking
- Persistent coughing
- Repetitive heavy lifting
- Aging
- Long hours of cycling
- Anxiety
- Sexual abuse
- Certain medical conditions
- Abdominal surgeries

Fecal leakage is common in constipation. Chronic straining during bowel movements in case of constipation, weakens PF muscles. Hemorrhoids and fissures affect evacuation. It adversely affects quality of life (QOL), mood and self-esteem. Patients start planning/rerouting their day to accommodate their bowel movements and avoid accidents. Many patients limit their social life, outdoor activities or restrict food intake when outside the house. Bowel urgency and urinary urgency may exist together. If a patient comes with diagnosis of fecal incontinence but has history of constipation, treatment should start with addressing constipation first. Food diary, daily bowel regimen, defecation posture modification, healthy diet, improving transfer/gait/balance, urge control strategy instructions, PF muscle exercises, relaxation exercises and medical management of diarrhea can help with it. Rectal prolapse is not very common in men, can be present in the patient suffering from constipation.

Pain Related Conditions

Pain can be in low back, lower abdomen, hips, sacroiliac (SI) joint, groin, perineal, pubic, scrotal, penis, bladder, urethra, or thigh area. Acute pain can be because of infection, trauma or neurological conditions. Acute pain needs medical attention first.

Classification of Pelvic Pain Related Conditions

Box 36.1 enlists the pelvic pain related conditions commonly seen in males.

Causes for Pelvic Pain

Causes for pelvic pain are multifactorial:

- **Musculoskeletal:** Causes can include trauma, poor posture, poor body mechanics, muscle tightness, muscle weakness, muscle imbalance, trigger points, hypertonic pelvic floor muscles. Examples of referred pain from trigger points:
    - *Iliacus and psoas:* Abdominal region, groin, thigh, testicles, quadratus lumborum and rib cage area
    - *Levator ani:* Tip of penis, discomfort in lower abdomen, prostate and urethral pain, "sitting on golf ball/rectal sensation", frequency and urgency
    - *Deep PF muscles:* Pelvic pain, ilium, sacral pain
    - Abdominal wall: Testicular pain

Box 36.1: Pelvic pain related conditions.

Pelvic pain related conditions can be divided into:
- **Bladder conditions:** Bladder spasms, interstitial cystitis
- Chronic prostatitis
- **Bowel conditions:** Anal/rectal spasms (proctalgia fugax), fissures
- **Sexual pain:** Painful ejaculation
- Pain in lumbar region, SI joints, hips, coccyx or scrotum, rectum, penis or groin.

- **Visceral:** Pain may refer from surrounding organs. Examples include:
    - Referred pain to lower lumbar region, sacral area or testes due to prostate
    - Referred pain to lower abdomen or sacral area due to testes
    - Referred pain to groin, lower abdomen, scrotum, suprapubic, proximal thigh, thoracolumbar area from the urethra.
- **Neurological:** Nerve injury, nerve entrapment
- **Urological:** Kidney stones, interstitial cystitis, recurrent UTIs, prostatitis
- **Gastrointestinal:** Irritable bowel syndrome (IBS), constipation, diverticulitis
- **Psychological:** Post-traumatic stress disorder (PTSD), anxiety, depression
- Cancer related pain
- Scar adhesions.

Since pelvic pain is multifactorial, it requires multidisciplinary approach:

- Pain medication
- Pelvic floor physical therapy (PFPT)
- Psychological approach
- GI and urology care

Clinical Pointer

Chronic pain may require diagnostic tests to rule out red flags. Along with pain, patient may have associated symptoms like dysuria, voiding dysfunction, erectile dysfunction, bladder, or rectal spasms.

It is important to understand driving force at the time of onset of pain, referred pain, centralization of pain, and emotional pain.

Social and psychological perspective can flare up the symptoms of mechanical dysfunction. Two aspects of pelvic floor require consideration:

1. Pelvic floor plays a role in emotional processing
2. Activity in all muscles, including the pelvic floor, increases with exposure to stress and during anxiety evoking experiences.

Pain by nature is inhibitory so it can inhibit core muscles. For example, inhibited diaphragm function in case of abdominal pain, or inhibited transverse rectus and multifidus in case of chronic LBP. When there is increased sensitivity at the tip of penis or glans, it can create significant discomfort.

Simple triggers like clothing touching the area can worsen symptoms.

Common Painful PF Conditions in Males

Genitofemoral neuralgia (GFN): Because the genitofemoral nerve also passes through inguinal canal, it can be susceptible to injury during hernia repair surgery. Sensory innervation to the penis and testes is by genitofemoral nerve and when it is affected, it can cause penis or testes pain, numbness, hypersensitivity, and sexual dysfunction.

Vasectomy: The cause for postvasectomy pain could be because of fibrosis or genitofemoral nerve irritation. A patient who has lower back/abdominal/groin or hip pain prior to the vasectomy may have increased chances of pain. Any type of increase in tissue tension or mechanical loading may increase the symptoms.

Interstitial cystitis (IC)/painful bladder syndrome: IC patients do present with comorbid autoimmune conditions, central and autonomic nervous system disorders affecting multiple organs besides bladder. IC bladder is more common in females but men often get delayed in diagnosis and treatment as symptoms are similar to prostatitis. According to the American Urological Association, physical therapy is the most proven treatment and recommended along with the first line of medical treatment. In controlled clinical trials, manual physical therapy has shown significant benefits in both men and women. Manual therapy techniques include trigger point release, myofascial release, muscle energy techniques, passive stretches, and strain counterstrain amongst other.

Some other pain related conditions include:

- Posthernia repair, penis or testes pain.
- Scar and adhesion in the area causing GF nerve entrapment. Scar and adhesions get dense over the years.
- Mesh placement can cause GF nerve injury/tethering.
- GFN can also result from other surgeries in the area like appendectomies, femoral catheters for heart procedures and occasionally during vasectomy.

Other Pelvic Floor Conditions

- **Benign prostate hypertrophy (BPH):**
  - The prevalence of BPH increases with age.
  - Common symptoms are increased frequency, slow stream, hesitancy and postvoid dribble.
  - Medical and surgical management: TURP does not cause UI unless there is a surgical complication.
  - Common tests performed: Urinalysis, ultrasound, urodynamics, X-ray, MRI, prostate-specific antigen (PSA) blood test, biopsy, cystoscopy and digital rectal examination.
- **Prostatitis:**
  - It can be acute, chronic, or inflammatory.
  - **Common complaints:** Pain in rectal or pubic area, dysuria, urgency, frequency and voiding dysfunction.
- **Prostate cancer:**
  - In the United States, prostate cancer is the second most common cancer among men after skin cancer.
  - Sudden change in PSA value is important.
  - Treatment options include radiation (brachytherapy), hormone therapy, chemotherapy, cryotherapy, radical prostatectomy (incision can be suprapubic or perineal), laparoscopic radical prostatectomy, and pelvic rehabilitation. The treatment options depend on the tumor size, location, or stage.
  - Side effects include urinary incontinence, erectile dysfunction, urethral stricture, fibrosis/scar tissues, lymphedema and pelvic pain. Less common side effects include scarring in the penis (Peyronie syndrome) and climacturia (releasing a small amount of urine during ejaculation).
  - Neurovascular damage, sphincter damage and muscular damage can cause PF conditions.
  - Comorbidity, age, obesity, previous TURP surgery, extent of surgery, intraoperative techniques and pre-existing pelvic issues affect prognosis of rehabilitation. Most men will have some form of leakage immediately after the surgery but will improve over time and with rehabilitation. Fecal incontinence is rare, and it depends on the spread of cancer and radiation.

Types of UI after prostatectomy:

- Stress UI due to sphincter incompetence
- Urge UI from bladder dysfunction
- Mixed UI: Stress and urge UI
- Postvoid dribble
- Functional incontinence due to physical and environmental factors
- Overflow incontinence from stricture or recurrent obstruction
- Chronic retention of urine (urodynamic study is done to determine postvoid residual volume along with bladder diary).

Medical and surgical approaches for postprostatectomy UI:

- Incontinence pads
- Intermittent self-catheterization
- Penile clamp—it can cause pressure necrosis
- Artificial urinary sphincter
- Male slings
- Adjustable balloon device
- Sacral neurostimulation device

Preoperative rehabilitation can be helpful:

- To establish baseline/understand comorbidity
- For patient education
- For learning PF muscle exercises
- To establish patient therapist relationship

Rehabilitation outcome does depend on comorbidity, pre-existing PF weakness or UI.

Postprostatectomy PFPT rehabilitation includes:

- Patient education
- Behavior modification/bladder irritants control
- Posture modification—correct way of transfers, good body mechanics

- Timed voiding
- Bladder retraining
- Constipation management
- Core activation
- Avoiding Valsalva
- Diaphragmatic breathing exercises
- PF exercises (goal—hypertrophy of external urethral sphincter)
- Hypopressive exercises to reduce downward pressure on pelvic organs and pelvic floor.

Sexual Dysfunction

- It can be due to infection, inflammation, hormonal deficiency, certain medical conditions (diabetes mellitus, hypertension), certain medicines, BPH, vascular insufficiency, weak pelvic floor muscles, nerve damage, age related changes and psychological factors. Other factors include trauma, radiation, smoking, certain activities like cycling/horseback riding.
- It affects mood, self-esteem and relationships.
- Ischiocavernosus and bulbocavernosus play important role in penile erection.
- Pelvic floor exercises are significantly effective in the treatment for erectile dysfunction (ED).

Andropause

- Changes occur due to drop in testosterone level. Drop in testosterone starts after age of 30 years and increased symptoms with age advancement.
- It is usually insidious onset and slow progressing.
- Unlike menopause, changes are gradual and do not affect all men.
- Factors influencing andropause are obesity, high stress, certain medical conditions, certain medicines.
- Besides decline in sexual functions, decrease in bone density, increased risk of cardiovascular diseases, obesity, impaired glucose metabolism, impaired memory, mood swings, decreased muscle mass and low energy level may be found.
- Besides testosterone therapy, management of existing medical conditions and healthy lifestyle can help.

Diastasis Recti

- Usually found in men of age 30–40 years.
- Factors influencing are high intensity core exercises, history of myofascial weakness, fluctuations in body weight, advancing age and abdominal distension.

Voiding issues due to injuries to nerves, spinal cord or neurological conditions.

Some of the common ones are:

- Multiple sclerosis (MS)
- Parkinson's disease
- Spinal cord injuries
- Stroke
- Diabetes mellitus (DM)
- Brain tumors

Symptoms depend on the type of neurological damage and hence symptoms differ. Common symptoms are:

- Urinary incontinence (UI)
- Urine dribble
- Overactive bladder (OAB)
- Urinary tract infection (UTI)
- Hesitancy

Treatments include:

- Medical and surgical management
- Self-catheterization
- Sacral nerve stimulator, posterior tibial nerve stimulation
- Lifestyle modification
- Pelvic floor exercises if motor control is available

PHYSICAL THERAPY EVALUATION AND EXAMINATION

History

Good history-taking is very important to create a treatment hypothesis. Important components of history should include:

- **Onset of condition:** Understand driving force/what was going on in patient's life at the time of onset of symptoms. Onset-duration/mechanism of injury/progression of symptoms/aggravating and relieving factors/occupation/exercise-sports-hobby/previous treatment/smoking/daily fluid intake/pain level-location-description
- **Bladder history:** Voiding dysfunction/postvoid dribble/pain with urination/number of daily voids and night voids/frequency of UI/amounts of leakage/urgency present?/Number of incontinence pads needed
- **Bowel history:** Constipation/straining during bowel movements/stool consistency/hemorrhoids/fecal urgency/fecal incontinence/number of bowel movements per week
- **Sexual history:** Erectile dysfunction/pain during ejaculation
- **Past medical/surgical history**
- **Medications**
- **Special tests** (diagnostic)
- **Patient's goals**
- **Barrier to learning:** Hearing vision, cognitive status
- **Functional outcome scale:** International prostate symptom score (IPSS), ICS male short form, Patient Specific Functional Scale (PSFS).

Examination

Thorough examination helps to understand contributing factors and put together an algorithm for treatment. Important components of examination include:

- **Observation:**
  - *Sitting/standing posture:* Change in posture changes pressure on pelvic floor. Poor posture inhibits core muscles. Look for forward head, elevated shoulders, rounded shoulders, slouched or slanted sitting posture, increased anterior pelvic tilt in standing
  - *Breathing:* Apical, diaphragmatic, or abdominal.

- **Transfers/gait:** Sit to stand test, gait speed test, assistive device use—these are important in patients with functional UI or with OAB
- **Thoracic/lumbar/SI/hip screening:** Alignment, flexibility, strength, reproduction of symptoms, "pattern of holding"—back gripper (compresses lumbar area), butt gripper—forces femoral head forward in the socket, chest gripper—restricts diaphragm movement
- **Neurological:** Reflexes/nerve tension tests/knee and ankle reflexes/anal wink/cremasteric reflex
- **Palpation:** Trigger points in abdominal wall, diaphragm, thigh and low back muscles
- **Scars:** Mobility, sensation, pain
- **Functional movements:** Single leg stance, squat
- **Pelvic floor muscle assessment:** External and internal.
  - *External PF assessment:* Includes perineal, anal, scrotal and penile area; observation for redness/rashes/hemorrhoids/fissures/any congenital abnormalities; check sensation, palpation for tenderness, anal wink, cremasteric reflex, cough reflex, whether subject is able to demonstrate PF contraction and relaxation.
  - *Internal PF muscle assessment:* Hands on training is required for internal PF muscle assessment. Patient's consent and chaperone are required. Digital examination (gloved lubricated finger) is done through rectal area. Check tone, sensation, tenderness, muscle strength, coordination, and assessment of reproduction of symptoms. It includes assessment of external anal sphincter, puborectalis, pubococcygeus, iliococcygeus and ischiococcygeus muscles. At external sphincter level, check the tone of contraction and ability to perform fast contractions. Check puborectalis pull which can be graded as 0–5/5 PERFECT scheme (*See* Chapter 4: Assessment in Women's Health).
- **Functional urine stop test:**
  - Able to stop completely
  - Dribbles
  - Able to slow down
  - Not able to stop at all

PHYSICAL THERAPY TREATMENT

Management of PF dysfunction includes medical, surgical, pharmacological interventions, alternative medicine and physical therapy. For OAB, nocturnal enuresis and severe urge UI, anticholinergic drugs may help while receiving pelvic floor physical therapy (PFPT). Acupuncture can also help.

Physical Therapy Management

- **Patient education:** About relevant anatomy/physiology/factors influencing/pain mechanism
- Bladder/bowel symptom diary for 3–5 days
- Behavioral modification and lifestyle changes: adequate water intake/eliminate bladder irritants/timing and amount of fluid intake/respond urge to void/weight reduction
- Awareness of good sitting and standing posture/body mechanics/transfers
- Diaphragmatic breathing with variations as needed like exhale > inhale
- Skin care instructions/information on available incontinence products
- Constipation management instructions/toileting techniques instructions
- KNACK maneuver training: Intentionally engaging pelvic floor muscles while coughing up and out
- Strong repetitive superficial PF contractions and instruct about postvoid dribble
- Urge control strategy instructions: Strong PF muscle contractions help detrusor muscles relax by perineo-pudendal facilitative reflex
- Home management instructions

Manual Therapy

Soft tissue mobilization, joint mobilization, myofascial release, passive stretches, muscle energy techniques, trigger point release, abdominal massage, scar release, K taping can be used.

Exercises

- Goal is to improve flexibility, strength, endurance, neuromuscular reeducation and balance.
- Abdominal pressure system **(Fig. 36.4)** plays important role in pelvic floor issues. Top of the system is diaphragm, front is transverse rectus abdominus, bottom is pelvic floor muscles and back is multifidus muscles. Increase in abdominal pressure (during coughing, sneezing, lifting, straining, and Valsalva) will pass through the weak area of the system.

Below are some examples of the exercises that can be useful for PF dysfunction rehabilitation:

- Pelvic floor exercises
- Transversus abdominis (TrA) activation, core stabilization exercises
- Diaphragmatic breathing
- Stretches to improve hip muscle flexibility **(Figs. 36.5 to 36.7)**
- Multifidus activation
- Global hip muscle strengthening **(Figs. 36.8 and 36.9)**
- Posture exercises and scapular muscles strengthening **(Figs. 36.10 and 36.11)**
- Bridging, squats, lunges with good core control since they are functional positions
- Jaw relaxation exercises if patient has history of clenching/grinding teeth
- Swiss ball exercises
- Water exercises—easier on joints
- Pelvic floor exercises: Also known as Kegels exercises. Most find it challenging as it requires mind body connection. Some of the cueing that can help to teach PF exercises in men are:
  - Visualize stopping "your urine flow", it should not be done by actually stopping the urine flow while urinating as that can cause PF dysfunction

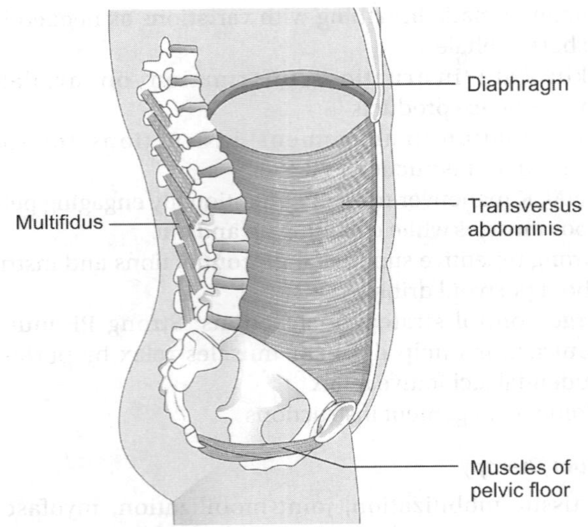

Fig. 36.4: Abdominal pressure system.

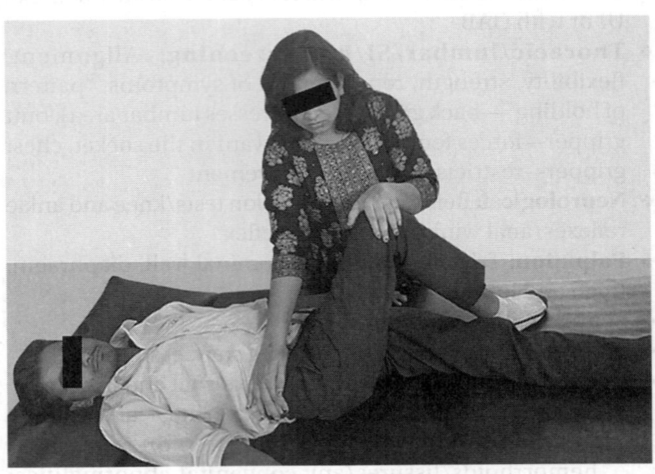
Fig. 36.5: Stretching for piriformis.

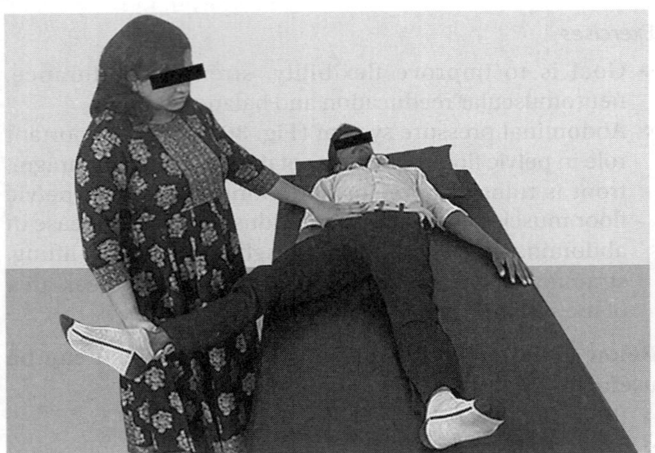
Fig. 36.6: Stretching for hip adductors.

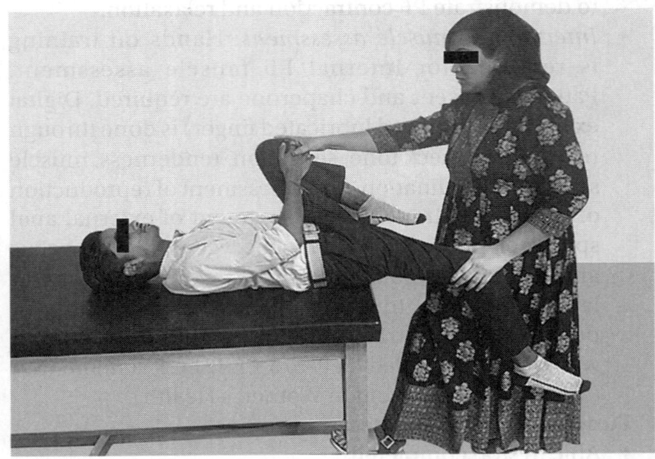
Fig. 36.7: Stretching for hip flexors.

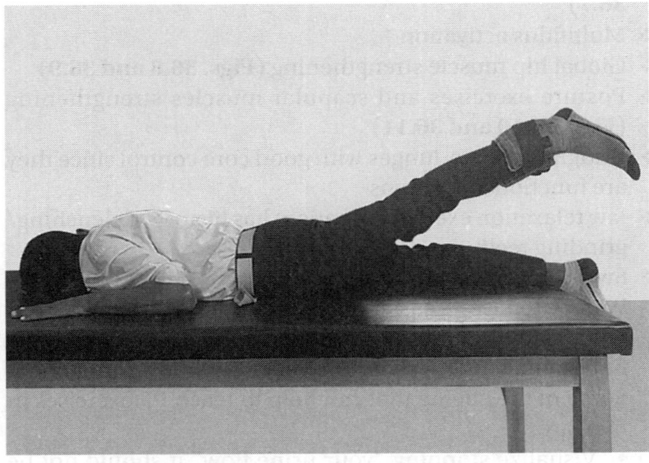
Fig. 36.8: Strengthening of hip extensors.

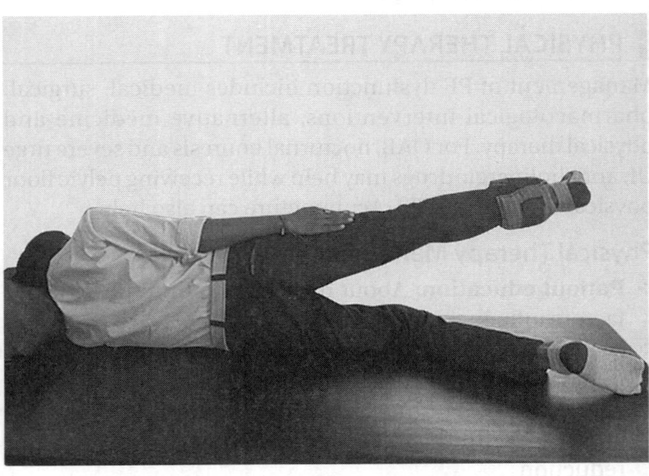
Fig. 36.9: Strengthening of hip abductors.

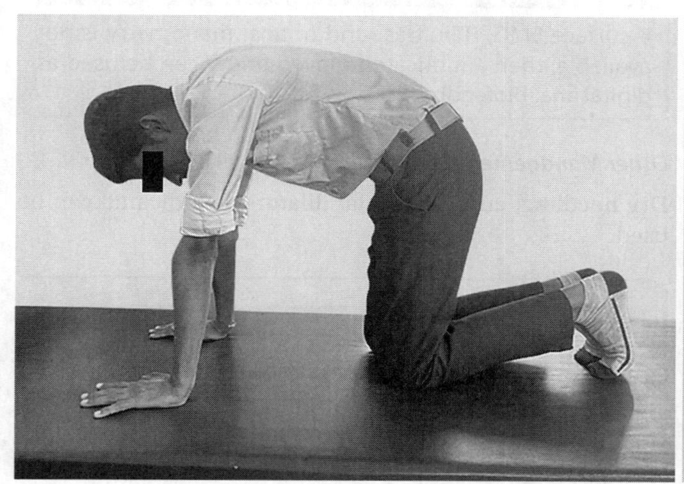

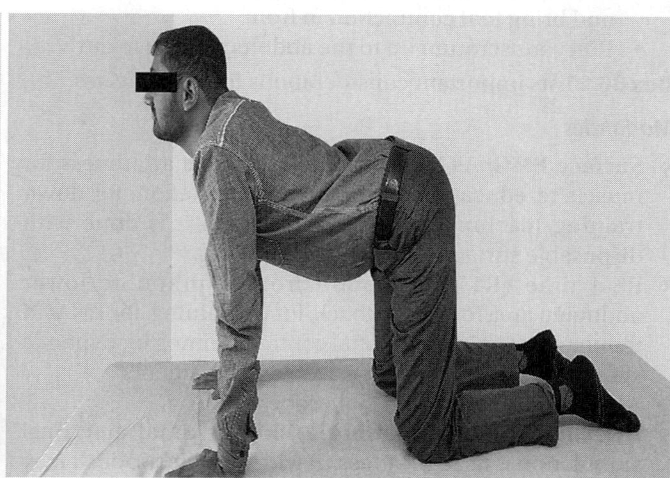

Fig. 36.10: Cat and cow exercises.

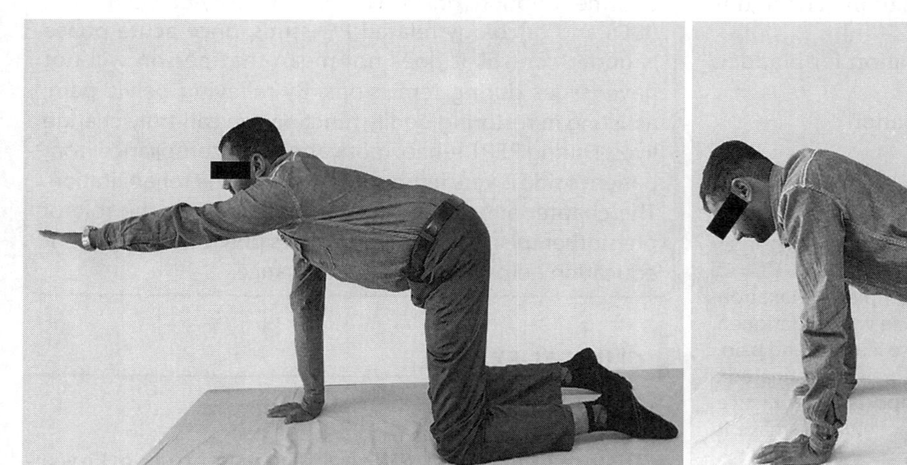

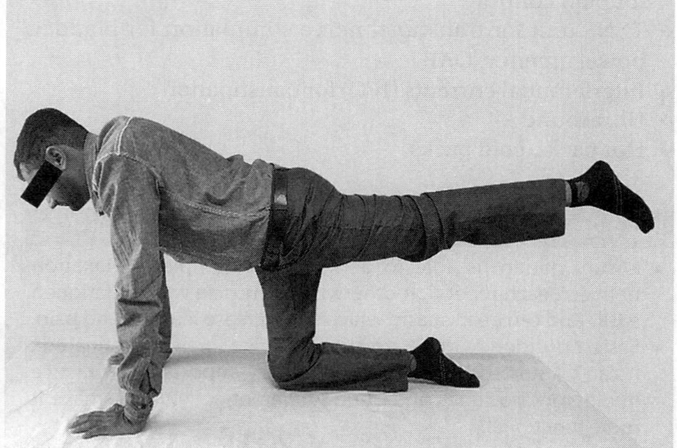

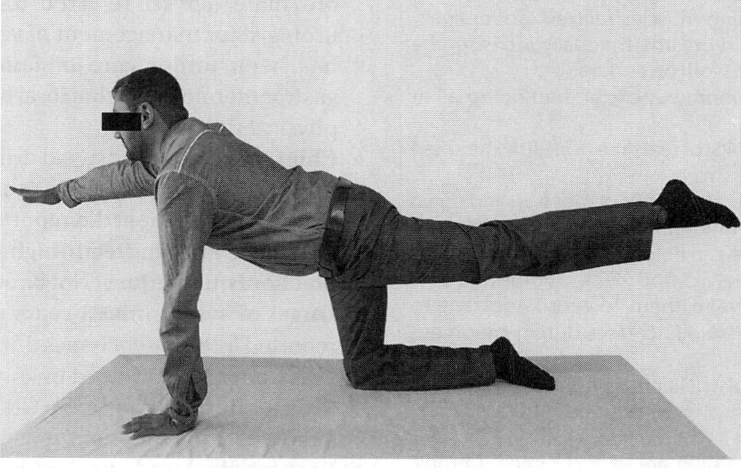

Fig. 36.11: Posture exercises.

- Visualize shortening your penis
- Pretend you are "holding the gas in/avoid passing it" and bring that contraction in front
- Pull your scrotum up to the abdomen "nuts to gut".

Box 36.2 lists important considerations for PF exercises.

Modalities

- **Surface EMG:** As biofeedback to improve awareness for muscle re-education, to improve coordination, for down training/teaching to relax PF muscles. It is done with disposable surface skin electrodes.
- Real time (RT) ultrasound from suprapubic/lower abdomen area for biofeedback, for up training, for KNACK maneuver training, for glottal control, training for dynamic stabilization during lower extremity movements
- Anal manometry with rectal probe
- **Internal PF muscle stimulation:** Maximal electrical stimulation is used for stress UI with anal electrode. It may help with very weak PF muscles to facilitate the contraction. There is not enough evidence on use of it. Low intensity stimulation is used for Urge UI. Along with all precautions of any electrical stimulation, patient's consent is needed.
- Transcutaneous electrical nerve stimulation (TENS) unit for pain control
- TENS unit for transtibial nerve stimulation for bladder/bowel urgency, OAB
- Interferential currents (IFC) for constipation
- Ultrasound
- Hot packs/cold packs

Box 36.2: Important considerations for pelvic floor exercises.

- Ensure patient is able to demonstrate complete relaxation between each repetition otherwise PF muscle will get fatigued easily and can go in spasm which will increase leakage and pain.
- Easiest position to do PF exercise is supine (gravity eliminated). It can be started in supine, but it is very important to practice in different positions and during different activities to make it more functional.
- Once patient has better understanding of PF contractions, bring awareness to keep surrounding muscles relaxed (abdominals, adductors, gluteal, not to hold breath). Gradually increase "the hold" length of contraction to work on endurance.
- Short frequent sessions are more beneficial than doing all at once.
- Surface electromyography (EMG) or real time (RT) ultrasound can help as biofeedback.
- Since respiratory diaphragm and pelvic floor move up and down together, breath work—"activation/lift of PF during exhale and relaxation of PF during inhale" can help.
- Core muscles consist of pelvic floor, TrA, multifidus and diaphragm. Teamwork between them is very important to manage intra-abdominal pressure (increases during coughing/sneezing/lifting/straining).
- TrA and PF muscles are synergists. Diaphragm is the driving force in PF conditions. It is not only a respiratory but also a postural muscle.
- Shallow and paradoxical breathing are very common. Chronic stress, poor posture, certain lung conditions affect diaphragm mobility.

 **Clinical Pointer**

If surface EMG, RT ultrasound or anal manometry is not available, then a lubricated gloved finger can be used as digital anal biofeedback.

Other Management Techniques

Dry needling, cupping, rectal dilators as indicated can be used.

 **Summary**

Anyone who has pelvic floor (PF) can have PF issues. PF issues adversely affect quality of life (QOL) and functions. Several research studies have demonstrated a correlation between urinary incontinence (UI) and the occurrence of depression and anxiety. Pelvic floor physiotherapy (PFPT) can be part of multidisciplinary approach to PF dysfunction. Lack of success in treating PF issues is due to "compartmentalization" and lack of awareness of available treatment options. In case of inflammatory bowel disease (IBD) and oncology related PF issues, once acute phase is under control, it does not mean that person will not have issues during remissions. By relieving pelvic pain, assisting in restoring bodily function, we can truly change lives. During PFPT rehab, motivation and compliance from patient's side is very important like any other rehabilitation. The chapter aims to introduce the readers to the role of physiotherapists in the area of men's pelvic health. Patient education helps to improve compliance.

CLINICAL EXAMPLE

History

- **History of presenting illness:** The patient was a 35-year-old/male dentist referred to physical therapy by his urologist for management of voiding dysfunction. Patient has been under care of family physician, urologist, gastroenterologist, behavioral health and musculoskeletal physical therapist.
- **Chief complaints:** Postvoid dribble, pain with ejaculation, rectal spasms, chronic thoracic/lumbar pain and constipation. Patient did report fall on coccyx, tendency of clenching/grinding teeth, high stress level job and anxiety.
- **Mechanism of injury:** Not known; Major changes at work
- **Onset of symptoms:** 3 years ago. Upon asking, patient reported intermittent issues during high school and college years, but these resolved in few weeks.
- **Progression of symptoms:** Gradually getting worse in last 3 months, more frequent spasms and dribbles
- **Past medical and surgical history:** Chronic back pain, allergic rhinitis, anxiety. Had received orthopedic physiotherapy and chiropractic care in past.

- **Drugs:** Pain medications [nonsteroidal anti-inflammatory drugs (NSAIDs)] as indicated, cetirizine, stool softener and fiber supplements
- **Fluid intake:** 24–30 oz coffee, 30–32 oz water, alcohol 3–4 times/week
- **Hobbies:** Gym workouts—weight lifting (for stress relief)
- **Aggravating factors/symptom patterns:** Increased episodes during evening hours, stress relieving factors: not known
- **Sleep:** Poor, difficulty falling asleep
- **Pain level:** Chronic dull back pain, painful rectal spasms—last for few seconds to minutes
- **Bladder concerns:** Postvoid dribbles, feeling of incomplete emptying of the bladder; night voids—3 times
- **Prostate issues:** None
- **Bowel concerns:** Constipation present, straining present, Hemorrhoids present, stool consistency on Bristol stool scale 1–3/7 weekly bowel movements: 3x
- **Expected goals:** Not to have rectal spasms and to address erectile dysfunction. Patient did mention that his urologist recommended PFPT 6 months ago, he was not sure if PT can help with his issues so did not consider.

Investigations

- **Lumbar X-rays:** Normal
- **Anorectal manometry (ARM) test:** PF dyssynergia

Objective Assessment

- Oriented to person, place and time
- Sitting posture slanted, constantly changing positions
- **Standing:** Elevated shoulders, "clenched butt/gluteal", "clenched teeth"
- **Breathing:** Shallow, decreased use of diaphragm
- **Transfers and gait:** Within normal limits
- **Lumbar range of motion:** Decreased core control, end range movements restricted
- **Single leg stance:** Increased work to balance, improved with gentle exhale (core activation)
- **Squats:** Decreased core control, end range restricted, improved when done against wall
- **Neurologic examinations:** Sensation intact
- **Slump test:** Negative, anal wink-present, cremasteric reflex-present
- **Muscle tightness:** Hip flexors, adductors, piriformis
- **Gross hip manual muscle testing (MMT):** 5/5
- **Abdominals:** Good strength except difficulty with TrA activation
- **Tenderness:** Lower thoracic and lumbar paravertebral muscles, hip flexors, adductors, obturator internus, sacrotuberous ligament area, no tenderness over external perineal muscles
- No internal PF muscle palpation done as per patient's request
- **Surface EMG:** Done with surface electrodes around perianal area. It was practiced in supine/sitting /standing/ full squats/sitting with step stool under feet. It demonstrated elevated resting tone, difficulty relaxing, intermittent Valsalva while trying to relax PF, able to demonstrate normal resting tone with full squats, and with breath work.

PT Assessment

- **Diagnosis:**
  - PF dysfunction
  - Constipation
  - Postvoid dribble
  - Coccyx pain
  - Erectile dysfunction
- **Prognosis:** Good
- **Factors influencing:** Fall on coccyx, anxiety/high stress, water: bladder stimulants ratio, decreased core control, long hours of sitting/patient care.

Goals

Short-term goals (1–4 visits):

- Patient education on relevant anatomy/physiology
- Patient education on factors influencing, symptom log instructions, habit modification, diaphragmatic breathing, relaxation technique instruct, good posture and body mechanics
- About 50% decrease in rectal spasm episodes.

Long-term goals (5–8 visits):

- Independent with home program and able to manage symptoms with it
- Able to have bowel movement every 1–2 days without straining
- Able to sit for couple hours at a time with minimum to no soreness
- Able to void every couple hour without any discomfort
- Able to have ejaculation without any pain
- Improve lumbopelvic stability during functional activities

Treatment

- **Frequency:** Total 8 visits/once every 2 weeks
- Patient education on relevant anatomy/physiology, factors influencing his PF issues; patient instructed to sit down on toilet seat to void, bend over and give few extra seconds to complete voiding
- **Habit and lifestyle modification:** Increase water intake, decrease intake of bladder irritants
- **Symptom log:** Instruct to write down about symptoms, to improve awareness of triggers for rectal spasms and postvoid dribble.
- **Constipation management:** Abdominal massage, diet modification, defecation posture modification, daily bowel regimen, daily brisk walk
- Sitting posture modification, posture breaks/posture exercises, instructed on correct body mechanics during lifting and avoiding Valsalva

- Diaphragmatic breathing and guided meditation
- Breath work while sitting on Swiss ball
- Jaw relaxation exercises
- TrA activation in functional positions followed by core stabilization exercises
- **Yoga poses:** Pavan muktasana, malasana, happy baby pose, baddhakonasana
- Exercises in quadruped position for spinal mobility and lumbopelvic stability
- Squats with good core control
- **Manual therapy:** Trigger point release, myofascial release in thoracic and lumbar area, passive hip muscle stretches, abdominal massage for constipation
- Home TENS unit use at sacral borders in supine hook lying with hip/knee at 90/90
- Surface EMG for biofeedback

Outcome

Patient reported all his personal goals were met. He reported improved awareness of his triggers, improved mind body connection, able to have bowel movements every other day without straining, no complaints of postvoid dribbles, significant decrease in rectal spasms and able to manage the rectal spasms with breath work when he had them. Patient reported no pain with ejaculation. Did report noticing the correlation between stress and ED. Patient reported back pain is much better and have not taken pain meds in last 3 weeks. Biofeedback with surface EMG, yoga stretches, breath work while sitting on the Swiss ball and home TENS treatment for back pain have been very useful.

Functional outcome scale forms used: patient specific functional scale (0–5/5; 5 is the worst)

At initial evaluation: (1) Rectal spasms 4/5; (2) Postvoid dribble 4/5; (3) Erectile dysfunction 4/5.

At discharge evaluation: (1) Rectal spasms 1/5; (2) Postvoid dribble 0/5; (3) Erectile dysfunction 1/5.

ACKNOWLEDGMENTS

I would like to thank my husband, Dr Amit Mehta for his support and faith in me. I would also like to thank the editors for this opportunity.

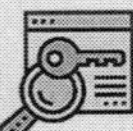

Review Questions

1. Describe the differences in male and female pelvic anatomy in brief.
2. What are the different pelvic floor conditions in men?
3. Explain physiotherapy management for pelvic floor conditions in men in detail.
4. Write short notes on:
   a. Urinary incontinence in men
   b. Pelvic floor muscles in men
   c. Examination of the male pelvic floor

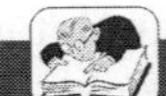

Bibliography

1. Abelson B, Sun D, Que L, Nebel RA, Baker D, Popiel P, et al. Sex differences in lower urinary tract biology and physiology. Biol Sex Differ. 2018;9(1):45. doi:10.1186/s13293-018-0204-8. PMID: 30343668; PMCID: PMC6196569.
2. Chelimsky G, Heller E, Buffington CA, Rackley R, Zhang D, Chelimsky T. Co-morbidities of interstitial cystitis. Front Neurosci. 2012;6:114. doi:10.3389/fnins.2012.00114. PMID: 22907988; PMCID: PMC3415690.
3. Clemens JQ, Nadler RB, Schaeffer AJ, Belani J, Albaugh J, Bushman W. Biofeedback, pelvic floor re-education, and bladder training for male chronic pelvic pain syndrome. Urology. 2000;56(6):951-5. doi:10.1016/S0090-4295(00)00796-2. PMID: 11113739.
4. de Santana Santos NA, de Lima Saintrain MV, Regadas RP, da Silveira RA. Assessment of physical therapy strategies for recovery of urinary continence after prostatectomy. Asian Pac J Cancer Prev. 2017;18(1):81-6. doi:10.22034/APJCP.2017.18.1.81. PMID: 28239914; PMCID: PMC5563211.
5. Dorey G, Speakman M, Feneley R, Swinkels A, Dunn C, Ewings P. Randomised controlled trial of pelvic floor muscle exercises and manometric biofeedback for erectile dysfunction. Br J Gen Pract. 2004;54(508):819-25. PMID: 15527607; PMCID: PMC1324914.
6. FitzGerald MP, Anderson RU, Potts J, Payne CK, Peters KM, Clemens JQ, et al. Randomized multicenter feasibility trial of myofascial physical therapy for the treatment of urological chronic pelvic pain syndromes. J Urol. 2009;182(2):570-80. doi:10.1016/j.juro.2009.04.022. PMID: 19535099; PMCID: PMC2872169.
7. Lee KS, Choi JD. Chronic prostatitis: approaches for best management. Korean J Urol. 2012;53(2):69-77. doi:10.4111/kju.2012.53.2.69. PMID: 22379583; PMCID: PMC3285711.
8. Lirette LS, Chaiban G, Tolba R, Eissa H. Coccydynia: an overview of the anatomy, etiology, and treatment of coccyx pain. Ochsner J. 2014;14(1):84-7. PMID: 24688338; PMCID: PMC3963058.
9. Lockwood T. Rectus muscle diastasis in males: primary indication for endoscopically assisted abdominoplasty. Plast Reconstr Surg. 1998;101(6):1685-91. doi:10.1097/00006534-199805000-00042. PMID: 9583506.
10. Masterson TA, Masterson JM, Azzinaro J, Manderson L, Swain S, Ramasamy R. Comprehensive pelvic floor physical therapy program for men with idiopathic chronic pelvic pain syndrome: a prospective study. Transl Androl Urol. 2017;6(5):910-15. doi:10.21037/tau.2017.08.17. PMID: 29184791; PMCID: PMC5673826.
11. Myers C, Smith M. Pelvic floor muscle training improves erectile dysfunction and premature ejaculation: a systematic review. Physiotherapy. 2019;105(2):235-43. doi:10.1016/j.physio.2019.01.002. PMID: 30979506.
12. Newman DK, Guzzo T, Lee D, Jayadevappa R. An evidence-based strategy for the conservative management of the male patient with incontinence. Curr Opin Urol. 2014;24(6):553-9. doi:10.1097/MOU.0000000000000115. PMID: 25232762.
13. Padoa A, Rosenbaum T. The overactive pelvic floor. 1st ed. Cham: Springer; 2016.
14. Poylin VY, Irani JL, Rahbar R, Kapadia MR. Rectal-prolapse repair in men is safe, but outcomes are not well understood. Gastroenterol Rep. 2019;7(4):279-82. doi:10.1093/gastro/goz016. PMID: 31798934; PMCID: PMC6939070.
15. Sapsford R. Rehabilitation of pelvic floor muscles utilizing trunk stabilization. Man Ther. 2004;9(1):3-12. doi:10.1016/j.math.2003.06.001. PMID: 14723873.
16. Scott KM. Pelvic floor rehabilitation in the treatment of fecal incontinence. Clin Colon Rectal Surg. 2014;27(3):99-105. doi:10.1055/s-0034-1384662. PMID: 25320568; PMCID: PMC4174224.

17. Singh P. Andropause: Current concepts. Indian J Endocrinol Metab. 2013;17(Suppl 3):S621-9. doi:10.4103/2230-8210.123552. PMID: 24910824; PMCID: PMC4046605.
18. Singla N, Singla AK. Post-prostatectomy incontinence: Etiology, evaluation, and management. Turk J Urol. 2014;40(1):1-8. doi:10.5152/tud.2014.222014. PMID: 26328137; PMCID: PMC4548645.
19. Soliman Y, Meyer R, Baum N. Falls in the elderly secondary to urinary symptoms. Rev Urol. 2016;18(1):28-32. PMID: 27162509; PMCID: PMC4859925.
20. Stafford RE, Ashton-Miller JA, Constantinou C, Coughlin G, Lutton NJ, Hodges PW. Pattern of activation of pelvic floor muscles in men differs with verbal instructions. Neurourol Urodyn. 2016;35(4):457-63. doi:10.1002/nau.22745. PMID: 25727781.
21. Talasz H, Kofler M, Kalchschmid E, Pretterklieber M, Lechleitner M. Breathing with the pelvic floor? Correlation of pelvic floor muscle function and expiratory flows in healthy young nulliparous women. Int Urogynecol J. 2010;21(4):475-81. doi:10.1007/s00192-009-1060-1. PMID: 19911197.

Multiple Choice Questions (MCQs)

To test your understanding and recall of key concepts.

1. **A 35-year-old male presents with post-void dribble, pain during ejaculation, and chronic constipation. His history reveals a fall on the coccyx and high levels of job-related stress. As a physiotherapist, which combination of interventions is the most appropriate initial management strategy?**
   A. Initiate pelvic floor strengthening exercises and prescribe a stool softener
   B. Teach diaphragmatic breathing techniques, defecation posture modification, and address lifestyle factors
   C. Perform manual therapy for coccygeal realignment and recommend surgical evaluation
   D. Focus on myofascial release techniques for abdominal tension and schedule an anorectal manometry
2. **A male patient reports frequent nocturia, urgency, and weak urine stream. His physical examination reveals pelvic floor muscle weakness and tenderness in the suprapubic area. Which condition is the most likely contributing factor to his symptoms?**
   A. Benign prostatic hypertrophy (BPH)
   B. Overactive bladder syndrome
   C. Chronic prostatitis
   D. Pelvic floor dyssynergia
3. **A patient undergoing rehabilitation after prostatectomy exhibits stress urinary incontinence. Which exercise program would best address his symptoms in the initial phase?**
   A. High-intensity pelvic floor contractions in functional standing positions
   B. Hypopressive exercises and Transversus Abdominis (TrA) activation
   C. Supine pelvic floor exercises focusing on endurance and relaxation
   D. Progressive overload training targeting the multifidus and gluteal muscles
4. **A 40-year-old male complains of persistent pelvic pain exacerbated by prolonged sitting and cycling. Which combination of referrals and interventions is most appropriate?**
   A. Neurologist for pudendal neuralgia and urologist for interstitial cystitis
   B. Physical therapy for pelvic floor relaxation techniques and dietary adjustments for constipation
   C. Psychologist for stress management and physiotherapist for trigger point release
   D. Multidisciplinary approach involving physical therapy, pain management, and psychosocial support
5. **Which muscle is primarily responsible for penile rigidity during an erection?**
   A. Bulbospongiosus
   B. Ischiocavernosus
   C. Superficial transverse perineal muscle
   D. External anal sphincter
6. **Which of the following is *not* a primary function of pelvic floor muscles in males?**
   A. Providing bladder and bowel continence
   B. Supporting pelvic organs
   C. Regulating blood glucose levels
   D. Enhancing sexual function

ANSWERS

1. B	2. A	3. C	4. D	5. B
6. C				

Index

Page numbers followed by *b* refer to box, *f* refer to figure, and *t* refer to table.

B

C

I

J

K

L

M

Q

U

V